Color Atlas of
Clinical Hematology
Third Edition

A Victor Hoffbrand MA DM DSc FRCP FRCPath FRCP (Edin)

Emeritus Professor of Hematology
The Royal Free and University College Medical School
Honorary Consultant Hematologist
Royal Free Hospital
London, UK

John E Pettit MD (Otago) FRCPA FRCPath

Director and Hematologist
Medlab South Ltd
Christchurch, New Zealand
Formerly Associate Professor of Hematology
University of Otago Medical School
Dunedin, New Zealand

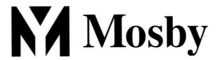

London   Edinburgh   New York   Philadelphia   St Louis   Sydney   Toronto   2000

MOSBY
An imprint of Harcourt Publishers Limited

© Harcourt Publishers Limited 2000

M is a registered trademark of Harcourt Publishers Limited

First published 2000

Reprinted 2000

ISBN 07234 31159

British Library Cataloguing in Publication Data
A catalogue record for this book is available from the British Library

Library of Congress Cataloging in Publication Data
A catalog record for this book is available from the Library of Congress

Note
Medical knowledge is constantly changing. As new information becomes available, changes in treatment, procedures, equipment and the use of drugs become necessary. The editors/authors/contributors and the publishers have taken care to ensure that the information given in this text is accurate and up to date. However, readers are strongly advised to confirm that the information, especially with regard to drug usage, complies with the latest legislation and standards of practice.

Printed and bound by Grafos, SA Arte Sobre papel, Barcelona, Spain

Publisher: Serena Bureau
Project Managers: John Ormiston, Briony Short
Production: Yolanta Motylinska, Mark Sanderson
Design and Illustration: Designers Collective Limited

The
Publisher's
policy is to use
**paper manufactured
from sustainable forests**

Preface

In the 5 years since the second edition of this *Clinical Atlas* appeared major advances have occurred in the understanding of the etiology and treatment of disorders of the blood. For the third edition we have added much of the new information on these aspects to our previous illustrations of the clinical, microscopic and radiographic appearances of blood disorders. For some diseases, such as primary hemochromatosis, pyridoxine-responsive congenital sideroblastic anemia, α-thalassemia with mental retardation, Fanconi anemia, dyskeratosis congenita and chronic granulomatous disease, some of the underlying genetic abnormalities have been elucidated and are now illustrated. We have also included a number of diseases that were barely recognized in 1994 e.g. hereditary hyperferritinemia with cataract, autoimmune lymphoproliferative disease, new variant Creutzfeld–Jakob disease and ALK-positive large cell lymphoma. Newly discovered disease mechanisms, such as that for thrombotic thrombocytopenic purpura, have been added. A new chapter is devoted to stem cell transplantation, and the Revised European–American Lymphoma (REAL) and World Health Organization classifications of malignant lymphomas and other malignant blood disorders are now included and illustrated. The chronic lymphoproliferative disorders have been given a chapter separate from the other forms of chronic leukemia. New diagnostic procedures have also been added, including an increased emphasis on fluorescent *in-situ* hybridization, magnetic resonance imaging of the bone marrow, diagnostic methods for deep vein thrombosis and molecular methods of HLA typing. As previously, the first chapter provides the background to the subsequent clinical sections, with discussion and illustration of normal blood and bone marrow appearances, normal hemopoiesis, as well as new sections on apoptosis, thrombopoietin, dendritic and mesenchymal cells.

We are pleased to be joined by Professor Kevin Gatter, Professor Kenneth MacLennan and Professor David Mason, who have contributed substantially to the major chapter that deals with malignant lymphomas. We are also grateful to the many colleagues from all over the world who have kindly provided slides and diagrams suitable for reproduction in the *Atlas*. Each of these has been acknowledged in the caption to the relevant figure. We are also grateful to the many colleagues and publishers who have given us permission to reproduce previously published scientific diagrams and tables. This has enabled the *Atlas* to become more comprehensive. We would nevertheless be grateful to receive suggestions for new material to be included in future editions. In this way we hope the *Atlas* will continue to provide an up-to-date illustrated 'encyclopedia' of the blood and its disorders.

We are most grateful to the Publishers, in particular John Ormiston and Mark Willey, for expert and enthusiastic help in assembling the material (often given to them in a state of disorder) in a clear and beautifully presented form, drawing new scientific diagrams and tables and accommodating all our various additions and changes throughout the proof stages.

Victor Hoffbrand
John Pettit
March, 2000

Contents

Normal Haemopoiesis and Blood Cells

HAEMOPOIETIC STEM AND PROGENITOR CELLS

Haemopoietic stem cells have the property of self-renewal and also, through cell division and differentiation, form populations of progenitor cells which are committed to the main marrow cell lines: erythroid, granulocytic and monocytic; megakaryocytic; and lymphocytic (*Fig. 1.1*). The earlier progenitor cells are multipotent but, as division and differentiation proceed, later progenitors are formed that are committed to three, two or one cell line. Most evidence suggests that the haemopoietic stem and progenitor cells morphologically resemble small and intermediate-sized lymphocytes (*see Fig. 14.6*).

The marrow contains a stromal matrix that provides the correct microenvironment for stem cell growth (*Figs 1.2 and 1.3*). A stromal layer can be grown *in vitro* in long-term cultures on which haemopoietic cells grow. The yolk sac in the embryo and the fetal spleen and liver provide the correct environment for stem cells to grow and replicate.

Although progenitor cells are not distinguishable from other lymphocyte-like cells morphologically, they can be revealed by marrow culture techniques. The human pluripotent stem cells are difficult to culture *in vitro* but, in the mouse, stem cells form colonies in the spleen of an irradiated recipient. A number of culture systems have been developed that permit proliferation of the committed progenitor cells for the major marrow cell lines (*Figs 1.3–1.7*). In culture media the progenitor cells are defined as 'colony forming units' (CFUs). Thus, the earliest detectable haemopoietic progenitor cell that gives rise to granulocytes, erythroblasts, monocytes and megakaryocytes is termed CFU_{GEMM} or CFU_{mix}. More mature and specialized precursor cells are termed CFU_{GM} (granulocytes and monocytes), CFU_{Eo} (eosinophils), CFU_{Ba} (basophils), CFU_E (erythroid) and CFU_{Meg} (megakaryocytes). The burst-forming unit, erythroid (BFU_E) is an earlier erythroid progenitor than the CFU_E (*Fig. 1.7*). It is now thought likely that a common stem cell gives rise to haemopoietic and mesenchymal stem cells (*see page 39*).

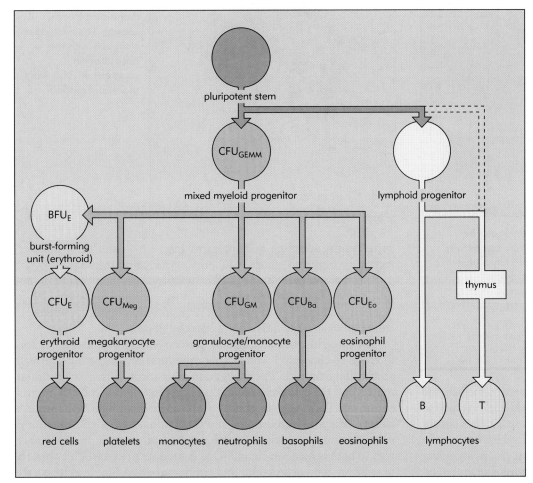

Fig. 1.1 Haemopoietic stem and progenitor cells: bone marrow pluripotent stem cell and the cell lines that arise from it. The various progenitor cells can be identified by culture in semisolid media by the type of colony they form. (CFU, colony-forming unit; GEMM, mixed granulocyte–erythroid–monocyte–megakaryocyte; E, erythroid; Meg, megakaryocyte; GM, granulocyte–monocyte; Eo, eosinophil; Ba, basophil; BFU, burst-forming unit.)

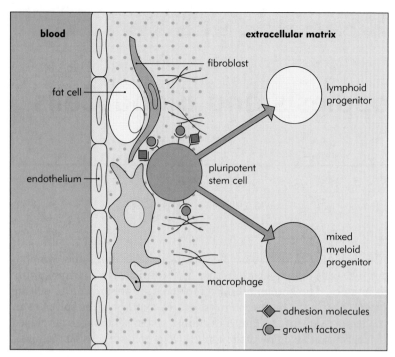

Fig. 1.2 Haemopoiesis: a suitable microenvironment for haemopoiesis is provided by a stromal matrix on which stem cells grow and divide. Adhesion molecules and growth factors bound to stromal cells or extracellular matrix provide attachment sites for the stem cells.

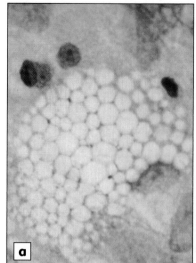
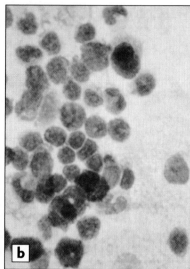

Fig. 1.3a and b Bone marrow cultures: (a) stromal cells present in long-term haemopoietic cultures of marrow. The main cellular components are fibroblasts, fat cells and macrophages; (b) a focus of haemopoietic cells deep in the adherent layer of a long-term haemopoietic culture. Each focus forms from a single 'long-term culture-initiating cell' (LTC-IC) as a result of cell–cell interactions and production of haemopoietic growth factors by stromal cells. The LTC-ICs have 'stem' cell characteristics in that they can self-replicate, as well as proliferate and differentiate into mature haemopoietic cells. (Courtesy of Prof. JM Hows.)

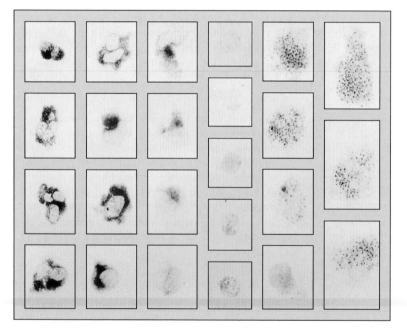

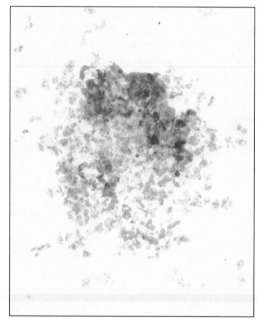

Fig. 1.5 Bone marrow culture: mixed granulocyte–erythroid (GE) colony. Haemoglobin-containing cells are stained with o-dianisidine (reddish brown). The neutrophils stain only with the haematoxylin counterstain. (Courtesy of Dr GE Francis.)

Fig. 1.4 Bone marrow culture: cells in diffuse GM colonies can be identified using a dual esterase method. Chloracetate esterase activity, present in cells of the granulocytic series, is demonstrated by a blue-staining reaction; non-specific esterase, present in cells of the macrophage lineage, is demonstrated by an amber-staining reaction. (Courtesy of Dr GE Francis.)

ADHESION MOLECULES

A large family of molecules termed cell adhesion molecules mediate the attachment of various body cells to each other and to extracellular matrix. The adhesion molecules on leucocytes and other haemopoietic cells are termed receptors and they bind with molecules (termed ligands) on the surface of target cells. Adhesion molecules include six groups according to their molecular structure, three main groups – immunoglobulin (Ig) superfamily, selectins and integrins (*Fig. 1.8*) – and three smaller, recently recognized groups (cadherins, syndecams and ADAMs).

Selectins recognize a sialylated carbohydrate on their counter-receptor. They mediate attachment of circulating leucocytes to the vessel wall. L-Selectin is expressed in nearly all circulatory leucocytes. D-Selectin is stored in Weibel–Palade bodies of endothelial cells.

The integrins mediate cell adhesion essential for adhesion of granulocytes to the vessel wall during migration and signals for growth and differentiation. They integrate activation of the extracellular matrix and the cytoskeleton and take part in cell–cell and cell–matrix communication (e.g. to collagen, fibronectin, or von Willebrand's factor). Integrins consist of α and β subunits, with eight different β subunits and more than 20 different αβ combinations. Integrins take part in both outside-in signalling (e.g. binding to extracellular matrix may affect gene expression) and inside-out signalling (e.g. leucocyte

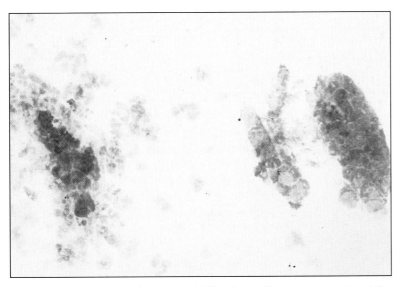

Fig. 1.6 Bone marrow culture: mixed GE colony adjacent to an eosinophil colony. (Luxol-fast blue stain; courtesy of Dr GE Francis.)

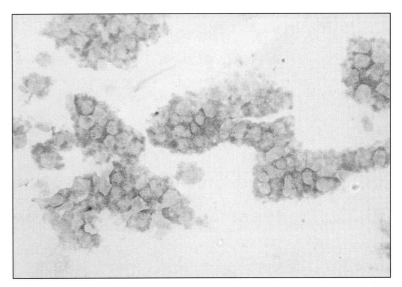

Fig. 1.7 Bone marrow culture: an erythroid 'burst'. This type of multicentre colony develops from a single BFU$_E$ cell. The cultures are stimulated by both erythropoietin and multicolony stimulating factor [burst-promoting activity (BPA, IL-3)] derived from phytohaemagglutinin-stimulated lymphocytes or other sources. (Courtesy Dr GE Francis.)

Adhesion molecules		
Family	**Function**	
Immunoglobulin superfamily	Antigen receptors	T-cell receptors, immunoglobulins
	Growth factor receptors	For example KIT, FMS
Selectins	Leucocyte and platelet adhesion to endothelium during inflammation or coagulation	
Integrins	Important in immune function, tissue repair, tumour spread and invasion, and platelet aggregation	

Fig. 1.8 Adhesion molecules: main. Three other families exist: cadherins, syndecans (receptors for extracellular matrix protein and growth factors) and ADAMs, which have a role in membrane fusion.

Stromal calls and extracellular matrix	
Stromal cells	**Extracellular matrix**
Macrophages	Fibronectin
Fibroblasts	Haemonectin
Reticulum ('blanket') cells	Laminin
Fat cells	Collagen
Endothelial cells	Proteoglycans (acid mucopolysaccharides; e.g. chondroitin, heparan)

Fig. 1.9 The stromal cells and extracellular matrix: haemopoiesis depends upon these.

recruitment in inflammation). Deficiency of β_2 integrins leads to leucocyte adhesion deficiency Type 1, which is severe if CD8 expression is 0–1% and moderately severe if CD8 expression is 2–5%; deficiency of $\alpha_{11}\beta_3$ integrin causes Glanzmann's disease (*see* page 276).

HAEMOPOIETIC GROWTH FACTORS

Proliferation of the stem and progenitor cells is under the control of the hormone-like inducers of growth and differentiation, produced by stromal cells of the microenvironment (*Fig. 1.9*) and by the haemopoietic cells themselves, such as the colony-stimulating factors, interleukins (ILs), the kidneys (erythropoietin) or liver (thrombopoietin). These may act locally or via the systemic circulation.

Haemopoietic growth factors are glycoproteins involved in the self-renewal of stem cells and the proliferation and differentiation of lineage-committed progenitor cells (*Fig. 1.10*). They also affect the functions of mature cells and are involved in the amplification of production of leucocytes in response to infection, red cells in response to anaemia, and platelets in response to thrombocytopenia. Several of them are termed colony-stimulating factors (CSFs), since they stimulate colony formation of progenitors *in vitro*; a prefix is added according to the major type of colony produced (e.g. G-CSF for granulocyte colonies), although it is now clear that the factors have a broad spectrum of overlapping activities (*Fig. 1.11*). Thrombopoietin (c-Mpl ligand) is a glycoprotein with some homology to erythropoietin. It stimulates

proliferation and maturation of megakaryocytes and greatly increases platelet production (*Fig. 1.12*).

Stem cell factor (SCF, KIT ligand) is a growth factor for the pluripotential stem cell (PSC) and also acts synergistically with other factors on later cells; Flt-3 ligand also acts as on stem and progenitor cells. IL-6 acts synergistically with the other factors on early cells and may be specifically involved in megakaryopoiesis (*see Fig. 1.12*). The growth factors G-CSF, GM-CSF and M-CSF have been used clinically to stimulate white cell production (e.g. post-chemotherapy; *Fig. 1.13*) in bone marrow transplantation, in the treatment of acquired immunodeficiency syndrome, myelodysplasia and aplastic anaemia, and for idiopathic and drug-induced neutropenia or agranulocytosis. They are also used to mobilize multipotent progenitors into peripheral blood to improve the harvest of these cells prior to autologous stem cell transplantation.

Neither IL-3 nor GM-CSF are lineage-specific; they are required throughout haemopoiesis, acting on pluripotent and early progenitor cells, and are required for self-renewal as well as differentiation. G-CSF, M-CSF, IL-5, thrombopoietin and erythropoietin act on more mature cells of a specific lineage, but they also act synergistically with other growth factors on early cells. The sources of the CSFs are marrow stromal cells (fibroblasts and endothelial cells), lymphocytes and macrophages. Monocyte-derived IL-1 and tumour necrosis factor (TNF; see below) probably induce fixed marrow stromal cells, as well as T lymphocytes and macrophages, to produce G-CSF and GM-CSF (*see Fig. 1.11*). All these cell types are also capable of producing G-CSF,

Biological aspects of the cytokines and haemopoietic growth factors

Cytokine	Molecular weight (Da)	Cell sources	Target cells	Main effects	Chromosome
IL-1αβ	17,500	Macrophages, somatic cells	Haemopoiesis, immune system	Inflammatory (see Fig. 1.14)	2q12–21
IL-2	15,500	T lymphocytes	T and B cells	T-cell growth factor	4q26–27
IL-3	28,000	T lymphocytes	Early haemopoietic cells	Haemopoietic growth factor	5q23–31
IL-4	19,000	T cells, mast cells	T and B cells, early haemopoietic cells	Immune and haemopoietic growth factor	5q31
IL-5	40,000–50,000 homodimer	T cells, mast cells	Eosinophils	Eosinophil growth and differentiation factor	5q23–31
IL-6	21,000–28,000	Fibroblasts, T cells, macrophages, somatic cells	B cells, megakaryocytes	Immunoglobulin production, hepatic acute phase protein platelet production	7p21–14
IL-7	25,000	Stromal cells	Early B and T lymphocytes	Growth factor for B and T cells	8q12–13
IL-8	6000–8000	Ubiquitous: macrophages, endothelial cells, fibroblasts, somatic cells	Chemoattractant for neutrophils and T lymphocytes	Neutrophil and basophil migration	4q12–21
IL-9	35,000	TH2 cells	Mast cells, erythroid progenitors	Haemopoiesis and T-cell development	5q31.1
IL-10	35,000–40,000	T helper and B cells, keratinocytes, macrophages	B and T cells, monocytes, macrophages	Mast cell and B-cell proliferation and antibody production; suppresses cytokine production from monocytes, T helper cells	1
IL-11	23,000	Fibroblasts, stromal cells	Megakaryocytes, early haemopoietic cells, B cells	Haemopoiesis and thrombopoiesis, B-cell immunoglobulin secretion	19q13.3–13.4
IL-12	70,000 heterodimer	Macrophages, B cells	T cells, NK cells	Induces IFNγ and cell-mediated immunity	19p13.1 and 1p31.2
IL-13	10,000	T cells	Monocytes, B cells	Promotes IgE production	5q31
IL-14	60,000	T cells, some B cells	Growth factor	Inhibits Ig synthesis	
IL-15	14,000	Monocytes, granulocytes, fibroblasts	T cells	Growth and proliferation of T cells	4q31
IFNαβ	18,000–20,000	Leucocytes, fibroblasts	Macrophages, NK cells	Antiviral, antiproliferative and immunomodulating; induces Class I MHC antigens	
IFNγ	20,000–25,000	T lymphocytes, NK cells	T and B cells	Immunomodulating antiproliferative (inhibits apoptosis) and antiviral; induces cell membrane antigens (e.g. MHC Class I or II)	12q24.1
TNFα	17,000	Macrophages, somatic cells, T and B lymphocytes	Ubiquitous	Inflammatory, immunoenhancing and induces apoptosis; secondary production of cytokines by stromal cells	6p21.3
TNFβ (lymphotoxin)	18,000	T lymphocytes	Ubiquitous	Inflammatory, immunoenhancing and induces apoptosis; secondary production of cytokines by stromal cells	
TGFβ	25,000	Platelets, T cells, somatic cells	Fibroblasts, many other cells	Anti-inflammatory, wound healing, bone remodelling	19q13
MIP-1α	7500	T and B cells, neutrophils, macrophages	B cells, progenitor cells, macrophages	Inhibitory factor	17q11–21
SCF (KIT ligand)	20,000–35,000	Stromal cells, fibroblasts, liver cells	Mast cells, early pluripotent cells, and myeloid, lymphoid or erythroid progenitors	Growth factor for stem cells, early lymphoid and myeloid progenitors, mast cells	12q22–24
Flt-3L	ca. 30,000	Stromal fibroblasts	Stem and progenitor cells	Growth factor for stem and progenitor cells	
LIF	20,000	Stromal cells	Early haemopoietic cells	Growth factor for stem cells	22q14
GM-CSF	14,000–35,000	Stromal cells, T lymphocytes, mast cells	Haemopoietic progenitors and late cells in granulocytic, monocytic lineages	Stimulates early haemopoiesis, mast cell granulopoiesis, monocyte formation and function	5q31–32
G-CSF	18,000	Stromal cells, macrophages, monocytes	Granulocyte progenitors and granulocytes	Early haemopoiesis, granulocyte production and function	17q21–22
M-CSF	40,000–70,000	Stromal cells, macrophages, monocytes	Monocyte progenitors and monocytes	Monocyte production and function	5q33.1
Erythropoietin	34,000–39,000	Kidney, liver	Erythroid progenitors (late BFUE, CFUE) and erythrocyte precursors to reticulocyte stage	Growth factor for red cells	7pterq22
Thrombopoietin	35,000	Liver, kidney	Stem cells, megakaryocytes, BFUE	Growth factor for platelets	3q26–27

Fig. 1.10 The cytokines and haemopoietic growth factors: biological aspects. (IL, interleukin; IFN, interferon; TNF, tumour necrosis factor; TGF, transforming growth factor; MIP, macrophage inflammatory protein; SCF, stem cell factor; Flt-L, ligand for stem cell tyrosine kinase-1; LIF, leucocyte inhibitory factor; NK, natural killer; MHC, major histocompatibility complex.)

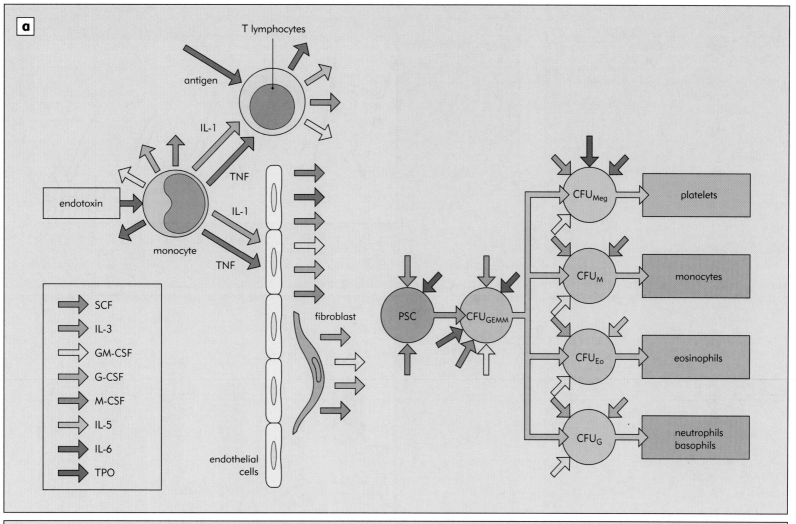

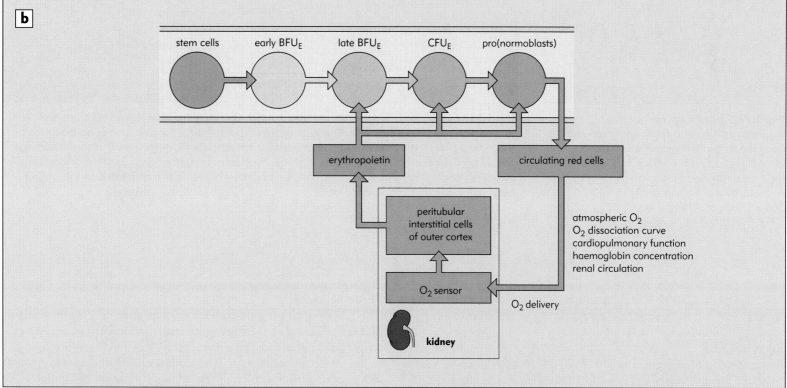

Fig. 1.11a and b Regulation of haemopoiesis: (a) pathways of stimulation of leucopoiesis by endotoxin (e.g. from infection). It is likely that endothelial and fibroblast cells release basal quantities of GM-CSF and G-CSF in the normal resting state and that this is enhanced substantially by the monokines TNF and IL-1 released in response to infection. Also, IL-1 and TNF stimulate T cells, and antigen may stimulate T cells directly. The action of IL-3 on human PSCs has not been proved (TPO, thrombopoietin). (b) The production of erythropoietin by the kidney in response to its oxygen (O_2) supplies is shown. Erythropoietin stimulates erythropoiesis and so increases O_2 delivery; O_2 delivery may also be affected by other factors, as shown. (From Erslev AJ, Gabuzda TG. *Pathology of Blood*, 3rd edn. Philadelphia: WB Saunders; 1985.)

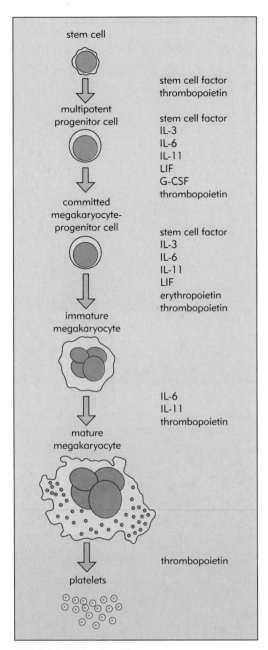

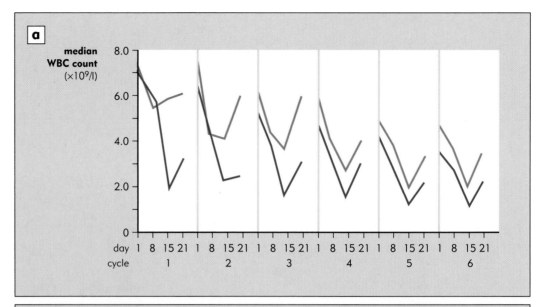

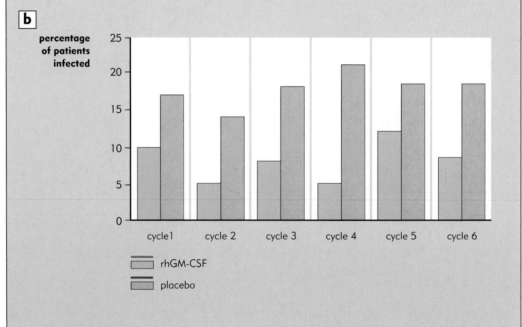

Fig. 1.12 Role of cytokines in megakaryocytopoiesis: many cytokines have been shown to affect megakaryocyte and platelet production *in vivo*, but only SCF and thrombopoietin seem essential. (Adapted with permission from Kaushansky K. Thrombopoietin. *N Engl J Med*. 1998;339:746–54.)

Fig. 1.13a and b GM-CSF response: the effect of GM-CSF on (a) median leucocyte counts and (b) infection rates in patients who receive six cycles of chemotherapy for high-grade non-Hodgkin lymphoma. (Adapted with permission from Gerhartz HH, Engelhard M, Meusers P, *et al*. Randomized, double-blind, placebo-controlled, phase III study of recombinant human granulocyte–macrophage colony-stimulating factor as adjunct to induction treatment of high-grade malignant non-Hodgkin's lymphomas. *Blood*. 1993;82:2329–39.)

M-CSF and Eo-CSF. IL-8 is a chemoattractant for neutrophils and T lymphocytes and plays an important role in neutrophil migration.

Erythropoietin

Erythropoietin of molecular weight (MW) 34–39 kDa, when fully glycosylated (polypeptide MW 18.4 kDa), derives from the kidney and, to a small extent, the liver, and is secreted in response to anoxia caused, for example, by anaemia or high altitude (*Fig. 1.11*). It stimulates erythropoiesis largely at the committed CFU_E stage; also, a proportion of BFU_E progenitors are sensitive to it and it acts on later cells (up to the reticulocyte stage) to stimulate haemoglobin synthesis. The progenitor cells are stimulated to proliferate and differentiate terminally.

Thrombopoietin

The thrombopoietin gene encodes a polypeptide of 353 amino acids, including a 21 amino acid secretory leader sequence. The mature protein of 332 amino acids has a predicted MW of 38 kDa. The amino terminal 155 residues have a 21% sequence identity and 46% overall sequence similarity with erythropoietin. The carboxyl 177 amino acids have multiple N- and O-linked carbohydrate residues. The gene is expressed mainly in the liver, with some expression in the kidney. It stimulates survival and proliferation of haemopoietic stem and megakaryocyte colony-forming cells (*Fig. 1.12*). It also stimulates formation of megakaryocytes, including endomitosis and polyploidy, megakaryocyte maturation, expression of platelet markers CD41 and CD61 and release of platelets into the blood. After daily administration, a 7–10 day delay in the rise of platelets occurs, and platelets remain increased for 6–16 days after discontinuation of thrombopoietin therapy. Thrombopoietin has an elimination half-life of 30 hours, the longest of any of the haemopoietic growth factors. It also, with erythropoietin stimulates the growth of erythroid progenitor cells.

LYMPHOKINES AND MONOKINES

Lymphokines and monokines are glycoproteins that are released by lymphocytes and monocytes (macrophages) and have wide-ranging effects on haemopoiesis, the immune response, and the response to infection and to invasion by tumours (see Fig. 1.10). They have a complex network of interactions and are described here only briefly.

Interleukin-1

Activated macrophages produce IL-1 in two forms, alpha and beta, in the ratio 1:10, as do endothelial cells, astrocytes, fibroblasts and T cells,. Both α and β IL-1 are biologically active, with widespread participation in the recruitment and activation of cells involved in the inflammatory response, in wound healing, in the immune response and in early stages of haemopoiesis. Fig. 1.14 illustrates some of the functions of IL-1, which:
- acts as an endogenous pyrogen;
- activates lymphocytes, neutrophils, other macrophages and natural killer (NK) cells;
- induces proliferation of osteoclasts, fibroblasts, epithelial, endothelial and synovial cells; and
- enhances major histocompatibility complex (MHC) Class II antigen expression.

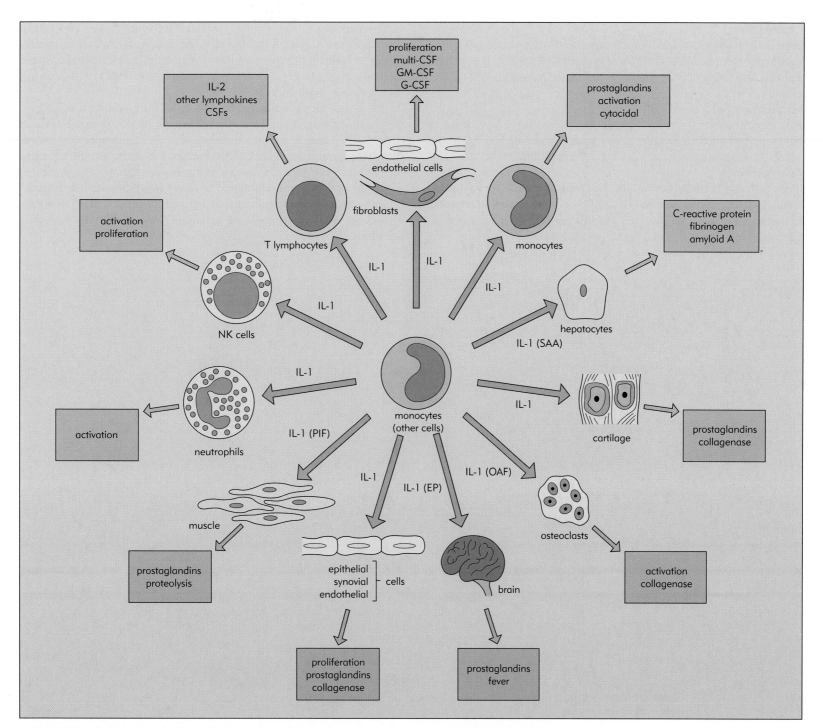

Fig. 1.14 Interleukin 1: some of its effects on target cells and tissues. Osteoclast activating factor (OAF) may be TNFα induced by IL-1. (SAA, serum amyloid A; PIF, proteolysis inducing factor; EP, endogenous pyrogen; modified from Oppenheim, et al. Immunol Today. 1986;7:45–56.)

Prostaglandin and collagenase syntheses are increased by IL-1. It plays an important role in haemopoiesis by stimulating marrow stromal cells to secrete CSFs.

Interleukin-2

The proliferation of T lymphocytes is promoted by IL-2, as is, to a lesser extent, that of B cells and monocytes. It promotes cytotoxic function by stimulating the proliferation and activity of NK cells. The IL-2 receptor consists of two proteins, one of which is detected by monoclonal antibodies of the CD25 group.

Interleukin-4

IL-4 has a wide variety of effects both in haemopoiesis and in development of both B and T cells. It is required for the development of B cells to switch expression of Ig class.

Interleukin-6

Like IL-1, IL-6 has a wide variety of effects in haemopoiesis, the immune system and as an acute phase protein (*Fig. 1.15*). It may have a particular role in platelet production, but is not essential for this.

Interleukins 7–15

The more recently discovered cytokines IL-7 to IL-15 have roles in haemopoiesis and immune development and function (*see Fig. 1.10*).

Apoptosis

Cell death can occur by necrosis or by a physiologically active mechanism (apoptosis, programmed cell death). Necrosis occurs in response to ischaemia, chemical trauma or hyperthermia. It affects many adjacent cells, and is characterized by cell swelling, with early loss of plasma membrane integrity and swelling of organelles and nucleus. There is usually an inflammatory infiltrate of phagocytic cells in response to spillage of cell contents into surrounding space.

Programmed cell death occurs by an active process that requires calcium ions. Nuclear condensation, nuclear fragmentation, and cytoplasmic vacuolation occur early, with later changes in the organelles and plasma membrane (*Fig. 1.16*). Apoptosis also involves digestion of cell DNA by an endonuclease to produce on a gel a ladder of regular bands 180 base pairs apart (*see Fig. 10.20*). Cleavage occurs by double-stranded breaks on linker regions between nucleosomes (*see Fig. 10.20*). The final part of the apoptosis pathway involves caspase enzymes. The executioner caspase 3 cleaves a restricted set of cellular proteins, including polyadenosine diphosphate–ribose polymerase, laminin and gelsolin. Caspase 3 is activated by caspase 9. This in turn is activated by the apoptotic protease 1 (APAF-1), which itself is activated by cytochrome c. Cytochrome c is released from mitochondria when the pro-apoptotic protein BAX is in excess and forms homodimers. Cells are protected from apoptosis by BCL-2, which binds to BAX and thereby inhibits cytochrome c release and caspase activation (*Fig. 1.17*). Apoptosis is promoted by BAD, which forms heterodimers with BCL-2.

Apoptosis may be triggered by extracellular ligands such as TNF or the ligand of the FAS pathway that activates the ICE protease cascade (*Fig. 1.17*). There is a direct association of their receptors with a caspase family protease, FLICE. Oligomerization of the receptors consequent on ligand binding results in direct activation of the protease. Apoptosis may also be stimulated by direct DNA damage (e.g. by radiation or drugs) or by withdrawal of a growth factor (e.g. IL-3) that promotes survival by stimulating phosphorylation of BAD by protein kinase B, thus preventing its association with BCL-2.

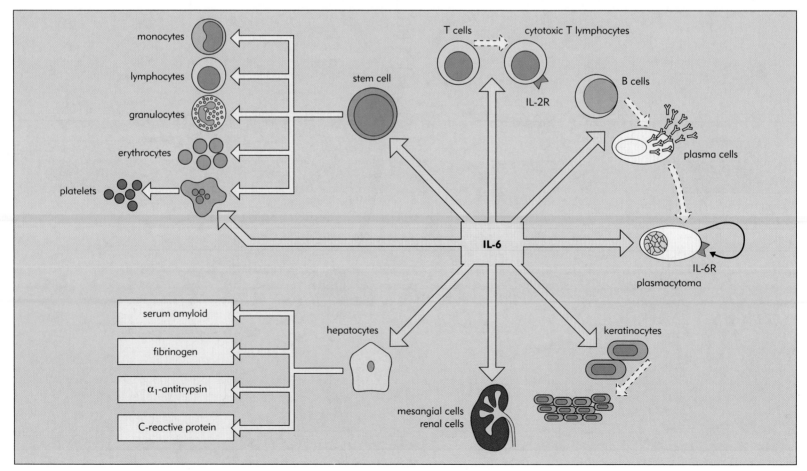

Fig. 1.15 Interleukin 6: pleiotropic functions. (Modified with permission from Hirano T, Akira S, Taga T, *et al.* Biological and clinical aspects of interleukin-6. *Immunol Today.* 1990;11:443–9.)

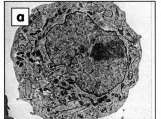 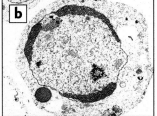 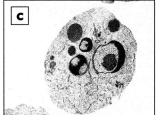 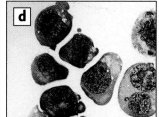 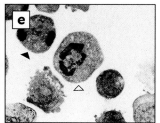

Fig. 1.16a–e Apoptosis: (a–c) electron microscopic and (d, e) light microscopic appearances. (a) Normal K562 cell line; (b) early apoptotic cell showing chromatin condensation at the nuclear periphery; (c) later apoptotic cell showing both chromatin condensation and nuclear fragmentation; (d) normal K562 cell line; and (e) early apoptotic cell (open arrowhead) with peripheral chromatin condensation and late apoptotic cell (solid arrowhead) with both chromatin condensation and nuclear fragmentation. (Reproduced with permission from Riordan FA, Bravery CA, Mengubas K, *et al*. Herbimycin A accelerates the induction of apoptosis following etoposide treatment or gamma-irradiation of bcr/abl-positive leukaemia cells. *Oncogene*. 1998;16:1533–42.)

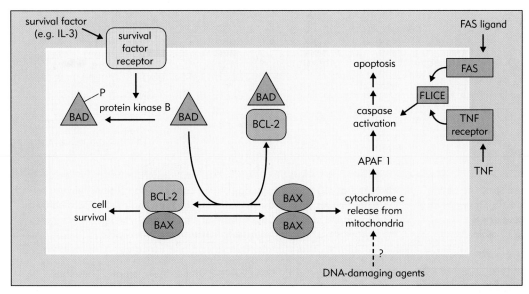

Fig. 1.17 Apoptosis: regulation by BCL-2, BAX and BAD proteins. A predominance of BAX results in cytochrome c release, caspase activation and apoptosis. BCL-2 prevents apoptosis by dimerization with BAX, and BAD promotes apoptosis by sequestration of BCL-2. Phosphorylation of BAD by protein kinase B neutralizes its pro-apoptotic function by preventing its association with the anti-apoptotic BCL-2 protein. The mechanisms by which DNA-damaging agents (e.g. radiation and drugs) cause cytochrome c release are unclear. Cytokines regulate apoptosis both positively and negatively. FLICE is a caspase family protease (caspase 8). [Adapted with permission from Wickremasinghe RG, Hoffbrand AV. The molecular basis of leukaemia and lymphoma. In: Hoffbrand AV, Lewis SM, Tuddenham EGD (eds). *Postgraduate Haematology*, 4th edn. Oxford: Butterworth–Heinemann; 1999:354–72.]

Interferons

Interferons are proteins synthesized by a wide variety of cells in response to viral infections. They inhibit viral replication in other cells by inducing new cellular RNA and protein synthesis. Interferon-α has a MW of 18–20 kDa and consists of a family of proteins encoded by separate genes. The biological effects are mediated through activation of the enzyme 2′,5′-oligoadenylate synthase and induction of protein phosphokinase and other proteins. Interferon-α has a variety of effects on the immune system, enhancing NK and other cytotoxic effector activity while depressing lymphocyte proliferation, inhibiting apoptosis and altering cell surface antigen expression (*see also Fig. 1.91*).

Interferon-γ is produced by T lymphocytes in response to stimulation by IL-1 and IL-2. It activates NK cells and has widespread activity in promoting Class II antigen expression on B and T cells, antigen-presenting cells (APCs), endothelial and epithelial cells and other cells outside the immune system. It activates macrophages to phagocytose and to secrete IL-1. Also, it has potent direct-growth inhibitory properties, and inhibits apoptosis of B lymphocytes.

Tumour necrosis factor (α) and lymphotoxin (tumour necrosis factor β)

A protein of MW 17 kDa, TNFα is produced by macrophages and NK cells and is capable of causing lysis of some malignant cells (with less effect on normal equivalent cells) and also of some parasites and early marrow precursor cells. Like IL-1, it may also act as a mediator of inflammation, causing production of collagenase and prostaglandins and activation of neutrophils, eosinophils and monocytes, and it is a mediator of endotoxin shock and cachexia ('cachectin'). A substance with close homology to TNFα and produced by CD4+ and CD8+ lymphocytes has been called lymphotoxin or TNFβ; it has similar activities to TNFα.

Migration inhibition factor

Migration inhibition factor (MIF), released by T lymphocytes, decreases the migration of macrophages, arresting them at the site of inflammation or tumour. Related factors released by lymphocytes include a macrophage activating factor and a chemotactic factor for macrophages.

MEMBRANE–GROWTH FACTOR INTERACTIONS

Growth factor receptors

The mechanism by which the signal to proliferate or differentiate, carried by an extracellular factor, is transmitted from the cell membrane to the cell nucleus is becoming apparent. Binding of the growth factor to a specific receptor on the cell surface causes a transmembrane signal. All the cytokine receptors are transmembrane glycoproteins with an extracellular amino-terminal ligand-binding domain, a short hydrophobic transmembrane domain and a carboxy-terminal intracellular domain. The receptors share common structural motifs and fall into different families (*Fig. 1.18*). Most of the interleukins and growth factor receptors are members of the cytokine-receptor superfamily, Class I or Class II. For Class I there are one or two conserved cytokine receptor domains (CRDs) in the extracellular region. The CRD includes two repeats of a fibronectin Type III-like domain, one with four regularly spaced cysteine residues, and the other with the WSXWS motif (*Fig. 1.18*). The Class II receptors do not include WXSWS motifs. Both Class I and II receptors include a conserved cytoplasmic domain, known as a Box I region, that is important in signal transduction. They do not include intrinsic enzymatic activities.

The Ig superfamily contains two classes, those with an intrinsic tyrosine kinase domain (e.g. M-CSFR, SCFR) and those which activate

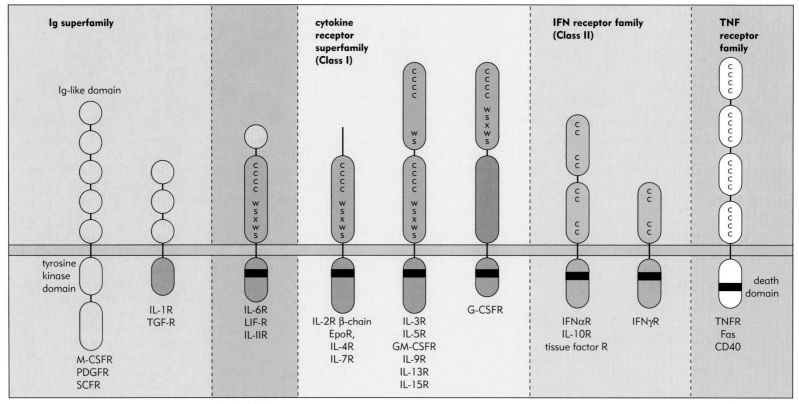

Fig. 1.18 Receptors for growth factors and other cytokines: structure of the different families. Receptors for M-CSF, PDGF and SCF (c-KIT), shown by an R at the end of each symbol, act as tyrosine kinases to achieve signal transduction. Receptors for the other cytokines include a 210 amino acid homologous region in the ligand-binding portion. This contains four conserved cysteine residues (c) and a tryptophan–serine repeated motif separated by a random amino acid (Trp–Ser–X–Trp–Ser etc., shown by wsxws). The intracytoplasmic regions are usually rich in serine and proline.

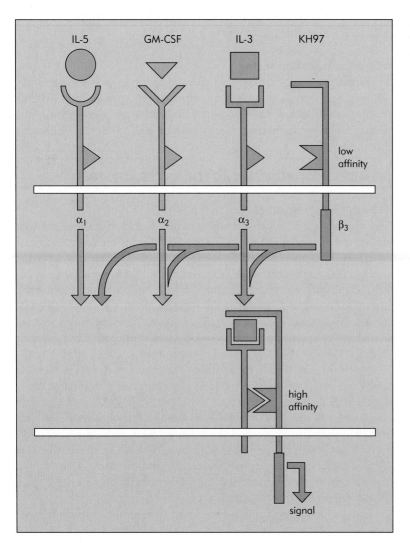

Fig. 1.19 Receptors for GM-CSF, IL-3 and IL-5: structures. These have different α chains but a common β chain (KH97) that, after binding to the α chain in the presence of the growth factor forms a high-affinity receptor and is subsequently responsible for signal transduction to the cell interior. The receptors for IL-2, IL-4, IL-6, IL-7, erythropoietin and G-CSF all consist of heterodimers with different α and β chains. (Modified from Nicola NA, Metcalf D. Subunit promiscuity among haemopoietic growth factor receptors. *Cell.* 1991;67:1–4.)

associated serine–threonine kinases (e.g. TGFR, IL-1R). Activation of signal transduction often occurs by dimerization of two receptors after ligand binding, or by activation of one chain of the receptor to transmit the signal after binding of the growth factor to a heterodimer receptor (*Fig. 1.19*).

Signal transduction

A cascade of phosphorylation events has been proposed to link receptors to activation of transcription factors in the nucleus, which then activate genes involved in the cell cycle (*Figs 1.20 and 1.21*). In some cases (e.g. the receptors for SCF, M-CSF) the intracellular domain of the receptor acts as a tyrosine kinase, which phosphorylates itself on tyrosine residues following ligand binding. These phosphotyrosine residues now bind signal-transducing proteins that contain SRC homology 2 (SH2) domains, thereby initiating cascades of biochemical events (*Fig. 1.22*). RAF-1 and a series of MAP-kinases (ERKs) have major roles in transmitting the signal to the nucleus and activating transcription factors. RAS proteins are activated by a complex of proteins called Grb-2 and Sos (*Fig. 1.20*). In one pathway, the enzyme phospholipase Cγ (PLCγ), which cleaves phosphatidyl inositol bisphosphate, is activated to break down membrane lipid, releasing two secondary messengers, diacylglycerol (DG) and inositol triphosphate (IP3; *Fig. 1.22*). Activation of PLCγ occurs by binding to phosphotyrosine residues of the activated receptor (*Fig. 1.22*). The

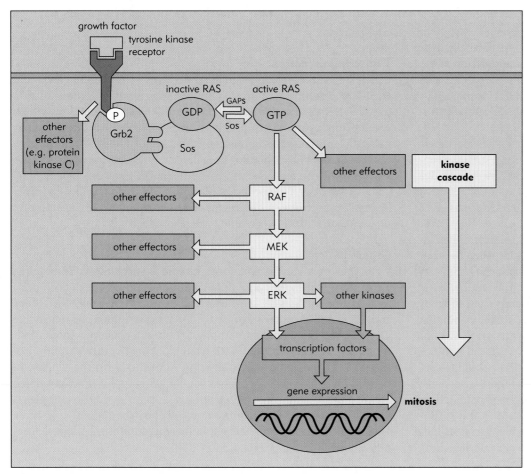

Fig. 1.20 The RAS pathway: this is central to growth control in organisms as diverse as humans, fruitflies, nematode worms and yeast. It runs from the cell surface to the nucleus, where genes are turned on or off in response to the incoming signal. The process starts with the binding of a growth factor, such as stem cell factor or M-CSF, to its tyrosine kinase receptor, which results in autophosphorylation of the receptor's tyrosine residues. Controllers of RAS exchange factors, such as Grb2, then come into operation. They recruit exchange factors (or activators, Sos being an example) to interact with RAS; the activators function as guanine nucleotide releasing agents that convert RAS-GDP, the inactive form, into active RAS-GTP. Downstream of RAS, a principal target is the RAF protein, also the product of a proto-oncogene. Once activated, RAF phosphorylates a second kinase (MAP kinase kinase, or MEK). After mediation by other kinases, signals pass into the cell nucleus through phosphorylation of transcription factors that regulate gene expression. Active RAS-GTP is returned to RAS-GDP by an intrinsic GTPase which is activated by GTPase-activating protein (GAP). Not shown are other signalling routes that interact with this pathway, or details of branch or feedback points. (Modified from Egan SE, Weinberg RA. The pathway to signal achievement. *Nature*. 1993;365:781–2.)

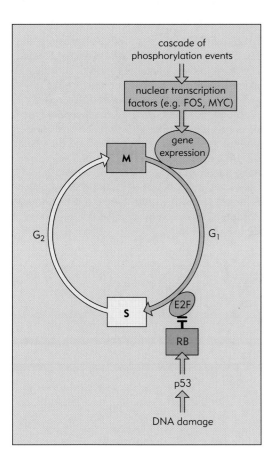

Fig. 1.21 The cell cycle: E2F is a transcription factor needed for cell transition from G1 to S. E2F. is inhibited by the tumour suppressor gene RB (retinoblastoma), which can be indirectly activated by p53.

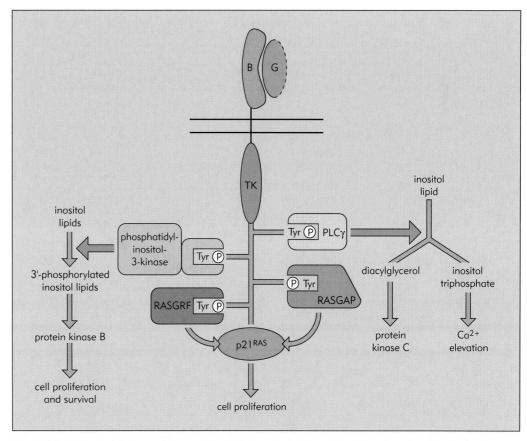

Fig. 1.22 SH2 domain-containing proteins: binding to activated, tyrosine phosphorylated growth factor receptors. For clarity, only one partner of the receptor dimer is shown. [PLCγ, phospholipase Cγ; RASGAP, RAS GTPase-activating protein; RASGRF, guanine nucleotide releasing factor, shown as Grb2–Sos complex in *Fig. 1.20*; adapted with permission from Wickremasinghe RG, Hoffbrand AV. The molecular basis of leukaemia and lymphoma. In: Hoffbrand AV, Lewis SM, Tuddenham EGD (eds). *Postgraduate Haematology*, 4th edn. Oxford: Butterworth–Heinemann; 1999:354–72.]

enzyme protein kinase C (PKC) is activated by DG and, in turn, phosphorylates proteins mainly on threonine and serine residues. Release of intracellular calcium ions is caused by IP3. The exact way in which these two biochemical changes subsequently cause signal transduction to the nucleus is unclear. Phosphatidyl inositol 3'-kinase (PI-3 kinase) is also activated by binding to activated receptor. It phosphorylates inositol lipids, which activate protein kinase B (AKT), which signals for cell proliferation and survival.

For those receptors (cytokine superfamily) that do not possess inherent protein kinase activity, the JAK–STAT system links cell surface receptors with transcription factor genes. The JAK kinase family includes JAK1, JAK2, JAK3 and TYK2. They are cytoplasmic, of MW 130 kDa and possess a conserved region at the N-terminal end, a kinase-like domain and a tyrosine kinase domain at the C-terminal end (Fig. 1.23). The JAK kinases are activated by ligand binding and receptor dimerization. Box 1 and Box 2, conserved regions on the cytokine receptor intracytoplasmic regions, are involved in binding and activation of JAKs. The JAK kinases then phosphorylate tyrosine residues in latent cytokine transcription factors, the signal transducers and activators of transcription (STATs). The STATs, of MW 80–100 kDa, are DNA-binding proteins with an SH2 domain and tyrosine phosphorylation sites at the C-terminal region (Fig. 1.23). The activated STATs form a homo- or heterodimer and translocate to the nucleus, where they bind to specific DNA motifs, positive promoter elements for cytokine-responsive genes. In addition to STAT activation, JAK kinases also phosphorylate additional proteins, including insulin-receptor substrate 1 and 2 (IRS-1, 2) and GAB2. The resultant phosphotyrosine residues serve as binding sites for SH2 domain-containing proteins which activate signalling pathways that lead to ERK activation, essentially as shown in Figs 1.20 and 1.22.

Transcription factors

The response to cytokine signalling involves activation of genes that encode transcription factors. These belong to six different families (Fig. 1.24) and contribute to the changes in gene expression which results from cytokine receptor activation. The genes are activated by intranuclear phosphorylation (e.g. by STATs or ERKs). The transcription factor has a DNA-binding domain that binds a factor-specific DNA sequence, the enhancer element E (Fig. 1.25). The transactivation domain binds to the general transcription machinery (RNA polymerase and other factors) and facilitates binding of this machinery to TATA promoter sequences upstream of the gene to be transcribed.

Cell cycle

Cytokines may activate cells into a cycle (see Fig 1.21). The cyclins are proteins the expression of which differs throughout the cell cycle by periodic changes in synthesis and degradation (Fig. 1.26). They activate a set of protein kinases (CDKs) which then phosphorylate various proteins. Phosphorylation of the retinoblastoma susceptibility gene product RB prevents RB from blocking the transcription factors (e.g. E2F) essential for transition from the G_1 to the S phase of the cell cycle (see Fig 1.21). The cyclin CDK complexes are regulated by inhibitors. Thus, cyclin D–CDK4 and cyclin D–CDK6 complexes are inhibited by a 16 kDa protein encoded by the INK4a gene and a 15 kDa protein encoded by the INK4b gene, inhibiting progress from mid to late G_1.

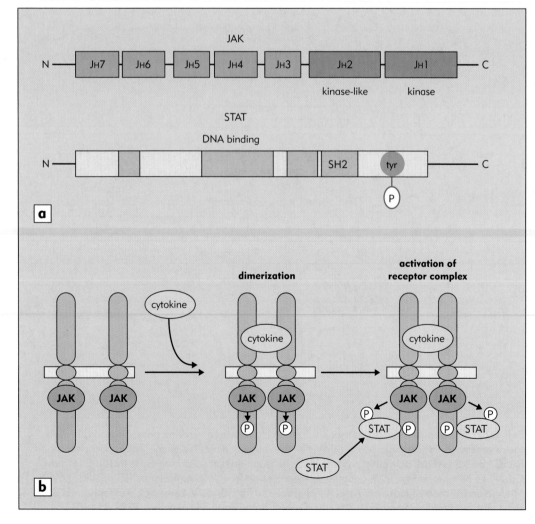

Fig. 1.23a and b JAKs and STATs: (a) structure and (b) a model of their activation by a cytokine. Binding of a cytokine to the receptor results in dimerization or oligomerization of the receptor, which leads to activation of the receptor-associated JAK kinases. The receptors are then tyrosine-phosphorylated, and STATs are recruited to the phosphorylated tyrosine residues of the receptors through the SH2 domain of STATs. JAKs then activate STATs. [JH, JAK homology domain; adapted with permission from Hara T, Miyajima A. Cytokine receptors and signal reduction. In: Degos L, Linch DC, Löwenberg B (eds). *Textbook of Malignant Haematology*. London: Martin Dunitz; 1999:111–32.]

Families of transcription factors	
Family	**Examples**
Leucine zipper	FOS, JUN
Helix–loop–helix	MYC, TAL-1
Helix–turn–helix	PBX-1
Zinc finger	PML, RAR
LIM	Rhombotin 1 and 2
REL	NF-KB

Fig. 1.24 Transcription factors involved in haemopoietic cell signalling: these occur in six families.

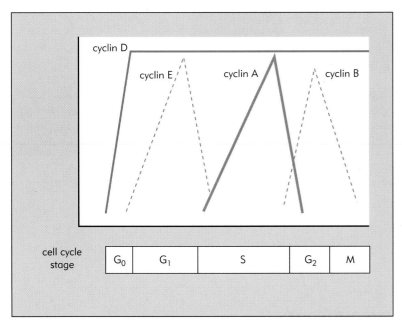

Fig. 1.26 Cell cycle: synthesis and degradation of specific cyclins. [Adapted with permission from Wickremasinghe RG, Hoffbrand AV. The molecular basis of leukaemia and lymphoma. In: Hoffbrand AV, Lewis SM, Tuddenham EGD (eds). *Postgraduate Haematology*, 4th edn. Oxford: Butterworth–Heinemann; 1999:354–72.]

Three classes of gene whose mutation, translocation or abnormal expression may lead to malignant transformation	
Cellular oncogenes	
Extracellular growth factor	SIS
Membrane-associated tyrosine kinases (including growth factor receptors)	FMS, KIT, ERB-B
Intracellular signal transducers:	
GTP binding	H-RAS, K-RAS, N-RAS
Serine/threonine kinases	RAF, MOS
Tyrosine kinase	ABL
Nuclear:	
transcriptor factors	JUN, FOS, MYC, ETS,
hormone/vitamin receptor	ERB-A, RARA-α
Tumour suppressor genes	p53, RB
Inhibition of apoptosis	BCL-2

Fig. 1.27 Abnormal gene expression: three classes of gene that may lead to malignant transformation.

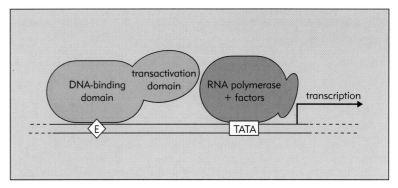

Fig. 1.25 Transcription activation by a transcription control factor: simplified model. The DNA-binding domain of the factor binds a factor-specific chromosomal DNA sequence, the enhancer element (E). The transactivation domain binds the general transcription machinery (RNA polymerase and associated factors) and facilitates binding of the latter to nucleotide (TATA) promoter sequences upstream of the structural gene, which is consequently transcribed to generate mRNA. [Adapted with permission from Wickremasinghe RG, Hoffbrand AV. The molecular basis of leukaemia and lymphoma. In: Hoffbrand AV, Lewis SM, Tuddenham EGD (eds). *Postgraduate Haematology*, 4th edn. Oxford: Butterworth–Heinemann; 1999:354–72.]

Cell cycle checkpoints: role of p53 gene

The p53 gene codes for a 53 kDa transcription control factor that mediates a block in the cell cycle at the G_1–S phase boundary (*Fig 1.21*). This is mediated by a p21 cyclin CDK inhibitor, $p21^{CIPI}$. Expression of p53 is induced by DNA damage that results from radiation or drugs. The cell is therefore held up in G_1 and may repair the damage. If the damage is extensive, p53 induces apoptosis by increased expression of BAX.

ONCOGENES AND TUMOUR SUPPRESSOR GENES

Changes in the function of certain normal genes that have been well-conserved throughout mammalian and other species may lead to malignant transformation (*Fig. 1.27*). Most of these genes, called cellular oncogenes or proto-oncogenes, code for proteins involved in cell proliferation or differentiation (*Fig. 1.28*). The first examples of these genes to be discovered were named after the vertebrate species in which acute transforming viruses carrying closely homologous genes caused tumours. Cellular oncogenes may be activated in human tumours by chromosome translocations, point mutations or amplification.

In haematological malignancies, oncogenes are activated most frequently by translocation, which affects the expression of the gene either *quantitatively* (especially frequent in acute lymphoblastic leukaemia) or *qualitatively*. Quantitative effects usually occur by translocation adjacent to an Ig gene (IgH, κ or λ light chain) or T-cell receptor gene (α, β, γ or δ). Qualitative effects occur by forming a fusion gene with part of an adjacent gene to which the gene is translocated (*Fig. 1.29*). For example, BCR-ABL in chronic myeloid leukaemia, PML-RARA in acute myeloid leukaemia M₃ or PBX-EHA in pre B-ALL (*see* Chapters 8 and 9).

Another set of genes, tumour suppressor genes, are normally involved in the negative control of cell proliferation (*see Fig. 1.21*). Loss of activity of these genes because of deletion or mutation on both alleles may therefore contribute to uncontrolled cell proliferation. The inappropriate expression of a third group of genes may lead to malignancy by inhibiting programmed cell death; this group is represented by BCL-2, a gene whose protein product is normally expressed in the outer membrane of mitochondria.

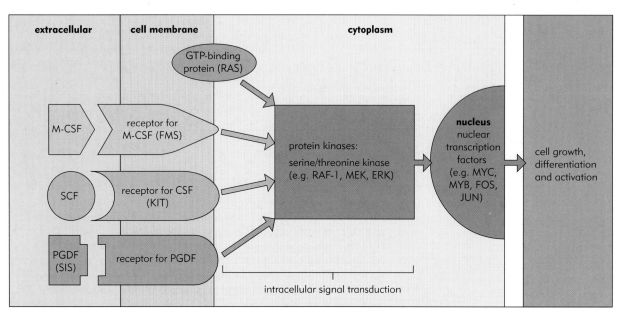

Fig. 1.28 Cellular proto-oncogene products: examples of those that act at different stages of the pathways by which growth signals are transduced through the cell membrane to the nucleus.

Lineage	Malignancy	Translocation	Genes	Mechanism
T cell	T-cell ALL	t(1;14), t(1;7), t(1;3)	SCL	Dysregulation
		t(7;9)	TAL-2	
		t(7;19)	LYL-1	
		t(11;14)	LMO-1	
		t(11;14), t(7;11)	LMO-2	
		t(10;14), t(7;10)	HOX11	
		t(8;14)	MYC	
	ALL	t(1;19)	PBX-1, E2A	
		t(17;19)	HLF, E2A	
		t(12;21)	TEL, AML-1	
B cell	Burkitt's lymphoma	t(8;14), t(2;8), t(8;22)	MYC	
	NHL, CLL	t(10;14)	LYT-10	
		3q27 rearrangements	BCL-6	
Myeloid	AML	t(15;17)	PML, RARα	Fusion protein
		t(11;17)	PLZF, RARα	
		t(5;17)	NPM, RARα	
		t(8;21)	AML-1, ETO	
		t(12;22)	TEL, MN1	
		t(8;16)	MOZ, CBP	
		Inv 16	CBFβ, SMMHC	
		11q23 rearrangements	MLL	
	MDS	t(3;21)	AML-1, MDS-1	
	CMML	t(3;21)	AML-1, EAP	
		t(5;12)	TEL, PDGFR	
	CML (myeloid blast crisis)	t(3;21)	AML-1, EVI-1	

Transcription factor genes adjacent to the breakpoints of translocations associated with haematological malignancies

ALL, acute lymphoblastic leukaemia; NHL, non-Hodgkin's lymphoma; CLL, chronic lymphocytic leukaemia; AML, acute myeloid leukaemia; MDS, myelodysplastic syndrome; CMML, chronic myelomonocytic leukaemia; CML, chronic myeloid leukaemia.

Fig. 1.29 Transcription factor genes: haematological malignancies are associated with transcription factor genes adjacent to the breakpoints of translocations. At least one of the two genes disrupted by the translocation is a transcription factor. [Adapted with permission from Green AR. Transcription factors in haemopoietic differentiation and leukaemia. In: Degos L, Linch DC, Löwenberg B (eds). *Textbook of Malignant Haematology*. Martin Dunitz; 1999:165–86.]

CHROMOSOMES

A map of the normal human karyotype is shown in *Fig 1.30*. Chromosomes may be identified by the chromosome painting technique and visualized by fluorescent *in situ* hybridization (FISH; *Fig. 1.31*).

TELOMERES

Telomeres are repetitive sequences at the ends of chromosomes that decrease with each round of replication. For cells that need to self-renew and maintain a high proliferative potential (e.g. germ and other stem cells), the enzyme telomerase can extend the repetitive sequences and compensate for loss at replication. The degree of maintenance of telomeres determines the number of generations a cell can produce and is often increased above normal in malignant cells (*Fig. 1.32*).

BONE MARROW EXAMINATION

Bone marrow aspirates provide films on which the cytological details of developing cells can be examined (*Figs 1.33 and 1.34*). The proportions of different cells are assessed (*Fig. 1.35*), appearances of the individual cells noted and a search made for the presence of cells foreign to the normal marrow, such as metastatic deposits from carcinoma. Iron stores may also be assessed (*see Fig. 1.56*).

Bone marrow trephine biopsies produce cores of bone and marrow which are decalcified and processed for histological assessment (*Figs 1.36–1.38*). The trephine provides an excellent sample for examination of marrow architecture and cellularity. It is the most reliable method of detecting marrow infiltrates.

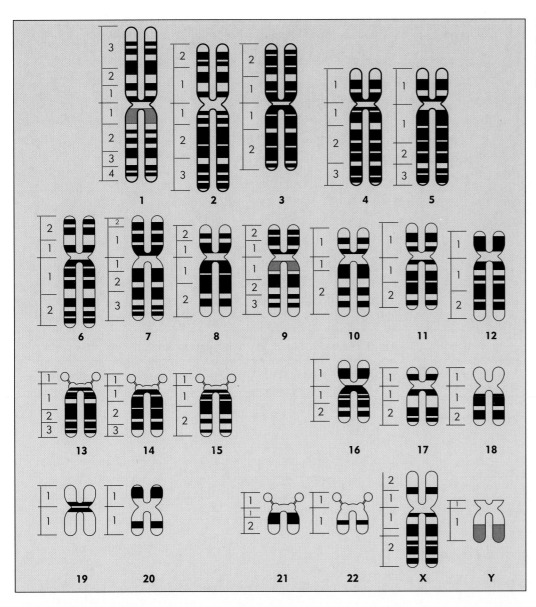

Fig. 1.30 Normal chromosomes: banding patterns as seen on Giemsa staining. Hypervariable (heterochromatin) regions are coloured red. (Adapted from Heim S, Mitelman F. *Cancer Cytogenetics*. New York: Alan R Liss; 1987.)

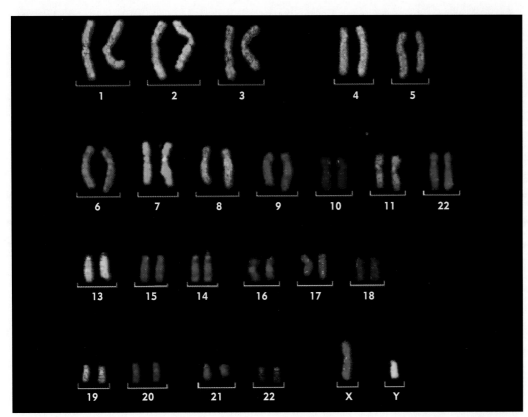

Fig. 1.31 Normal male metaphase: multiple fluorescence *in situ* hybridization (M-FISH). This employs 24 differentially human painting probes, labelled in combinatorial fashion with five fluorochromes such that no two chromosome pairs have the same combination. These are applied to the cells in a single hybridization to produce a 24-colour karyotype. Although some of the colours appear identical to the eye they can be discriminated by the appropriate computer software. This technique allows chromosomal rearrangements to be characterized accurately and cryptic rearrangements to be revealed. (Courtesy of Dr CJ Harrison.)

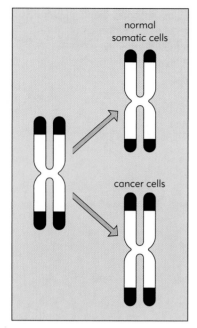

Fig. 1.32 Telomerase: in most normal cells, telomerase is not present, so the telomeres shorten with each replication; in cancer cells, telomerase activity is present or an alternative mechanism maintains telomere length, so there is no telomere shortening at replication.

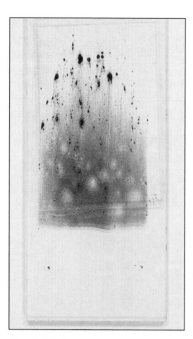

Fig. 1.33 Bone marrow aspirate: this normal aspirate has been spread, allowed to dry, and stained by the May–Grünwald/Giemsa technique. Bone marrow fragments are clearly visible at the tail end of the smear.

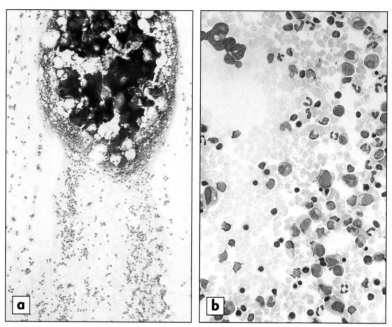

Fig. 1.34a and b Normal marrow fragment and cell trails: the marrow fragment (a) contains haemopoietic cells, supporting reticuloendothelial cells and some fat spaces. During the spreading procedure, representative cells of each haemopoietic cell line spill out into 'trails' behind the marrow fragments; (b) higher magnification.

Percentage of cells of various categories in bone marrow films			
Cells		**Observed range**	**95% range (mean)**
Blast cells		0.0–3.2	0.0–3.0 (1.4)
Promyelocytes		3.6–13.2	3.2–12.4 (7.8)
Neutrophil myelocytes		4.0–21.4	3.7–10.0 (7.6)
Eosinophil myelocytes		0.0–5.0	0.0–2.8 (1.3)
Metamyelocytes		1.0–7.0	2.3–5.9 (4.1)
Neutrophils	males	21.0–45.6*	21.9–42.3 (32.1)
	females	29.6–46.6*	28.8–45.9 (37.4)
Eosinophils		0.4–4.2	0.3–4.2 (2.2)
Eosinophils plus eosinophil myelocytes		0.9–7.4	0.7–6.3 (3.5)
Basophils		0.0–0.8	0.0–0.4 (0.1)
Erythroblasts	males	18.0–39.4*	16.2–40.1 (28.1)
	females	14.0–31.8*	13.0–32.0 (22.5)
Lymphocytes		4.6–22.6	6.0–20.0 (13.1)
Plasma cells		0.0–1.4	0.0–1.2 (0.6)
Monocytes		0.0–3.2	0.0–2.6 (1.3)
Macrophages		0.0–1.8	0.0–1.3 (0.4)
Myeloid:erythroid ratio	males	1.1–4.0†	1.1–4.1 (2.1)
	females	1.6–5.4†	1.6–5.2 (2.8)
Significance of difference between men and women: *$P < 0.001$; †$P < 0.01$.			

Fig. 1.35 Bone marrow films: the percentage of cells of various categories from 50 subjects. (Adapted with permission from Bain BJ. The bone marrow aspirate of healthy subjects. *Br J Haematol.* 1996;94:206–9.)

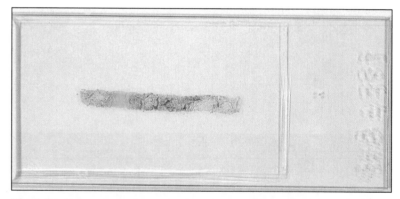

Fig. 1.36 Normal trephine biopsy: gross appearance of a section prepared from a trephine biopsy of the posterior iliac crest. (H & E stain.)

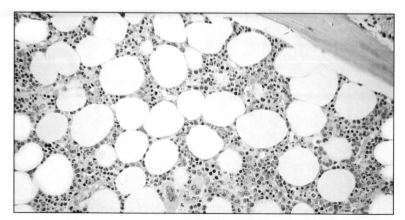

Fig. 1.37 Normal trephine biopsy: representative histology taken from the posterior iliac crest. Approximately half the intertrabecular space is occupied by haemopoietic tissue and half by fat. (H & E stain.)

Erythropoiesis

A representation of the nuclear and cytoplasmic changes during erythropoiesis is given in *Fig. 1.39*. The earliest recognizable erythroid cell in the marrow is the proerythroblast, a large cell with dark blue cytoplasm and a primitive nuclear chromatin pattern (*Fig. 1.40*). Kinetic studies have identified four cell cycles between the proerythroblast and the late non-dividing erythroblast.

The more differentiated erythroblasts are progressively smaller and contain increasing amounts of haemoglobin, to give a polychromatic cytoplasm; the nuclear chromatin becomes progressively more condensed. Basophilic (early), polychromatic (intermediate) and pyknotic (late) stages of erythroblast development are recognized (*Figs 1.41 and 1.42*).

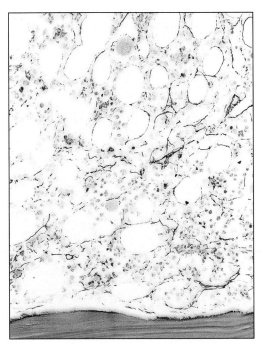

Fig. 1.38 Normal trephine biopsy: the reticulin fibres are thin and delicate, and form a network around the haemopoietic cells. (Silver impregnation stain.)

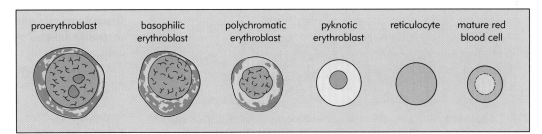

Fig. 1.39 Red cells: differentiation and maturation.

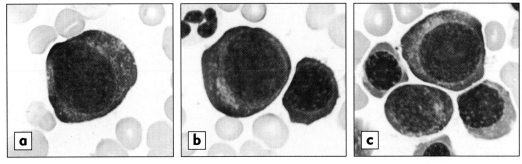

Fig. 1.40a–c Erythropoiesis: (a–c) proerythroblasts and smaller basophilic and polychromatic erythroblasts.

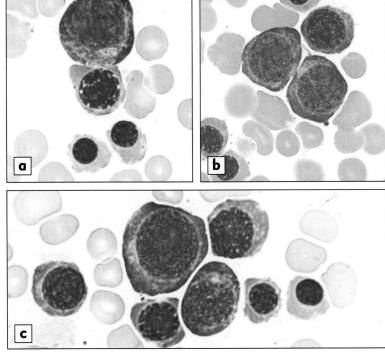

Fig. 1.41a–c Erythropoiesis: (a) from top to bottom, basophilic, polychromatic and two pyknotic erythroblasts; (b, c) further examples of basophilic, polychromatic and pyknotic erythroblasts.

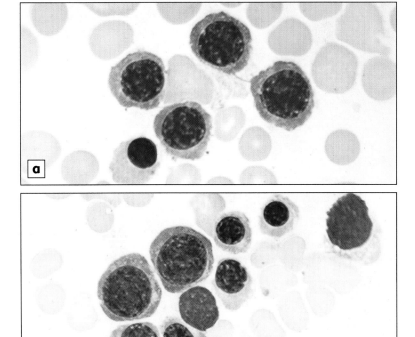

Fig. 1.42a and b Erythropoiesis: (a, b) polychromatic and pyknotic erythroblasts.

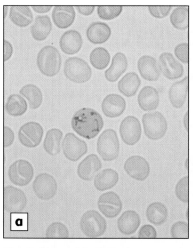
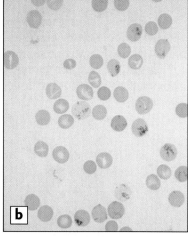

Fig. 1.43a and b Reticulocytes: reticular material (precipitated RNA and protein) is shown clearly (a) in normal blood by supravital staining with new methylene blue, and (b) in autoimmune haemolytic anaemia.

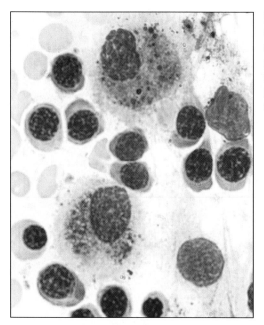

Fig. 1.44 Bone marrow macrophages: close association of polychromatic normoblasts with two pigmented macrophages.

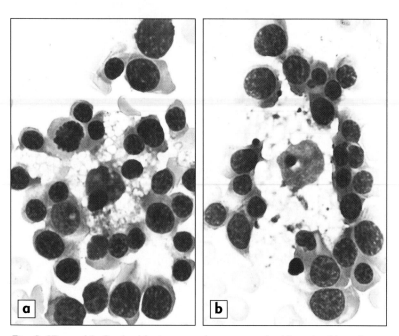

Fig. 1.45a and b Erythroblast–macrophage nests: (a, b) erythroblasts in tight clusters around central macrophages with lipid-laden cytoplasm.

The nucleus is finally extruded from the late erythroblast within the marrow, to produce a reticulocyte that still contains some ribosomal RNA (*Fig. 1.43*) and is capable of synthesizing haemoglobin. This cell spends 1–2 days in the marrow and then a further 1–2 days in the peripheral blood and spleen, in which the RNA is completely lost and an orthochromatic or pink-staining erythrocyte (red cell, RBC) results. In the marrow, erythroblasts are associated closely with their supportive macrophages (*Figs 1.44 and 1.45*).

Granulopoiesis and monocyte production

In granulopoiesis (*Fig. 1.46*) the first recognizable cell of the granulocytic series is the myeloblast. Following division and differentiation, the following sequence of cells may be seen (*Figs 1.47–1.50*):

- promyelocyte (which contains primary granules);
- myelocyte;
- metamyelocyte;
- band cell; and
- segmented or mature granulocyte.

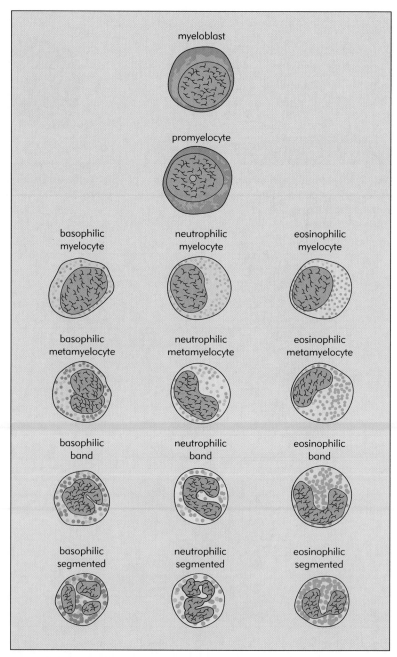

Fig. 1.46 Granulocyte differentiation and maturation: the myeloblast and promyelocyte give rise to three different cell lines, according to the type of secondary granules and nuclear morphology.

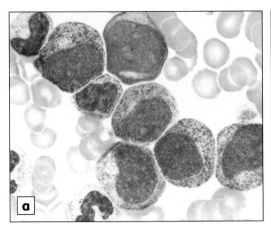

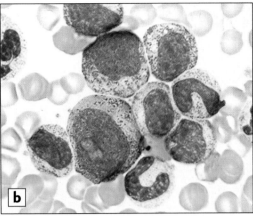

Fig. 1.47a and b Granulopoiesis: (a) a myeloblast, late promyelocytes and myelocytes; (b) a promyelocyte, myelocytes and metamyelocytes.

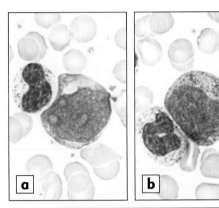

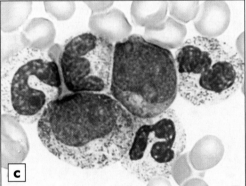

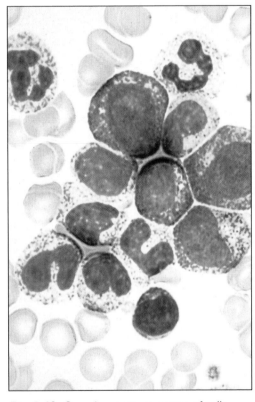

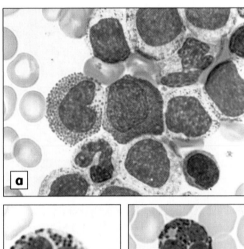

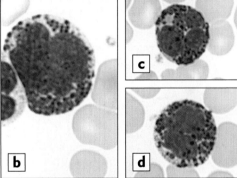

Fig. 1.48a–c Granulopoiesis: (a) myeloblast and (b) promyelocyte; (c) early promyelocyte, myelocyte, metamyelocyte and band neutrophils.

Fig. 1.49 Granulopoiesis: sequence of cells from myelocytes through metamyelocytes and band forms, and a single segmented neutrophil.

Fig. 1.50a–d Granulopoiesis: (a) eosinophilic myelocyte and metamyelocyte; (b) basophilic myelocyte; (c, d) more mature basophils.

Specific (secondary) granules (neutrophilic, eosinophilic or basophilic) appear from the promyelocyte stage onwards.

In line with the dominance of neutrophils among the granulocytes of the peripheral blood, neutrophil precursors form the majority of granulocyte precursors in the marrow, with a few eosinophil precursors and rare basophil precursors present. Only small numbers of monocytes and their precursors, the monoblasts and promonocytes, are seen in normal marrow.

Megakaryocyte and platelet production

The earliest small progenitor cells of the megakaryocytic line are not easily differentiated from myeloblasts. They may be identified by electron microscopic or immunological techniques. The megakaryocyte matures through endomitotic synchronous nuclear replications, which enlarge the cytoplasmic volume as the number of nuclei increases in multiples of two.

These polyploid cells contain the equivalent of 4, 8,16 or 32 sets of chromosomes. At a variable stage of development, usually at the 4N, 8N or 16N stage, further nuclear replication and cell growth cease; the cytoplasm becomes granular and platelets are produced (*Figs 1.51–1.53*).

Lymphocytes and plasma cells

Although the marrow remains the principal site of 'virgin' lymphocyte formation, the majority of circulating lymphoid cells (mature T and B cells) are produced in peripheral lymphoid tissue – lymph nodes, spleen, thymus and lymphoid tissues of the gastrointestinal and respiratory tracts. Lymphocytes usually comprise less than 10% of the normal myelogram, and the progenitor lymphoblasts are difficult to differentiate from other blast cells. Isolated plasma cells (*Figs 1.54 and 1.55*) are generally not difficult to find in marrow cell trails, and comprise up to 4% of the normal marrow cell population.

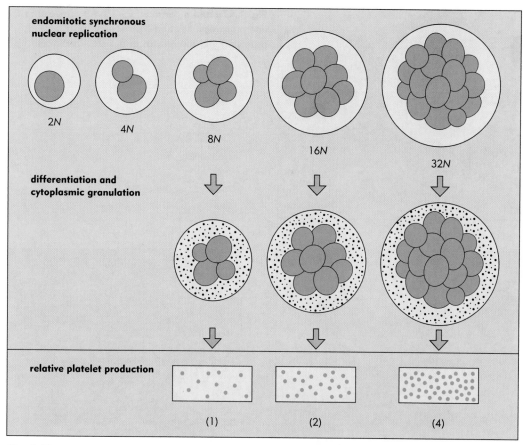

endomitotic synchronous
nuclear replication

2N

4N

8N

16N

32N

differentiation and
cytoplasmic granulation

relative platelet production

(1)   (2)   (4)

Fig. 1.51 Megakaryocyte development and platelet production: each nuclear unit has two sets of chromosomes. (*N*, number of sets of chromosomes or 'ploidy'.)

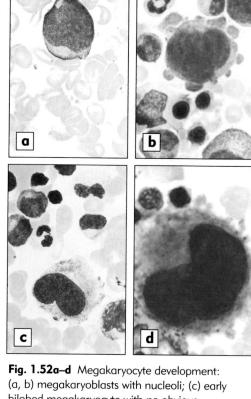

Fig. 1.52a–d Megakaryocyte development: (a, b) megakaryoblasts with nucleoli; (c) early bilobed megakaryocyte with no obvious cytoplasmic granulation; (d) larger megakaryocyte with obvious early granulation of cytoplasm.

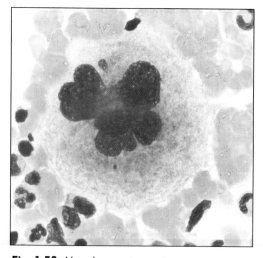

Fig. 1.53 Megakaryocyte: mature megakaryocyte with many nuclear lobes and pronounced granulation of its cytoplasm.

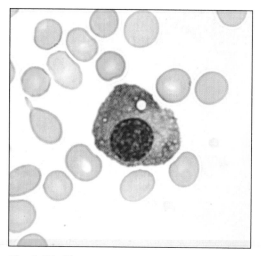

Fig. 1.54 Plasma cell: typical eccentric nucleus with basophilic cytoplasm, prominent perinuclear clearing and a single vacuole.

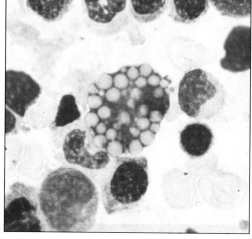

Fig. 1.55 Plasma cell: this type contains many spherical cytoplasmic inclusions and is sometimes referred to as a 'Mott' cell.

Assessment of iron status

In the assessment of iron status, marrow films are stained by the Perls' reaction. Tissue (macrophage) stores are observed in the marrow fragments, and one or two siderotic granules are normally present in about a third of developing erythroblasts (*Fig. 1.56*).

Osteoblasts and osteoclasts

Osteoblasts and osteoclasts are occasionally seen during bone marrow examination (*Figs 1.57 and 1.58*). When they are present in significant numbers, it is important not to confuse them with metastatic malignant cells.

Cells in mitosis

Although bone marrow is one of the most rapidly dividing tissues in the body, only small numbers of dividing cells are seen in normal marrow aspirate cell trails (*Fig. 1.59*).

PERIPHERAL BLOOD CELLS

The usual initial diagnostic approach to blood disorders is blood counting and blood film examination. Various parameters make up the normal blood count (*Fig. 1.60*). Blood films on glass slides (*Fig. 1.61*)

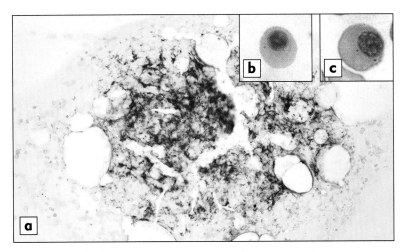

Fig. 1.56a–c Bone marrow iron assessment: bone marrow fragment stained for iron by the Perls' reaction. (a) Abundant Prussian blue positivity indicates iron as haemosiderin in reticuloendothelial cell macrophages; (b, c) in the cell trails, some of the erythroblasts contain one, two or three Prussian blue-positive 'siderotic' granules.

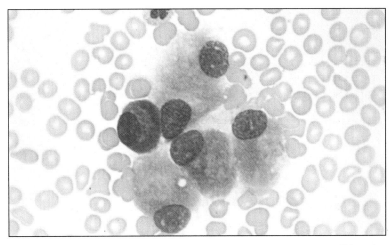

Fig. 1.57 Osteoblasts: a group of five osteoblasts and a plasma cell (on the left). The osteoblasts are large cells that resemble plasma cells, but their chromatin pattern is more open, their cytoplasm less basophilic and they tend to occur in clumps.

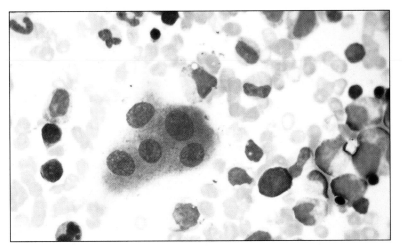

Fig. 1.58 Osteoclasts: these multinucleate cells are occasionally seen in normal marrow aspirates. In contrast to megakaryocytes, the nuclei of osteoclasts are usually discrete, round or oval, and often contain nucleoli.

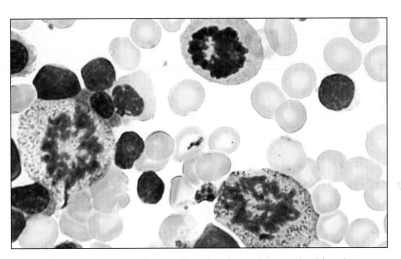

Fig. 1.59 Mitotic figures: three cells, a late basophilic erythroblast (upper field) and two myelocytes, in metaphase. Only a small fraction of the cells seen in normal marrow are undergoing mitosis.

Normal blood count		
Haemoglobin (Hb)	male	13.5–17.5 g/dl
	female	11.5–15.5 g/dl
Red cells (RBC; erythrocytes)	male	4.5–6.5 /l
	female	$3.9–5.6 \times 10^{12}$/l
Packed cell volume (PCV; haematocrit)	male	40–52%
	female	36–48%
Mean corpuscular volume (MCV)		80–95 fl
Mean corpuscular haemoglobin (MCH)		27–34 pg
Mean corpuscular haemoglobin concentration (MCHC)		30–35 g/dl
Reticulocytes		0.5–20%
White cells (WBC; leucocytes)	total	$4.0–11.0 \times 10^9$/l
	neutrophils	$2.5–7.5 \times 10^9$/l
	lymphocytes	$1.5–3.5 \times 10^9$/l
	monocytes	$0.2–0.8 \times 10^9$/l
	eosinophils	$0.04–0.44 \times 10^9$/l
	basophils	$0.01–0.1 \times 10^9$/l
Platelets		$150–400 \times 10^9$/l

Fig. 1.60 Blood count: normal adult values.

Fig. 1.61 Peripheral blood film: glass slide of a well spread blood film stained by the May–Grünwald/Giemsa technique.

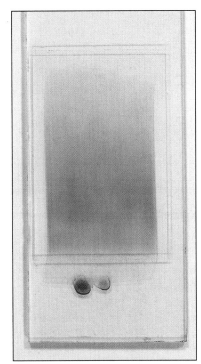

are usually stained with one of the Romanowsky stains (for example, May–Grünwald/Giemsa or Wright's).

Red cells in normal peripheral blood are circular and fairly uniform in size with a mean cell diameter of 8 μm. Only mild variations in size (anisocytosis) and shape (poikilocytosis) are seen (*Fig. 1.62*). In the ideal part of the blood film for examination, which is where the red cells are just beginning to touch and overlap, their biconcave shape produces a central pallor.

Platelets appear as granular basophilic forms with a diameter of 1–3 μm (*Figs 1.62 and 1.63*). Small numbers of large platelets with diameters up to 7 μm may also be found (*Fig. 1.64*). The volume of platelets diminishes as they mature and age in the circulation.

During blood film examination, the white cell numbers and morphology are assessed and a differential count is performed, if this has not been provided by an electronic laboratory blood counter. Representative examples of white cells found in normal blood are shown in *Figs 1.65–1.71*.

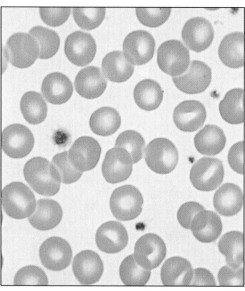

Fig. 1.62 Normal red cells: mean 8 μm in diameter with minor variations in size and shape. The majority show a central pale area of diminished staining. Platelets, 1–3 μm across, are also evident.

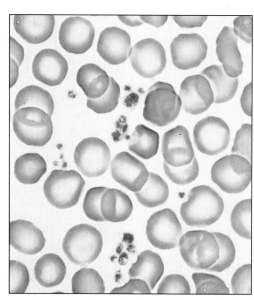

Fig. 1.63 Normal platelets: in this blood film, made from a finger-prick sample, the platelets have agglutinated into small clumps. This is a regular feature of blood films prepared from blood that has not been collected into an anticoagulant.

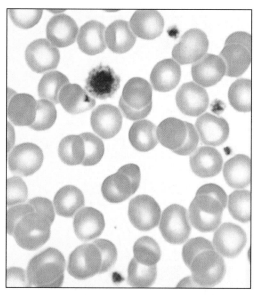

Fig. 1.64 Normal platelets: these platelets show more variation in size than those in *Fig. 1.63*, the largest measuring approximately 6 μm in diameter. Platelets of this size are seen only rarely in normal blood films.

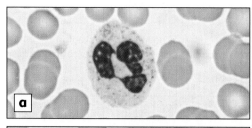
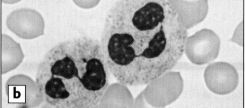
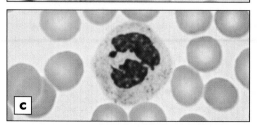

Fig. 1.65a–c Normal neutrophils: (a–c) mature forms showing typical nuclear lobe separation by fine filaments; normal segmented neutrophils may show up to five lobes; (c) a 'Barr body' is attached to a lobe of the nucleus, which is typical of a female neutrophil and results from the possession of two X chromosomes.

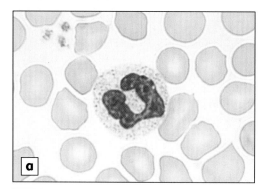
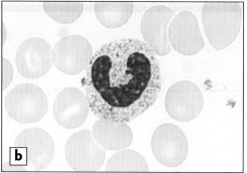

Fig. 1.66a and b Normal neutrophils: (a, b) stab or band forms. The nuclear segmentation of these less mature cells is incomplete.

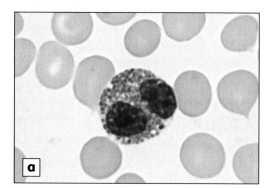
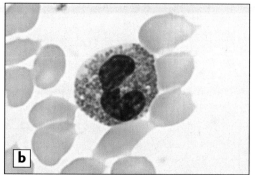

Fig. 1.67a and b Normal eosinophils: (a, b) each of these cells shows two nuclear segments and the typical coarse eosinophilic granulation of the cytoplasm.

Very occasionally, either epithelial (*Fig. 1.72*) or endothelial (*Fig. 1.73*) cells are seen during blood film examination. It is likely that these have been aspirated from the skin or the blood vessel wall during venepuncture. Other rare appearances include neutrophil–platelet rosetting (*Fig. 1.74*) and neutrophil aggregation (*Fig. 1.75*), neither of which is usually of clinical significance.

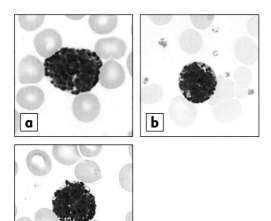

Fig. 1.68a–c Basophils: (a–c) the coarse basophilic granules of these cells often overlie the nucleus, thus obscuring the detail of its segmented structure. Only small numbers of basophils are found in the normal blood film.

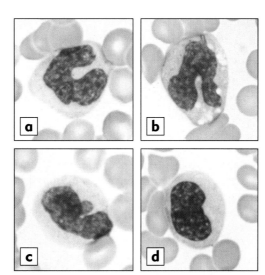

Fig. 1.69a–d Monocytes: (a–d) these cells are usually the largest white cells found in normal blood. The nucleus is usually folded or convoluted, with a moderately fine chromatin pattern. The cytoplasm typically has a grey 'ground-glass' appearance with fine azurophilic granules. Some (b) have rather prominent cytoplasmic vacuoles.

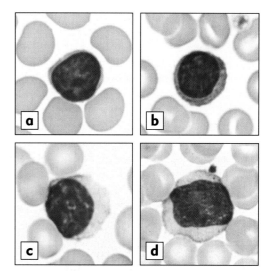

Fig. 1.70a–d Lymphocytes: (a, b) normal small lymphocytes are 7–12 μm in diameter with light blue scanty cytoplasm and a central round nucleus with a condensed amorphous chromatin pattern. (c, d) Some lymphocytes have diameters up to 20 μm, and even larger forms are found during viral and other infections.

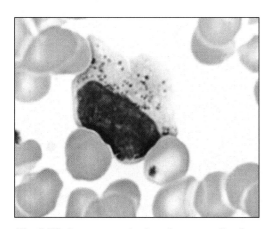

Fig. 1.71 Large granular lymphocyte: cells of lymphoid appearance with multiple azurophilic granules probably include cells of both lymphocyte (CD8$^+$) and myeloid origin and have NK activity.

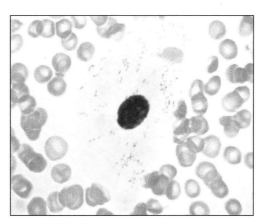

Fig. 1.72 Epithelial cell: occasional isolated squamous cells are found in normal blood films. These very large cells are an artefact collected from the epidermis during venepuncture.

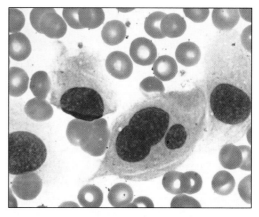

Fig. 1.73 Endothelial cells: isolated clusters of vascular endothelial cells are a rare finding in normal blood films. These cells are dislodged from the intima of the vein during venepuncture.

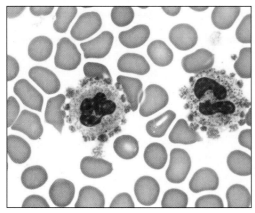

Fig. 1.74 Neutrophil–platelet adhesion: rosetting of platelets around neutrophils is an occasional interesting, but unexplained, finding in blood films. It only occurs in the presence of the anticoagulant, ethylenediamine tetra-acetic acid.

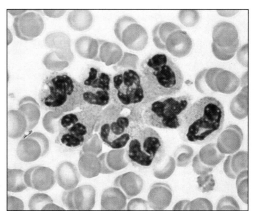

Fig. 1.75 Neutrophil agglutination: clusters of aggregated neutrophils are also an occasional and unexplained finding during blood film examination. The phenomenon is sometimes seen in patients with viral infections.

RED CELLS

The main function of red cells is to carry oxygen to the tissues and return carbon dioxide from the tissues to the lungs. The protein haemoglobin is responsible for most of this gaseous exchange. The principal adult haemoglobin molecule (Hb A) has a MW of 68,000 and comprises two alpha and two beta polypeptide chains (α_2, β_2), each with its own haem group.

There are small quantities of Hb F (α_2, γ_2) and Hb A_2 (α_2, δ_2; *Fig. 1.76*). In the embryo, haemoglobins Gower 1 (ζ_2, ϵ_2), Portland (ζ_2, γ_2) and Gower 2 (α_2, ϵ_2) are formed and, in the fetus, Hb F predominates. Two types of γ chain exist ($^A\gamma$ and $^G\gamma$), according to whether alanine or glycine, respectively, is present at position 136 (*see Fig. 5.1*).

Haem synthesis occurs mainly in the mitochondria by a series of biochemical reactions, commencing with the substrates glycine and succinyl coenzyme A, and globin chains are assembled on polyribosomes (*see Fig. 2.1*). Two-thirds of the total cell content of haemoglobin is synthesized in erythroblasts, and the remainder at the reticulocyte stage.

As the haemoglobin molecule takes up and releases oxygen, the individual globin chains move on each other. When oxygen is released, the β chains are pulled apart, permitting the entry of the glycolytic metabolite 2,3-diphosphoglycerate (2,3-DPG; *Fig. 1.77*). This results in a lower affinity of haemoglobin for oxygen and improved delivery of oxygen to

the tissues. It is also responsible for the sigmoid form of the oxygen dissociation curve (*Fig. 1.78*).

For successful gaseous exchange, the flexible biconcave red cell, 8 μm in diameter, has to pass through the microcirculation, whose diameter is only 3.5 μm; it has to maintain haemoglobin in a reduced state and maintain osmotic equilibrium, despite having an inherently leaky membrane and an osmotic pressure approximately five times that of plasma. Devoid of mitochondria and the enzymes required for oxidative phosphorylation, the mature red cell is dependent on the glycolytic pathway (*see Fig. 4.27*) to provide adenosine triphosphate (ATP) for its energy requirements to maintain its volume, shape and flexibility. It is also able to generate reducing power as reduced nicotinamide–adenine dinucleotide (NADH) by this pathway and as reduced nicotinamide–adenine dinucleotide phosphate (NADPH) by the pentose phosphate shunt pathway (*see Fig. 4.27*). The iron atoms in normal haemoglobin are in the ferrous (iron II) form. The methaemoglobin reductase enzymes use NADH or NADPH to reduce methaemoglobin [which contains ferric (iron III) ions] formed normally during the lifespan of the red cell. Deficiency of NADH–methaemoglobin reductase leads to cyanosis with up to 30% methaemoglobin present and consequent deoxygenation of the haemoglobin (*Fig. 1.78b*).

The Rapoport–Luebering shunt (*see Fig. 4.28*) regulates the concentration of 2,3-DPG vital to the release of oxygen from the haemoglobin tetramer. As enzymes cannot be replaced in the mature red cell, a gradual deterioration occurs in the red cell metabolism and the

Globin chain synthesized		
Embryo	ζ_2, ϵ_2	Gower 1
	ζ_2, γ_2	Portland
	α_2, ϵ_2	Gower 2
Fetus	α_2, γ_2	Hb F
Adult	α_2, δ_2	Hb A_2
	α_2, β_2	Hb A

Fig. 1.76 Haemoglobins in the embryo, fetus and adult: there are two genes each on chromosome 16 for the ζ and α chains, and genes on chromosome 11 for Aγ and Gγ chains, as well as one each for ϵ, δ and β chains. (*See also* Chapter 5.)

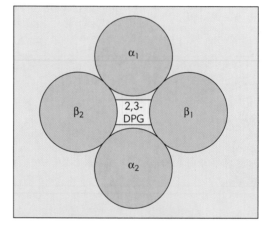

Fig. 1.77 Normal adult haemoglobin A: there are two α and two β chains, and 2,3-DPG fits into a pocket between the β chains and displaces oxygen.

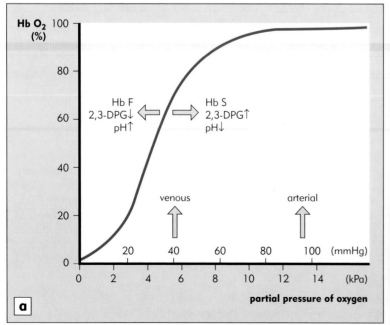

a

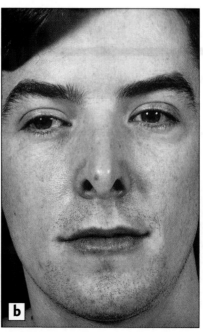

b

Fig. 1.78a and b
Haemoglobin–oxygen dissociation: (a) normal sigmoid curve relating Hb saturation to the partial pressure of oxygen (PaO$_2$) to which it is exposed. The curve is shifted to the left (less oxygen is released at any given PaO$_2$) by a fall in 2,3-DPG, by a rise in pH (Bohr effect), or if Hb A is replaced by Hb F or by a high-affinity Hb. The curve is shifted to the right by a rise in 2,3-DPG attached to the Hb, by a fall in pH, if Hb A is replaced by Hb S or an Hb M (in which the haem iron is stabilized in the ferric form), or if Hb is oxidized to methaemoglobin. (b) Cyanosis caused by NADH–methaemoglobin reductase deficiency shows a typical slate-grey appearance in this 22-year-old man whose blood count was normal.

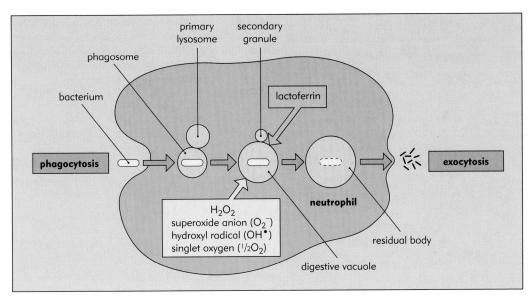

Fig. 1.79 Phagocytosis and bacterial destruction: the neutrophil surrounds the bacterium with an invaginated surface membrane to form a phagosome by fusion with a primary lysosome. The lysosomal enzymes attack the bacterium. Secondary granules also fuse with the phagosomes, and new enzymes and lactoferrin attack the organism. Various types of activated oxygen generated by glucose metabolism also help to kill bacteria. Undigested residual bacterial products are excreted by exocytosis.

cells become less viable with age. After a mean lifespan in the circulation of 120 days and an estimated vascular journey of about 300 miles, ageing red cells are destroyed extravascularly by macrophages of the reticuloendothelial system (RES; *see Fig. 4.1*).

GRANULOCYTES

All cells of this group (neutrophils, eosinophils and basophils) play an essential role in inflammation. They are primarily phagocytes and, with lymphocytes, antibodies and complement, are responsible for the defence against microorganisms.

Neutrophils (polymorphs)

Neutrophil production and differentiation in the bone marrow takes from 6 to 10 days. Large numbers of band and segmented neutrophils are held in the marrow as a 'reserve pool' which, in the normal state, contains 10–15 times the number of neutrophils in the peripheral blood. Following their release from the marrow, they spend 6–12 hours in the circulation before migrating into tissues where they perform their phagocytic function. They survive 2–4 days in the tissues before being destroyed during defensive action or as a result of senescence.

Following chemotactic attraction of phagocytic cells to sites of inflammation, offending microorganisms are ingested and contained within phagosomes (*Fig. 1.79*). The neutrophil granule enzyme contents are released into these spaces. The primary azurophilic granules contain lysozyme and other enzymes (*Fig. 1.80*). These enzymes are partly responsible for bacterial destruction; a second killing mechanism consists of oxidant damage by hydrogen peroxide and superoxide generated by glucose metabolism through NADH and NADPH. Lactoferrin, secreted by granulocytes, leads to bacteriostasis by depriving infected cells of iron.

Eosinophils

Although less is known about the kinetics of eosinophil production, differentiation, circulation and migration, it is likely that the mechanism is similar to that for neutrophils. Eosinophils are also capable of phagocytosis. The granules are membrane bound organelles with a 'crystalloid' core (*Fig. 1.81*). These cells are particularly important in allergic and parasitic diseases. Following appropriate stimulation, the granule contents may be released outside the cell at large targets, such as helminth parasites. Eosinophils release histaminase and aryl sulphatase, which inactivate histamine and a slow-reacting substance of anaphylaxis (SRS-A) released from mast cells.

Granule contents of human neutrophils		
Primary (azurophil) granules	**Specific granules**	**Other organelles**
Microbicidal proteins		
Myeloperoxidase		
Lysozyme	Lysozyme	Lysozyme
Bactericidal–permeability inducing factor/CAP57		
Defensins		
Serprocidins (serine proteases): cathepsin G proteinase 3 azurocidin/CAP37		
elastase	Collagenase	Alkaline phosphatase
	Gelatinase	Gelatinase
		Tetranectin
Acid hydrolases		
β-Glucuronidase		
β-Glycerophosphatase		
N-Acetyl-β-glucosaminidase		
α-Mannosidase		
Cathepsin B		
Cathepsin D	Other neutrophil gelatinase-associated lipocalin	
Aryl sulphatase	Lactoferrin	
	Transcobalamin I and III	
	Plasminogen activator	
	Histaminase	
	β$_2$-Microglobulin	
	Cytochrome b$_{559}$	
	Receptors	**Receptors**
	α$_{2M}$β$_2$ integrin = complement receptor 3 (C3bi)	α$_M$β$_2$ integrin
	Bacterial tripeptide receptor (formyl-methionyl-leucyl-phenylalanine)	Complement receptor 1 = CD35
	Laminin receptor	FcγRIIIB
	α$_2$β$_2$ integrin = Victronectin R	

Fig. 1.80 Human neutrophils: granule contents. [Adapted with permission from Roberts PJ, Linch DC, Webb DKH. Phagocytes. In: Hoffbrand AV, Lewis SM, Tuddenham EGD (eds). *Postgraduate Haematology*, 4th edn. Oxford: Butterworth–Heinemann; 1999:235–66.]

Eosinophil granule contents		
Granule type/protein	**Function**	**Downstream physiological role**
Primary granule		
Charcot–Leyden crystal protein	Cleaves fatty acids from lysophospholipids (lysophospholipase)	Phospholipid mechanism
		Neutralizes pulmonary surfactants
Eosinophil peroxidase	Generates hypothiocyanous acid from H_2O_2	Kills microorganisms (*Escherichia coli*, schistosomes, microfilariae, trypanosomes, *Toxoplasma* spp. and mycobacteria
		Toxic to mammalian cells – mast cells and tumours
	Allosteric inhibitor of muscarinic receptors	Bronchoconstriction
Specific/secondary granule		
Eosinophil peroxidase	As above	As above
Major basic protein (forms crystalline core of the granule)	Binds to acidic lipids, disrupts membranes (non-enzymatic activity)	Widespread toxicity to parasites
		Toxic to mammalian cells – desquamation and hypertrophy of lung epithelium (bronchospasm)
Eosinophil cationic protein	Forms transmembrane pores	Bactericidal – *E. coli* and *Staphylococcus aureus*
		Toxic to parasites
		Damage to lung epithelium (as above)
		Stimulates mast cell degranulation
	Ribonuclease	
	Neurotoxin (*in vitro*)	
	Neutralizes heparin	Effects on coagulation and fibrinolysis
Eosinophil-derived neurotoxin (eosinophil protein X)	Ribonuclease	Toxic to parasites
	Neurotoxin	
Gelatinase	Metalloproteinase	Damage to extracellular matrix

Fig. 1.81 Eosinophils: granule contents. [Adapted with permission from Roberts PJ, Linch DC, Webb DKH. Phagocytes. In: Hoffbrand AV, Lewis SM, Tuddenham EGD (eds). *Postgraduate Haematology*, 4th edn. Oxford: Butterworth–Heinemann; 1999:235–66.]

Basophils

Although both basophils and tissue mast cells are of bone marrow origin, their relationship is not entirely clear. The granules of both cell types contain heparin and pharmacological mediators such as SRS-A and histamine (*Fig. 1.82*). Release of these substances follows an allergen–IgE complex binding to the cell surface via Fc receptors for IgE. Mast cells may be important in the defence against parasites; they are also responsible for many of the adverse symptoms in allergic disorders.

MONONUCLEAR PHAGOCYTIC SYSTEM

Monocytes

Monocytes spend only a short time in the marrow. Their precursors (monoblasts and promonocytes) are difficult to distinguish from myeloblasts and monocytes.

Monocytes are active phagocytes. Both ingestion and adherence to microorganisms are facilitated by special surface receptors for the Fc portion of IgG and for complement (e.g. C3b) with which the microorganisms may be coated. Monocytes carry other surface markers including HLA-DR and receptors for lymphokines, such as interferon-γ and migration inhibition factor. Monocytic lysosomes contain acid hydrolases and peroxidase, which are important in the intracellular destruction of microorganisms. They also produce complement components, prostaglandins, interferons, monokines, such as IL-1 and TNF, and haemopoietic growth factors, such as CSFs (see *Figs 1.11 and 1.14*).

After circulating for 20–40 hours, monocytes leave the blood to enter the tissues, where they mature and carry out their principal functions. Their extravascular lifespan may be as long as several months or sometimes years. These cells are divided into the phagocytic macrophages, which remove particulate antigens, and the APCs, the main function of which is to present antigens to lymphocytes (*Figs 1.83 and 1.84*).

Reticuloendothelial system: phagocytes and dendritic cells

In addition to the wandering or free tissue macrophages, the monocyte-derived phagocytic cells form a network known as the RES and are found in many organs (*Fig. 1.83*). This system includes the Kupffer cells in the liver, alveolar macrophages in the lung, macrophages of various serosal surfaces, mesangial cells of the kidney, brain microglia and macrophages of the bone marrow, splenic sinuses and lymph nodes.

Dendritic cells (DCs), specialized APCs, are found primarily in the skin, lymph nodes, spleen and thymus (*Fig. 1.84*). They have an irregular shape, numerous cell-membrane processes, spiny dendrites and bulbous pseudopods (*Figs 1.85–1.87*). There is a paucity of intracellular organelles with prominent mitochondria, endosomes and lysosomes. The DCs are able to take up and process antigen, to migrate to tissues and to interact with, stimulate and direct T-cell responses. They include Langerhans cells, myeloid- and monocyte-derived DCs and lymphoid-derived DCs (*Fig. 1.88*). One subset (myeloid) originates from bone marrow precursors, and comprises 1–2% of the blood

Basophil and mast cell granule contents				
Component	**Function**	**Downstream physiological role**	**Other properties**	**Cell specificity**
Protein				
Histamine	Binds to H1, H2 and H3 receptors	Major inducer of hypersensitivity reactions and inflammation		Basophils, mast cells
Proteoglycan				
Heparin	Packages basic proteins into granules		Binds and stabilizes proteases	Predominant in MC$_{CT}$
Chondroitin sulphates	Same function		Same function	Predominant in basophils
Enzymes: neutral proteases				
Chymase	Inactivates bradykinin	Affects microcirculation		MC$_{CT}$
	Injures lamina lucida of basement membrane at dermal–epidermal junction			
	Activates angiotensin I	Modulates microcirculation		
	Activates precursor IL-1β	Modulates skin inflammation		
Tryptase	Cleaves C3 into C3a + C3b	Proinflammatory; stimulates neutrophil chemotaxis and adherence	Tetrameric when bound to heparin; monomer active	Mast cells
	Cleaves C3a into inactive peptides		Restricted substrate specificity	
	Activates metalloproteinase 3	Regulates collagenase	Raised levels in mast cell disorders; anaphylaxis, mastocytosis	
	Inactivates fibrinogen	Attenuates fibrin deposition		
	Degrades calcitonin gene-related peptide			
Cathepsin G-like protease				MC$_{CT}$
Carboxypeptidase B				MC$_{CT}$
Other				
Charcot–Leyden crystal protein	Cleaves fatty acid from lysophospholipid (lysophospholipase)	Phospholipid mechanism		Basophils
		Neutralizes pulmonary surfactants		
Major basic protein		Disrupts membranes		
Sulphatase, exoglycosidase				
Mast cells = both connective tissue and mucosal mast cells; MC$_{CT}$ = connective tissue mast cell.				

Fig. 1.82 Basophils and mast cells: granule contents. [Adapted with permission from Roberts PJ, Linch DC, Webb DKH. Phagocytes. In: Hoffbrand AV, Lewis SM, Tuddenham EGD (eds). *Postgraduate Haematology*, 4th edn. Oxford: Butterworth–Heinemann; 1999:235–66.]

mononuclear cells. They are negative for lineage markers, but are HLA-DR positive. A separate lineage is derived from CD34$^+$ cells and populates the skin epidermis (where they are called Langerhans cells) and liver sinusoids, and may migrate via lymph to lymph nodes. They also occupy interstitial spaces in solid organs (e.g. the heart and kidney). A subset of dendritic cells may be of lymphoid origin (*see Fig. 1.88*) and within the thymus may be involved in the induction of tolerance to autoantigens.

Follicular dendritic cells (FDCs), also called germinal centrodendritic cells, form a dense network in germinal centres (GCs) of lymph nodes (B cell areas). They are derived from bone marrow and are able to take up antigen–antibody complexes and retain antigen for months. They do not degrade the antigen but hold it on the surface, presumably to maintain B cell activation and, indirectly, T cell activation.

Following stimulation, the Langerhans cells of the skin migrate via the afferent lymphatics into the paracortical areas of draining lymph nodes where they 'interdigitate' with T cells, presenting them with antigens carried from the skin (*see Fig. 1.84*).

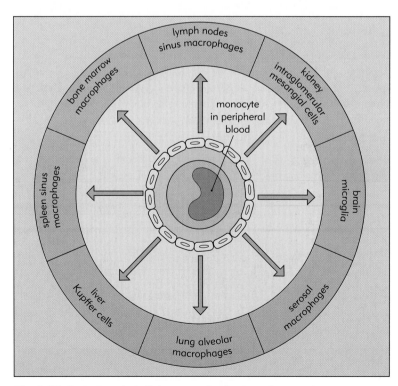

Fig. 1.83 Reticuloendothelial system: distribution of macrophages.

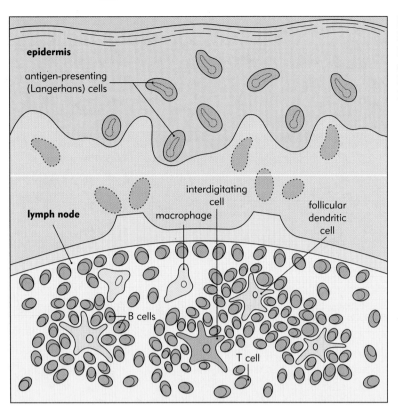

Fig. 1.84 Dendritic (antigen-presenting) cells in the skin and lymph nodes: Langerhans cells in the epidermis are characterized by the presence of Birbeck bodies (tennis racquet-shaped collections of granules; *see Fig. 7.35*). These antigen-carrying cells migrate via afferent lymphatics to the neighbouring lymph nodes and become interdigitating cells in the T-cell paracortical zone. Follicular DCs are found in the B-cell germinal centres (GCs).

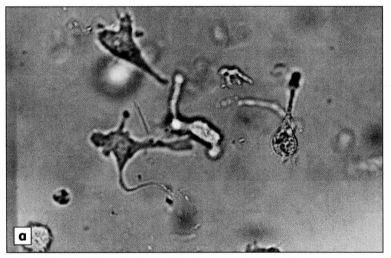

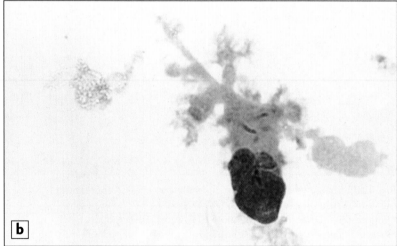

Fig. 1.85a, b Dendritic cells: (a) DCs developing in methylcellulose culture from CD34+ bone marrow progenitors after 14 days in TNFα and GM-CSF. Note the fine, long dendritic processes characteristic of DCs under these conditions. These cells generally have the appearance and phenotype of skin Langerhans cells, are CD1a+, CD14− and HLA-DR+, but lack Birbeck granules. (b) Giemsa-stained DC from 14 day cultures of CD34+ as shown in (a). Note the fine, long dendritic processes and eccentric lobed nucleus characteristic of DCs under these conditions. [(a, b) Courtesy of Dr CDL Reid.]

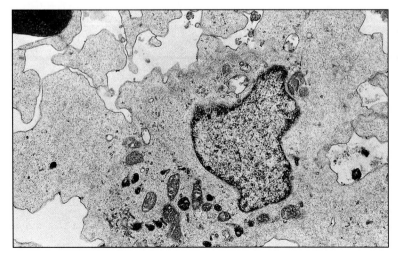

Fig. 1.86 Dendritic cells: electron microscopic appearances of DCs from 14 day cultures of CD34+ cells (as shown in *Fig. 1.85a*). Note the many blunt pseudopodia and dendritic processes, the pale rather featureless cytoplasm with little endoplasmic reticulum and many free ribosomes and polyribosomes. (Courtesy of Dr CDL Reid.)

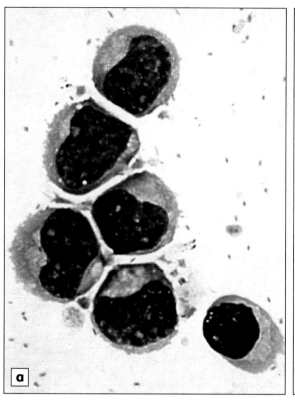

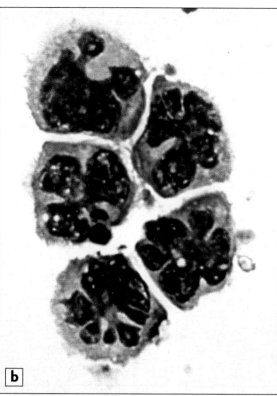

Fig. 1.87a, b Dendritic cells: (a, b) morphology of DC freshly isolated from peripheral blood. These cells are separated on the basis of strong Class II (HLA-DR) expression, but are lineage negative (CD3⁻, CD19⁻, CD20⁻, CD14⁻, CD16⁻, CD34⁻) and are allostimulatory in mixed lymphocyte cultures with T lymphocytes. The appearances of the two major subclasses of these cells differ according their expression of the β_2 integrin CD11c: (a) CD11c⁻; (b) CD11c⁺. [(a, b) Courtesy of Dr S Robinson and Dr CDL Reid.]

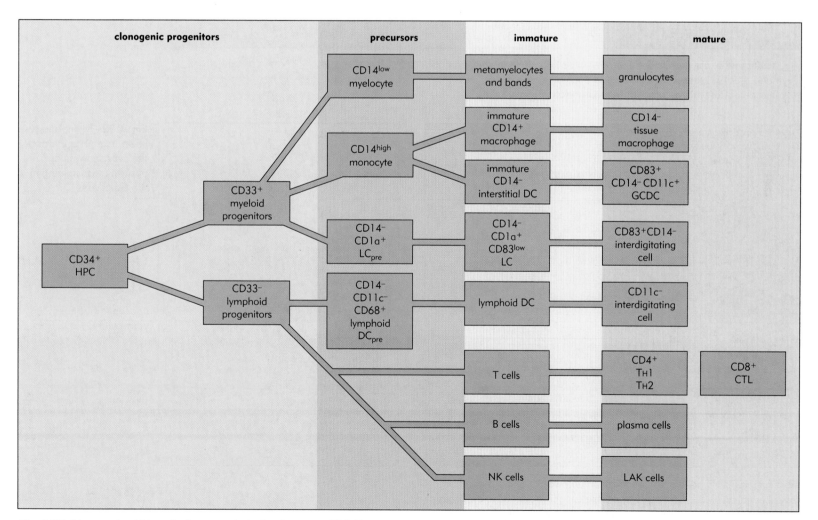

Fig. 1.88 Human dendritic cells: haemopoietic development. CD34⁺ haemopoietic progenitor cells (HPCs) give rise to clonogenic myeloid or lymphoid progenitors. Regardless of the type of DC (myeloid versus lymphoid, monocyte-derived versus CD34⁺ haemopoietic progenitor cell derived, or Langerhans cell (LC)-like or interstitial type), DCs exist in both immature and mature, terminally differentiated forms. The CD34⁺ bipotential intermediate, generated *in vitro* from CD34⁺ HPCs, is the presumed equivalent of circulating monocyte precursors of DCs. (CD, cluster differentiation; CTL, cytolytic T lymphocyte; GCDC, germinal centre dendritic cell; TH1, T helper 1; TH2, T helper 2; adapted with permission from Young JW. Dendritic cells: expansion and differentiation with hemopoietic growth factors. *Curr Opin Hematol.* 1999;6;135–44.)

LYMPHOCYTES

Lymphocytes assist the phagocytes in the defence of the body against infection and other foreign invasion, and add specificity to the attack. They are produced in the bone marrow from pluripotent stem cells and fall into two main groups with different functions, T cells and B cells, indistinguishable by traditional Romanowsky staining. T cells are processed initially in the thymus; B cells are so called because in birds they differentiate in an organ known as the bursa of Fabricius.

T cells

Mature T cells, which comprise 65–80% of the circulating lymphocyte population, carry a marker (antigen CD2) that binds sheep erythrocytes

(*Fig. 1.89*). Other surface markers may be defined by indirect immunofluorescence or by immunoperoxidase-linked specific antibodies (*Fig. 1.90*), some of which define subpopulations of T cells.

T cells are subdivided into two major subsets that are detected by monoclonal antibodies to CD8 and CD4 surface membrane antigens. CD8$^+$ cells, the major subpopulation of T cells in the marrow, include the suppressor and/or cytotoxic cells, while CD4$^+$ (helper) cells predominate in the peripheral blood. CD4$^+$ cells are in turn subdivided into TH1 and TH2 cells, which secrete different cytokines in response to stimulation by IL-2 and IFNγ or IL-4, respectively (*Fig. 1.91*). T cells also contain a number of lysosomal acid hydrolases, such as β-glucuronidase, and acid phosphatase, which may be detected cytologically as discrete masses in the Golgi zone in the cytoplasm (*Fig. 1.92*).

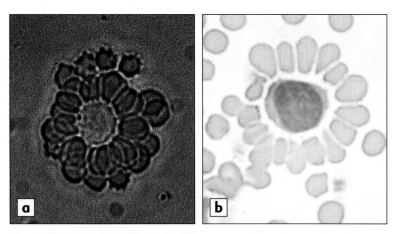

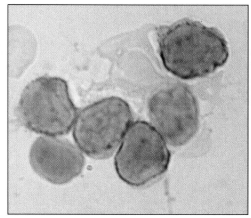

Fig. 1.90 T lymphocytes: human T cells identified by (brown) staining of surface antigen (four of the central cells are T cells). (Immunoperoxidase technique using anti-CD5 monoclonal antibody.)

Fig. 1.89a and b T lymphocytes: following centrifugation together, human T lymphocytes and sheep red cells bind to each other in rosettes. [(a) Phase-contrast microscopy; (b) May–Grünwald/Giemsa stain].

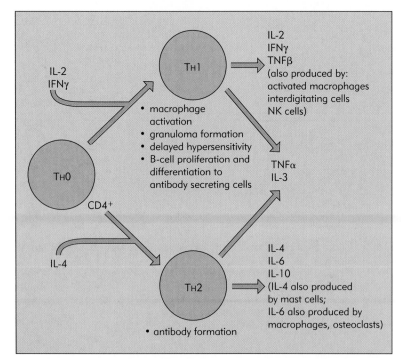

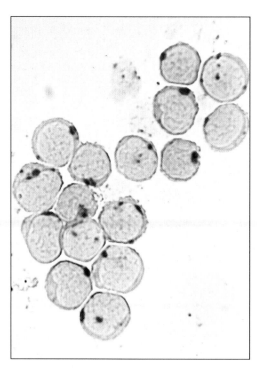

Fig. 1.92 T lymphocytes: using acid phosphatase, the cells show polar positive (red) staining in the Golgi zone.

Fig. 1.91 CD4$^+$ T helper cells: maturation pathways. CD4$^+$ T cells that have been activated by antigen acquire the capacity to produce cytokines. The cytokines produced depend on the environment in which activation occurs. Two main types of cytokine-producing TH cell are recognized – TH1 and TH2 cells. The cytokines produced by TH1 cells tend to promote further TH1 cell formation and inhibit TH2 cell formation, and IL-4 produced by TH2 cells promotes further differentiation towards TH2 cells. TH1-promoting cytokines are also produced by activated macrophages, interdigitating cells and NK cells, while mast cells also produce IL-4.

The T-cell surface contains an antigen receptor that consists of α and β chains, each with variable and constant portions (*Fig. 1.93*). A receptor coded for by γ and δ genes exists in a minority of T cells. The genes for these polypeptide chains, on chromosomes 14 and 7 (*Fig. 1.94*), are rearranged in T cells in a manner similar to the rearrangement of Ig genes in B cells (*Fig. 1.95*), which results in a wide diversity among T lymphocytes. Close by the T cell receptor on the cell surface membrane is a complex of proteins termed the CD3 complex, which consists of γ, δ and ε chains (*see Fig. 1.93*). This complex is responsible for transducing signals derived from interaction of antigen with the T-cell receptor to the cell interior.

The sequence of events in T-cell development appears to be initial expression of nuclear terminal deoxynucleotide transferase (TdT) and the surface antigen CD7 followed by CD2 (*Fig. 1.96*). Rearrangement of the T-cell receptor genes occurs in the sequence δ, γ, β and, finally, α. The CD2 and CD3 antigens are expressed on the surface later, although intracytoplasmic CD3 is one of the earliest markers. The CD4 and CD8 antigens are expressed in medullary thymocytes after T-cell receptor gene rearrangement is complete (*Fig. 1.96*).

B cells

This subpopulation of lymphocytes comprises 5–15% of the circulating lymphocyte population. Mature B cells are defined by the presence of endogenously produced Ig molecules inserted into the surface membrane, where they act as receptors for specific antigens. Fluorescein-labelled specific antibodies may be used to demonstrate these surface-bound Ig molecules (*Fig. 1.97*) and B cells can be identified by monoclonal antibodies to certain surface cell antigens [e.g. CD10, CD19

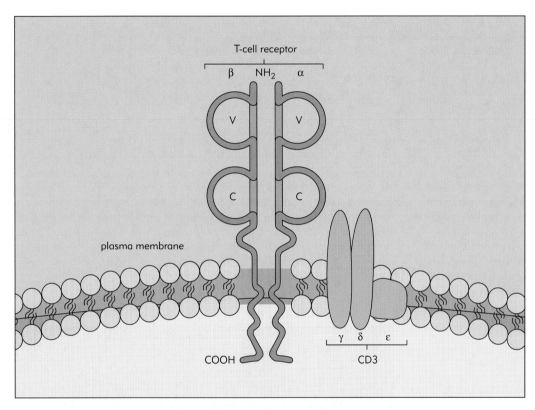

Fig. 1.93 The T-cell antigen receptor: this consists of α and β chains, each of which has a variable (V) and a constant (C) segment. The chains have transmembranous portions, but very short intracytoplasmic domains. The associated CD3 complex is involved in signal transduction to the cell interior.

Fig. 1.94 Antigen receptor genes: organization.

Gene	Chromosome localization	V	D	J	C	Additional diversity	Complementarity determining region 3 diversity	Clonal rearrangement in (%) acute lymphoblastic leukaemia	
								B lineage	T Lineage
IgH	14q32	~50	30	6	10	N regions	V-N1-D1-N2-J	100	15–20
							V-N1-D1-N2-D2-N3-J		
IgLκ	2p12	~40	–	5	1	N regions	V-N-J/V-J	20	0
IgLγ	22q11	~29	–	6	6	None	V-J	5	0
TCRα	14q11	~70	–	~90	1	N regions	V-N-J	NT	70
TCRδ	14q11	~4	3	3	1	N regions	V-N1-D1-N2-D2-N3-J	40–50	95*
TCRγ	7p15	12	–	5	2	N regions	V-N-J	40–50	95
TCRβ	7q32	~50	2	13	2	N regions	V-N1-D-N2-J	0	80

*At least 30% of these cases show deletion of TCRδ

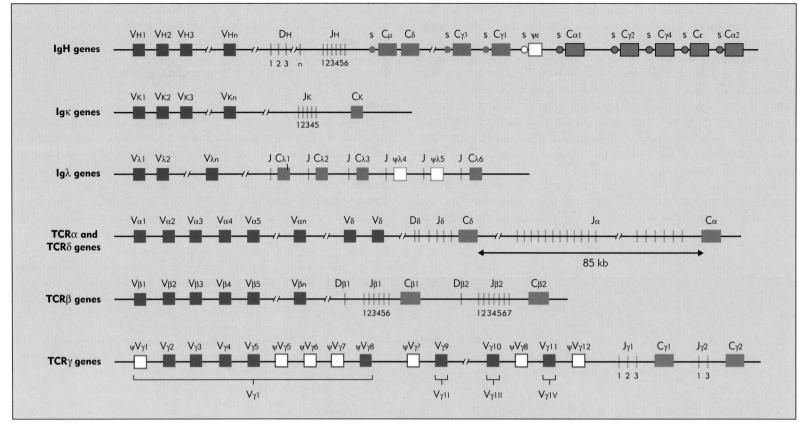

Fig. 1.95 Human Ig genes: the IgH genes consist of many V genes, at least 30 D genes, about six J genes and ten C genes for the various IgH classes and subclasses. Most C genes are preceded by a switch (s) gene, which plays a role in IgH (sub)class switch. The Igκ gene complex consists of a series of V genes, about five J genes and one C gene, while the Igλ gene complex consists of many V genes and six C genes, all of which are preceded by a J gene. Pseudo genes (ψ) are indicated with open symbols. The TCRα genes consist of many V genes, a remarkably long stretch of J genes and one C gene. The TCRβ gene complex consists of a series of V genes and two C genes, both of which are preceded by one D gene and six or seven J genes. The TCRγ genes consist of a restricted number of V genes (12 functional Vγ genes and seven pseudo genes) and two C genes, each preceded by two or three J genes. Interestingly, the TCRδ genes are located between the Vα and Jα genes and probably consist of a few V genes, three D genes, three J genes and one C gene. (Modified with permission from Van Dongen JJM, Wolvers-Tettero ILM. Analysis of Ig and T-cell receptor genes. Part 1: basic and technical aspects. *Clin Chim Acta*. 1991;198:1–92.)

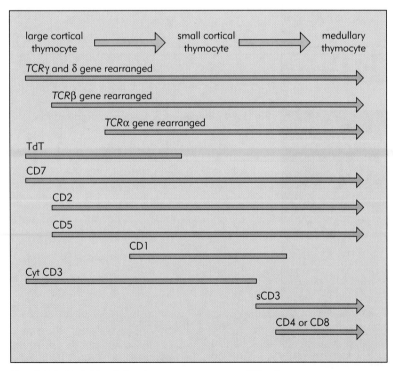

Fig. 1.96 Early T-cell development: sequence of T-cell receptor gene rearrangements and antigen expression. (s, surface; cyt, cytoplasmic.)

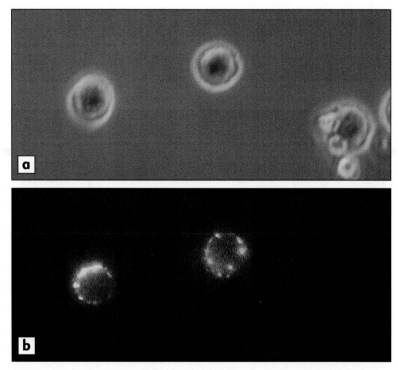

Fig. 1.97a and b B lymphocytes: (a) three peripheral blood lymphocytes seen by phase contrast microscopy; (b) patchy fluorescence under ultraviolet light using fluoresceinated anti-human Ig shows that only two of the cells carry surface Ig.

(*Fig. 1.98*), CD20 and CD22]; B cells also express HLA-DR. B cells that have matured and secrete Ig are termed plasma cells (*Fig. 1.99*).

The surface Igs are individual to each clone of B cells and are identical to those secreted as antibodies by the B lymphocyte or plasma cell. The Ig may be one of five classes – IgM, IgD, IgG (divided into four subtypes), IgE or IgA (divided into two subtypes). Each Ig molecule consists of light chains (κ or λ) and heavy chains (μ, δ, γ, ε or α) which determine

the class of Ig (*Fig. 1.100*). Both heavy and light chains contain constant and variable regions. The heavy chain genes are on chromosome 14 and the light chain genes on chromosomes 2 (κ) and 22 (λ) (*see Fig. 1.94*).

The sequence of antigen expression and gene rearrangements in early B-cell development, which occurs in the bone marrow, is illustrated in *Fig. 1.101*. Some surface antigens may be detected before surface Ig. The Igs are expressed in the cytoplasm (in pre-B cells; *Fig. 1.102*) before they

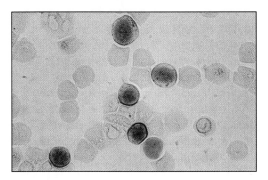
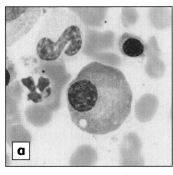
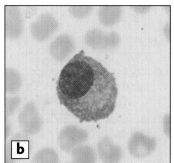
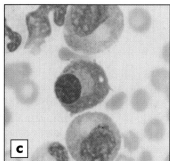

Fig. 1.98 B lymphocytes: identification by (brown) staining of antibody fixed to a surface antigen using the immunoperoxidase technique and CD19 monoclonal antibody.

Fig. 1.99a–c Plasma cells: (a–c) these occur in bone marrow and in other tissues of the RES, including the intestine. They are not found in normal peripheral blood. The cells are usually oval. They show a deeply basophilic cytoplasm with a perinuclear halo, and an eccentric nucleus with coarse chromatin condensation ('clockface' pattern).

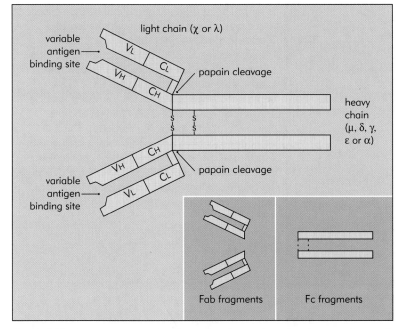

Fig. 1.100 Basic structure of an Ig molecule: each molecule is made up of two light (κ or λ) and two heavy chains, and each chain is made up of variable (V) and constant (C) portions; the V portions include the antigen binding site. The heavy chain (μ, δ, γ, ε or α) varies according to the Ig class. IgA molecules form dimers, while IgM forms a ring of five molecules. Papain cleaves the molecules into an Fc fragment and two Fab fragments.

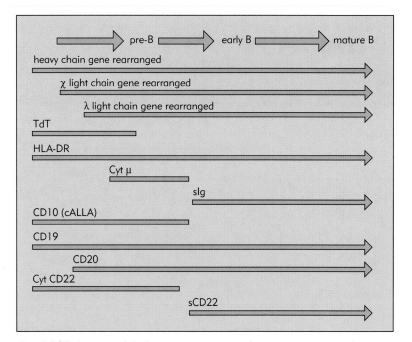

Fig. 1.101 Immunoglobulin gene: sequence of rearrangement, and antigen and Ig expression during early B-cell development. Intracytoplasmic CD22 is also a feature of very early B cells. (s, surface; Cyt, cytoplasmic; cALLA, common acute lymphoblastic leukaemia antigen; *see* Chapter 7.)

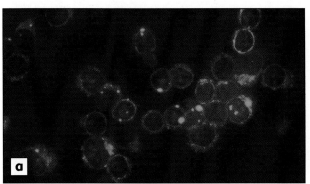
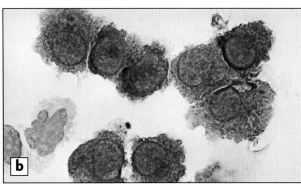

Fig. 1.102a and b Pre-B lymphoid cells: peripheral blood cells expressing intracytoplasmic IgM (a) seen with a crystalline appearance using indirect immunofluorescence, from a patient with chronic lymphocytic leukaemia, and (b) seen using the indirect immunoperoxidase method, from a case of hairy cell leukaemia. (Courtesy of Dr JV Melo.)

can be detected on the surface, while the nuclear enzyme TdT is expressed early in B-cell ontogeny. Diversity is produced by differences in the rearrangement of the genes for the variable (V), diversity (D), joining (J) and constant (C) regions of the Ig molecules they secrete (*Figs 1.95 and 1.103*), and also by insertions of a variable number of random bases in 'N' regions of TdT. Gene rearrangement processes are mediated by a recombinase enzyme system that recognizes specific joining sequences, which consist of a palindromic heptamer and nonamer sequences separated by spacer regions of 12 or 23 base pairs. The sequence starts with the heptamers that border the 3' side of each V and D segment and the 5' side of each D and J segment. The gene rearrangement first requires back-to-back fusion of the heptamer–nonamer sequences. These sequences and a circular intervening sequence, including the sequences to be deleted, are excised and the ends of two gene segments joined up (*Fig. 1.103*). Class switching is achieved by deletion of the constant region genes upstream from the gene to be expressed. The process is similar to that of Ig variable gene rearrangement. The order of the heavy chain constant region genes downstream from the

variable region genes is μ, δ, γ_3, γ_1, α_1, γ_2, γ_4, ϵ, α_2. Class switching is triggered by interactions between T and B cells in the T-cell zone of secondary lymphoid organs. Both CD40 and the CD40 ligand are essential to the signalling of class switching (*Fig. 1.104*). The majority of B cells carry HLA-DR antigens, which are important in the regulation of the immune response. Complement receptors for C3b and C3d are also found on more mature B cells.

Natural killer cells

A minor population of 'lymphocytic' cells do not carry markers of either T or B cells and are known as 'non-T, non-B' cells or 'third population' cells. The sequence of differentiation of these cells is given in *Fig. 1.88*. The majority of 'null' cells appear as large granular lymphocytes (*see Fig. 1.71*) in the peripheral blood. This population of cells contains the majority of NK cells, which can kill target cells without MHC restriction, and antibody-dependent cellular cytotoxic cells, which are able to kill tumour and virus-infected cells. They are also involved in graft rejection. Small numbers of circulating 'null' cells are immature T or

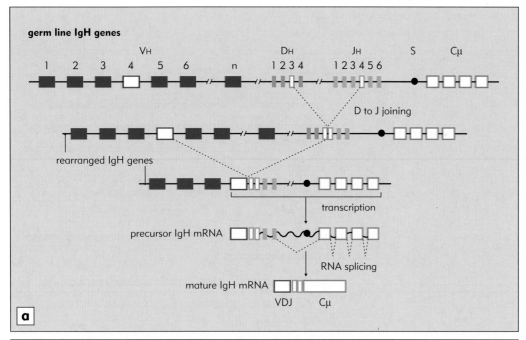

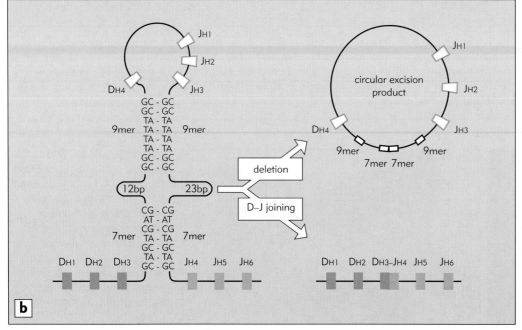

Fig. 1.103a and b Gene rearrangement: (a) rearrangement and transcription of IgH genes. First D to J joining occurs, followed by V to D–J joining. The rearranged genes can be transcribed into a precursor IgH mRNA, which becomes a mature IgH mRNA after splicing all non-coding intervening sequences. (b) Function of the joining sequences during gene rearrangement. In this typical rearrangement the 3' DH3 and 5' JH4 heptamer–nonamer sequences fuse back to back. This is followed by a DH3–JH4 joining and the deletion of a circular excision product. The heptamer–nonamer sequences shown are not those exactly associated with DH3 and JH4, but represent consensus sequences well-conserved in Ig as well as TCR genes. (Modified with permission from Van Dongen JM, Wolvers-Tettero ILM. *Clin Chim Acta.* 1991;198:1–92.)

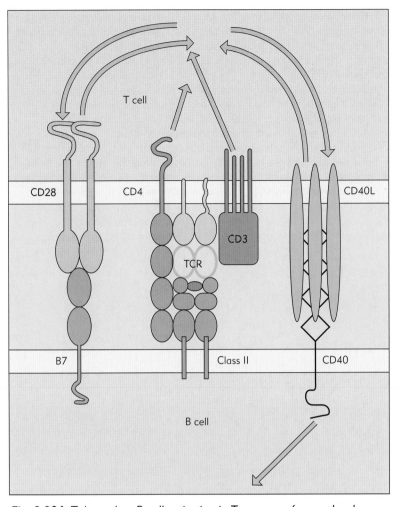

Fig. 1.104 T-dependent B-cell activation in T zones: surface molecule involvement. B cells take up antigen which they bind specifically through their surface Ig. This is internalized and broken down into peptides, which are presented on the B-cell surface, held in the peptide-binding grooves of MHC Class II molecules. Cross-linking of surface Ig by antigen induces endocytosis of the antigen–antibody complex and signals upregulation of CD40 expression and *de novo* B7.1 and B7.2 expression. If this B cell interacts with a primed T cell that recognizes the peptide complex with Class II MHC molecules, there will be costimulation through a molecule CD28, which is constitutively expressed by CD4 T cells. This can result in further signalling through co-stimulatory molecules that are transiently expressed on the T cell surface. CD40 ligand exemplifies these transiently expressed signalling molecules. These interactions can lead B and T cell proliferation and differentiation and may also induce cytokine secretion by the cells. Cytokine receptor expression by the B and T cells is initiated or upregulated. The arrows indicate that TCR engagement induces CD40-ligand expression, and that engagement of these molecules by their counterstructures on the B cell delivers further signals to the T cell. CD40 ligation induces Ig class switching in the B cell and migration. [Adapted with permission from MacLennan ICM, Drayson MT. Normal lymphocytes and non-neoplastic lymphocyte disorders. In: Hoffbrand AV, Lewis SM, Tuddenham EGD (eds). *Postgraduate Haematology*, 4th edn. Oxford: Butterworth–Heinemann; 1999:267–308.]

Lymphocyte proliferation and differentiation

T and B cells proliferate and develop in reactive lymphoid tissue (e.g. lymph nodes, and lymphoid tissues of the alimentary and respiratory tracts and spleen). Both T and B cells acquire receptors for antigens, which commit them to a single antigenic specificity, and are activated

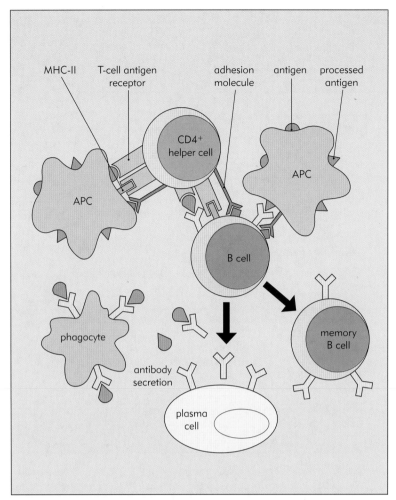

Fig. 1.105 The immune response: there is interaction between an APC and a CD4[+] (helper) T cell, with MHC-II and antigen T-cell receptor recognition, and both cells interact with a B cell, with recognition between its surface Ig and the antigen. T cells and B cells interact with different epitopes of the antigen. As a result, clones of T cells and B cells are stimulated to proliferate (see Fig. 1.107), the B cells becoming either plasma cells (secreting antibody to the antigen) or memory B cells. A phagocyte takes up the antigen–antibody complex.

when they bind their specific antigen in the presence of accessory cells.

Provided there is MHC (see below) recognition (Class I for CD8[+] and class II for CD4[+] cells), APCs interact with T cells bearing the appropriate receptor for that particular antigen. B cells with the appropriate surface receptor (Ig) for the antigen are also stimulated (*Fig. 1.105*). Adhesion molecules are involved in the cell–cell binding (*see Fig. 1.104*). Subsequently, these stimulated T and B cells proliferate and differentiate under the stimulus of factors released from APCs (IL-1, IL-6 and IL-7) and activated T helper cells (IL-2, IL-4, IL-6, IL-10, interferon-γ, and TNF; *see Fig. 1.91*). The B cells are also stimulated to secrete antibody. Clones of both effector and memory T and B cells are produced (*Figs 1.106 and 1.107*). When the memory cells are stimulated at a later date by their specific antigen, they are able to proliferate again in an accelerated fashion (secondary response).

Activated TH1 cells become responsible for cell-mediated immunity (*see Fig. 1.91*). Other lymphokines activate killer T cells, enabling them to attack an invading organism or cell, and induce macrophages to stay at the site of infection and help to digest the cells they have phagocytosed. They may also have a direct action on organisms by inhibiting proliferation or activating apoptosis.

B cells and myeloid or erythroid progenitor cells. NK cells include cells of mainly T cell (CD8[+]) and myeloid cell lineages. Their proliferation is stimulated by IL-2 and interferon-γ.

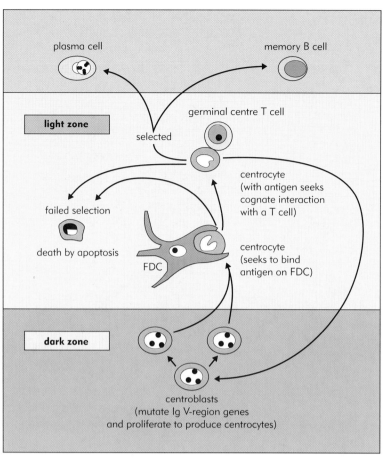

Fig. 1.106 Hypermutation: selection of cells that have undergone Ig V-region hypermutation in GCs. The hypermutation mechanism is active in centroblasts, which are the rapidly dividing cells of the dark zone that give rise to centrocytes. Centrocytes die by apoptosis unless they pick up and process antigen held on FDC, and find a T cell in the GC that recognizes the peptides from this antigen presented on centrocytes in association with self-MHC class II. The T-cell dependent selection mechanism makes it unlikely that centrocytes with mutated Ig V-region genes that encode self-reactive antibody will be selected. Most B cells that are selected leave the GC either to migrate to distant sites of antibody production (the gut or bone marrow) where they differentiate to become plasma cells, or to differentiate into memory B cells (see Fig. 1.107). Some selected cells remain within the GC and return to the dark zone as centroblasts. [Adapted with permission from MacLennan ICM, Drayson MT. Normal lymphocytes and non-neoplastic lymphocyte disorders. In: Hoffbrand AV, Lewis SM, Tuddenham EGD (eds). *Postgraduate Haematology*, 4th edn. Oxford: Butterworth–Heinemann; 1999:267–308.]

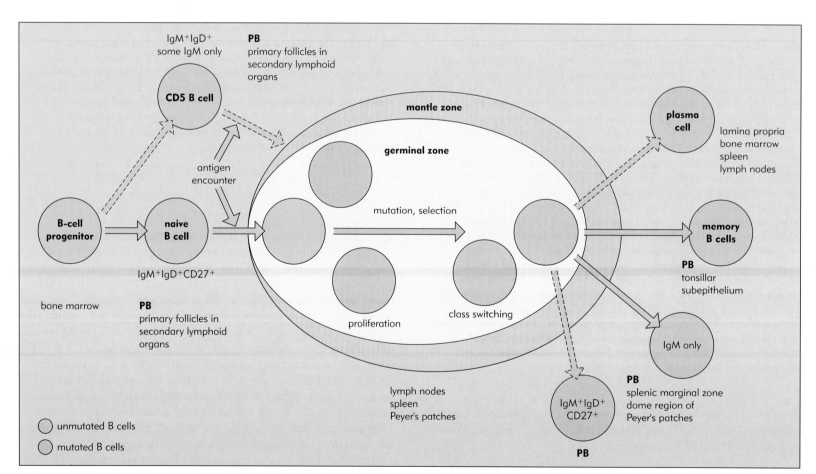

Fig. 1.107 Molecularly defined human B-lineage subsets: these have been characterized by V-gene sequence analysis, and their location in the human body is shown. Hypothetical differentiation pathways are indicated by dashed arrows. (PB, peripheral blood; adapted with permission from Klein U, Goossens T, Fischer M, *et al*. Somatic hypermutation in normal and transformed human B cells. *Immunol Rev.* 1998;162:261–80.)

Thus, T helper cells are important in the initiation of a B-cell response to antigens; T suppressor cells reduce the B lymphocytic response; and T cytotoxic cells are capable of directly damaging cells recognized as foreign or virus-infected (*Fig. 1.108*).

Activated B cells are responsible for humoral immunity. Many B-cell blasts mature into plasma cells, which produce and secrete antibodies of one specificity and Ig class (*Fig. 1.109*). B lymphocytes at different stages of differentiation and activation are shown in *Fig. 1.110*.

Somatic hypermutation in normal B cells

B cells released from the bone marrow into the peripheral blood have generated a functional non-autoreactive antigen receptor. They remain 'naive' until they encounter antigen, whereupon the antibody expressed by the B cell may be modified, both by class-switch recombination and somatic hypermutation (*Figs 106 and 107*). Somatic hypermutation is restricted to B cells that proliferate in the GC microenvironment. Somatically mutated V-region genes therefore characterize GC B cells or post-GC B cells. B-lineage derived lymphoma can thus be characterized as arising from GC or post-GC somatically hypermutated cells (*see* page 209).

Lymphocyte circulation

Lymphocytes from the primary lymphoid organs of the marrow and thymus migrate via the blood through postcapillary venules into the substance of lymph nodes, into unencapsulated lymphoid collections of the body and into the spleen. T cells home to the paracortical areas of these nodes and to the periarteriolar sheaths of the spleen. B cells accumulate selectively in germinal follicles of lymphoid tissue, in the subcapsular periphery of the cortex and in the medullary cords of the lymph nodes (*Figs 1.111 and 1.112*). Lymphocytes return to the peripheral blood by the efferent lymphatic system and the thoracic duct. The median duration of a complete circulation is about 10 hours. The majority of recirculating cells are T cells. B cells are mainly sessile and spend long periods in lymphoid tissue and the spleen. Many lymphocytes have long lifespans and may survive as memory cells for several years.

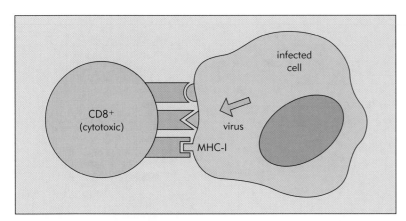

Fig. 1.108 Interaction between a CD8+ (cytotoxic) T cell and a virus-infected cell: when there is MHC-I recognition between the two cells, as well as correspondence between the antigens of the virus expressed on the cell surface and the T-cell antigen receptor on the surface of the CD8+ cell, the CD8+ cell kills the virus-infected cell.

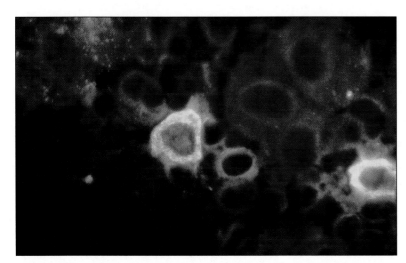

Fig. 1.109 Plasma cells: two plasma cells from a bone marrow aspirate show intense intracytoplasmic fluorescence. (Fluoresceinated anti-IgG, Evans blue counterstain.)

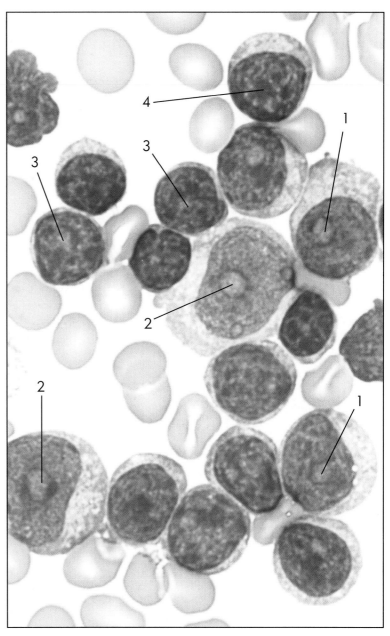

Fig. 1.110 B lymphocytes: peripheral blood film of a patient with chronic lymphocytic leukaemia with prolymphocytoid transformation shows B cells at various stages of development (1, prolymphocytes; 2, immunoblasts; 3, small lymphocytes; 4, large lymphocytes). Prolymphocytes probably represent a stage of activated B cell. (Courtesy of Dr JV Melo.)

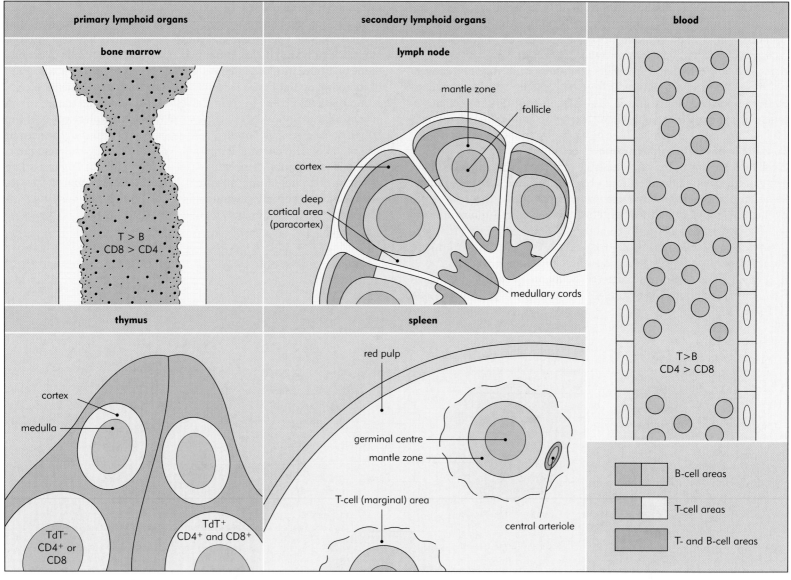

| primary lymphoid organs | secondary lymphoid organs | blood |

bone marrow

T > B
CD8 > CD4

thymus

cortex
medulla

TdT⁻
CD4⁺ or
CD8

TdT⁺
CD4⁺ and CD8⁺

lymph node

mantle zone
follicle
cortex
deep cortical area (paracortex)
medullary cords

spleen

red pulp
germinal centre
mantle zone
T-cell (marginal) area
central arteriole

T > B
CD4 > CD8

B-cell areas
T-cell areas
T- and B-cell areas

Fig. 1.111 Lymphocyte distribution: primary and secondary lymphoid organs and blood. Aggregates of secondary lymphoid tissue are found elsewhere in the body (e.g. Peyer's patches of the small intestine). The mantle zones of the lymph nodes and spleen also contain macrophages and APCs, and the paracortex also contains many interdigitating reticulum cells.

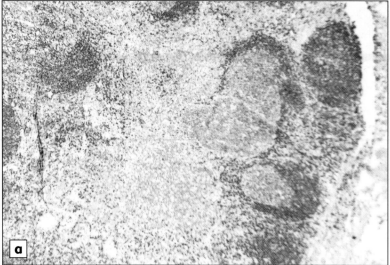

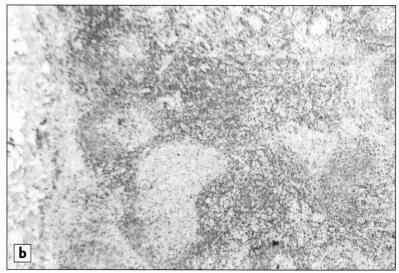

Fig. 1.112a and b B- and T-lymphocyte distribution: lymph node section showing (a) B cells in the GCs, their coronas (heavy staining) in the subcapsular cortex and medullary cords; (b) T cells, most numerous in perifollicular areas of the deeper cortical region. [Immunoperoxidase technique using (a) pan-B monoclonal antibody (anti-CD19) and (b) pan-T (anti-CD3) monoclonal antibody.]

MESENCHYMAL CELLS

Bone marrow contains precursors of mesenchymal tissues including bone, cartilage and muscle. This has been demonstrated in humans by allogeneic bone marrow transplantation, which has been shown to correct the mesenchymal disorder osteogenesis imperfecta (*Fig. 1.113*). In this disorder, mutation occurs of one of the two genes that encode Type I collagen, the main structural protein of bone, which results in generalized osteopenia with bone deformities, pathological fractures and short stature. In culture, depending on the conditions, mesenchymal stem cells (MSCs) can differentiate into osteoblasts and osteocytes, cartilage or tendon (*Fig. 1.114*). It is likely that a common pluripotential stem cell can give rise either to mesenchymal stem cells or to haemopoietic stem cells (*Fig. 1.115*). Also, recent evidence suggests that, given the correct culture conditions, certain types of nerve cells, muscle cells, and other body cells can transform into haemopoietic stem cells.

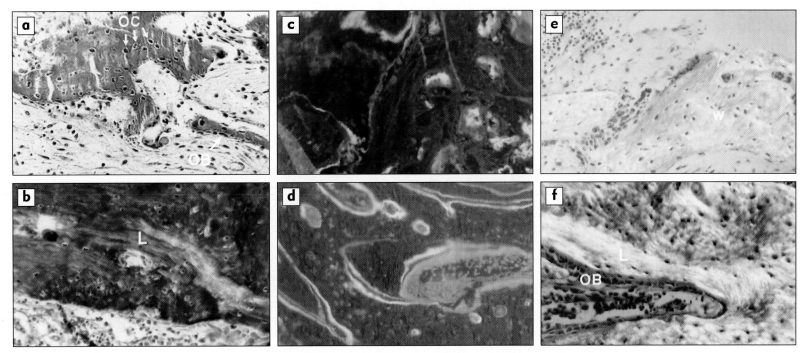

Fig. 1.113a–f Mesenchymal cells: allogeneic bone marrow transplantation in osteogenesis imperfecta. (a) Biopsy specimen of trabecular bone before transplantation. The calcified tissue appears blue–green and the uncalcified tissue is red–brown. Numerous, randomly arranged osteocytes (OC) are present in large lacunae. Peritrabecular marrow fibrosis is also present, and there is a paucity of osteoblasts (OB) relative to the specimens after transplantation and an incompletely calcified area of bone marrow. (b) A specimen after transplantation taken near to the site shown in (a). Osteocytes are fewer and a small section of lamellar bone (L) indicates normalization of the remodelling process. (c) Fluorescence photomicrograph of the trabecular bone specimen [same section as shown in (a)]. The poorly defined labelling indicates disorganized formation of new bone and abnormal mineralization. (d) A contrasting specimen to that shown in (c) after transplantation, with definitive, crisp, single and double tetracycline labelling, indicative of considerably improved new bone formation and mineralization. (e) Trabecular bone specimen before transplantation that shows the woven (w) texture of the bone, a characteristic feature of patients with osteogenesis imperfecta. (f) Bone specimen after transplantation that demonstrates lamellar (L) bone formation and linearly arranged osteoblasts (OB) in areas of active bone formation along the calcified trabecular surface. [(a, b) Goldners–Masson trichrome; (c, d) fluorescent tetracycline labelling; (e, f) toluidine blue under polarized light; reproduced with permission from Horwitz EM, Prockop DJ, Fitzpatrick LA, et al. Transplantability and therapeutic effects of bone marrow-derived mesenchymal cells in children with osteogenesis imperfecta. *Nature Med.* 1999;5:309–13.]

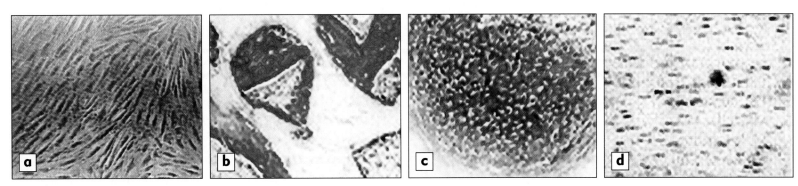

Fig. 1.114a–d Differentiation of mesenchymal stem cells in culture: (a) undifferentiated human MSCs; (b) bone formation by osteoblasts and osteocytes into which human MSCs have differentiated when grown on ceramic tubes and placed in severe combined immunodeficiency mice; (c) cartilage derived from human MSCs grown from a cell pellet; (d) rabbit MSCs form tendon when placed in a ruptured tendon sheath. (Reproduced with permission from Gerson SL and Mesenchymal stem cells: no longer second class marrow citizens. *Nature Med.* 1999;5:262–4.)

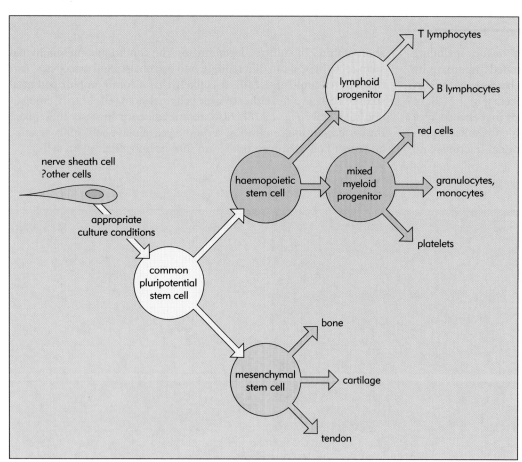

Fig. 1.115 Mesenchymal cells: these cells and haemopoietic cells probably have a common precursor pluripotential cell. Under appropriate culture conditions, muscle cells (and nerve sheath cells) may be transformed into common pluripotential haemopoietic stem cells.

Hypochromic Anaemias and Iron Overload

The hypochromic anaemias are characterized by hypochromic cells in the peripheral blood with a mean cell haemoglobin (MCH) of <27 pg. The cells are also usually microcytic, with a mean cell volume (MCV) of <80 fl. With manual methods of haemoglobin and haematocrit (packed cell volume, PCV) estimation, the mean corpuscular haemoglobin concentration (MCHC) is also reduced (to <32 g/dl), but this estimation is not of value when using modern electronic counters.

The hypochromasia is caused by failure of haemoglobin synthesis, the mechanism of which is shown in *Fig. 2.1*. This failure occurs most commonly as a result of iron deficiency, but it may also arise from a block in iron metabolism as in the anaemia of chronic disorders, from failure of protoporphyrin and haem synthesis as in the sideroblastic anaemias, from failure of globin synthesis as in the thalassaemias (*see* Chapter 5), or from crystallization of haemoglobin in some of the other haemoglobin disorders, for example, haemoglobin C (*see* Chapter 5). Lead inhibits both haem and globin synthesis and may cause a hypochromic anaemia, but it also causes haemolysis, probably because of failure of RNA breakdown.

IRON METABOLISM

Most body iron present in haemoglobin is found in circulating red cells. The macrophages of the reticuloendothelial system store iron, released from haemoglobin, as ferritin and haemosiderin. They also release iron to plasma, where it attaches to transferrin which takes it to tissues with transferrin receptors, especially the bone marrow, where the iron is incorporated by erythroid cells into haemoglobin. There is a small loss of iron each day in urine, faeces, skin, nails, and in menstruating females via blood. This loss (1–2 mg daily) is replaced by iron absorbed from the diet. Iron absorption is discussed on page 55.

Iron uptake via the transferrin receptor, intracellular storage of iron in ferritin and the incorporation of iron into haem in mitochondria are all coordinated in response to iron supply at the transcriptional and translational levels. This is achieved by the presence of iron-responsive elements (IREs) located in the upstream untranslated regions of the messenger RNAs (mRNAs) for ferritin and the erythroid haem synthetic enzyme δ-aminolaevulinic acid synthase (ALA-S), or in the downstream region for the transferrin receptor in untranslated regions of the mRNAs (*Fig. 2.2*). The IREs consist of both a double-stranded stem and single-stranded loop RNA structure (resembling a hairpin; *see Fig. 2.61*).

IRON-DEFICIENCY ANAEMIA

Iron deficiency usually results from haemorrhage since most body iron is present in circulatory haemoglobin (*Fig. 2.3*). The symptoms of iron deficiency are caused by anaemia (if sufficiently severe) as well as, in some cases, by damage to epithelial tissues. Also, symptoms of the underlying disease may cause the deficiency. On rare occasions, the patient has a bizarre craving to eat items such as ice, chalk or paper – known as pica. In infants, impairment of psychomotor development and cognitive function may occur, especially in the first 2 years of life.

The patient with iron-deficiency anaemia may show pallor of the mucous membranes, which is usually only recognized clinically if the haemoglobin is less than about 9 g/dl. There is pallor of the conjunctivae, lips, palm creases and nail beds (*Figs 2.4–2.6*). Skin colour,

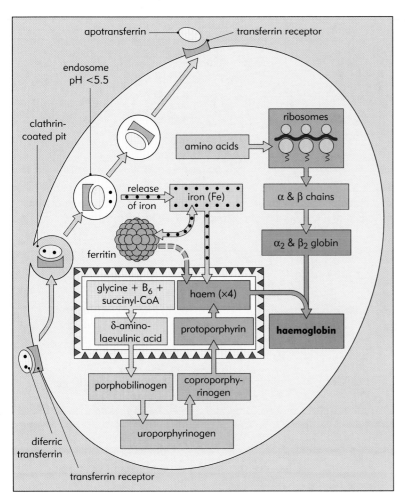

Fig. 2.1 Haemoglobin synthesis in the developing red cell: iron enters the cell with transferrin and is combined with protoporphyrin, synthesized largely from glycine and succinyl-CoA in mitochondria, to form haem. One molecule of haem attaches to one of the globin polypeptide chains to form a unit of haemoglobin, and one haemoglobin molecule is made up of four haemoglobin units. Transferrin together with its receptor enters the cell by receptor mediated endocytosis. Iron is released by a fall in pH and the apotransferrin and receptor are recycled to plasma and membrane, respectively. Hypochromic anaemias arise from lack of iron or failure of haem synthesis for other reasons.

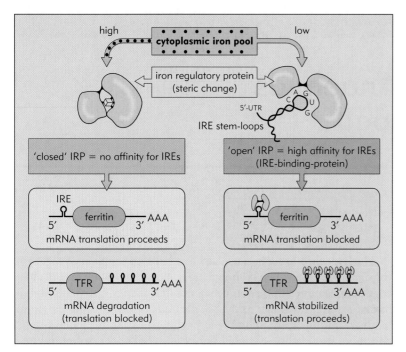

Fig. 2.2 Cellular iron homeostasis: the synthesis of ferritin, the transferrin receptor (TFR), erythroid ALA-synthase (ALA-S) and possibly other proteins involved in iron metabolism is regulated at the level of RNA translation by cytoplasmic iron regulatory proteins (IRP). These proteins can bind to mRNAs that contain a stem and loop structure – an iron-responsive element (IRE). When iron is plentiful, it has a low affinity for IRE, resulting in less transferrin receptor but more ferritin and erythroid ALA-S synthesis. When iron supply is low, binding to the IRE is increased with increased synthesis of transferrin receptor and less ferritin and ALA-S synthesis. (Courtesy of Dr D Girelli.)

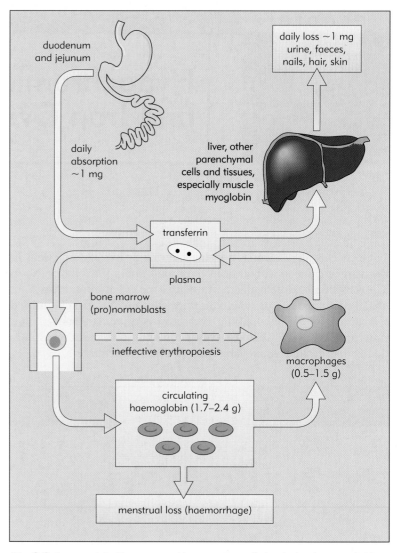

Fig. 2.3 Iron metabolism: normal iron content of circulating haemoglobin and macrophages is indicated as well as the approximate amount of iron absorbed and lost from the body each day (*see also Fig. 2.59*).

however, is not a reliable sign of anaemia, since it depends on the state of the skin circulation as well as on the haemoglobin content of the blood. The patient's nails are frequently ridged and brittle (*Fig. 2.7*) or may show spoon nails, known as koilonychia (*Fig. 2.8*). There may be angular cheilosis (stomatitis; cracking at the corners of the mouth), especially in those with badly fitting false teeth (*Fig. 2.9*).

In severe cases, especially in older patients, an atrophic glossitis with loss of filiform papillae (*Fig. 2.10*) may be present.

There may also be dysphagia due to postcricoid webs (Plummer–Vinson or Paterson–Kelly syndrome), especially in middle-aged women (*Fig. 2.11*).

The biochemical explanation for these epithelial cell abnormalities is unclear; they may be related to a reduction in haem-containing enzymes, for example, cytochromes, cytochrome *c* oxidase, succinic dehydrogenase, catalase, peroxidase, ribonucleotide reductase, xanthine oxidase and aconitase. When the anaemia is very severe and of rapid onset, there may be retinal haemorrhages (*Fig. 2.12*).

Blood and bone marrow appearances

The blood film shows the presence of hypochromic microcytic red cells (*Figs 2.13–2.15*) with abnormally shaped cells ('pencil' or cigar-shaped poikilocytes) and occasional target cells. The severity of the blood film changes and of the fall in the MCH and MCV is related to the degree of anaemia. The platelet count is often raised, particularly if haemorrhage is occurring. A typical blood count for a patient with iron-deficiency anaemia is shown in *Fig. 2.16*.

The bone marrow is of normal cellularity, sometimes with normoblastic hyperplasia, and the developing erythroblasts show a ragged vacuolated cytoplasm (*Fig. 2.17*). Perls' staining shows a complete absence of iron stores (*Fig. 2.18*) and of siderotic granules from developing erythroblasts (*Fig. 2.19*).

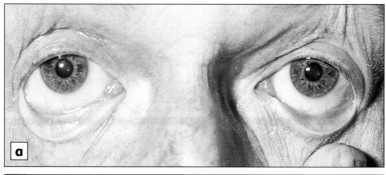

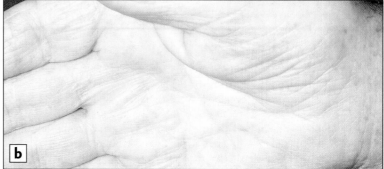

Fig. 2.4a and b Iron-deficiency anaemia: (a) pallor of conjunctival mucosa; mucous membrane pallor becomes clinically apparent when the haemoglobin concentration is below 9 g/dl; (b) pallor of palmar skin creases.

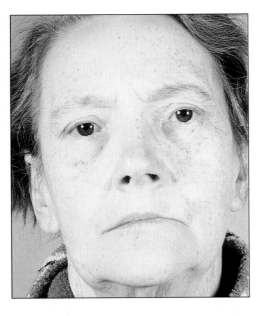

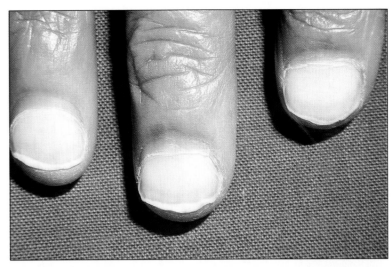

Fig. 2.5 Iron-deficiency anaemia: pallor of mucous membranes (lips) and skin in a 69-year-old woman. (Hb, 8.1 g/dl; RBC, $4.13 \times 10^{12}/1$; PCV, 26.8%; MCV, 65 fl; MCH, 19.6 pg.)

Fig. 2.6 Iron-deficiency anaemia: marked pallor of the nail beds in a dark-skinned patient. The nails are flattened.

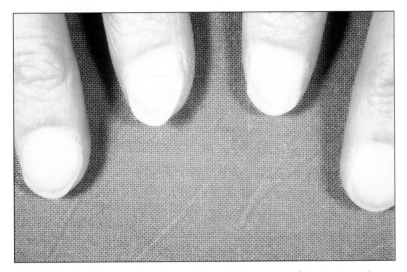

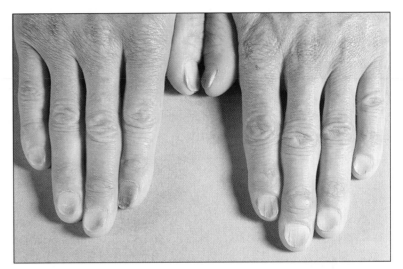

Fig. 2.7 Iron-deficiency anaemia: although there is no obvious concavity, these nails are flattened and brittle with marked pallor of the nail beds.

Fig. 2.8 Iron-deficiency anaemia: koilonychia. The nails are concave, ridged and brittle. This patient's anaemia had been rapidly corrected by blood transfusion prior to an operation for caecal carcinoma. The cause of the nail changes in iron deficiency is uncertain, but may be related to the iron requirement of many enzymes present in epithelial and other cells. (Courtesy of Dr SM Knowles.)

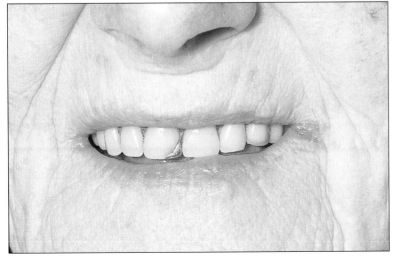

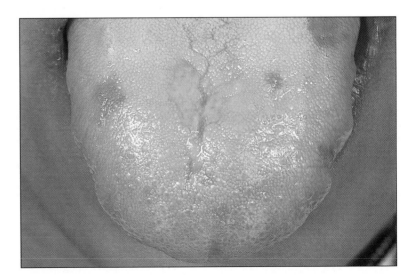

Fig. 2.9 Iron-deficiency anaemia: angular cheilosis. There is fissuring and ulceration at the corners of the mouth. The biochemical mechanism is uncertain but may be similar to that for nail, mucosal and pharyngeal changes.

Fig. 2.10 Iron-deficiency anaemia: glossitis. The bald, fissured appearance of the tongue is caused by flattening and loss of papillae.

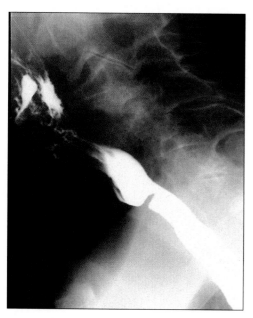

Fig. 2.11 Iron-deficiency anaemia: barium swallow radiograph showing a postcricoid web causing a filling defect in a 50-year-old woman with the Plummer–Vinson (Paterson–Kelly) syndrome who complained of dysphagia.

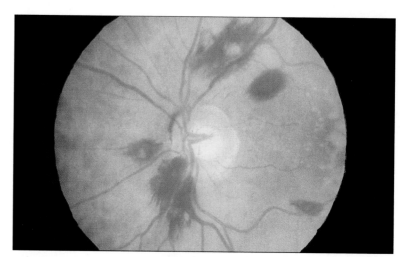

Fig. 2.12 Iron-deficiency anaemia; multiple retinal haemorrhages in a 25-year-old woman with chronic iron deficiency because of severe haemorrhage (menorrhagia; Hb, 2.5 g/dl). These appearances may occur in other severe anaemias.

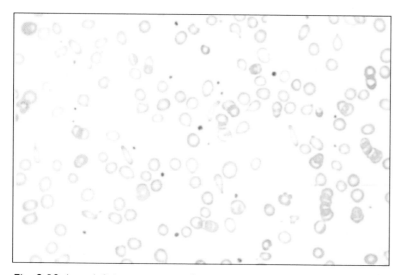

Fig. 2.13 Iron-deficiency anaemia: low power view of peripheral blood film. The red cells are hypochromic and microcytic. Some poikilocytes are present, including thin elongated ('pencil') cells and occasional target cells. Platelets are plentiful. (Hb, 7.5 g/dl.)

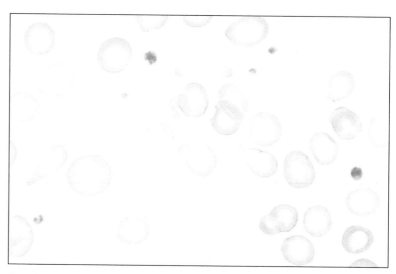

Fig. 2.14 Iron-deficiency anaemia: high power view of peripheral blood film shows hypochromic cells and poikilocytes.

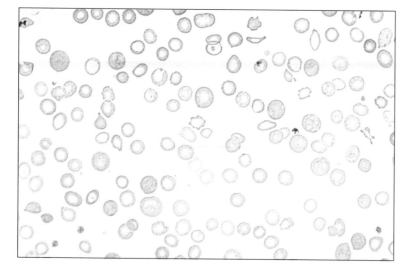

Fig. 2.15 Iron-deficiency anaemia: low power peripheral blood film taken during therapy with oral iron. There is a dimorphic population of hypochromic microcytic cells and target cells, and well-haemoglobinized cells of normal size but with some large polychromatic cells (newly formed well-haemoglobinized reticulocytes).

Blood count in iron-deficiency anaemia	
Hb	7.5 g/dl
RBC	4.05×10^{12}/l
PCV	26%
MCV	64 fl
MCH	18.5 pg
reticulocytes	2.6%
WBC	7.5×10^9/l
differential	normal
platelets	530×10^9/l

Fig. 2.16 Iron-deficiency anaemia: blood count in moderately severe iron-deficiency anaemia (same case as for *Fig. 2.13*).

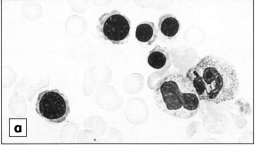
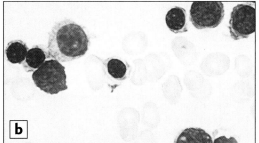
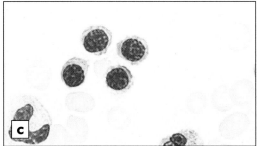
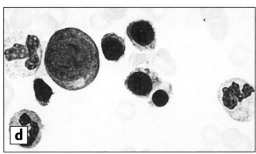

Fig. 2.17a–d Iron-deficiency anaemia: bone marrow aspirate. (a)–(d) The cytoplasm of polychromatic and pyknotic erythroblasts is scanty, vacuolated and irregular in outline. This type of erythropoiesis has been described as 'micronormoblastic'.

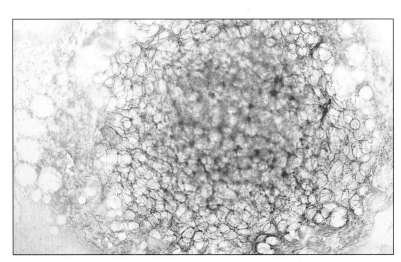

Fig. 2.18 Iron-deficiency anaemia: bone marrow aspirate showing absence of stainable iron in a bone marrow fragment. The appearances are similar in iron-deficiency anaemia and latent iron deficiency (absent iron stores without anaemia). Compare with the appearances of normal iron stores in *Fig. 1.56*. (Perls' stain, methyl red counterstain.)

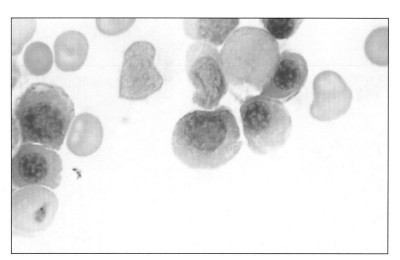

Fig. 2.19 Iron-deficiency anaemia: bone marrow aspirate showing lack of siderotic granules in developing erythroblasts. Compare with the normal appearance of isolated Prussian blue-positive granules in the erythroblast cytoplasm in *Fig. 1.56*. (Perls' stain, methyl red counterstain.)

Fig. 2.20 Iron-deficiency anaemia: causes.

Causes of iron-deficiency anaemia				
Haemorrhage	Gastrointestinal hiatus hernia oesophageal varices peptic ulcer aspirin ingestion hookworm neoplasm ulcerative colitis telangiectasia angiodysplasia diverticulosis haemorrhoids	Pulmonary pulmonary haemosiderosis Uterine menorrhagia ante- and postpartum Renal tract haematuria chronic dialysis Self-induced	**Transfer to fetus**	pregnancy
			Haemosiderinuria	Chronic intravascular haemolysis paroxysmal nocturnal haemoglobinuria heart valve haemolysis
			Malabsorption	Atrophic gastritis Gluten-induced enteropathy Partial gastrectomy
			Poor diet	Poor quality diet, especially if mostly vegetable Infants fed on cow's milk with late weaning

Causes of iron deficiency

The causes of iron-deficiency anaemia are listed in *Fig. 2.20*. About two-thirds of body iron is circulating in red cells as haemoglobin, one litre of blood containing about 500 mg of iron. The next biggest store, which varies between 0 and 2 g, is within the macrophages of the reticuloendothelial system in the form of the storage proteins haemosiderin (visible on light microscopy) and ferritin (seen only by electron microscopy). The absence of iron stores, with a fall in serum iron and serum ferritin and a rise in total iron-binding capacity (transferrin), but without anaemia and without a fall in red cell indices, is termed 'latent iron deficiency'. Iron in myoglobin and a variety of enzymes (see page 42) make up the rest of the body iron.

Daily iron losses and, thus, requirements for iron in adults, are normally small in relation to body stores, about 1 mg daily in males and postmenopausal females, and 1.5–3.9 mg in menstruating females. Requirements are also increased in children (to provide for growth and increase in red cell mass) and during pregnancy for transfer to the fetus.

Iron deficiency is usually the result of haemorrhage, the most common cause in many countries being hookworm infestation (*Fig. 2.21*); the loss is related to the worm load. In females, menorrhagia or repeated pregnancy without iron supplementation is a frequent cause. In men and postmenopausal women iron deficiency is usually caused by chronic gastrointestinal blood loss which in Western countries is often the result of hiatus hernia (*Fig. 2.22*), peptic ulceration (*Fig. 2.23*), chronic aspirin ingestion, colonic or caecal carcinoma (*Fig. 2.24*), angiodysplasia (*Fig. 2.25*), colonic diverticulosis or haemorrhoids. Rare causes or iron deficiency are pulmonary haemosiderosis (*Fig. 2.26*), chronic intravascular haemolysis as in paroxysmal nocturnal haemoglobinuria, and self-inflicted venesection.

A normal Western diet contains 10–15 mg of iron daily, of which 5–10% is absorbed. Iron absorption is increased in iron deficiency but reduced by some food substances, such as phytates and phosphates. Poor dietary intake of iron may be the sole cause of iron deficiency if present for many years. However, more often it provides a background of reduced iron stores on which other causes of iron deficiency, such as

heavy menstrual loss, or increased requirements for pregnancy or for growth in infants and children, may lead to iron-deficiency anaemia.

Malabsorption alone is also an unusual cause of iron deficiency. Even in patients with atrophic gastritis or gluten-induced enteropathy, loss

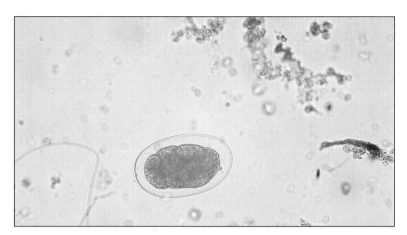

Fig. 2.21 Iron-deficiency anaemia: an ovum of the hookworm. *Ancylostoma duodenale*, a frequent cause of iron-deficiency anaemia in many parts of the world, is present. Blood loss and therefore severity of anaemia are related to the degree of parasitization.

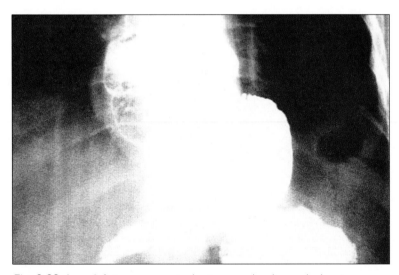

Fig. 2.22 Iron-deficiency anaemia: barium meal radiograph showing a gross hiatus hernia in a 55-year-old patient. Endoscopy showed a small ulcerated area of bleeding.

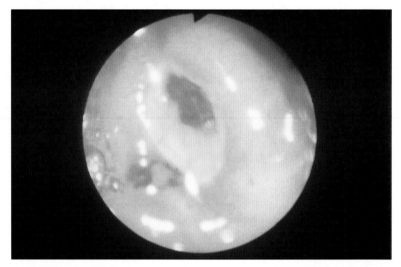

Fig. 2.23 Iron-deficiency anaemia: endoscopic appearance of a bleeding duodenal ulcer in a 45-year-old man who presented with symptoms of anaemia. (Courtesy of Prof. RE Pounder.)

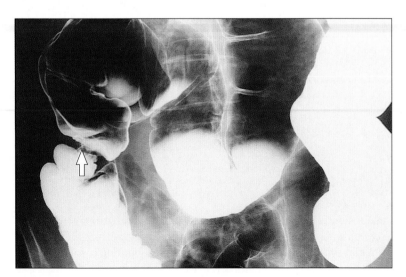

Fig. 2.24 Iron-deficiency anaemia: barium enema radiograph showing an annular filling defect (arrow) of the ascending colon due to adenocarcinoma.

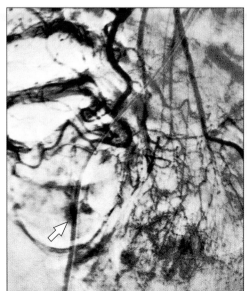

Fig. 2.25 Iron-deficiency anaemia: angiogram of coeliac axis showing numerous 'blushes' (arrow) that result from angiodysplasia of the terminal ileum and ascending colon. (Courtesy of Dr R Dick.)

resulting from an increased turnover of cells and exudation of transferrin iron may be as important as the malabsorption. Following gastrectomy, the two main factors are blood loss and malabsorption, more marked for food iron than for inorganic iron.

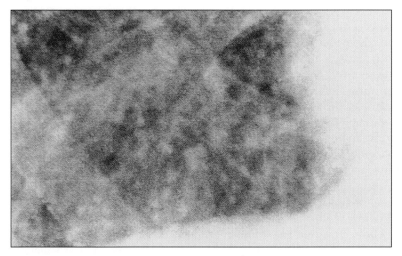

Fig. 2.26 Iron-deficiency anaemia: chest radiograph showing diffuse mottled appearance caused by pulmonary haemosiderosis. The lesions consist of aggregates of iron-laden macrophages with surrounding fibrosis. (Courtesy of Dr R Dick.)

There are two main aims in the management of iron deficiency. The first is to identify the cause and wherever possible to eliminate this. The second is to give iron in sufficient quantities to correct the anaemia and replenish tissue iron stores. This is best achieved with oral iron, although in occasional cases parenteral iron, such as total dose infusion of iron–dextran, is necessary. The rise in haemoglobin with adequate iron therapy is of the order of 2 g/dl every 3 weeks.

SIDEROBLASTIC ANAEMIA

Sideroblastic anaemia is characterized by the presence of ring sideroblasts in the bone marrow. The iron is deposited in the mitochondria of the erythroblasts. The disorder is classified into congenital and acquired types; the acquired type is further subdivided into primary and secondary types, including some types associated with other bone marrow disorders (*Fig. 2.27*). In the secondary types, the proportion of ring sideroblasts is usually <15% and the anaemia has other causes.

The congenital type usually occurs in males (*Fig. 2.28*), indicating a sex-linked pattern of inheritance; but it is also seen, though rarely, in females (*Fig. 2.29*). The blood film is hypochromic and microcytic, or dimorphic of varying severity (*Fig. 2.30*). About a third of congenital cases respond to pyridoxine (vitamin B₆), a greater percentage than in the other types of sideroblastic anaemia.

Causes of ring sideroblast formation
Congenital*
Hereditary sex-linked occurring most frequently in males Autosomal Mitochondrial DNA defects
Acquired
Primary*
Classified as one of the myelodysplastic syndromes; also termed 'idiopathic acquired sideroblastic anaemia' (see Chapter 9)
Associated with malignant marrow disorders†
Acute myeloid leukaemia Polycythaemia vera Myelofibrosis Myeloma Myelodysplastic syndromes
Secondary†
Drugs, e.g. isoniazid and cycloserine Toxins, e.g. lead and alcohol Megaloblastic anaemia Haemolytic anaemia Pregnancy Rheumatoid arthritis Carcinoma

*In these disorders the proportion of sideroblasts in the marrow is usually >15%.
†In these disorders, the proportion of ring sideroblasts is usually <15%.

Fig. 2.27 Sideroblastic anaemia: causes.

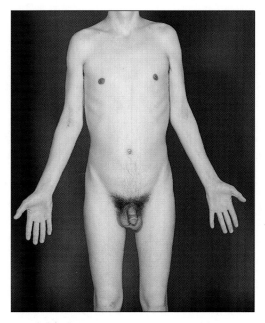

Fig. 2.28 Sideroblastic anaemia: this 18-year-old male with hereditary (congenital) sideroblastic anaemia presented with symptoms of anaemia at the age of 16 and was found to have a microcytic hypochromic anaemia (Hb, 9.8 g/dl; MCV, 75 fl; MCH, 23.1 pg) with many ring sideroblasts in the bone marrow. His height (1.75 m) and sexual development are normal. Pallor of the mucous membranes and early melanin skin pigmentation resulted from iron overload arising from blood transfusions given over a 2-year period, and commenced soon after presentation because his haemoglobin had fallen spontaneously to <6 g/dl. He subsequently died of infection with *Yersinia enterocolitica*, having received over 500 units of blood. The patient's elder brother was also affected (*see Figs 2.34 and 2.35*).

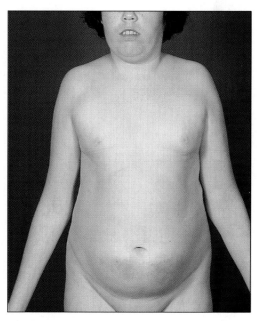

Fig. 2.29 Sideroblastic anaemia: a 17-year-old girl with congenital sideroblastic anaemia, a rare occurrence. Iron overload developed because of the need for regular blood transfusions from the age of 3 years. She failed to commence menstruation and shows delayed puberty, absence of axillary and pubic hair, and minimal breast development. She also has a thalassaemic facies with a bossed skull, prominent maxilla and abnormally widened spaces between the teeth. The lower abdominal bruising is from the regular insertion of needles for subcutaneous desferrioxamine infusions.

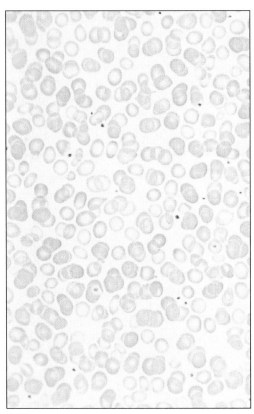

Fig. 2.30 Sideroblastic anaemia (hereditary): peripheral blood film from a 19-year-old man shows a dimorphic anaemia with a mixture of poorly haemoglobinized microcytic cells and well-haemoglobinized normocytic cells. (Hb, 11.5 g/dl; MCV, 78 fl; MCH, 25.3 pg.)

The congenital type of sideroblastic anaemia includes a group with mutations in the gene on the X-chromosome coding for the erythroid specific enzyme, ALA-S (*Fig. 2.31*). It usually affects men and presents in the third decade of life. Women are rarely affected. Presentation in both sexes in old age has been described. The mutations identified have been missense, affecting exons 5, 7, 8 and 9. Pyridoxine responsiveness correlates with mutations affecting exon 9, the region that codes for the pyridoxal-5-phosphate binding site. Exon 5 may also code for sequences involved in pyridoxal-5-phosphate binding.

Some of the congenital types are now thought to result from a fault in mitochondrial DNA, including that in Pearson syndrome, which causes a defect in one or more enzymes in the respiratory chain generating ATP and coded for by mitochondrial DNA (*Fig. 2.32*).

Pearson syndrome consists of neutropenia, thrombocytopenia, sideroblastic anaemia, exocrine pancreatic dysfunction and hepatic dysfunction. There is vacuolation of marrow erythroid and myeloid precursors (*Fig. 2.33a*). The syndrome may be accompanied by neurological and muscle disorders. The bone marrow and skeletal muscle findings of a 42-year-old man with the combination of congenital sideroblastic anaemia and a proximal myopathy are shown in *Figs. 2.33b and 2.34*. The bone marrow shows ring sideroblasts and vacuolation of normoblasts (*Fig. 2.33b*). Electron microscopy of a skeletal muscle biopsy shows crystalline deposits in mitochondria (*Fig. 2.34*). The exact defect is unclear despite analysis of ALA-S and mitochondrial DNA. This patient does not fit precisely into any clear phenotype.

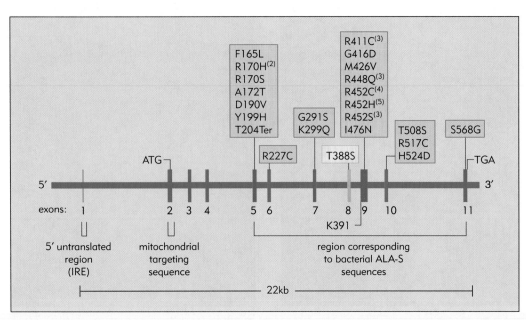

Fig. 2.31 Sideroblastic anaemia: mutations in the ALA-S gene in patients with X-linked sideroblastic anaemia. (The superscript numbers in brackets refer to the number of cases described at the time of writing; courtesy of Prof. DF Bishop.)

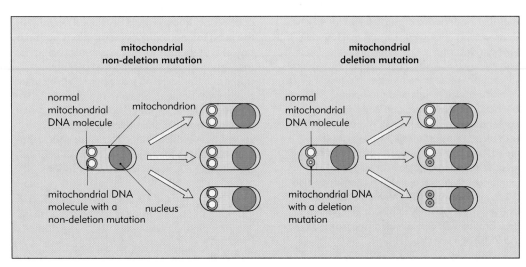

Fig. 2.32 Mitochondrial DNA: this consists of a circular loop of DNA coding for enzymes in the mitochondrial respiratory chain. Mitochondrial DNA is inherited from the cytoplasm of the maternal ovum. Multiple copies (50–1000) are present in each cell. The relative proportions of a mutant (deletional or non-deletional) and wild-type mitochondrial DNA that occur in the individual cells of a particular tissue determine the phenotype when a mitochondrial defect is inherited.

The DIDMOAD (Wolfram) syndrome consists of diabetes insipidus, diabetes mellitus, optic atrophy and sensorineural deafness. It may be accompanied by megaloblastic and sideroblastic anaemia, in some cases responding to thiamine. As in other forms of sideroblastic anaemia, there is iron loading of erythroblast mitochondria (*Fig. 2.35*). A less common triad of thiamine responsive megaloblastic anaemia, diabetes mellitus and sensorineural deafness has been described. A defect in thiamine phosphorylation has been identified. The patient illustrated in *Fig. 2.36* resembles one with the DIDMOAD syndrome most closely.

In primary acquired sideroblastic anaemia, there is usually macrocytosis and gross anisocytosis and poikilocytosis (*Fig. 2.37*). This disease is classified by the French–American–British group as a type of myelodysplasia (*see* Chapter 9). In a proportion of patients the disease transforms, after a variable number of years, into acute myeloid leukaemia. In many cases careful examination reveals white-cell or platelet abnormalities in the peripheral blood or in their precursors in the bone marrow. These cases with trilineage dysplasia have a much higher incidence of transformation in acute myeloid leukaemia.

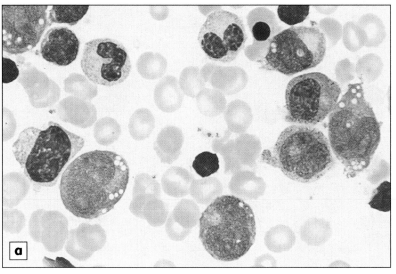
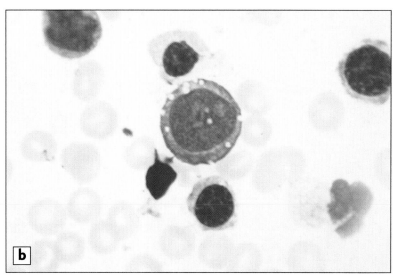

Fig. 2.33a and b Congenital sideroblastic anaemia: (a) bone marrow of a baby with Pearson syndrome showing vacuolated proerythroblasts and dysplastic neutrophils.

(b) bone marrow of a 42-year-old man showing vacuolation of blast cells.

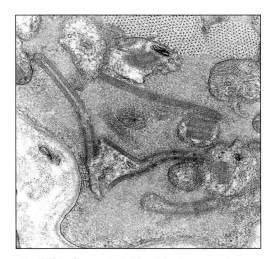
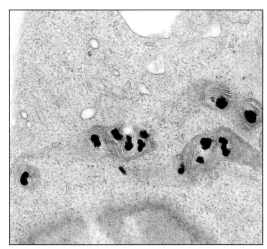
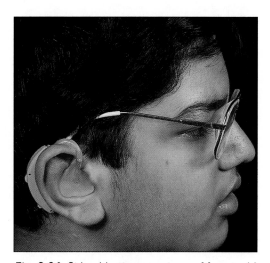

Fig. 2.34 Congenital sideroblastic anaemia: electron micrograph of skeletal muscle of a 42-year-old man, showing bizarrely shaped mitochondria with abnormal cristae and intramitochondrial paracrystalline inclusions. The changes are typical of a mitochondrial respiratory chain defect. (Courtesy of Prof. AHV Schapira.)

Fig. 2.35 Hereditary sideroblastic anaemia: electron microscopy of erythroblast showing iron-laden mitochondria. The patient, a 13-year-old male, presented with diabetes mellitus, deafness and optic atrophy (Hb, 10.3 g/dl; RBC, 3.47 × 10^{12}/l). Peripheral blood showed macrocytes and hypochromic and microcytic red cells; bone marrow showed megaloblastic and dyserythropoietic changes and ringed sideroblasts. There was no response to folic acid or pyridoxine, but a reticulocytosis with a rise in haemoglobin to 12.9 g/dl occurred in response to thiamine therapy. (From Haworth C, Evans DJ, Mitra J, *et al.*, Thiamine responsive anaemia: a study of two further cases. *Br J Haematol* 1982;50:549–61; courtesy of Prof. SN Wickramasinghe.)

Fig. 2.36 Sideroblastic anaemia: an 11-year-old boy with congenital deafness, optic atrophy, diabetes mellitus, and megaloblastic and sideroblastic anaemia (a variant of DIDMOAD syndrome). His older sister showed the same syndrome, but in her case the anaemia responded to thiamine. In this patient, the anaemia is refractory to thiamine, pyridoxine and folic acid, and regular blood transfusions are needed. (Courtesy of Dr JZ Wimperis.)

Siderotic granules are frequently seen in the peripheral blood red cells following splenectomy (*Fig. 2.38*). The bone marrow shows erythroid hyperplasia (*Fig. 2.39*) with vacuolated erythroblasts (*Fig. 2.40*).

In contrast to the inherited form, in primary acquired sideroblastic anaemia (*see Fig. 9.25*) the erythroblasts are megaloblastic in about 50% of cases (*Fig. 2.41*). Iron staining shows many ring sideroblasts (*Fig. 2.42*) and iron stores may be increased (*Fig. 2.43*). In the primary forms of acquired sideroblastic anaemia, 15–50%, or often more, of the erythroblasts show partial or complete rings. In the secondary forms, ring sideroblasts are usually less common.

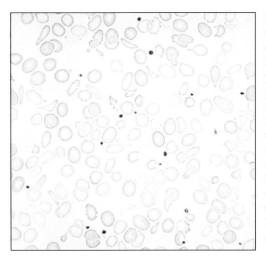

Fig. 2.37 Sideroblastic anaemia (primary acquired): peripheral blood film from a 65-year-old man who presented with a predominantly hypochromic anaemia with numerous poikilocytes. In most such cases, the anaemia is dimorphic with an overall increase in MCV to above normal. (Hb, 7.2 g/dl; MCV, 82 fl; MCH, 26.8 pg.)

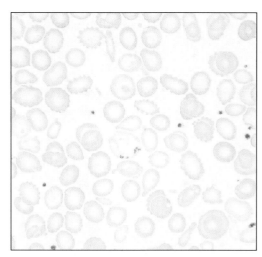

Fig. 2.38 Sideroblastic anaemia (primary acquired): peripheral blood film following splenectomy showing Pappenheimer bodies in the red cells. Their iron content is demonstrated by Perls' staining (siderotic granules). In addition, Howell–Jolly bodies (DNA remnants) were present and the platelet count was raised (652 × 10⁹/l).

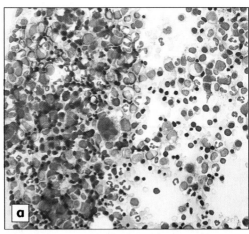
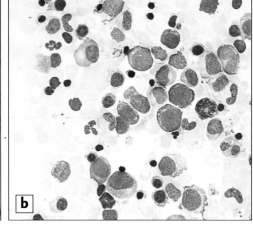

Fig. 2.39a and b Sideroblastic anaemia (primary acquired): (a) low power view of bone marrow aspirate shows increased cellularity of the fragment and trails; (b) at higher power, erythroid hyperplasia is also seen.

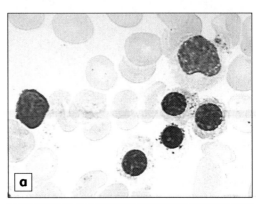
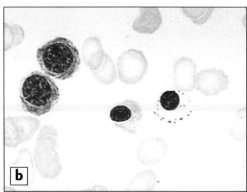
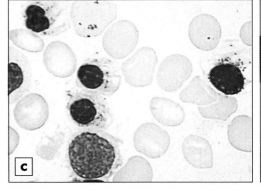
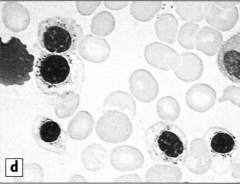

Fig. 2.40a–d Sideroblastic anaemia (primary acquired): (a–d) bone marrow aspirate showing vacuolation of erythroblasts with intact cytoplasmic margins. In some cells the vacuoles are surrounded by heavily stained cytoplasmic granules (punctate basophilia). Contrast the appearances with those in iron-deficiency anaemia (*see Fig. 2.17*) and thalassaemia major (*see Fig. 5.23*).

Sideroblastic anaemia, especially the inherited form, occasionally responds to vitamin B$_6$ (pyridoxine) therapy. Other therapy may include folic acid, blood transfusion and iron chelation. Thiamine may produce a response in rare cases. In primary acquired sideroblastic anaemia, treatment resembles that for other myelodysplastic syndromes.

ALCOHOL

Excessive ingestion of alcohol may cause a variety of haematological abnormalities, including macrocytosis, megaloblastic and sideroblastic changes, and thrombocytopenia. In some cases vacuolation of erythroblasts is apparent (*Fig. 2.44*).

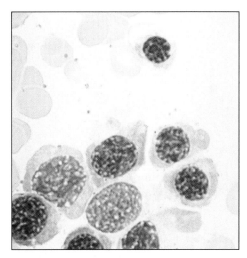

Fig. 2.41 Sideroblastic anaemia (primary acquired): bone marrow showing mildly megaloblastic erythroblasts. Serum vitamin B$_{12}$ and folate levels were normal; the deoxyuridine suppression test was normal; giant metamyelocytes and hypersegmented polymorphs were absent. Megaloblastic change is found in 50% of patients with this type of anaemia. The biochemical mechanism is uncertain.

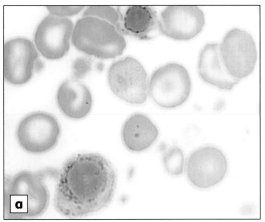

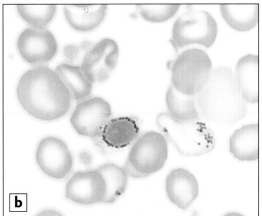

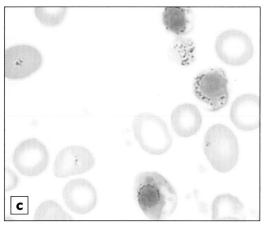

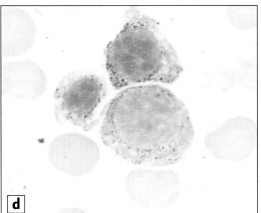

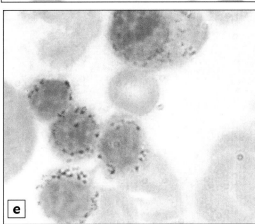

Fig. 2.42a–e Sideroblastic anaemia (primary acquired): (a–e) bone marrow aspirate showing erythroblasts with complete or nearly complete rings (or collars) of iron granules around their nuclei. The rings are best seen in late erythroblasts but, in severe cases, also occur in the earliest recognizable erythroblasts. (Perls' stain.)

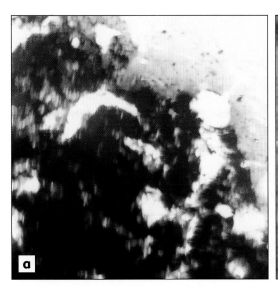

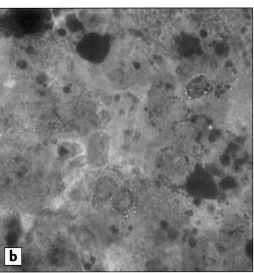

Fig. 2.43a and b Sideroblastic anaemia (hereditary): bone marrow fragments stained for iron show (a) a gross increase in iron in a patient who had been transfused for many years before the diagnosis was made. Treatment with pyridoxine allowed a satisfactory rise in haemoglobin, enabling subsequent venesections for reduction of iron overload. The high power view (b) shows multiple ring sideroblasts and increased iron (haemosiderin) in macrophages.

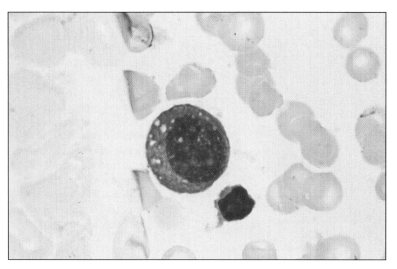

Fig. 2.44 Alcohol-related bone marrow toxicity: vacuolation of a pronormoblast can be seen.

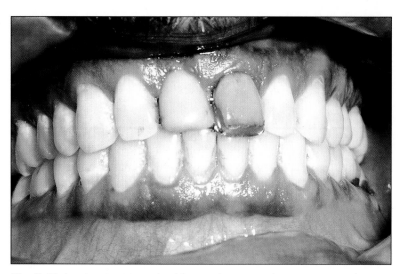

Fig. 2.45 Lead poisoning: a lead line in the gums of a young man who presented with abdominal colic. The poisoning was from prolonged occupational exposure to molten lead.

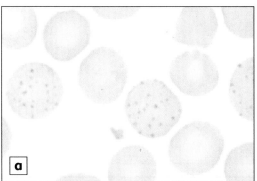

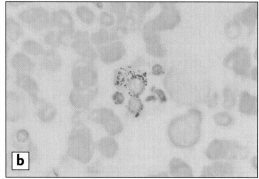

Fig. 2.46a and b Lead poisoning: (a) peripheral blood film showing punctate basophilia. This is caused by precipitates of undegraded RNA, the result of inhibition by lead of pyrimidine 5′-nucleotidase, one of the enzymes responsible for RNA degradation. Similar appearances occur in hereditary pyrimidine 5′-nucleotidase deficiency (*see Fig. 4.35*). (b) bone marrow aspirate showing coarse siderotic granules in a ring around the nucleus of an erythroblast. (Perls' stain.)

Causes of punctate basophilia
Thalassaemia (α and β)
Acquired sideroblastic anaemia and other myelodysplasias
Lead poisoning
Severe megaloblastic anaemia
Pyrimidine 5′-nucleotidase deficiency
Congenital dyserythropoietic anaemia

Fig. 2.47 Punctate basophilia: causes.

LEAD POISONING

Clinically, lead poisoning presents with abdominal colic and constipation, a peripheral neuropathy and anaemia. Two important enzymes in haem synthesis, δ-aminolaevulinic acid (ALA) dehydratase and ferrochelatase are inhibited. There may be a lead line visible in the gums (*Fig. 2.45*), marked punctate basophilia in the peripheral blood (*Fig. 2.46a*), a mild hypochromic anaemia with haemolysis, and ring sideroblasts in the marrow (*Fig. 2.46b*). Lead poisoning may result from excessive exposure to lead paints, or to lead in industry. It may also occur because of ingestion of herbal medicines containing excess lead. The punctate basophilia is caused by aggregates of undegraded RNA, a result of inhibition of the enzyme pyrimidine 5′-nucleotidase (*Figs 2.46 and 2.47*).

DIFFERENTIAL DIAGNOSIS OF HYPOCHROMIC MICROCYTIC ANAEMIAS

The causes of hypochromic microcytic anaemias include iron deficiency, thalassaemias and other haemoglobinopathies, the anaemias of chronic disorders, sideroblastic anaemia and lead poisoning. These causes may be differentiated by special tests, including measurement of serum iron, total iron-binding capacity or serum ferritin; by haemoglobin electrophoresis; or, if necessary, by studies of globin α- and β-chain synthesis or by DNA analysis. Bone marrow examination is necessary to diagnose sideroblastic anaemia. In thalassaemia trait, the disorders may be suspected from the presence of a high red cell count (more than 5.5×10^{12}/l) with relatively low MCV and MCH values (*see* Chapter 5).

THE PORPHYRIAS

The main types of inherited defect of porphyrin synthesis associated with light sensitivity affect the haemopoietic system: congenital erythropoietic porphyria (CEP, known as Günther's disease) and congenital erythropoietic protoporphyria (CEPP). Although not associated with a hypochromic anaemia, they are discussed here for convenience.

Congenital erythropoietic porphyria

Inherited as an autosomal recessive trait, CEP is characterized by excessive production of uroporphyrinogen I, which forms the pigments uroporphyrin I and coproporphyrin I. There is deficiency of the haem synthetic enzyme uroporphyrin III cosynthase. The plasma and erythrocytes contain excessive quantities of uroporphyrin I, coproporphyrin I and protoporphyrin.

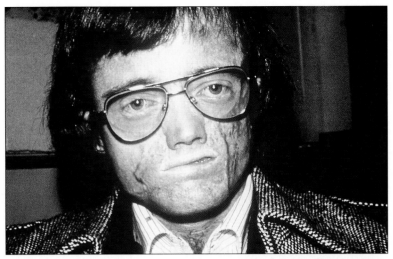

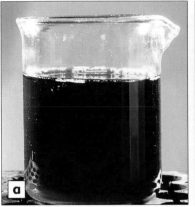 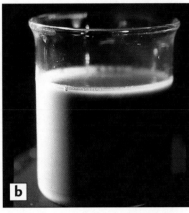

Fig. 2.48 Congenital erythropoietic porphyria: this 22-year-old man was first diagnosed to have this condition (Günther's disease) at 6 years of age, although skin changes had been noted from the age of 2 years, especially in the summer. These changes of blistering and susceptibility to mechanical injury were found on exposed areas of skin and led to mutilation of the extremities, including the nose, ears and hands. He has erythrodontia, splenomegaly and increased erythropoiesis with red cells which fluoresce. Haemolysis increased with age and is associated with a reticulocytosis. In this case, increased activity of ALA-S and decreased activity of uroporphyrinogen cosynthase were demonstrated, with increased excretion of uroporphyrin I and coproporphyrin I in the urine, together with increased concentrations of these porphyrins in erythrocytes and plasma. (Courtesy of Dr MR Moore.)

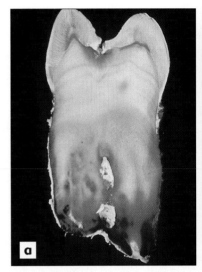 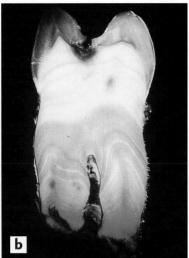

Fig. 2.49a and b Congenital erythropoietic porphyria: urine sample (a) in daylight and (b) in ultraviolet light. [(a, b) Courtesy of Dr MR Moore.]

Fig. 2.50a and b Congenital erythropoietic porphyria: molar tooth in (a) ordinary light, with brown discoloration, and (b) ultraviolet light, with fluorescence most marked in the cortical bone. [(a, b) Courtesy of Dr MR Moore.]

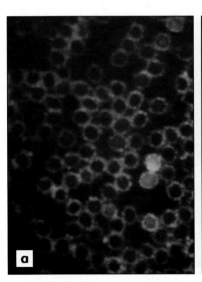 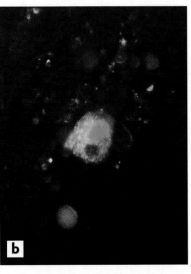

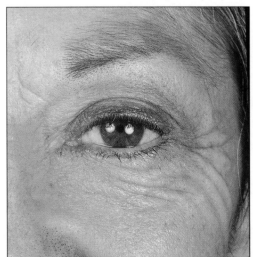

Fig. 2.52 Porphyria cutanea tarda: this 55-year-old woman presented with bullous eruptions on exposed skin surfaces. (Courtesy of Dr M Rustin.)

Fig. 2.51a and b Congenital erythropoietic porphyria: peripheral blood film (a) and bone marrow aspirate (b) viewed in ultraviolet light show nuclear fluorescence of erythroblasts caused by the presence of large amounts of uroporphyrin I. [(a, b) Courtesy of Dr I Magnus.]

The patient shown in *Fig. 2.48* has bullous ulcerating lesions on light-exposed skin, hirsutism and a haemolytic anaemia associated with splenomegaly. The urine is red and fluorescent (*Fig. 2.49*), and the bones and teeth are discoloured and also fluorescent (*Fig. 2.50*). The nucleated red cells fluoresce when exposed to ultraviolet light (*Fig. 2.51*).

For contrast, a patient with porphyria cutanea tarda is also shown (*Fig. 2.52*). A bullous eruption occurs on exposure to sunlight. There is a defect of hepatic uroporphyrinogen decarboxylase, which may be genetic or acquired as a result of alcohol, iron or oestrogen in excess. Iron loading may be a result as well as a cause of the syndrome.

Congenital erythropoietic protoporphyria

In CEPP, which is inherited as autosomal dominant, the underlying defect is one of ferrochelatase (haem synthase), the final enzyme in haem synthesis. There is excess production of protoporphyrin, which accumulates in erythrocytes, the liver and other tissues. The erythroblasts fluoresce when exposed to ultraviolet light.

Patients with CEPP are also light-sensitive and develop pruritus, swelling and reddening of the skin. The urine and teeth are of normal colour and non-fluorescent, and haemolytic anaemia is not present. Cholestasis, hepatitis and cirrhosis may lead to death from liver failure.

IRON OVERLOAD: PRIMARY (GENETIC) HAEMOCHROMATOSIS

The causes of increased storage of iron are listed in *Fig. 2.53*. Transfusional iron overload is discussed in detail in conjunction with thalassaemia major in Chapter 5 and porphyria cutanea tarda is discussed above. The genetic basis for most cases of primary haemochromatosis has now been established and this disease is discussed briefly here.

The clinical features are largely similar to those of transfusional iron overload and include hyperpigmentation of the skin (*Fig. 2.54*) and endocrine abnormalities: diabetes mellitus; gonadal, pituitary, thyroid and parathyroid dysfunction. Liver parenchymal iron overload is invariable (*Figs 2.55 and 2.56*) and fibrosis, cirrhosis and hepatocellular carcinoma may develop. A cardiomyopathy may occur with arrhythmia, pericarditis or congestive heart failure. An asymmetric arthropathy principally affecting the distal interphalangeal joints with calcium pyrophosphate deposition is characteristic of primary haemochromatosis (*Fig. 2.57*) and is not seen in transfusional iron overload.

Causes of iron overload
Increased iron absorption
From diets of normal iron content
Primary (genetic) haemochromatosis
Iron loading anaemia (refractory anaemias with increased bone marrow erythroid cells)
Chronic liver disease (cirrhosis, porto-caval shunt)
Porphyria cutanea tarda
Rare congenital defects (atransferrinaemia, aceruloplasminaemia, Friedreich's ataxia, hyperferritinaemia with autosomal dominant congenital cataracts, other diseases)
From diets with increased iron content
African diet overload*
Medicinal iron
Transfusional iron overload
*A genetic abnormality may play a role

Fig. 2.53 Iron overload causes.

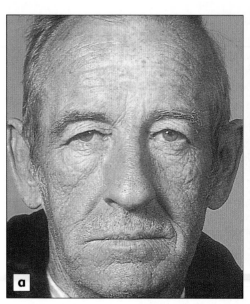
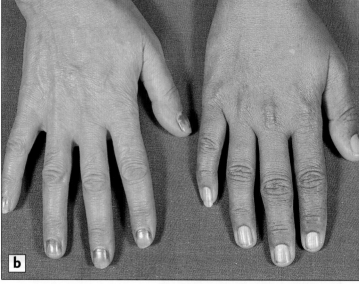

Fig. 2.54a and b Haemochromatosis: (a) the appearance of an adult male patient with primary haemochromatosis is shown. Note the characteristic bronze appearance. The hyperpigmentation results from melanin deposition in the skin. The patient also showed hepatic cirrhosis and diabetes mellitus. (b) For comparison, the hand (on the right) of a 16-year-old thalassaemia major patient shows heavy melanin pigmentation; in contrast, his mother's hand (on the left) shows normal colouration. [(a) Courtesy of Dr R Britt.]

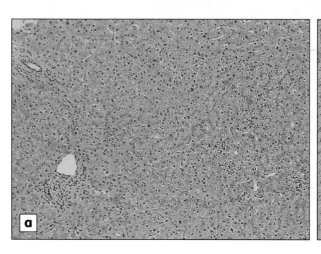
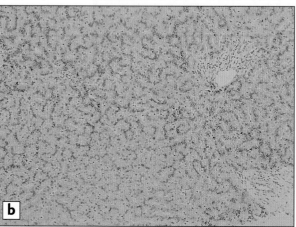

Fig. 2.55a and b Primary haemochromatosis: (a) needle biopsy of the liver in a 30-year-old woman. H & E stain showing normal architecture with golden brown deposits (haemosiderin) in parenchymal cells. (b) Perls' stain confirming heavy siderosis of parenchymal cells with sparing of Kupffer cells.

The gene responsible is known to be located on the short arm of chromosome 6, close to the HLA-A locus and to have an association with HLA-A3 and to a lesser extent with B7. A novel MHC class 1 like gene, termed HFE, has been identified 3 mb telomeric to the HLA-A locus (Feder *et al. Nat Genet* 1996;13:399–408). It contains seven exons; the putative protein structure is shown in *Fig. 2.58*. A homozygous missense G to A mutation at nucleotide 845 resulting in a cysteine to tyrosine substitution at amino acid 282 has been found in 83% to 100% of cases in most series studied. A second mutation, C to G in exon 2, results in a histidine to aspartic acid substitution at amino acid 63, and a small percentage of patients are compound heterozygotes. The possible role of HFE in iron absorption is shown in *Fig. 2.59*. There is evidence that the HFE mutation causes the duodenal enterocyte to behave as though it were iron deficient, with increased expression of *Nramp2* (DMT-1) causing increased transfer of iron from the lumen across the microvilli into the enterocyte (*Fig. 2.60*). Management consists in venesection to remove iron and appropriate treatment for dysfunction of damaged organs.

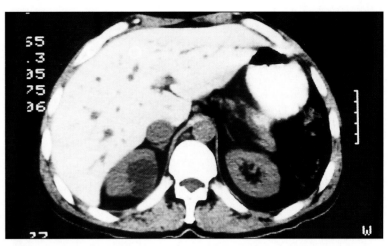

Fig. 2.56 Primary haemochromatosis: axial computed tomography (CT) scan showing increased density of the liver caused by iron overload. The patient, a man aged 50 years, has diabetes mellitus and also pyruvate kinase deficiency for which splenectomy had been performed.

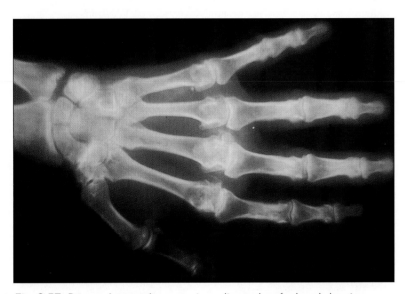

Fig. 2.57 Primary haemochromatosis: radiographs of a hand showing degenerative arthritis (caused by calcium pyrophosphate deposition) affecting the interphalangeal joints.

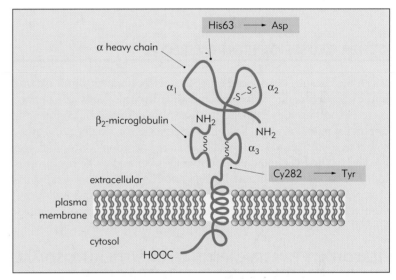

Fig. 2.58 Primary haemochromatosis: hypothetical model of the protein derived from the HFE gene based on its homology to the MHC class 1 molecule. The sites of the mutations found in primary haemochromatosis are shown. (Adapted with permission from Feder JN, Girke A, Thomas W, *et al*. A novel MHC class I-like gene is mutated in patients with hereditary haemochromatosis. *Nat Genet* 1996;13:399–408.)

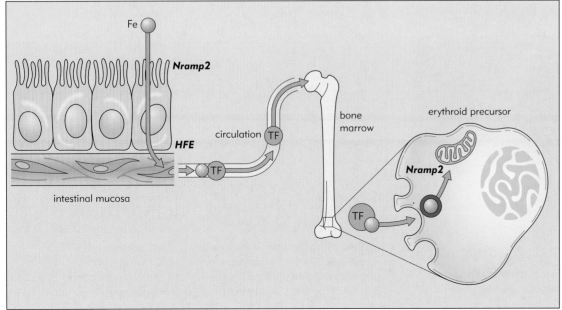

Fig. 2.59 Critical steps in mammalian iron transport: *Nramp2*(DMT-1) acts as an iron transporter at two steps. It is required for the transfer of iron across the intestinal brush border and for the export of iron from transferrin (TF) cycle endosomes in the bone marrow. HFE appears to regulate basolateral iron transfer from enterocytes to plasma. (Adapted with permission from Andrews NC, Levy JE. Iron is hot: an update on the pathophysiology of hemochromatosis. *Blood* 1998;92:1845–51.)

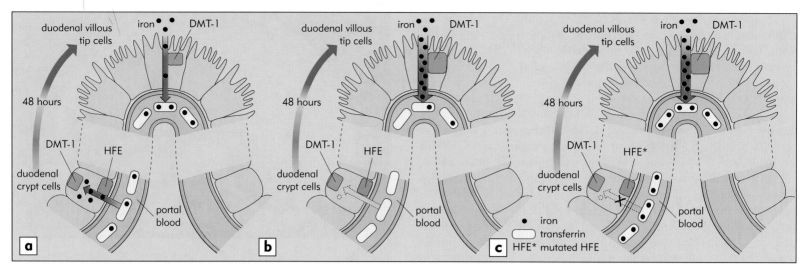

Fig. 2.60a–c Hereditary haemochromatosis: mechanisms for absorption of iron – (a) normal, (b) iron deficiency, (c) hereditary haemochromatosis. In primary (genetic) haemochromatosis it is postulated that the HFE mutation Cys 282 Tyr (HFE*) causes reduced iron supply to the duodenal crypt enterocyte from transferrin in portal blood. The enterocyte then behaves as though iron deficient with increased DMT-1 mRNA and protein expression (as in iron deficiency), which results in increased absorption of iron at the duodemal villous tip from the intestinal lumen into portal blood.

OTHER CAUSES OF IRON OVERLOAD

Porphyria cutanea tarda (*see Fig. 2.52*) is associated with iron loading in the liver. In the rare autosomal recessive disorder *atransferrinaemia*, there is a microcytic, hypochromic anaemia with excess iron deposition in the reticuloendothelial cells. In *aceruloplasminaemia*, also autosomal recessive, retinal and basal ganglia degeneration occurs with iron loading in the liver, pancreas, brain and other organs. Serum iron is low, total body iron content normal and ferritin raised. *Friedreich's ataxia* presents in middle age with spinocerebellar ataxia and a cardiomyopathy. There is a mutation in the gene for frataxin, a mitochondrial protein. Excess iron deposition is found in the heart. ·

HEREDITARY HYPERFERRITINAEMIA WITH AUTOSOMAL DOMINANT CONGENITAL CATARACT SYNDROME

Hereditary hyperferritinaemia–cataract syndrome (HHCS) presents with early onset cataract (caused by ferritin deposition in the lens; *Fig. 2.61*) and elevated serum ferritin (1000–2500 μg/l). The serum ferritin, normally composed of molecules with either light (L; molecular weight 19 kDa, coded for on chromosome 19) or heavy (H; molecular weight 21 kDa, coded for on chromosome 11) subunits (24 in total), is of L type only, the type mainly found in normal tissues of iron storage, e.g. liver and spleen (the H type is dominant in organs not normally iron storage sites, e.g. heart). There are mutations in the IRE of the L-ferritin mRNA (*Fig. 2.62*) that affect its binding to IRF (*see Fig. 2.2*). Iron stores, serum iron and transferrin levels are normal.

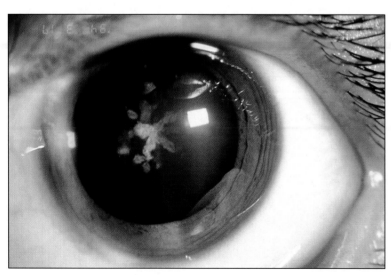

Fig. 2.61 Hereditary hyperferritinaemia–cataract syndrome (HHCS): the 'starring' lens opacity is characteristic. (Courtesy of Dr D Girelli and Prof. R Corrocher.)

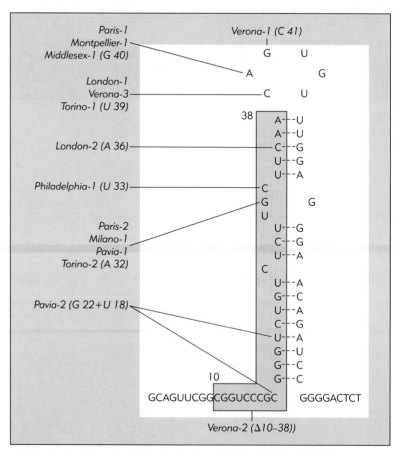

Fig. 2.62 Hereditary hyperferritinaemia–cataract syndrome (HHCS): representation of the iron-response element (IRE) located in the 5′ untranslated region (UTR) of L-ferritin mRNA and of the mutations associated with HHCS (updated September 1998), showing evidence for genetic heterogeneity of the disease. (Courtesy of Dr D Girelli and Prof. R Corrocher.)

Megaloblastic Anaemias

The megaloblastic anaemias are a group of disorders characterized by a macrocytic blood picture and megaloblastic erythropoiesis; causes are listed in *Fig. 3.1*. The underlying biochemical defect appears to be a fault in DNA synthesis, which may result from a lesion at some point in pyrimidine or purine synthesis or to inhibition of DNA polymerization. The anaemia is usually caused by deficiency of vitamin B_{12} (referred to simply as B_{12} hereafter) or folate. In most cases the site of the biochemical defect in DNA synthesis is known. In some types, however, particularly in myeloblastic leukaemia and myelodysplasia in which megaloblastic changes are unresponsive to B_{12} and folate therapy, the exact site of the defect remains obscure.

The roles of B_{12} and folate in DNA biosynthesis are shown in *Fig. 3.2*. Folate deficiency affects thymidylate synthesis, a rate-limiting step in pyrimidine synthesis, since a folate coenzyme, 5,10-methylene tetrahydrofolate–polyglutamate, is necessary for this reaction. Folate coenzymes are also required in two reactions in purine synthesis, but these are not normally thought to be rate-limiting for DNA synthesis in humans.

B_{12} is not required directly for DNA synthesis. It is needed to convert 5-methyltetrahydrofolate (methyl-THF), which enters cells from plasma, into other folate coenzyme forms (including all the polygluta-mate derivatives) through its involvement in the methionine synthase reaction in which homocysteine is methylated to methionine. In this reaction the removal of the methyl group from methyl-THF forms THF, which can be converted into folate polyglutamates by the addition of glutamate moieties. Methyl THF cannot act as substrate for the enzyme responsible for polyglutamate formation. The role of folate in the metabolism of homocysteine is shown in *Fig 3.10*.

B_{12} in food is released from protein binding by proteolytic enzymes and attached to a so-called R-binder (*Fig. 3.3*). B_{12} is released from this binding by pancreatic enzymes and transferred to intrinsic factor secreted by the parietal cells of the stomach. B_{12} in bile also attaches to intrinsic factor. Intrinsic factor-bound B_{12} is carried to the ileum, where it attaches to specific receptors; the intrinsic factor is digested and B_{12} appears in the portal blood attached to a polypeptide protein, transcobalamin II. In peripheral blood most B_{12} is attached to the glycoprotein transcobalamin I (derived from granulocytes, monocytes and their precursors), but it is transcobalamin II that is responsible for delivery of the vitamin to the tissues.

Dietary folate is deconjugated to the monoglutamate form, fully reduced and methylated in the upper intestinal epithelial cells, so that it is all absorbed in the form of methyl-THF (*Fig. 3.2*).

Causes of megaloblastic anaemia				
Causes of megaloblastic anaemia I	**Causes of megaloblastic anaemia II**		**Causes of megaloblastic anaemia III**	
Vitamin B_{12} deficiency	Folate deficiency		Abnormalities of	
Inadequate diet	**Inadequate diet**	**Malabsorption**	**Vitamin B_{12} metabolism**	**DNA synthesis**
Veganism	Poverty	Gluten-induced enteropathy	Congenital:	Congential:
Malabsorption	Institutions	Dermatitis herpetiformis	transcobalamin II deficiency	orotic aciduria
Gastric:	Goat's milk	Tropical sprue	homocystinuria with	Lesch–Nyhan syndrome
pernicious anaemia, acquired (autoimmune) and congenital partial or total gastrectomy	Special diets	Congenital specific	methylmalonic aciduria	dyserythropoietic anaemia
	Excess losses	**Increased utilization**	Acquired:	
Intestinal:	Dialysis	Pregnancy	nitrous oxide anaesthesia	thiamine-responsive
stagnant-loop syndrome (e.g. jejunal diverticulosis, ileocolic fistulae)	Congestive heart failure	Prematurity	**Folate metabolism**	etc.
	Drugs	Excess marrow turnover (e.g. in haemolytic anaemias)	Congenital:	Acquired:
chronic tropical sprue	Anticonvulsants	Malignancy (e.g. myeloma, carcinoma)	inborn errors (e.g. 5-methyltetra-hydrofolate transferase deficiency)	drugs (e.g. hydroxyurea, cytosine, arabinoside, 6-mercaptopurine, 5-azacytidine)
ileal resection and Crohn's disease	Barbiturates			
congenital-specific malabsorption with with proteinuria (Imerslund–Gräsbeck)	**Mixed**	Inflammatory disease (e.g. Crohn's, rheumatoid arthritis, widespread eczema)	Acquired:	
fish tapeworm	Alcohol		antifolate drugs (e.g. methotrexate, pyrimethamine)	
drugs (e.g. metformin)	Liver disease			

Fig. 3.1 Megaloblastic anaemia: causes.

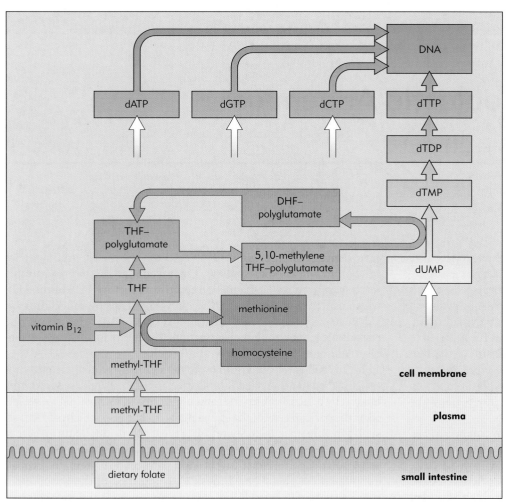

Fig. 3.2 Megaloblastic anaemia: suggested roles of B_{12} and folate in DNA biosynthesis. (THF, tetrahydrofolate; DHF, dihydrofolate; d, deoxyribose; UMP, uridine monophosphate; TMP, thymidine monophosphate; TDP, thymidine diphosphate; TTP, thymidine triphosphate; CTP, cytidine triphosphate; GTP, guanosine triphosphate; ATP, adenosine triphosphate.)

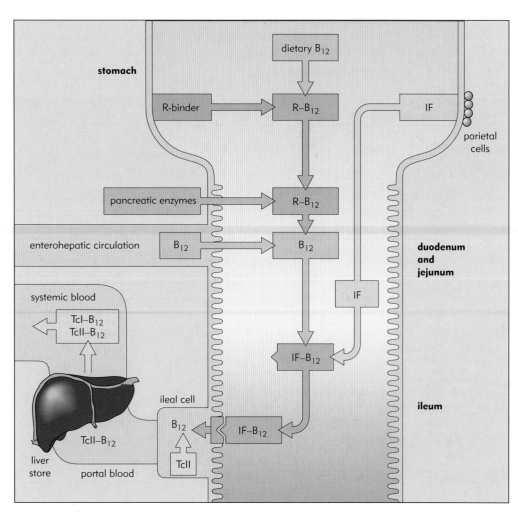

Fig. 3.3 Megaloblastic anaemia: absorption of B_{12}. (IF, intrinsic factor; R, R-binder; TcI, transcobalamin I; TcII, transcobalamin II.

CLINICAL FEATURES

Megaloblastic anaemia is usually of insidious onset, progressing so slowly that the patient has time to adapt. The patient may therefore not present until the anaemia is quite severe, unless diagnosed early through an incidental blood examination for other reasons. There is jaundice of varying degree in combination with anaemia, giving the patient a lemon-yellow tint (*Fig. 3.4*). The jaundice is caused by unconjugated bilirubin produced in excess because of severe intramedullary death of nucleated red cell precursors ('ineffective erythropoiesis') with reticuloendothelial breakdown of their haemoglobin. Also, a marked rise in serum lactate dehydrogenase concentration occurs because of excessive cell breakdown, and rapid clearance of injected radioiron with poor utilization for red cell formation.

Severe cases show features of intravascular breakdown of haemoglobin with methaemalbuminaemia and haemosiderinuria; pancytopenia often occurs and the patient may present with bruising from thrombocytopenia (*Fig. 3.5*). The white cell and platelet counts are rarely as low as in severe aplastic anaemia.

Disordered proliferation of the epithelial cell surfaces gives rise to glossitis (*Fig. 3.6*) and angular cheilosis (*Fig. 3.7*), and can also be seen microscopically in the buccal, bronchial, bladder and cervical mucosae.

In a small proportion of cases, melanin pigmentation of the skin is present (*Fig. 3.8*). A neuropathy of varying severity may occur with B$_{12}$

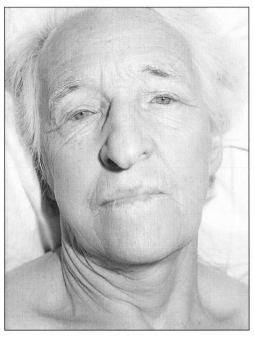

Fig. 3.4 Megaloblastic anaemia: typical lemon-yellow appearance of a 69-year-old woman with pernicious anaemia and severe megaloblastic anaemia (Hb, 7.0 g/dl; MCV, 132 fl). The colour is from the combination of pallor (from anaemia), and jaundice (from ineffective erythropoiesis).

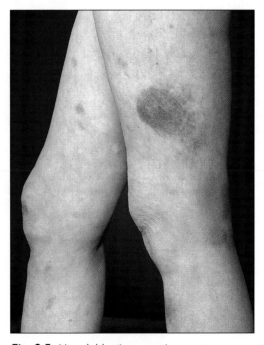

Fig. 3.5 Megaloblastic anaemia: spontaneous bruising on the thigh of a 34-year-old woman who presented with widespread purpura and menorrhagia. She was found to have megaloblastic anaemia as a result of nutritional folate deficiency and alcoholism. (Hb, 8.1 g/dl; MCV, 115 fl; platelet count, 2 × 10⁹/l.)

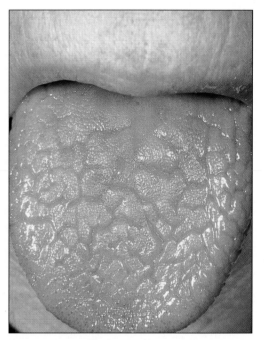

Fig. 3.6 Megaloblastic anaemia: glossitis caused by B$_{12}$ deficiency in a 55-year-old woman with untreated pernicious anaemia. The tongue is beefy red and painful, particularly with hot and acidic foods. An identical appearance occurs in folate deficiency because of impaired DNA synthesis in the mucosal epithelium.

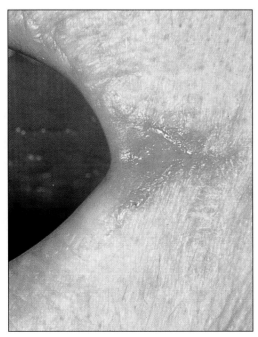

Fig. 3.7 Megaloblastic anaemia: angular cheilosis (same patient as in *Fig. 3.5*). This is also thought to result from impaired proliferation of epithelial cells. It is unusual for this abnormality to be so marked.

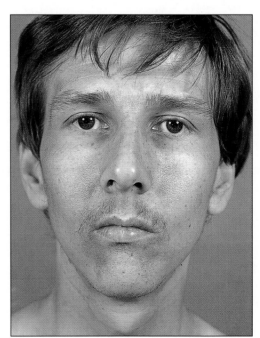

Fig. 3.8 Megaloblastic anaemia: melanin pigmentation of the skin in a 24-year-old man with B$_{12}$ deficiency caused by pernicious anaemia. Similar pigmentation affected the nail beds, skin creases and periorbital areas. Such pigmentation also occurs in patients with folate deficiency. In both, the pigmentation rapidly disappears with appropriate vitamin therapy. The biochemical basis for the melanin excess is unknown.

deficiency, such as subacute combined degeneration of the spinal cord which includes posterior and lateral column demyelination (*see Fig. 3.28*), and peripheral or optic neuropathy. The patient presents with bilaterally symmetrical symptoms which are usually most marked in the lower limbs and comprise tingling, unsteadiness of gait, falling over in the dark, altered sensation and reduced strength. Visual and psychiatric disturbances are less frequent.

Folic acid therapy before conception and in early pregnancy has been shown to reduce the incidence of neural tube defect (NTD) babies. The lesions may be spina bifida (*Fig. 3.9*), anencephaly or encephalocoele. This occurs even if the mother is not folate deficient, assessed haematologically or by serum or red cell folate (although the lower the serum folate or B_{12}, or red cell folate, the higher the incidence, even when the levels are in the accepted normal range). An association between NTD and a common mutation (nucleotide 677C→T) in the gene for the enzyme 5,10-methylene-THF reductase (*Fig. 3.10*) has been found. The mutated enzyme is thermolabile. It is considered that prophylactic folic acid overcomes this or other, as yet unidentified, abnormalities of folate or B_{12} metabolism. The mutation is associated with a raised homocysteine level. Folate or B_{12} aggravates the tendency for a rise in homocysteine level to occur in maternal plasma. Exactly how disturbed homocysteine metabolism leads to NTD is unclear.

Raised plasma homocysteine levels are also associated with an increased incidence of arterial and venous thrombosis (*see* Chapter 16). The levels may be raised because of B_{12} or folate deficiency, B_6 deficiency or through smoking or excess alcohol consumption. The levels are higher in males and postmenopausal women than in premenopausal women or those on hormone placement therapy, and rise with age. Congenital homocystinuria that results from an inherited defect of one of three enzymes cystathionine synthase, methionine synthase or 5,10-methylene-THF reductase is associated with the onset of cardiovascular disease in childhood or early adult life.

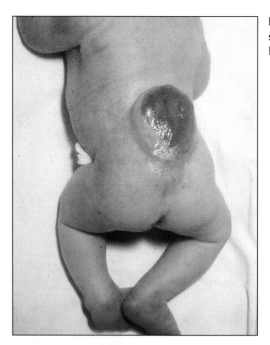

Fig. 3.9 Baby with spina bifida. (Courtesy of Prof. CJ Schorah.)

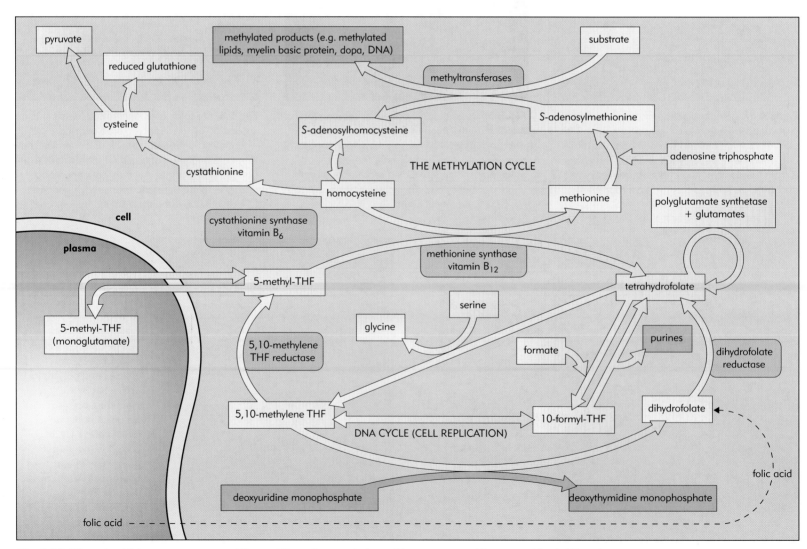

Fig. 3.10 The role of folate coenzymes, and B_{12} and B_6 in the metabolism of homocysteine. (Courtesy of Prof. J Scott.)

Blood count and blood film appearances

A typical blood count in megaloblastic anaemia is shown in *Fig. 3.11*. The blood film shows oval macrocytes, fragmented cells, poikilocytes of varying shapes (*Figs 3.12–3.14*) and hypersegmental neutrophils (showing more than five nuclear lobes, some of which may be macropolycytes; *Fig. 3.15*). The severity of these changes depends on the degree of anaemia. In the most anaemic patients, megaloblasts may circulate because of extramedullary haemopoiesis in the liver and spleen (*Fig. 3.16*). Cabot rings, which are acidophilic, arginine-rich and contain non-haemoglobin iron may also be seen (*Fig. 3.16* inset). If the spleen has been removed, as with a gastrectomy, or has atrophied, as in 15% of adult cases with gluten-induced enteropathy, changes caused by hyposplenism in the peripheral blood are particularly marked (*Fig. 3.17*). In some extremely anaemic cases, the mean cell volume is normal because of excessive fragmentation of red cells.

Blood count in severe megaloblastic anaemia	
Haemoglobin	5.1 g/dl
Red blood cell	$1.4 \times 10^{12}/l$
Packed cell volume	18%
Mean corpuscular volume	129 fl
Mean corpuscular haemoglobin	36.4 pg
Reticulocytes	2.5%
White blood cell	$1.9 \times 10^9/l$
Neutrophils	63%
Platelets	$53 \times 10^9/l$

Fig. 3.11 Typical blood count in severe megaloblastic anaemia (peripheral blood film from same patient shown in *Fig. 3.12*).

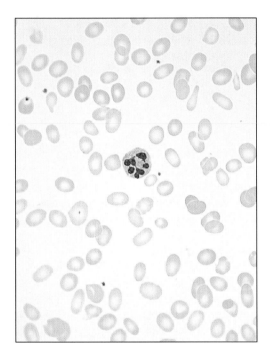

Fig. 3.12 Megaloblastic anaemia: peripheral blood film in a severe case, showing oval macrocytes, marked anisocytosis and poikilocytosis. There is a neutrophil with a hypersegmented nucleus (more than five lobes). (Hb, 5.1 g/dl; MCV, 129 fl.)

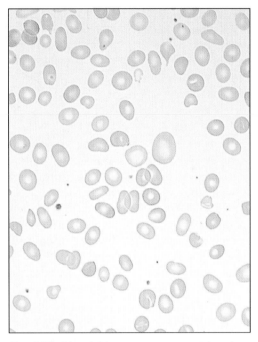

Fig. 3.13 Megaloblastic anaemia: peripheral blood film showing marked oval macrocytosis, anisocytosis and poikilocytosis. (Hb, 5.4 g/dl; MCV, 130 fl.)

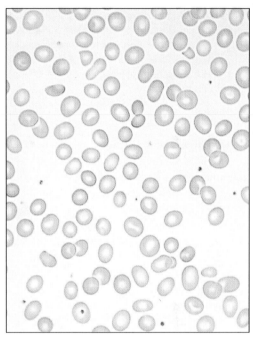

Fig. 3.14 Megaloblastic anaemia: peripheral blood film in a mild case showing moderate red cell macrocytosis, anisocytosis and poikilocytosis. (Hb, 10.5 g/dl; MCV, 112 fl.)

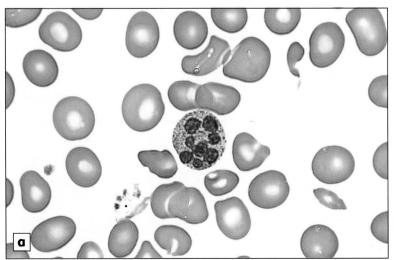

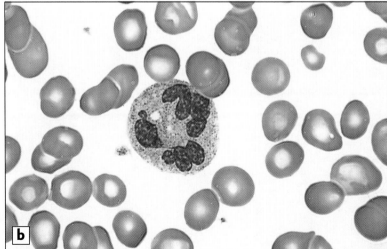

Fig. 3.15a and b Megaloblastic anaemia: higher power views showing (a) a hypersegmented neutrophil and (b) a hyperdiploid neutrophil or 'macropolycyte'.

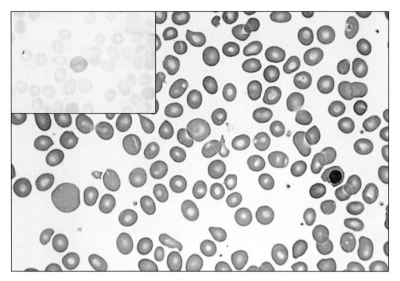

Fig. 3.16 Megaloblastic anaemia: peripheral blood film in a severe case showing a circulating orthochromatic nucleated red cell. The presence of such circulating megaloblasts may be the result of extramedullary haemopoiesis in the spleen and liver. The inset (upper left) shows a Cabot ring, which is occasionally seen in the peripheral blood in severe megaloblastic anaemia.

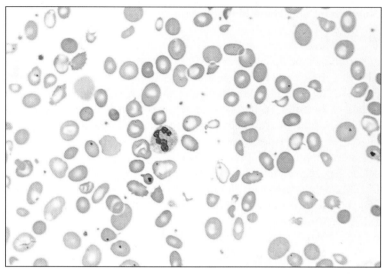

Fig. 3.17 Megaloblastic anaemia and splenic atrophy: peripheral blood film showing Howell–Jolly bodies (DNA remnants) and Pappenheimer bodies (iron- and protein-containing). The patient had severe folate deficiency and splenic atrophy caused by adult coeliac disease.

Bone marrow appearances

In severe cases, the bone marrow is markedly hypercellular with a relative increase in early erythroblasts caused by death of later cells (*Fig. 3.18*). The myeloid:erythroid ratio may be reversed, with an excess of erythroid precursors. Developing erythroblasts show asynchrony of nuclear and cytoplasmic maturation, the nucleus retaining an open, lacy or stippled appearance while the cytoplasm matures and haemoglobinizes normally. The developing (nucleated) red cells also show a variety of dyserythropoietic features with an excess of multinucleate cells, nuclear bridging and Howell–Jolly bodies; dying cells are also present (*Fig. 3.19*).

Giant and abnormally shaped metamyelocytes are found (*Fig. 3.20*), and the megakaryocytes show hypersegmented nuclei with an open chromatin network (*Fig. 3.21*).

In milder cases, megaloblastic changes in the red cell precursors are only identified in late erythroblasts with mild asynchrony of

nuclear–cytoplasmic development (*Fig. 3.22*). This is termed 'mild', 'transitional' or 'intermediate' megaloblastic change.

Where iron deficiency and megaloblastic anaemia coexist, a dimorphic anaemia occurs with two red cell populations in the peripheral blood, one of well-haemoglobinized macrocytes and the other of hypochromic microcytes (*Fig. 3.23a*). Megaloblastic changes may be masked in the erythroblasts, even though giant metamyelocytes are seen in the bone marrow (*Fig. 3.23b*). In patients with normal iron stores, there is usually excessive iron granulation of erythroblasts; in some cases, especially in association with alcohol, ring sideroblasts are frequent but disappear with appropriate therapy (*Fig. 3.24*). Trephine biopsy confirms the accumulation of early cells and excess mitoses (*Fig. 3.25*). It is of interest that erythropoiesis in early fetal life is also megaloblastic (*Fig. 3.26*).

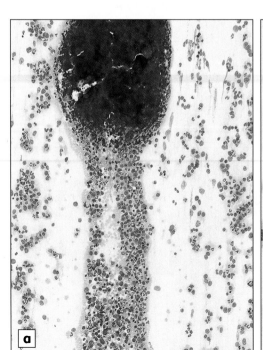

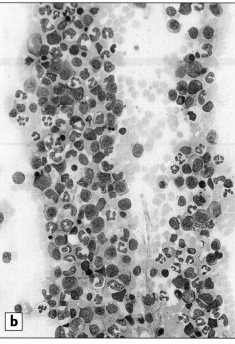

Fig. 3.18a and b Megaloblastic anaemia: (a) low power view of bone marrow fragments showing an increased cellularity with loss of fat spaces; (b) higher power view of cell trails showing accumulation of early cells, an increased proportion of erythroid precursors and the presence of giant metamyelocytes and hypersegmented neutrophils.

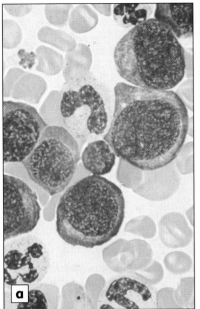
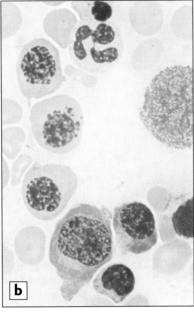
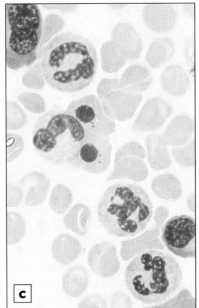
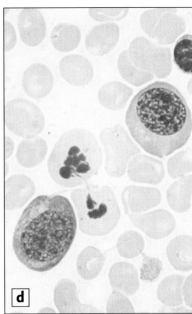

Fig. 3.19a–d Megaloblastic anaemia: high power views showing (a) accumulation of early cells, mainly promegaloblasts; (b) megaloblasts at all stages; the nuclei have primitive open (lacy) chromatin patterns despite maturation of the cytoplasm with haemoglobinization (pink staining) and two cells have nuclear (DNA) fragments (Howell–Jolly bodies) in their cytoplasm; (c) two late megaloblasts with fully orthochromatic (pink-staining) cytoplasm – two large band-form neutrophils are also present; (d) the central orthochromatic cells have karyorrhectic pyknotic nuclei linked by a thin chromatin bridge.

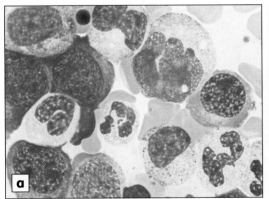
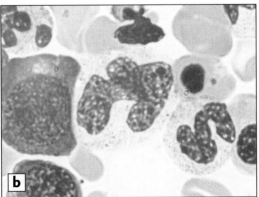
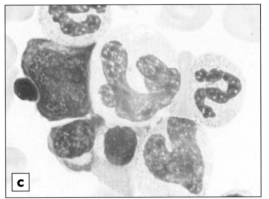

Fig. 3.20a–c Megaloblastic anaemia: (a–c) high power views showing a number of giant abnormally shaped metamyelocytes.

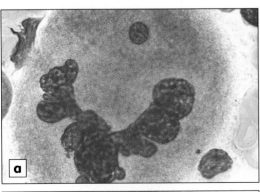
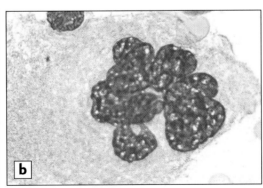

Fig. 3.21a–d Megaloblastic anaemia: megakaryocytes of variable maturity. (a–d) All show nuclei with abnormal open chromatin patterns.

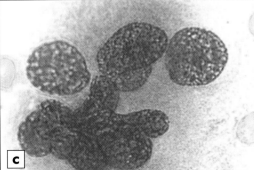
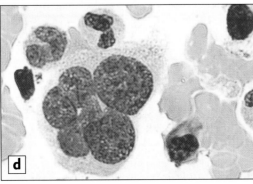

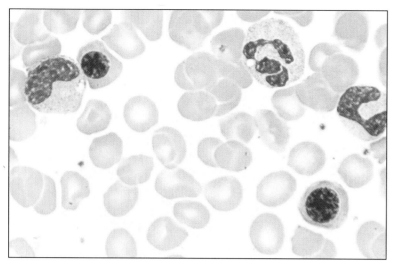

Fig. 3.22 Megaloblastic anaemia: mild marrow changes in B$_{12}$ deficiency following partial gastrectomy. The nucleated red cells show mild asynchrony of nuclear–cytoplasmic development with delay of nuclear maturation (lower right). Iron stores were present. [Hb, 12.4 g/dl; MCV, 105 fl; serum B$_{12}$, 80 ng/l (normal, 160–925 ng/l); serum folate, 10.3 μg/l (normal, 6.0–21.0 μg/l).]

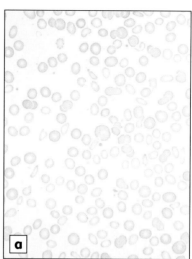
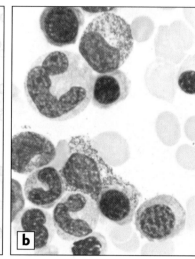

Fig. 3.23a and b Megaloblastic anaemia: (a) dimorphic peripheral blood film in iron and B$_{12}$ deficiencies following partial gastrectomy. There is a mixed population of microcytic hypochromic cells and well-haemoglobinized macrocytes (Hb, 8.0 g/dl; MCV, 87 fl; MCH, 27 pg). (b) In the bone marrow aspirate from the same case, giant metamyelocytes are present but megaloblastic changes in the erythroblasts are masked.

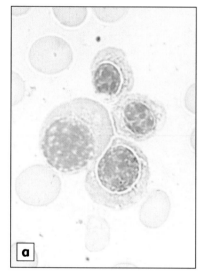
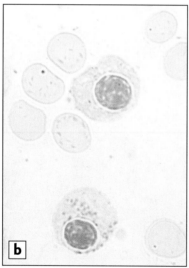

Fig. 3.24a and b Megaloblastic anaemia: (a, b) bone marrow aspirates in alcoholism and folate deficiency showing partial ring sideroblasts which rapidly disappeared on alcohol withdrawal and folic acid therapy. (Perls' stain.)

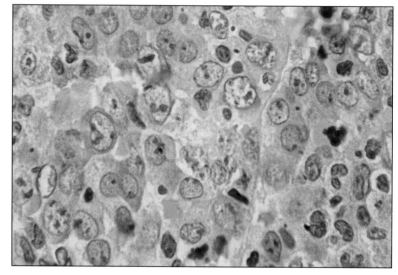

Fig. 3.25 Megaloblastic anaemia: trephine biopsy of iliac crest in untreated pernicious anaemia shows many megaloblasts with a fine open chromatin pattern and a number of mitotic figures.

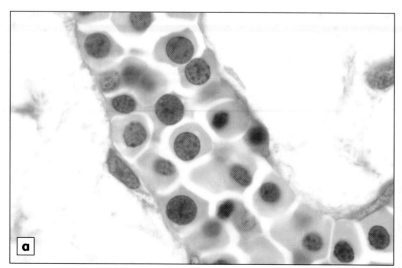
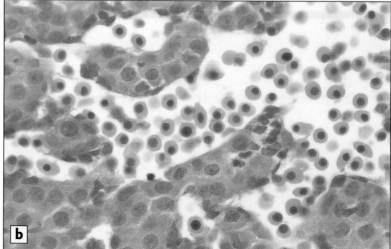

Fig. 3.26a and b Fetal erythropoiesis: sections of (a) placenta, showing circulating erythroblasts with a nuclear morphology similar to megaloblasts; (b) liver, showing extramedullary megaloblastic erythropoiesis.

CAUSES OF MEGALOBLASTIC ANAEMIA

Vitamin B$_{12}$ deficiency

As B$_{12}$ is stored in amounts of 2–3 mg, and daily losses and therefore requirements are 1–2 μg, it takes 2–4 years for B$_{12}$ deficiency to develop from dietary lack or malabsorption. Deficiency resulting from excessive losses or breakdown of B$_{12}$ has not been described. The anaesthetic gas nitrous oxide may rapidly inactivate body B$_{12}$ from the fully reduced cobalamin I state to the oxidized cobalamin II and cobalamin III forms; if exposure is prolonged, megaloblastic changes occur (*Fig. 3.27*).

While folate occurs in most foods, including fruit, vegetables and cereals as well as animal products, B$_{12}$ occurs only in foods of animal origin. Veganism may lead to B$_{12}$ deficiency, found most frequently in Hindus. Liver has the highest concentration of both folate and B$_{12}$, since it is the main storage organ.

Severe B$_{12}$ deficiency, assessed by serum B$_{12}$ levels, although not necessarily associated with severe anaemia, may cause demyelination of the posterior and lateral columns of the spinal cord (*Fig. 3.28*). It is often associated with a peripheral neuropathy and is found more frequently in males than in females; yet pernicious anaemia, the most common cause of severe B$_{12}$ deficiency, is more common in females.

Addisonian pernicious anaemia is the dominant cause of B$_{12}$ deficiency in Western countries. Although particularly common in northern Europe, it occurs in all races and countries. It is associated with early greying of the hair (*Fig. 3.29*), vitiligo (*Fig. 3.30*) and thyroid

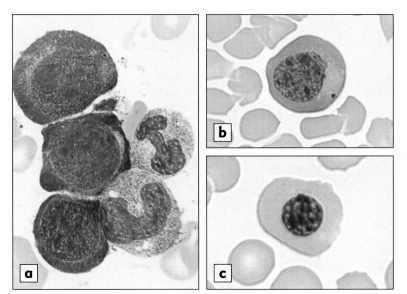

Fig. 3.27a–c B$_{12}$ oxidation: (a–c) bone marrow aspirate showing megaloblasts in a patient receiving prolonged nitrous oxide anaesthesia in intensive care following cardiac surgery.

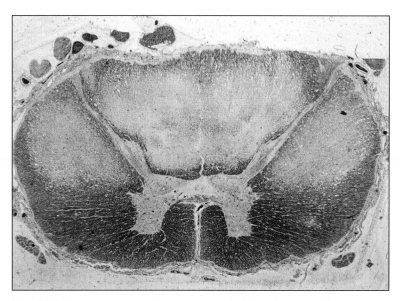

Fig. 3.28 Pernicious anaemia: cross-section of spinal cord of a patient who died with severe B$_{12}$ neuropathy (subacute combined degeneration of the spinal cord). There is demyelination of the lateral (pyramidal) and posterior columns. (Weigert–Pal stain.)

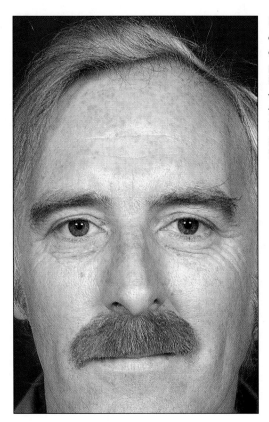

Fig. 3.29 Pernicious anaemia: this 38-year-old man shows premature greying and has blue eyes and vitiligo, three features that are more common in patients with pernicious anaemia than in control subjects.

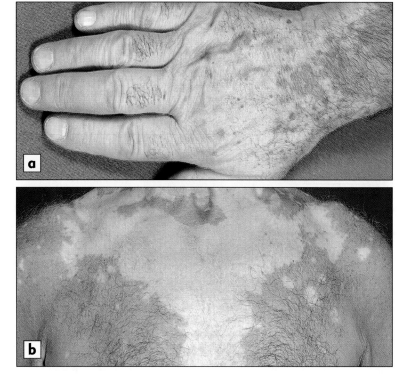

Fig. 3.30a and b Pernicious anaemia: (a, b) marked vitiligo in a 67-year-old man.

disorders (*Fig. 3.31*), as well as with other organ-specific autoimmune diseases such as Addison's disease and hypoparathyroidism. There is gastric atrophy (*Fig. 3.32*) with achlorhydria; also, parietal cell autoantibodies are present in the serum of 90% of patients (*Fig. 3.33*) and intrinsic factor autoantibodies in 50%. Gastric carcinoma develops two to three times more frequently than in control populations (*Fig. 3.34*).

Small intestinal causes of B_{12} deficiency include the stagnant-loop syndrome, for example jejunal diverticulosis (*Fig. 3.35*), ileocolic fistula (*Fig. 3.36*) and ileal resection.

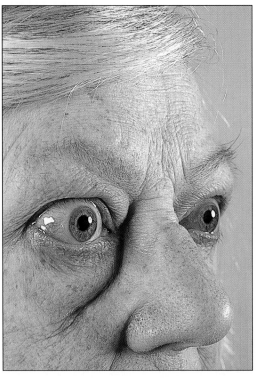

Fig. 3.31 Pernicious anaemia: exophthalmic ophthalmoplegia in a patient who developed myxoedema while receiving maintenance B_{12} therapy. She had presented with megaloblastic anaemia 6 years earlier.

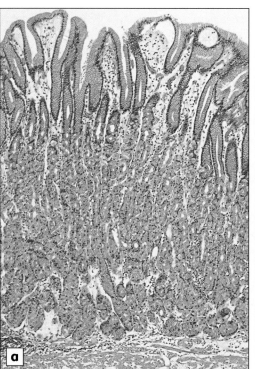
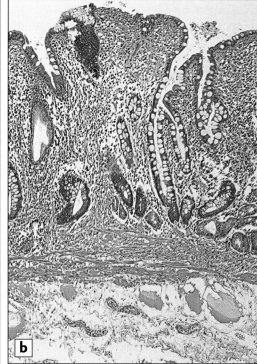

Fig. 3.32 Pernicious anaemia: sections of stomach – (a) normal and (b) in pernicious anaemia. There is atrophy of all coats, loss of gastric glands and parietal cells, and infiltration of the lamina propria by lymphocytes and plasma cells. [(a, b) Courtesy of Dr JE McLaughlin.]

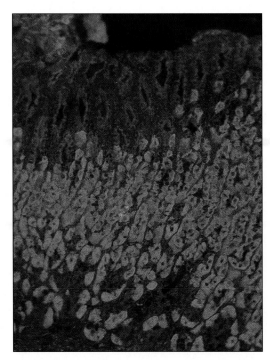

Fig. 3.33 Pernicious anaemia: positive indirect immunofluorescent test for parietal cell autoantibody. A frozen section of gastric mucosa (rat) has been layered with the patient's serum and washed, followed by the addition of rabbit anti-human immunoglobulin G conjugated with fluorescein.

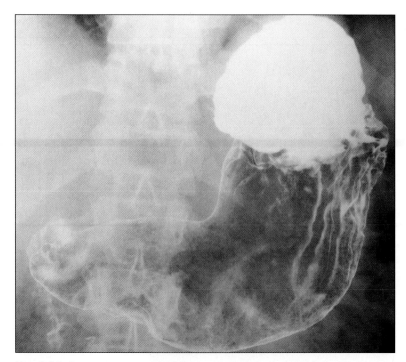

Fig. 3.34 Pernicious anaemia: barium meal radiograph showing gastric atrophy and carcinoma. There is thinning of the gastric wall and lack of mucosal pattern, and an ulcerated filling defect in the horizontal part of the greater curve.

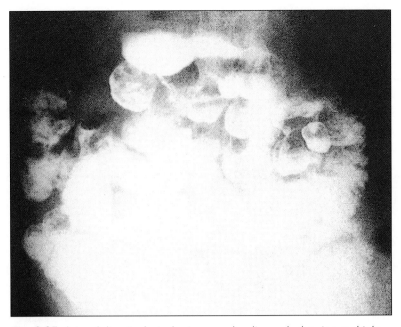

Fig. 3.35 Jejunal diverticulosis: barium meal radiograph showing multiple jejunal diverticula in a 71-year-old patient who presented with megaloblastic anaemia caused by B$_{12}$ deficiency. (Courtesy of Dr D Nag.)

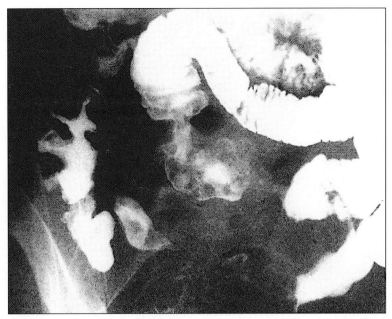

Fig. 3.36 Intestinal stagnant-loop syndrome: barium follow-through radiograph in Crohn's disease showing defective filling of the terminal ileum with a blind loop clearly visible. There is early filling of the ascending colon. The patient presented with megaloblastic anaemia caused by B$_{12}$ deficiency. (Courtesy of Dr R Dick.)

Folate deficiency

Since daily requirements of folate are 100–200 μg, body stores (10–15 mg) are sufficient for only a few months, a period which can be reduced in conditions of increased turnover and, hence, breakdown of folates.

Folate deficiency may result from inadequate dietary intake or malabsorption, as in gluten-induced enteropathy (*Figs 3.37–3.41*) and tropical sprue (*Fig. 3.42*).

Dermatitis herpetiformis is associated with gluten-induced enteropathy and, hence, with folate deficiency (*Fig. 3.43*). The most common cause of deficiency is pregnancy, when folate requirements rise from the normal 100–200 μg daily to about 350 μg daily.

However, the incidence of this complication is now reduced with prophylactic folic acid therapy. Other causes of increased folate utilization include diseases with increased bone marrow or other cell turnover (*see Fig. 3.1*). The excessive demands for folate in these conditions, combined with poor dietary intake, may lead to megaloblastic anaemia.

Abnormalities of vitamin B$_{12}$ or folate metabolism

These abnormalities may be inherited or acquired. Transcobalamin II deficiency is an autosomal recessive inherited trait leading, in the

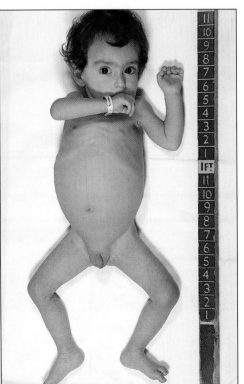

Fig. 3.37 Infantile coeliac disease: wasting and abdominal distension in a 2-year-old boy who developed megaloblastic anaemia as a result of folate deficiency. Coeliac disease was diagnosed by jejunal biopsy.

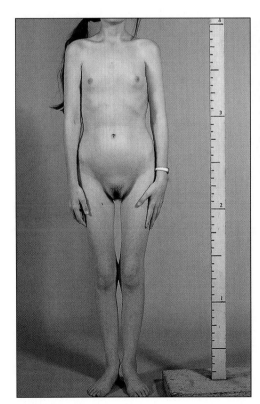

Fig. 3.38 Coeliac disease: a 16-year-old girl who presented with severe megaloblastic anaemia as a result of folate deficiency and was found, on jejunal biopsy, to have coeliac disease. There was no history of diarrhoea. She had delayed puberty and menarche.

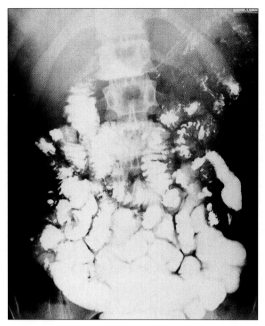

Fig. 3.39 Adult coeliac disease: barium follow-through radiograph of the small intestine showing flocculation of barium and lack of the normal fine mucosal pattern. (Courtesy of Dr D Nag.)

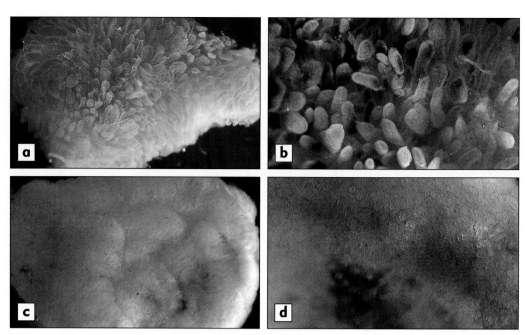

Fig. 3.40a–d Adult coeliac disease: low and medium power views of jejunal biopsies showing (a and b) normal villi in finger and leaf patterns; (c and d) abnormal mosaic pattern with obvious crypt openings. [(a–d) Courtesy of Dr JS Stewart.]

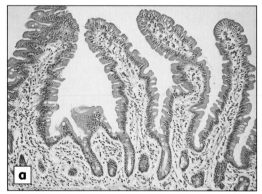

Fig. 3.41 and b Coeliac disease: histological sections of jejunal biopsies showing (a) normal mucosa with finger-like villi and (b) subtotal villous atrophy with absence of villi and hypertrophy of the mucosal crypts. [(b) Courtesy of Dr A Price.]

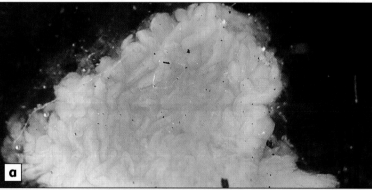

Fig. 3.42a and b Tropical sprue: jejunal biopsy showing (a) dissecting microscope appearance with typical convoluted mucosal pattern and (b) partial villous atrophy. [(a, b) Courtesy of Prof. V Chadwick.]

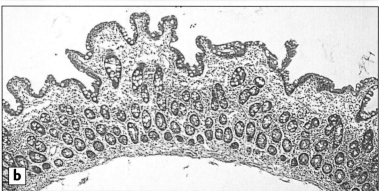

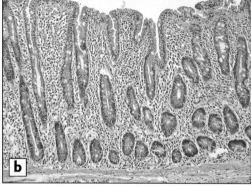

Fig. 3.43 Dermatitis herpetiformis: typical appearance of blisters on the extensor surfaces of the arms. This skin condition is associated with gluten-induced enteropathy and folate deficiency. (Courtesy of Prof. L Fry.)

homozygous state, to megaloblastic anaemia caused by failure of B_{12} transport into bone marrow and other cells. It presents in the first few months of life (*Fig. 3.44*). Nitrous oxide is discussed on page 65.

A number of rare abnormalities of folate metabolism have been described, and megaloblastic anaemia may also arise during therapy with the antifolate drugs that inhibit dihydrofolate reductase, such as methotrexate or pyrimethamine.

Other causes

Megaloblastic anaemia as a result of antimetabolite chemotherapy with, for example, hydroxyurea or cytosine arabinoside, shows similar mor-

phological features to those that result from B_{12} or folate deficiencies. However, dyserythropoietic changes are often more marked.

In acute myeloid leukaemia of the M_6 type or in myelodysplasia, megaloblastic changes are usually confined to the erythroid series. Giant metamyelocytes, hypersegmented polymorphs and other changes in leucopoiesis, or megakaryocytes seen in B_{12} or folate deficiency, are not present.

Rare inborn errors of metabolism other than those affecting B_{12} or folate metabolism, such as orotic aciduria in which there is a fault in pyrimidine synthesis, may also result in megaloblastic anaemia (*Fig. 3.45*).

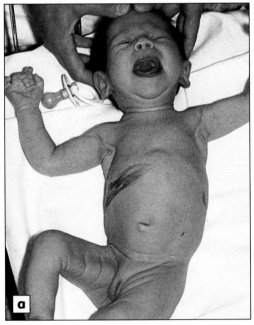
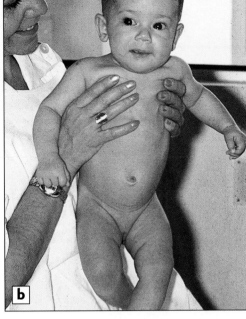

Fig. 3.44a and b Transcobalamin II deficiency: this child (a) before and (b) 6 months after therapy, presented at 20 days with weight loss, irritability, pallor, glossitis and hepatosplenomegaly. Tests showed a macrocytic anaemia and megaloblastic bone marrow. Serum B_{12} and folate levels were normal, but chromatography of serum showed absence of transcobalamin II. Treatment was 1 mg hydroxocobalamin intramuscularly twice weekly; the child remains well 18 years later. [(a, b) Courtesy of Dr MC Arrabel.]

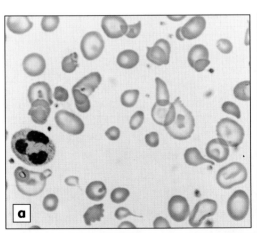
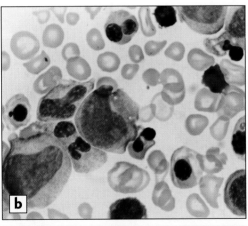
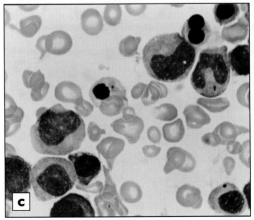
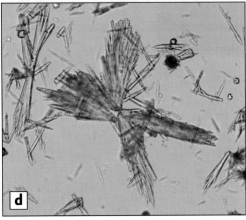

Fig. 3.45a–d Orotic aciduria: female who presented at 6 months with anaemia (Hb, 6.0 g/dl; MCV, 110 fl), and normal white cell and platelet counts. The serum B_{12} and folate levels were normal. (a) The peripheral blood film shows marked anisocytosis and poikilocytosis with macrocytic and microcytic cells. (b, c) Bone marrow shows megaloblastic erythropoiesis with a binucleate cell, Howell–Jolly body formation and giant metamyelocytes. (d) Crystals of orotic acid are present in the urine. The child responded haematologically to treatment with uridine 50 mg/kg daily orally with a reduction in orotic acid excretion. [(a–d) Courtesy of Dr J Price.]

TREATMENT OF MEGALOBLASTIC ANAEMIA

B_{12} deficiency is treated by intramuscular or subcutaneous hydroxo-cobalamin; for example, six injections each of 1 mg. Maintenance is with similar injections at 3-month intervals.

Folate deficiency may be corrected with daily oral folic acid given for 4 months. Long-term folic acid therapy may be needed when the cause of the deficiency, for example a severe haemolytic anaemia or myelosclerosis, cannot be corrected. In patients who present with severe megaloblastic anaemia and who need urgent therapy, both vit-amins may be given initially and continued until the cause of the anaemia has been established. Dietary fortification with folic acid has been introduced in several countries, including the US, in an attempt to reduce the incidence of renal tube defect babies.

CAUSES OF MACROCYTOSIS OTHER THAN MEGALOBLASTIC ANAEMIA

Macrocytosis may be caused by a number of marrow disorders that dis-turb erythropoiesis, cause lipid deposition on the red cell membrane or affect red cell size by other mechanisms (*Fig. 3.46*). When the cause is alcohol excess, the MCV is often raised, even though the haemoglobin level is normal.

Other causes of macrocytosis
Alcohol
Liver disease
Hypothyroidism
Myelodysplasia, including acquired sideroblastic anaemia
Aplastic anaemia and red cell aplasia
Raised reticulocyte count
Hypoxia
Myeloma and other paraproteinaemias
Cytotoxic drugs
Pregnancy

Fig. 3.46 Macrocytosis: causes other than megaloblastic anaemia.

4

Haemolytic Anaemia

The dominant cause of the anaemia in haemolytic anaemias is an increased rate of red cell destruction. This red cell destruction is usually extravascular (taking place in the macrophages of the reticuloendothelial system, as in normal individuals), although in some types of acute or chronic haemolysis red cell destruction occurs intravascularly (*Fig. 4.1*). The clinical and laboratory features differ according to whether the main site of destruction is extravascular or intravascular.

In addition to the clinical feature of pallor, many patients show mild fluctuating jaundice (*Figs 4.2 and 4.3*) and splenomegaly (*Fig. 4.4*).

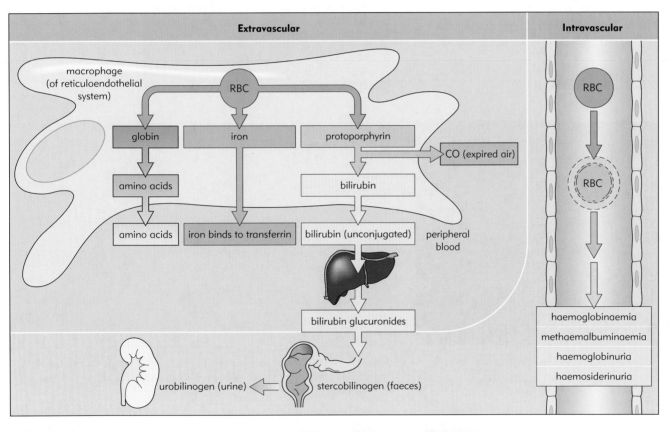

Fig. 4.1 Haemolytic anaemia: extravascular and intravascular mechanisms of red blood cell (RBC) breakdown.

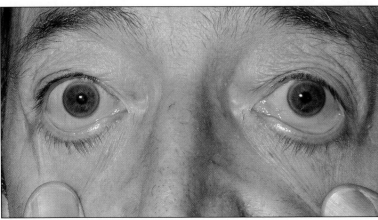

Fig. 4.2 Haemolytic anaemia (autoimmune): scleral jaundice.

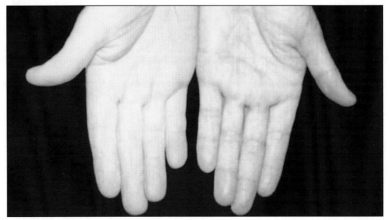

Fig. 4.3 Haemolytic anaemia (autoimmune): jaundice of the palmar skin (on the left) contrasted with normal skin colour.

Increased bilirubin production may result in pigment gallstones (*Figs 4.5 and 4.6*).

Laboratory findings in haemolytic anaemia include raised unconjugated serum bilirubin, and increased faecal stercobilinogen and urinary urobilinogen from accelerated red cell destruction; serum haptoglobins are absent. A reticulocytosis (*Fig. 4.7*) and bone marrow erythroid hyper-plasia (*Fig. 4.8*) are the result of compensatory increases in red cell production. Characteristic changes in red cell morphology occur in a number of haemolytic anaemias and, in the most severe, the peripheral blood film shows red cell polychromasia (caused by reticulocytosis) and occasional erythroblasts (as a result of extramedullary erythropoiesis; *Fig. 4.9*).

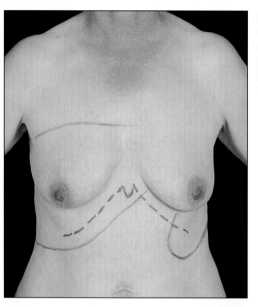

Fig. 4.4 Haemolytic anaemia: mild splenomegaly and jaundice in a delayed haemolytic transfusion reaction.

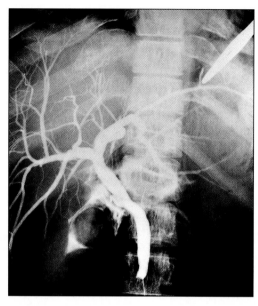

Fig. 4.5 Thalassaemia major: operative cholangiogram shows a distended biliary tree and failure of contrast to pass gallstone obstruction at the lower part of the common bile duct. (Courtesy of Dr R Dick.)

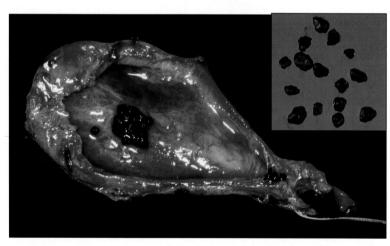

Fig. 4.6 Thalassaemia major: opened gall bladder and its bilirubin gallstones (inset).

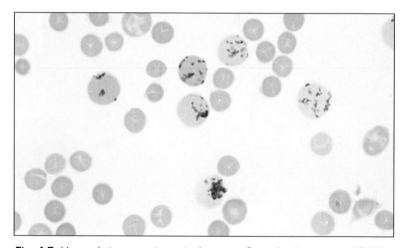

Fig. 4.7 Haemolytic anaemia: reticulocytosis. Reticular (precipitated RNA) material is seen in the larger cells. New methylene blue stain. (Giemsa counterstain.)

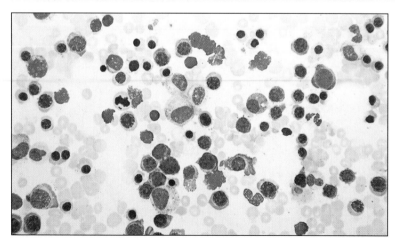

Fig. 4.8 Haemolytic anaemia: this bone marrow cell trail with erythroid hyperplasia shows a dominance of erythroblasts.

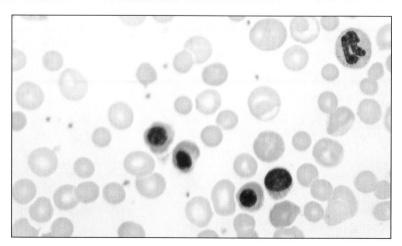

Fig. 4.9 Haemolytic anaemia (autoimmune): peripheral blood film showing erythroblasts, red cell polychromasia and spherocytosis.

In those anaemias caused by oxidant damage to haemoglobin and other red cell proteins, Heinz bodies may be found in reticulocyte preparations (*Fig. 4.10*). Intravascular red cell destruction is accompanied by haemoglobinaemia, haemoglobinuria (*Fig. 4.11*), plasma methaemoglobinaemia, methaemalbuminaemia and haemosiderinuria (*Fig. 4.12*). Jaundice is less common.

HEREDITARY HAEMOLYTIC ANAEMIA

The hereditary haemolytic anaemias are usually the result of intrinsic red cell defects. A simplified classification is shown in *Fig. 4.13*; thalassaemia and other genetic disorders of haemoglobin are discussed in Chapter 5.

Normal red cell membrane
Normal red cell membrane consists of a phospholipid bilayer, with hydrophilic phosphate residues on the external and inner surfaces and non-polar fatty acid side chains projecting into the centre (*Fig. 4.14*). The bilayer also contains a variable proportion of cholesterol. Proteins may be either transmembrane integral proteins, for example band 3 and glycophorins A or B, or peripheral (extrinsic) proteins, such as spectrin,

actin and bands 2.1 (ankyrin), 4.1 and 4.2, which form a scaffolding structure on the inner surface of the membrane. The band numbers refer to the Coomassie blue bands on sodium dodecyl sulphate plus polyacrylamide gel electrophoresis (SDS–PAGE; *Fig. 4.15*).

The phospholipids or proteins on the external surface may carry sugars which determine blood groups or may act as viral receptors. Spectrin consists of two forms, α and β, joined to form a heterodimer with a hairpin structure. The protein 2.1 (ankyrin) binds the spectrin β chains to band 3, a large integral membrane protein, while the tail end of spectrin binds to protein 4.1, thus forming spectrin tetramers. Protein 4.1 also binds to glycophorin A or aminophospholipids to serve as secondary attachment sites of the cytoskeleton to the inner surface of the bilayer.

Red cell blood group antigens
The red cell plasma membrane contains a large number of different antigens. Many of these have sugar residues attached to membrane proteins or lipids. The structure of the most important antigens, those of the ABO system, is discussed in Chapter 19.

Over 600 different antigens exist; the best characterized are listed in *Fig. 19.1*. Blood group antigens are important in blood transfusion

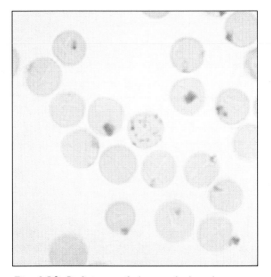

Fig. 4.10 Deficiency of glucose 6-phosphate dehydrogenase: peripheral blood film showing Heinz bodies in red cells and a single reticulocyte. (Supravital new methylene blue stain.)

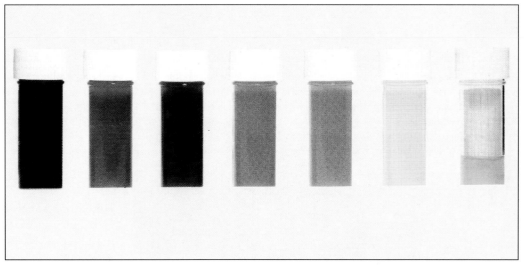

Fig. 4.11 Glucose 6-phosphate dehydrogenase deficiency: urine samples showing haemoglobinuria of decreasing severity following an episode of acute intravascular haemolysis.

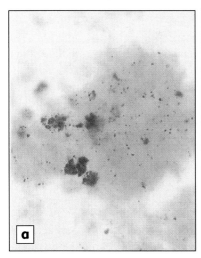 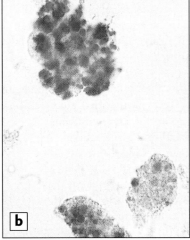

Fig. 4.12 Intravascular haemolysis in paroxysmal nocturnal haemoglobinuria (PNH): haemosiderinuria. (a) Prussian-blue positive material seen in urinary deposit and (b) at higher magnification in individual renal tubular cells. (Perls' stain.)

Hereditary haemolytic anaemia		
Membrane defects	**Metabolic defects**	**Haemoglobin defects**
Hereditary spherocytosis	Deficiency of:	Defective synthesis (e.g. thalassaemia α or β)
Hereditary elliptocytosis	pyruvate kinase	
	triose phosphate isomerase	Abnormal variants (e.g. HbS, HbC, unstable)
Hereditary stomatocytosis	pyrimidine 5-nucleotidase	
South-east Asian ovalocytosis	glucose 6-phosphate dehydrogenase	
	glutathione synthase	
etc.	etc.	

Fig. 4.13 Hereditary haemolytic anaemia: causes.

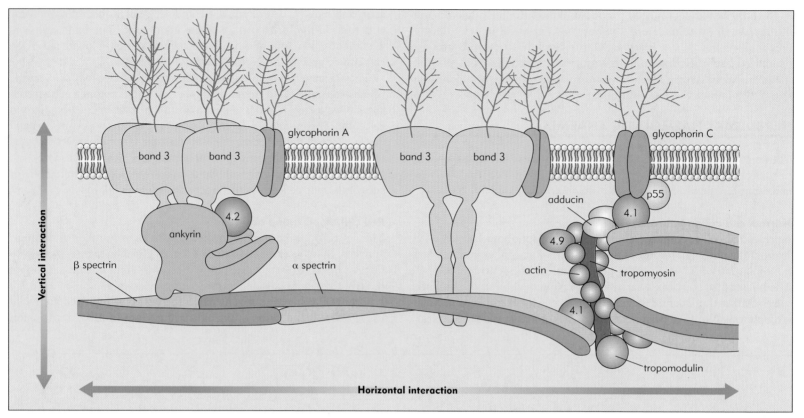

Fig. 4.14 Hereditary spherocytosis and hereditary elliptocytosis and/or pyropoikilocytosis: the red cell membrane with vertical and horizontal interactions of its components. Estimated frequencies of mutations in different membrane proteins are:
- vertical interaction – hereditary spherocytosis: band 3, about 20%; protein 4.2, about 5%; ankyrin, about 45%; and β spectrin, about 30%.
- horizontal interaction – hereditary elliptocytosis and/or pyropoikilocytosis: β spectrin, about 5%; α spectrin, about 80%; protein 4.1, about 15%;. The relative positions of the various proteins are correct, but the proteins and lipids are not drawn to scale. (Adapted with permission from Tse WT, Lux SE. Red blood cell membrane disorders (Review). *Br J Haematol.* 1999;104:2–13.)

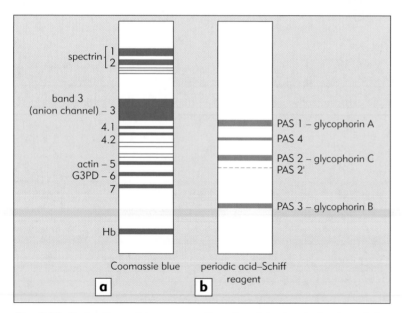

Fig. 4.15 Red cell membrane: separation of proteins by electrophoresis in SDS gels. (a) Staining for protein and (b) staining for carbohydrate. (Adapted with permission from Contreras M, Lubenko A. Immunohaematology: introduction. In: Hoffbrand AV, Lewis SM, Tuddenham EGD. *Postgraduate Haematology*, 4th edn. Oxford: Butterworth–Heinemann, 1999.)

and autoantibodies may be directed against them in autoimmune haemolytic anaemias (e.g. against specific Rhesus antigens in warm-type autoimmune haemolytic anaemia, and against the i antigen in infectious mononucleosis).

Hereditary spherocytosis

Hereditary spherocytosis may result from a variety of abnormalities of the cytoskeletal proteins involved in vertical interactions of the red cell membrane. Defects of ankyrin, spectrin, band 3 or other proteins have been described in various kindreds (*Fig. 4.16*). The cells are excessively permeable to sodium influx; glycolysis and adenosine triphosphate (ATP) turnover are increased. The marrow produces red cells of normal biconcave shape, but these lose membrane during passage through the spleen and the rest of the reticuloendothelial system. The resultant rigid and spherical cells have a shortened lifespan, the spleen being the principal organ of red cell destruction.

The condition is characterized by a dominant inheritance pattern. Typically, anaemia, jaundice and splenomegaly are present. The blood film from a patient with hereditary spherocytosis shows microsphero-cytes (*Fig. 4.17*); red cell osmotic fragility is characteristically increased (*Fig. 4.18*), and tests for autohaemolysis show increased lysis of red cells at least partly corrected by glucose (*Fig. 4.19*).

Splenectomy produces a considerable improvement in red cell survival and is associated with a rise in haemoglobin levels to normal. Sections of splenic tissue reveal many spherocytic red cells trapped in the splenic cords (*Fig. 4.20*).

Hereditary elliptocytosis

The characteristic feature in hereditary elliptocytosis is the presence of elongated red cells in the peripheral blood (*Fig. 4.21*). A number of inherited protein defects that affect horizontal interactions, especially of spectrin or band 4.1, may produce this condition (*Fig. 4.16*). A defective spectrin dimer–dimer interaction results in an increased proportion of dimers in relation to spectrin tetramers. The clinical expression in

Hereditary spherocytosis, hereditary elliptocytosis and South-east Asian ovalocytosis	
Hereditary spherocytosis (vertical interactions)	**Hereditary elliptocytosis (horizontal interactions)**
Ankyrin deficiency (>50%) Amino acid substitution Frame shift and nonsense mutations δ Untranslated region/promoter mutations Splicing defects Gene deletions Balanced translocations *Spectrin deficiency* α Chain defects (rare) β Chain defects (uncommon) *Pallidin (protein 4.2) abnormalities (5%)* *Band 3 deficiency (20%)*	*Spectrin abnormalities* α Chain defects (80%) β Chain defects (5%) *Protein 4.1 deficiency (15%)* *South-east Asian ovalocytosis* Band 3 defect (deletion of nine amino acids at junction of cytoplasmic and transmembrane domains)

Fig. 4.16 Hereditary spherocytosis, hereditary elliptocytosis and South-east Asian ovalocytosis: causes. The figures given in brackets indicate the approximate percentages of patients with hereditary spherocytosis or hereditary elliptocytosis with that abnormality.

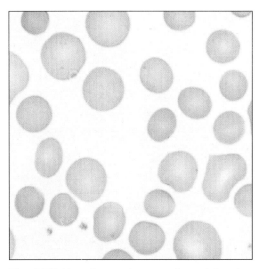

Fig. 4.17 Hereditary spherocytosis: peripheral blood film showing smaller spherocytes among larger polychromatic red cells.

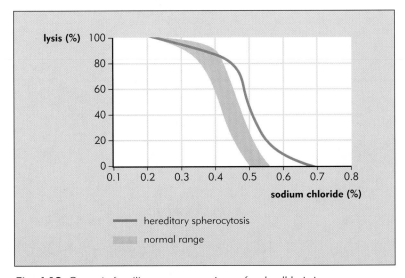

Fig. 4.18 Osmotic fragility test: comparison of red cell lysis in severe hereditary spherocytosis and in normal blood. The curve is shifted to the right of the normal range, but a tail of osmotically resistant cells (reticulocytes) is present.

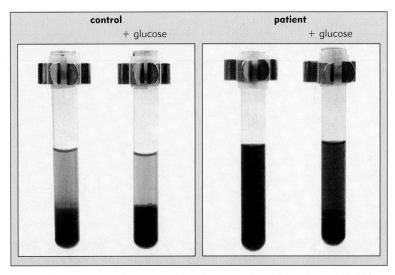

Fig. 4.19 Autohaemolysis test: red cells are incubated in saline at 37°C for 48 hours with and without additional glucose and the amount of lysis is determined. Autohaemolysis, particularly in the absence of an energy supply (glucose), is markedly increased in hereditary spherocytosis.

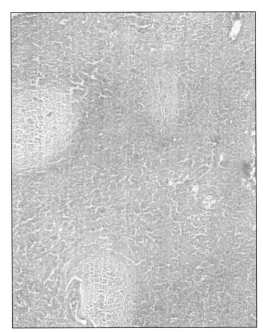

Fig. 4.20 Hereditary spherocytosis: section of spleen showing marked hyperplasia of reticuloendothelial cordal tissue and entrapment of large numbers of red cells.

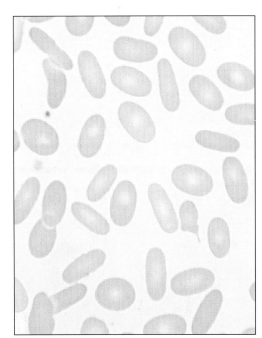

Fig. 4.21 Hereditary elliptocytosis: blood film showing characteristic elliptical red cells.

heterozygotes (elliptocytosis trait) is variable: while some have anaemia and splenomegaly, the majority have only minimal or no reduction in red cell survival with little or no anaemia. In rare homozygous patients, and occasional heterozygotes, there is severe anaemia with marked haemolysis and splenomegaly (*Fig. 4.22*) and bizarre red cell morphology termed pyropoikilocytosis (*Fig. 4.23*).

South-east Asian ovalocytosis (stomatocytic hereditary elliptocytosis)

South-east Asian ovalocytosis is an asymptomatic trait found in 30% of subjects in some coastal areas of New Guinea and Malaysia. The inheritance, whether dominant or recessive, is unclear (*Fig. 4.24*). Homozygosity is probably lethal; heterozygotes are relatively protected from malaria.

Other rare inherited defects of the red cell membrane

Other rare inherited defects of the red cell membrane include hereditary stomatocytosis (*Fig. 4.25*) and acanthocytosis associated with the McLeod blood group system (*Fig. 4.26*).

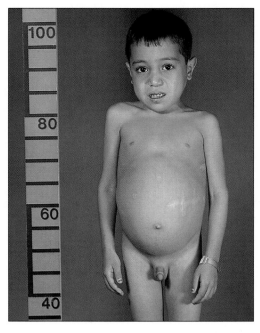

Fig. 4.22 Hereditary elliptocytosis: abdominal swelling caused by massive splenomegaly in a homozygous patient. The facies indicates expansion of haemopoietic tissue in the skull bones, particularly in the maxillae.

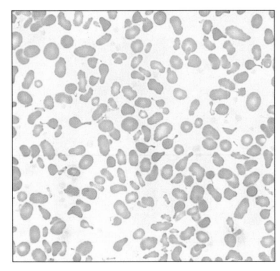

Fig. 4.23 Hereditary pyropoikilocytosis: blood film showing red cell anisocytosis and micropoikilocytosis (MCV, 61 fl; microspherocytosis).

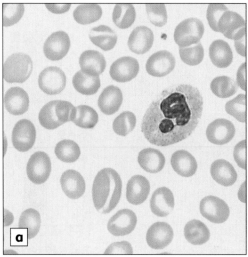

Fig. 4.24a and b South-east Asian ovalocytosis: (a, b) peripheral blood films showing ovalocytes and stomatocytes, some with a longitudinal or Y-shaped slit and others with a transverse ridge. The red cell membrane is rigid, conferring resistance to malaria. The cells may form abnormal rouleaux and have reduced deformability. The genetic defect is in band 3 protein in which there is deletion of nine amino acids and which binds tightly to ankyrin (*see Fig. 4.14*). (Courtesy of Dr BA Bain.)

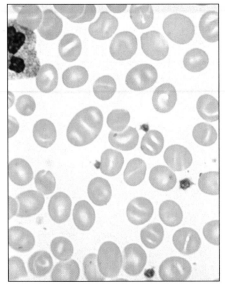

Fig. 4.25 Hereditary stomatocytosis: peripheral blood film showing many cells with the characteristic loosely folded appearance of the membrane. The membrane has increased passive permeability allowing excess sodium entry.

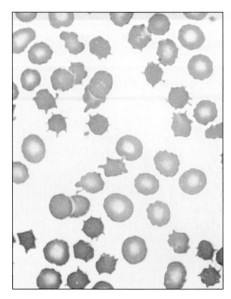

Fig. 4.26 McLeod phenotype: peripheral blood film showing marked acanthocytosis of red cells associated with the rare McLeod blood group. There is lack of the Kell antigen precursor (Kx).

Normal red cell metabolism

Normal red cells maintain themselves in a physiological state for about 120 days by metabolizing glucose through the glycolytic (Embden–Meyerhof) and pentose phosphate (hexose monophosphate shunt) pathways (*Fig. 4.27*). In this way the cells are able to generate the energy needed to maintain cell shape and flexibility as well as cation and water content through the action of sodium and calcium pumps. Although ATP acts as an energy store, it may also act as a substitute for 2,3-diphosphoglycerate (2,3-DPG) in maintaining the position of the oxygen dissociation curve. The most abundant red cell phosphate, 2,3-DPG is generated by the Rapoport–Luebering shunt of the glycolytic pathway (*Fig. 4.28*). The higher the 2,3-DPG content of red cells, the more easily is oxygen liberated from haemoglobin. Reducing power is also generated as the reduced forms of nicotinamide–adenine dinucleotide (NADH) and NAD phosphate (NADPH) and reduced glutathione (GSH), which protect the membrane, haemoglobin and other cell structures from oxidant damage.

Glucose 6-phosphate dehydrogenase deficiency

Glucose 6-phosphate dehydrogenase deficiency (G6PD) is a 'housekeeping gene' needed in all cells. Deficiency affects the red cells most severely, perhaps because they have no alternative source of NADPH and as a result of their long non-nucleated lifespan. The activity of G6PD diminishes as red cells age. The normal G6PD enzyme is genetically polymorphic and the most common form is Type B. In Africa, up to 40% of the population carry an electrophoretically different normal form, Type A.

Many of the several hundred inherited variants of the enzyme (*Fig. 4.29*) show less activity than normal. Worldwide, 400 million people are thought to be deficient. The G6PD abnormalities have been classified into five classes according to the activity of the enzyme:

- class I, severe deficiency associated with non-spherocytic haemolytic anaemia (NSHA);
- class II, <10% activity, includes the common Mediterranean and Oriental variants not associated with NSHA;
- class III, 10–60% of activity, includes the common A form;
- class IV, normal activity; and
- class V, raised activity.

The most frequent clinical syndrome is acute intravascular haemolysis caused by oxidant stress, drugs (*Fig. 4.30*), or fava beans, or during severe infection, diabetic ketoacidosis or hepatitis. Marked changes occur in red cell morphology (*Fig. 4.31*), with Heinz bodies (*see Fig. 4.10*) and haemoglobinuria (*see Fig. 4.11*). Neonatal jaundice may also occur and the most severe defects result in a chronic NSHA.

The gene is located on the X chromosome and is fully expressed in males, but only one X chromosome is active in each female cell. As a result of X-chromosome inactivation, female heterozygotes for G6PD deficiency have two populations of cells (on average 50% of each), either with or without the enzyme. As G6PD deficiency confers protection against *Plasmodium falciparum* malaria it has a high frequency in areas of the world where malaria is or was common. Rarely, lack of G6PD may be responsible for decreased leucocyte function and for hyperbilirubinaemia in some patients with neonatal jaundice or viral hepatitis.

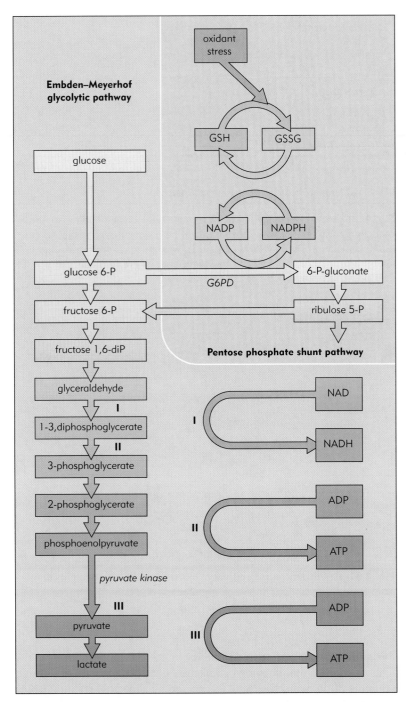

Fig. 4.27 Normal red cell metabolism: Embden–Meyerhof (glycolytic) and pentose phosphate (hexose monophosphate shunt) pathways. (P, phosphate; GSSG, oxidized glutathione; ADP, adenosine diphosphate; for other abbreviations see text.)

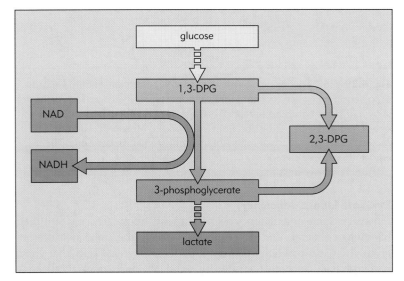

Fig. 4.28 Normal red cell metabolism: the Rapoport–Luebering shunt pathway for maintenance of red cell 2,3-DPG levels.

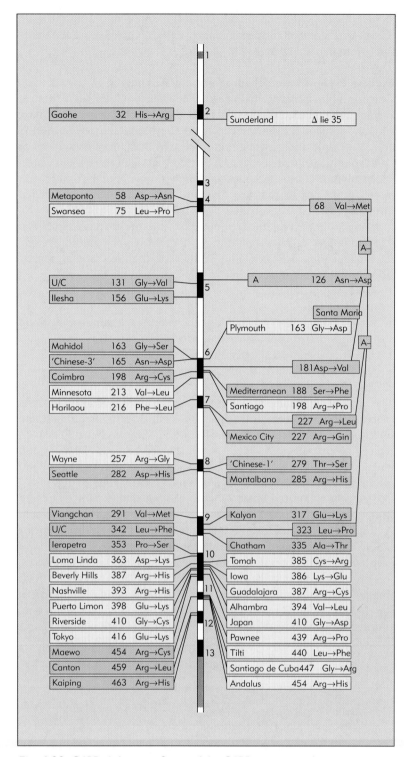

Fig. 4.29 G6PD deficiency: Some of the G6PD mutations that may cause drug sensitivity (green) or more rarely chronic NSHA (yellow). The exons are shown in black bands except exon 1, which is non-coding and shown in grey. (Adapted with permission from Vulliamy TJ, Mason PJ, Luzzatto L. Molecular basis of glucose-6-phosphate dehydrogenase deficiency. *Trends Genet.* 1992;8;138–43.)

Gaohe	32	His→Arg
Sunderland		Δ Ile 35
Metaponto	58	Asp→Asn
Swansea	75	Leu→Pro
	68	Val→Met
U/C	131	Gly→Val
Ilesha	156	Glu→Lys
A	126	Asn→Asp
Santa Maria		
Plymouth	163	Gly→Asp
Mahidol	163	Gly→Ser
'Chinese-3'	165	Asn→Asp
Coimbra	198	Arg→Cys
Minnesota	213	Val→Leu
Harilaou	216	Phe→Leu
	181	Asp→Val
Mediterranean	188	Ser→Phe
Santiago	198	Arg→Pro
	227	Arg→Leu
Mexico City	227	Arg→Gln
Wayne	257	Arg→Gly
Seattle	282	Asp→His
'Chinese-1'	279	Thr→Ser
Montalbano	285	Arg→His
Viangchan	291	Val→Met
U/C	342	Leu→Phe
Ierapetra	353	Pro→Ser
Loma Linda	363	Asp→Lys
Beverly Hills	387	Arg→His
Nashville	393	Arg→His
Puerto Limon	398	Glu→Lys
Riverside	410	Gly→Cys
Tokyo	416	Glu→Lys
Maewo	454	Arg→Cys
Canton	459	Arg→Leu
Kaiping	463	Arg→His
Kalyan	317	Glu→Lys
	323	Leu→Pro
Chatham	335	Ala→Thr
Tomah	385	Cys→Arg
Iowa	386	Lys→Glu
Guadalajara	387	Arg→Cys
Alhambra	394	Val→Leu
Japan	410	Gly→Asp
Pawnee	439	Arg→Pro
Tilti	440	Leu→Phe
Santiago de Cuba	447	Gly→Arg
Andalus	454	Arg→His

G6PD deficiency

Drugs that may cause haemolytic anaemia in subjects with G6PD deficiency	Drugs that can be given safely in therapeutic doses to subjects with G6PD deficiency without NSHA
Antimalarials Pyrimethamine with sulfadoxine (Fansidar) Pyrimethamine with dapsone (Maloprim) Primaquine ? Chloroquine	**Ascorbic acid** Aspirin Colchicine Isoniazid Menadiol Phenytoin Probenecid Procainamide Pyrimethamine Quinidine Quinine Trimethoprim
Sulphonamides Sulfamethoxazole Some other sulphonamides	
Sulphones Dapsone Thiazolesulphone	
Other antibacterial compounds Nitrofurans Nalidixic acid	
Anthelmintics Beta-naphthol	
Miscellaneous ? Vitamin K Naphthalene (moth balls) Methylene blue Doxorubicin	

? – there is some dispute with these compounds

Fig. 4.30 G6PD deficiency: drugs that cause haemolytic anaemia in association with G6PD, and those that can be given safely to subjects with G6PD deficiency without NSHA. (Adapted with permission from Beutler E. Glucose-6-phosphate dehydrogenase deficiency. *N Engl J Med.* 1991;324:169–74.)

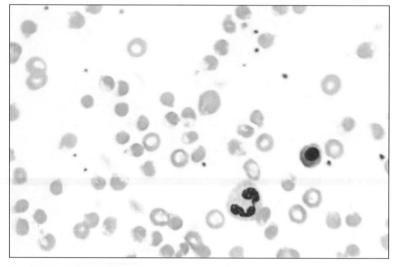

Fig. 4.31 G6PD deficiency: peripheral blood film following acute oxidant drug-induced haemolysis shows an erythroblast and damaged red cells, including irregularly contracted 'blister' and 'bite' cells.

Pyruvate kinase deficiency

Pyruvate kinase deficiency is the most frequently encountered haemolytic anaemia due to an inherited defect in the Embden–Meyerhof glycolytic pathway. The majority of patients have red cells that show no particular diagnostic features (*Fig. 4.32*), although 'prickle' cells may be found, especially following splenectomy (*Fig. 4.33*). The post-splenectomy reticulocyte count is often very high (*Fig. 4.34*). There is an abnormal autohaemolysis test not corrected by glucose, and diagnosis is made by a specific enzyme assay.

Pyrimidine 5-nucleotidase deficiency

This rare congenital haemolytic anaemia is associated with basophilic stippling of the red cells (*Fig. 4.35*) caused by abnormal residual RNA. This enzyme normally catalyses the hydrolytic dephosphorylation of pyrimidine 5'-ribose monophosphates to freely diffusible pyrimidine nucleosides, an important step in the breakdown of RNA at the reticulocyte stage. The enzyme is also inhibited by lead.

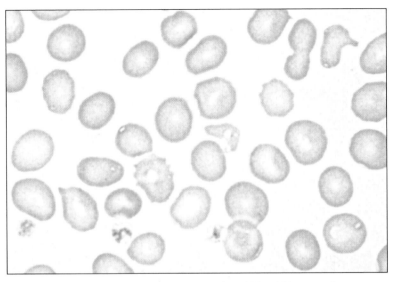

Fig. 4.32 Pyruvate kinase deficiency: peripheral blood film presplenectomy shows red cell anisocytosis and poikilocytosis.

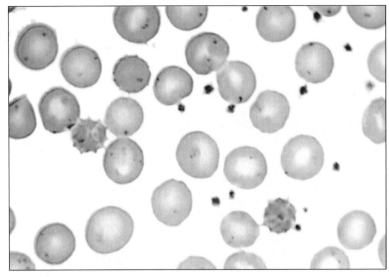

Fig. 4.33 Pyruvate kinase deficiency: peripheral blood film postsplenectomy with two small acanthocytes or 'prickle' cells.

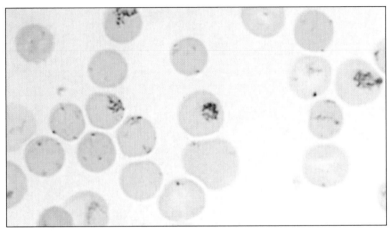

Fig. 4.34 Pyruvate kinase deficiency: gross reticulocytosis (over 90%) following splenectomy. (Supravital new methylene blue stain.)

ACQUIRED HAEMOLYTIC ANAEMIA

The majority of acquired haemolytic anaemias are caused by extracorpuscular or environmental changes. A simplified classification is given in *Fig. 4.36.*

Autoimmune haemolytic anaemias

Autoimmune haemolytic anaemias are characterized by a positive direct Coombs' (antiglobulin) test (*Fig. 4.37*) and are divided into 'warm' and 'cold' types, according to whether the antibody reacts better with red cells at 37°C or at 4°C. These acquired disorders occur at any age and produce haemolytic anaemias of varying severity, often with

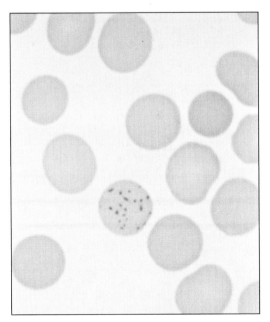

Fig. 4.35 Pyrimidine 5-nucleotidase deficiency: peripheral blood film showing basophilic stippling in the central red cell.

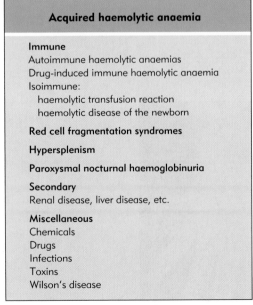

Acquired haemolytic anaemia

Immune
Autoimmune haemolytic anaemias
Drug-induced immune haemolytic anaemia
Isoimmune:
   haemolytic transfusion reaction
   haemolytic disease of the newborn

Red cell fragmentation syndromes

Hypersplenism

Paroxysmal nocturnal haemoglobinuria

Secondary
Renal disease, liver disease, etc.

Miscellaneous
Chemicals
Drugs
Infections
Toxins
Wilson's disease

Fig. 4.36 Acquired haemolytic anaemia: causes.

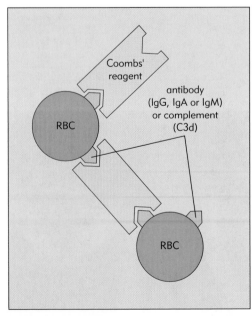

Fig. 4.37 Direct antiglobulin (Coombs') test: the Coombs' reagent may be broad spectrum or specifically directed against IgG, IgM, IgA or complement (C3d). The test is positive if the red cells agglutinate.

associated disease (*Fig. 4.38*). In the warm type, the peripheral blood usually shows marked red cell spherocytosis (*Figs 4.39 and 4.40*). In the cold type, the antibodies are usually IgM and may be associated with intravascular haemolysis. Marked autoagglutination of red cells may be seen in the blood film (*Fig. 4.41*). In many patients the haemolysis is aggravated by cold weather and it is often associated with Raynaud's phenomenon (*Fig. 4.42*). Rarely, the blood films show neutrophil–red cell rosettes (*Fig. 4.43*).

Autoimmune haemolytic anaemia	
Warm type	**Cold type**
Idiopathic	Idiopathic
Secondary	Secondary
Systemic lupus erythematosus, other connective tissue disorders	Mycoplasma pneumonia
	Infectious mononucleosis
Chronic lymphocytic leukaemia	Malignant lymphoma
	Ulcerative colitis
Malignant lymphoma	
Ovarian teratoma	Paroxysmal cold haemoglobinuria: rare; may be primary or associated with infection
Drugs (e.g. methyldopa, fluodarabine)	

Fig. 4.38 Autoimmune haemolytic anaemia: causes.

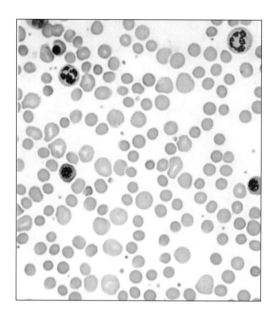

Fig. 4.39 Autoimmune haemolytic anaemia: peripheral blood film showing erythroblasts, polychromatic macrocytes and marked spherocytosis.

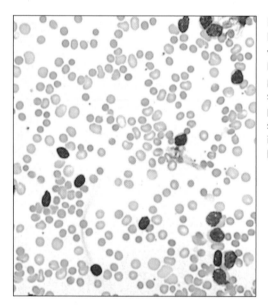

Fig. 4.40 Autoimmune haemolytic anaemia with associated chronic lymphocytic leukaemia: peripheral blood film showing red cell polychromasia spherocytosis and increased numbers of lymphocytes.

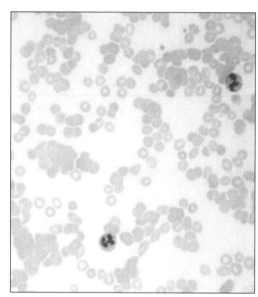

Fig. 4.41 Autoimmune haemolytic anaemia (cold type): peripheral blood film showing autoagglutination of red cells.

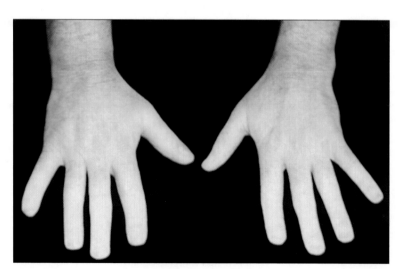

Fig. 4.42 Autoimmune haemolytic anaemia (cold type): Raynaud's phenomenon manifested by marked pallor of the fingers.

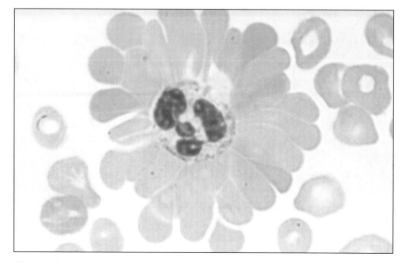

Fig. 4.43 Autoimmune haemolytic anaemia: peripheral blood film showing a neutrophil–red cell rosette.

In warm autoimmune haemolytic anaemia, high-dose corticosteroids often achieve a remission and splenectomy may be of value in those who do not respond satisfactorily. Patients with chronic cold autoimmune haemolytic anaemia should avoid the cold and some may benefit from therapy with alkylating agents.

Drug-induced immune haemolytic anaemia

Drugs cause immune haemolytic anaemia by three mechanisms:
- antibodies may be directed against a red cell membrane–drug complex (e.g. with penicillin);
- there may be deposition of a protein–antibody–drug complex on the red cell surface (e.g. with quinine, rifampicin); or
- occasionally an autoimmune process is involved, as with methyldopa or fludarabine.

Isoimmune haemolytic anaemia

Severe haemolysis follows transfusion of incompatible blood, particularly if the blood is of the wrong ABO group. There may be massive intravascular haemolysis and the blood film usually shows both autoagglutination and spherocytosis (*Fig. 4.44*). The other major cause of isoimmune haemolytic anaemia is haemolytic disease of the newborn, which may result from a number of different maternofetal blood group incompatibilities (*Figs 4.45–4.47; see also* Chapter 19).

Red cell fragmentation syndromes

Fragmentation arises from direct damage to red cells, either on abnormal surfaces, such as artificial heart valves, or when red cells pass through fibrin strands deposited in the microcirculation because of disseminated intravascular coagulation, as in mucin-secreting adenocarcinomas

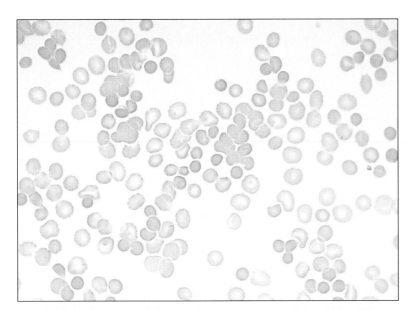

Fig. 4.44 ABO incompatibility transfusion reaction: peripheral blood film showing red cell autoagglutination and spherocytosis.

Isoimmune haemolytic anaemia		
Blood group system	Frequency of antibodies	Haemolytic disease of newborn
ABO	Very common	Causal
Rhesus	Common	Causal
Kell	Occasional	Causal
Duffy	Occasional	Causal
Kidd	Occasional	Causal
Lutheran	Rare	Causal
Lewis	Rare	Not causal
P	Rare	Not causal
MNSs	Rare	Not causal
Ii	Rare	Not causal

Fig. 4.45 Isoimmune haemolytic anaemia: the main blood group systems and their association with haemolytic disease in the newborn.

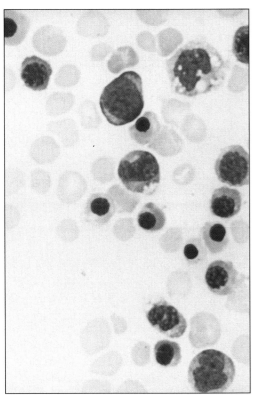

Fig. 4.46 Rhesus D haemolytic disease of the newborn (erythroblastosis fetalis); peripheral blood film from an infant born with severe anaemia showing large numbers of erythroblasts and microspherocytes.

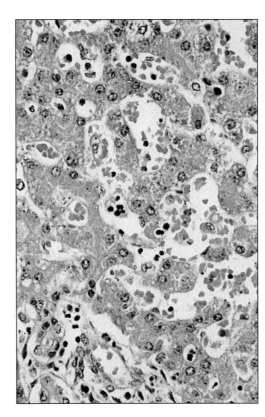

Fig. 4.47 Rhesus D haemolytic disease of the newborn: histological section of liver from a fatal case shows extramedullary haemopoiesis in the hepatic venous sinuses.

(*Fig. 4.48*), thrombotic thrombocytopenic purpura (*Fig. 4.49*) or in the haemolytic–uraemic syndrome (*Fig. 4.50*). Other causes of microangiopathic haemolytic anaemia include Gram-negative septicaemia (*Fig. 4.51*) and malignant hypertension.

Secondary haemolytic anaemias

In a number of systemic disorders, haemolysis may contribute to observed anaemia. In renal failure there may be crenated cells ('echinocytes'), including 'burr' cells and acanthocytes (*Fig.4.52; see also Fig. 6.40*). Red cell targeting is a feature of the haemolysis associated with liver disease, and with severe liver failure there is often marked haemolysis with prominent red cell acanthocytosis (*see Fig. 6.39b*).

Paroxysmal nocturnal haemoglobinuria

In paroxysmal nocturnal haemoglobinuria (PNH), an acquired clonal disorder, the bone marrow produces red cells with defective cell membranes that are particularly sensitive to lysis by complement. There is chronic intravascular haemolysis (*see Fig. 4.12*). The defect that results in complement sensitivity is in the formation of phosphatidyl inositol, which anchors a number of proteins via an intervening glycan structure to the red cell membrane (*Fig. 4.53*). The proteins anchored by glycosylphosphatidyl inositol (GPI) include membrane inhibitor of reactive lysis (MIRL = CD59), decay accelerating factor (DAF = CD55), C8 binding protein (C8B) – these three proteins all react with complement – leucocyte function antigen (LAF-3 = CD58), acetylcholinesterase, alkaline phosphatase and low affinity IgG receptor (FcRIII) (*Fig. 4.54*). Lack of MIRL appears to be responsible for the undue sensitivity to complement. The enzyme α-1,6-*N*-acetylglucosaminyltransferase is the enzyme involved in synthesis of the GPI anchor that is missing or defective because of different types of mutations in the PIG-A (phosphatidyl inositol glycan complementation class A) gene. The patients often develop iron deficiency. The bone marrow tends to be hypocellular and the reticulocyte count is lower than in other haemolytic anaemias of equal severity. The white cell and platelet counts are also often low. Many patients develop recurrent venous thromboses. Occasionally patients present with the Budd–Chiari syndrome (*Fig. 4.55*). The diagnosis of PNH is by finding positive acid lysis test (*Fig. 4.56*).

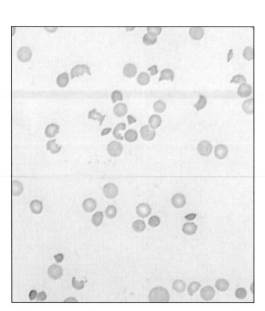

Fig. 4.48 Red cell fragmentation syndrome: peripheral blood film in widespread metastatic mucin-secreting adenocarcinoma showing deeply staining red cell fragments ('schistocytes') and anisocytosis.

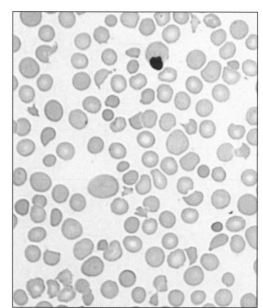

Fig. 4.49 Red cell fragmentation syndrome: peripheral blood film showing polychromatic and fragmented red cells in thrombotic thrombocytopenic purpura.

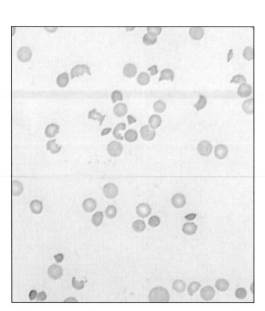

Fig. 4.50 Red cell fragmentation syndrome: peripheral blood film in haemolytic–uraemic syndrome.

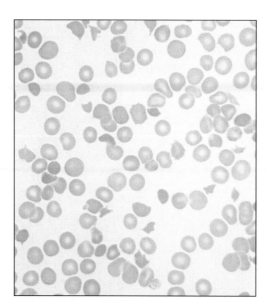

Fig. 4.51 Red cell fragmentation syndrome: peripheral blood film in Gram-negative septicaemia, showing red cell polychromasia, microspherocytes and fragmentation.

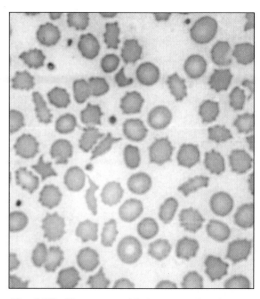

Fig. 4.52 Chronic renal failure: peripheral blood film showing red cell changes, including 'burr' cells and acanthocytes (coarse crenated cells).

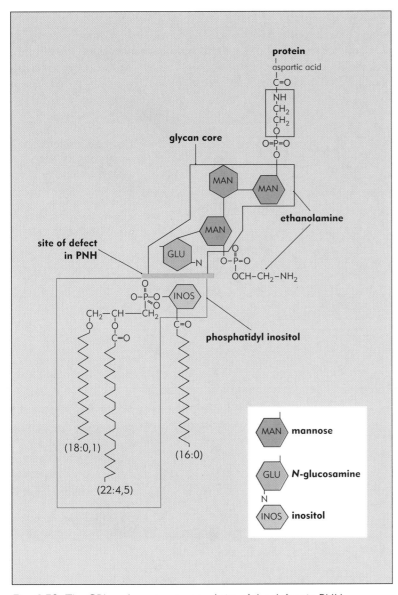

Fig. 4.53 The GPI anchor: structure and site of the defect in PNH. (Courtesy of Prof. Wendell Rosse.)

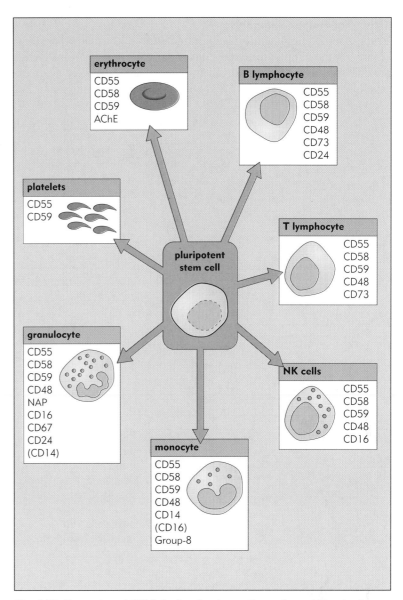

Fig. 4.54 Expression of GPI-linked molecules on the surface of blood cells: CD16 = FcRIII low affinity receptor for IgG; CD55 = DAF (see text); CD59 = MIRL (see text); AChE = acetylcholinesterase; NAP = alkaline phosphatase; Group-8 = monocyte activation antigen. (Adapted with permission from Rotoli B, Bessler M, Alfinito F, et al. Membrane proteins in paroxysmal nocturnal haemoglobinuria. Blood Rev. 1993;7:75–86.)

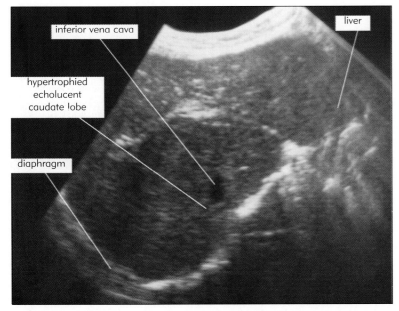

Fig. 4.55 PNH: ultrasound study of liver in Budd–Chiari syndrome. The caudate lobe is hypertrophied and spongy, and the inferior vena cava is compressed in its passage through it. (Courtesy of Dr L Berger.)

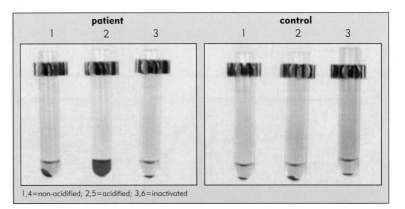

1,4=non-acidified; 2,5=acidified; 3,6=inactivated

Fig. 4.56 PNH: acid lysis test. The affected red cells (on the left) show marked complement-dependent lysis in acidified fresh serum at 37°C. Preheating the acidified serum inactivates complement, preventing lysis of the affected cells.

Other haemolytic anaemias

Severe haemolytic anaemia may be found during clostridial septicaemia (*Fig. 4.57*) and in other infections, including malaria and bartonellaemia (*see* Chapter 18). Haemolytic anaemias may also be caused by extensive burns (*Figs 4.58 and 4.59*), chemical poisoning, and snake and spider bites. Overdose with oxidizing drugs, such as sulfasalazine (*Fig. 4.60*) or dapsone (*Fig. 4.61*), may also cause severe haemolysis. Wilson's disease is also a cause of haemolysis, thought to result from oxidant damage to red cells caused by excess copper (*Fig. 4.62*).

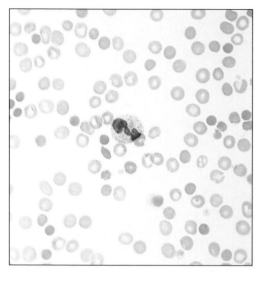

Fig. 4.57 Haemolytic anaemia in clostridial septicaemia: peripheral blood film showing red cell spherocytosis.

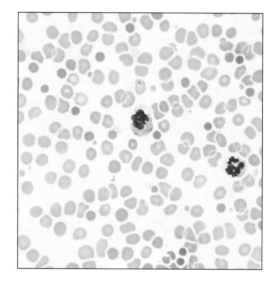

Fig. 4.58 Haemolytic anaemia following extensive burns: peripheral blood film showing marked spherocytosis, including microspherocytic cells.

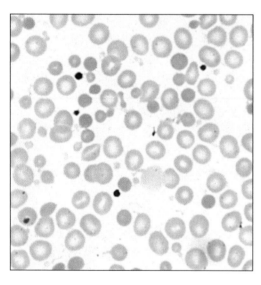

Fig. 4.59 Haemolytic anaemia following extensive burns: peripheral blood film showing microspherocytes, ghost cells, cells with membrane projections and 'dumb-bell' forms.

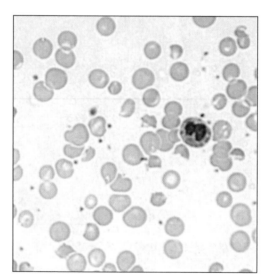

Fig. 4.60 Drug-induced haemolytic anaemia: peripheral blood film associated with overdose of sulfasalazine. The red cells show polychromasia, irregular contraction and some fragmentation.

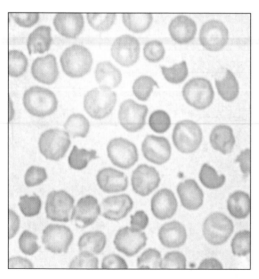

Fig. 4.61 Drug-induced haemolytic anaemia: peripheral blood film in a case associated with high-dosage dapsone therapy for dermatitis herpetiformis. The red cells show irregular contraction, target cells and cells with 'bites' out of the membrane. There is a single 'blister' cell in the lower central area of the field.

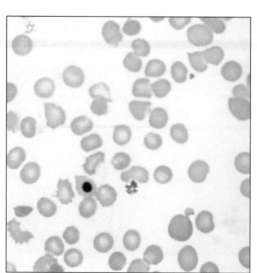

Fig. 4.62 Haemolytic anaemia in Wilson's disease: peripheral blood film showing polychromasia, target cells, spur cells (acanthocytes) and a normoblast. (Courtesy of Dr R Britt.)

chapter 5

Genetic Disorders of Haemoglobin

THALASSAEMIA

Globin synthesis depends on two gene clusters situated on chromosomes 11 and 16 (*Fig. 5.1*). Different haemoglobins dominate in the embryo, fetus and adult (*Fig. 5.2*). Each globin gene includes three coding regions, or exons, and two non-coding regions, called intervening sequences or introns. Globin molecules are synthesized from the appropriate genes via an RNA transcript. The genes all show two boxes, TATA and CCAAT, in the 5′ region, closely upstream in the flanking region, and further upstream sequences GGGGTG and CACCC; these all have important regulatory functions. There are promoter sequences involved in the initiation of transcriptions. At the 3′ non-coding region there is a sequence AATAAA, which is the signal for the mRNA to be cleaved. Further upstream of the β-globin cluster there is a key regulatory region, the locus control region (*Fig. 5.1*), which performs two functions. It

allows the β-globin cluster to transform from a transcriptionally inactive closed chromatin formation to an open transcriptionally active form. It also enhances transcription from the β-globin gene cluster. To do this, it binds erythroid specific (e.g. GATA-I, NF-E2) and ubiquitous trans-acting factors. The α-globin clusters also include an LCR-like region designated HS40, but it differs from the β LCR. Following transcription, the RNA is processed (spliced) to remove redundant RNA derived from introns situated within the coding part of each gene (*Fig. 5.3*). The exon–intron junctions have the sequence GT at their 5′ end and AG at their 3′ end; these sequences are essential for correct splicing. The messenger is modified by addition of a cap structure at the 5′ end and a series of adenylic acid residues [the poly(A)tail] at the 3′ end. The processed message moves to the cytoplasm, attaches to ribosomes and acts as a template for the addition of appropriate amino acids via their transfer RNAs. The amino acids link up to form the final polypeptide chain.

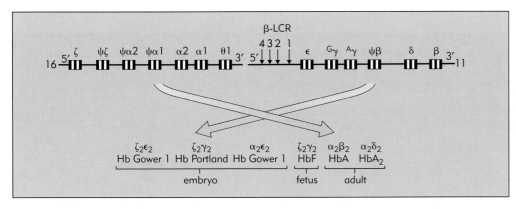

Fig. 5.1 Synthesis of haemoglobin: organization of the clusters of genes and their coding regions (exons, in black) for globin chain synthesis on chromosomes 11 and 16; non-coding regions (introns) occur between the exons. $^G\gamma$ and $^A\gamma$ are forms of the γ-globin gene that code for glutamic acid or alanine at position 136. (LCR, locus control region; adapted with permission from Weatherall DJ. Genetic disorders of haemoglobin. In: Hoffbrand AV, Lewis SM, Tuddenham EGD. *Postgraduate Haematology*, 4th edn. Oxford: Butterworth Heinemann, 1998:91–119.)

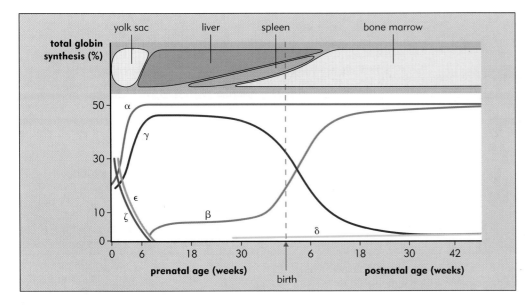

Fig. 5.2 Synthesis of haemoglobin: sites of globin chain synthesis in the embryo, fetus and adult. (Adapted with permission from Hoffbrand AV, Pettit JE. *Essential Haematology*, 3rd edn. Oxford: Blackwell Scientific Publications; 1993.)

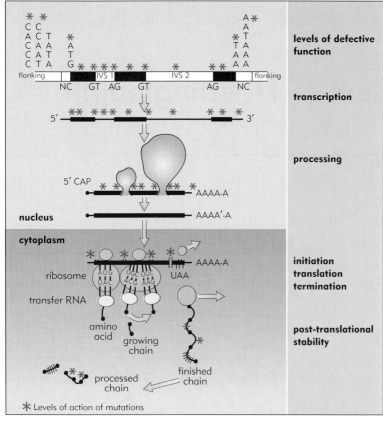

Fig. 5.3 Synthesis of haemoglobin: stages in the synthesis of β-globin from DNA to the final polypeptide chain. (IVS, intervening sequence; A, adenine; C, cytosine; G, guanine; T, thymine; adapted with permission from Weatherall DJ. Genetic disorders of haemoglobin. In: Hoffbrand AV, Lewis SM, Tuddenham EGD. *Postgraduate Haematology*, 4th edn. Oxford: Butterworth Heinemann, 1998:91–119.)

Each molecule of haemoglobin consists of four globin chains (*Fig. 5.4*). In normal adults, haemoglobin (Hb) A (α_2, β_2) forms 96–97% of the haemoglobin. The thalassaemias are a group of disorders in which the underlying abnormality is reduced synthesis of either the α or β chains of haemoglobin A (*Fig. 5.5*). The global distribution of thalassaemia and the frequency of different mutations in Mediterranean populations are shown in *Fig. 5.6*. The fall in the incidence of the disease following antenatal diagnosis is shown in *Fig. 5.7*.

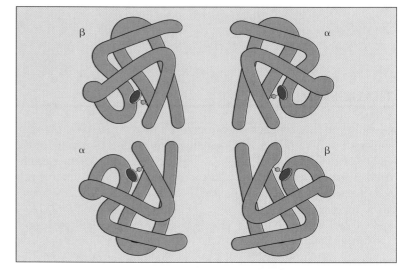

Fig. 5.4 Synthesis of haemoglobin: the haemoglobin tetramer – in this example, Hb A.

Classifications of thalassaemias

Classification of thalassaemias I	Classification of thalassaemias II			
Clinical	**α-Thalassaemias**			
Thalassaemia major	Designation	Haplotype	Heterozygous	Homozygous
Transfusion-dependent homozygous β⁰-thalassaemia	α⁰-Thalassaemia	– – /	α⁰-Thalassaemia; MCH, MCV low	Hydrops fetalis
Homozygous β⁺-thalassaemia (some types)	Dysfunctional α-thalassaemia	– α⁰/	α⁰-Thalassaemia; MCH, MCV low	Hydrops fetalis
Thalassaemia intermedia	α⁺-Thalassaemia	– α/	α⁺-Thalassaemia; minimal, if any, haematological abnormality	As heterozygous α⁰-thalassaemia
Mild forms of compound β⁺ α⁺ β⁰/β⁺ thalassaemia				
Haemoglobin Lepore syndromes	Non-deletion α-thalassaemia	α α̲/	Variable	Hb H disease in some cases
Homozygous δβ-thalassaemia and hereditary persistence of fetal haemoglobin	Hb-Constant Spring (CS)	α α̲/	0.5–1% Hb CS	More severe than heterozygous α⁰-thalassaemia
Combinations of α- and β⁺-thalassaemias	The combination of α⁰-thalassaemia (or dysfunctional α-thalassaemia) and α⁺-thalassaemia gives rise to Hb H disease			
Heterozygous β-thalassaemia with triplicated α genes				
Dominant β-thalassaemia	**Classification of thalassaemias III**			
Heterozygosity for β-thalassaemia and β chain variants (e.g. Hb E/β-thalassaemia)	**β-Thalassaemias**			
Haemoglobin H disease	Type	Heterozygous		Homozygous
Thalassaemia minor	β⁰	Thalassaemia minor; Hb A₂ >3.5%		Thalassaemia major; Hb F 98%; Hb A₂ 2%; no Hb A
β⁰-Thalassaemia trait	β⁺	Thalassaemia minor; Hb A₂ >3.5%		Thalassaemia major or intermedia; Hb F 70–80%; Hb A 10–20%; Hb A₂ variable
δβ-Thalassaemia trait				
Hereditary persistence of fetal haemoglobin	δβ hereditary persistence of fetal haemoglobin	Thalassaemia minor; Hb F >5–20%; Hb A₂ normal or low		Thalassaemia intermedia; Hb F 100%
β⁺-Thalassaemia trait				
α⁰-Thalassaemia trait	Hb Lepore	Thalassaemia minor; Hb A >80–90%; Hb Lepore 10%; Hb A₂ reduced		Thalassaemia major or intermedia; Hb F 80%; Hb Lepore 10–20%; Hb A, Hb A₂ absent
α⁺-Thalassaemia trait				

Fig. 5.5 Classification of the thalassaemia disorders: clinical, α-thalassaemias, and β-thalassaemias. (MCV, mean corpuscular volume; MCH, mean corpuscular haemoglobin; Hb, haemoglobin.)

The α-thalassaemias are classified according to the number of α genes affected There is duplication of the α-globin genes. In the α⁰ lesion, both α genes on one chromosome are deleted or ineffective; in the milder α⁺ lesion, only one of the two genes is deleted or defective (*Fig. 5.8*).

β-Thalassaemia is divided into three types:
- homozygous (major) form, in which there is complete or almost complete absence of β-globin chain synthesis;
- heterozygous (minor) or trait form, in which synthesis of only one β chain is reduced; and
- clinically intermediate form, which can be a mild form of homozygous β-thalassaemia, the result of interaction of β-thalassaemia

with other haemoglobinopathies, or an unusually severe form of β-thalassaemia trait.

In general, β-thalassaemias are the result of point mutations in or near the globin genes that cause, for example, defective splicing, premature stop codons, nonsense lesions and frameshift changes (*Fig. 5.9*). Gene deletion may also cause β-thalassaemias (*Fig. 5.10*), but is more common in the α-thalassaemias (*see Fig. 5.59*). Over 180 different genetic lesions have been detected in the β-thalassaemias.

β-Thalassaemia major

The clinical features of β-thalassaemia major result from a severe anaemia combined with an intense increase in erythropoiesis, largely

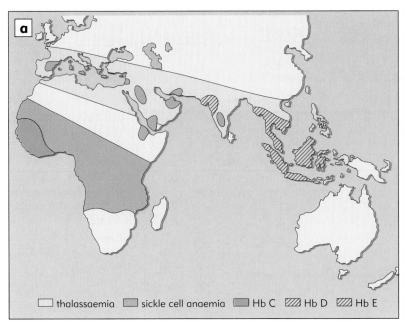

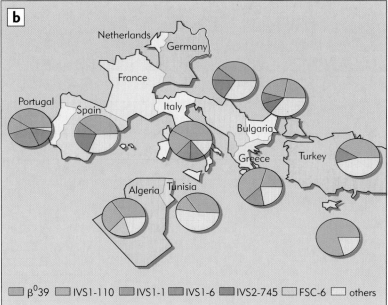

Fig. 5.6a and b Distribution of thalassaemia disorders: (a) The geographical distribution of thalassaemia, sickle cell anaemia, and the other common haemoglobin disorders. It is likely that the carriers of these disorders have a selective advantage against malaria compared with normal individuals. The disorders are also found in other parts of the world where emigrants from areas of higher incidence have settled. (b) Frequency of different mutations of β-thalassaemia in Mediterranean at-risk populations. (IVS 1, IVS 2, introns 1 or 2 of β-globin gene; 1, 6, 39, 110, 745, mutations of corresponding codons; FSC-6, frameshift mutation-6; courtesy of Prof. Anthony Cao.)

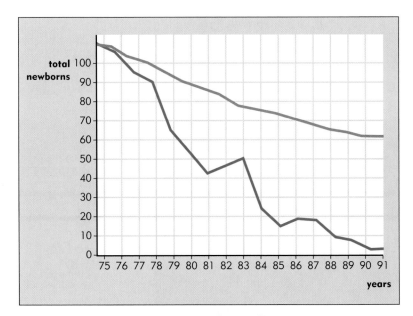

Fig. 5.7 β-Thalassaemia: fall in the birth rate of homozygous β-thalassaemia in Sardinia since the introduction of genetic counselling and antenatal diagnosis. The upper curve shows the predicted number of births without antenatal diagnosis, and the lower curve the actual number. (Courtesy of Prof. Anthony Cao.)

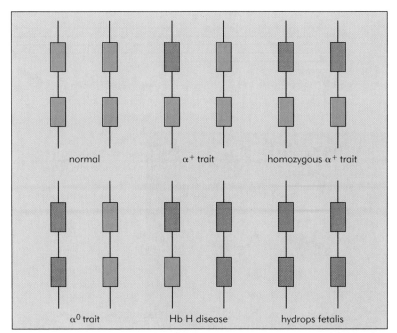

Fig. 5.8 α-Thalassaemia: the different types of α-thalassaemia. The purple boxes represent normal genes while the grey ones represent gene deletions or partially or completely inactivated genes.

ineffective, with excessive bone marrow activity and extramedullary haemopoiesis. In the poorly transfused patient there is expansion of the flat bones of the face and skull (*Figs 5.11–5 14*) and expansion of the marrow in all bones (*Fig. 5.15*). There may be gross osteoporosis and premature fusion of the epiphyses (*Fig. 5.16*). Even in well-transfused and -chelated patients, osteoporosis is frequent (*Figs 5.17* and *5.18*), especially in males and in association with diabetes mellitus and a failure of spontaneous puberty.

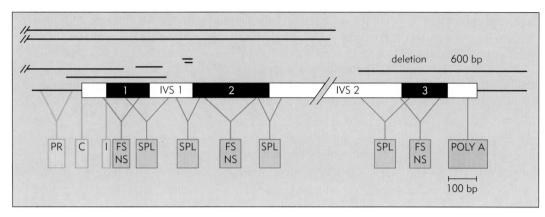

Fig. 5.9 β-Thalassaemia: the classes of mutations that underlie β-thalassaemia. The 600 base pair deletion may also cause β-thalassaemia. Other rare deletions may occur that affect the β-globin gene, the β and δ genes, or the γ, δ and β genes (*Fig. 5.10*). [PR, promoter; C, CAP site; I, initiation codon; FS, frameshift; NS, nonsense (premature chain termination) mutation; SPL, splicing mutation; POLY A, polyA addition site mutation; courtesy of Prof. DJ Weatherall.]

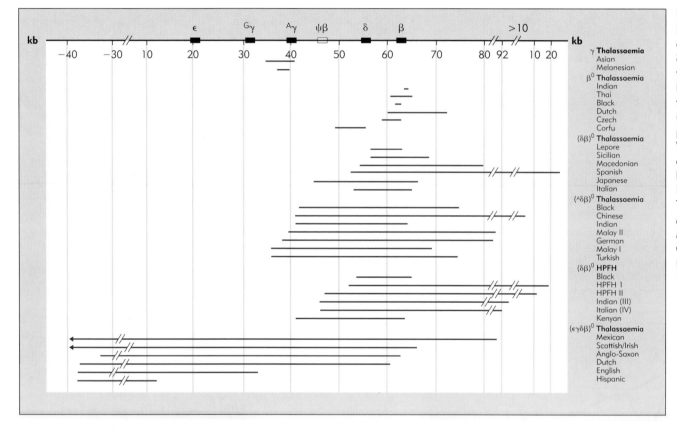

Fig. 5.10 β-Thalassaemia: the deletions that underlie δβ- and εγδβ-thalassaemias and hereditary persistence of fetal haemoglobin. (Adapted with permission from Weatherall DJ. Genetic disorders of haemoglobin. In: Hoffbrand AV, Lewis SM, Tuddenham EGD. *Postgraduate Haematology*, 4th edn. Oxford: Butterworth Heinemann, 1998:91–119.)

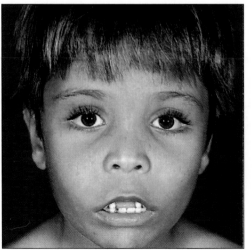

Fig. 5.11 β-Thalassaemia major: characteristic facies of a 7-year-old Middle Eastern boy includes prominent maxilla and widening of the bridge of the nose. There is also marked bossing of the frontal and parietal bones and zygomata, giving a mongoloid appearance.

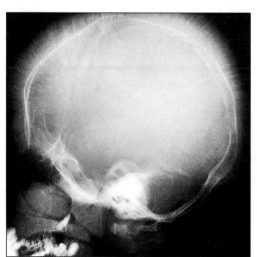

Fig. 5.12 β-Thalassaemia major: lateral radiograph of the skull (same case as shown in *Fig. 5.11*) shows the typical 'hair-on-end' appearance, with thinning of the cortical bone and widening of the marrow cavity.

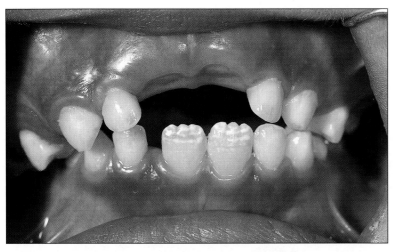

Fig. 5.13 β-Thalassaemia major: the teeth (same case as shown in *Fig. 5.11*) are splayed because of widening of the maxilla and mandible.

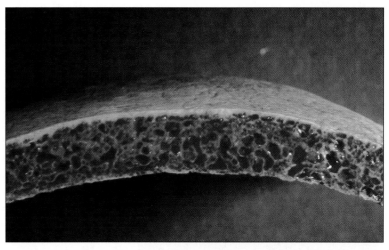

Fig. 5.14 β-Thalassaemia major: section through the skull at necropsy shows marked thinning of the cortices and an open porotic cancellous bone. The mahogany brown colour results from extensive iron deposition (haemosiderin), in the marrow. (Courtesy of Dr PG Bullough and Dr VJ Vigorita.)

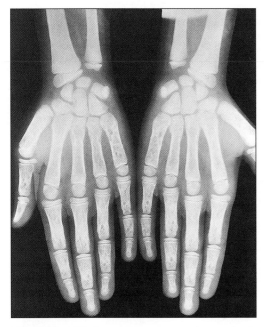

Fig. 5.15 β-Thalassaemia major: radiograph of the hands of an undertransfused 7-year-old child. Thinning of the cortical bone results from expansion of the marrow space.

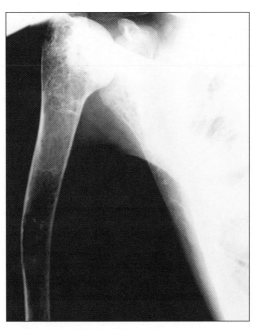

Fig. 5.16 β-Thalassaemia major: severe osteoporosis and premature fusion of humeral epiphysis in an undertransfused patient. (Courtesy of Dr B Wonke.)

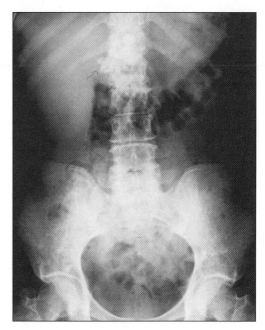

Fig. 5.17 β-Thalassaemia major: severe osteoporosis in a patient 30 years of age. Osteoporosis is more common in males, in patients with diabetes mellitus and in those with failed puberty. (Courtesy of Dr B Wonke.)

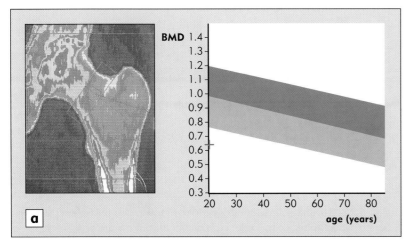

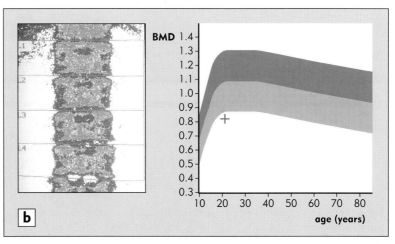

Fig. 5.18a and b β-Thalassaemia major: bone density scans of (a) hip and (b) lumbar vertebrae. The bands represent 1.5 standard deviation above and below the mean age-specific bone mineral density (BMD). The red crosses indicate the patient's results. (Courtesy of Dr B Wonke.)

Spontaneous fractures may occur. Another feature is enlargement of the liver and spleen (*Figs 5.19 and 5.20*), mainly because of extramedullary erythropoiesis, but also from excessive breakdown of red cells and iron overload.

The peripheral blood in the poorly transfused patient shows the presence of hypochromic cells, target cells and nucleated red cells (*Fig. 5.21*). Following splenectomy red cell inclusions increase (for example, iron granules and Howell–Jolly bodies) and the platelet count is high (*Fig. 5.22*). The bone marrow shows red cell hyperplasia with pink-staining inclusions of precipitated α-globin chains in the cytoplasm of erythroblasts (*Fig. 5.23*). Many of the erythroblasts die in the marrow and are digested by macrophages. There is increased iron in the macrophages and increased iron granules in developing erythroblasts (*Fig. 5.24*).

Much of the bone abnormality can be prevented by regular transfusions from the age of presentation (usually 6 months) to maintain the haemoglobin at all times at a level above 9–10 g/dl. However, these regular transfusions, together with increased iron absorption, lead to iron overload. Each unit of blood contains 200–250 mg iron. After 50 units have been transfused, or earlier in children, siderosis develops, with increased pigmentation of skin exposed to light (*Fig. 5.25*) and susceptibility to infection (*Fig. 5.26*), reduced growth and delayed sexual development and puberty (*Fig. 5.27*).

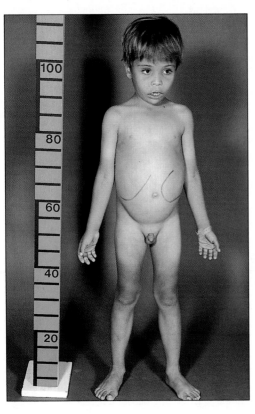

Fig. 5.19 β-Thalassaemia major: overall view of the boy shown in *Fig. 5.11*, showing enlargement of the liver and spleen, and stunted growth. The child had been inadequately transfused since presenting with anaemia at the age of 4 months.

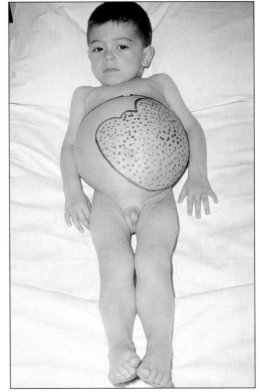

Fig. 5.20 β-Thalassaemia major: this 4-year-old, inadequately transfused Cypriot boy has enlargement of the spleen to an unusual degree, which may be partly reversed by adequate transfusion. Splenectomy is usually required, but should usually be delayed until the child is older than 6 years of age to reduce the incidence of postoperative fatal infection.

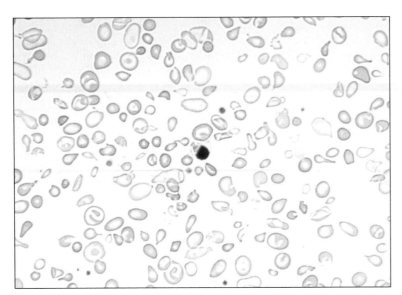

Fig. 5.21 β-Thalassaemia major: peripheral blood film showing prominent hypochromic microcytic cells, target cells and an erythroblast. Some normochromic cells are present from a previous blood transfusion.

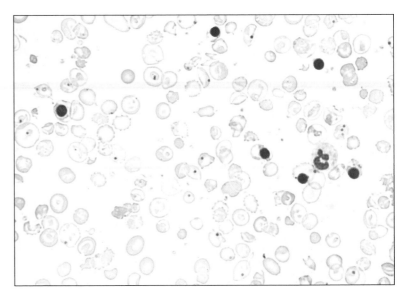

Fig. 5.22 β-Thalassaemia major: peripheral blood film postsplenectomy in which hypochromic cells, target cells and erythroblasts are prominent. Pappenheimer and Howell–Jolly bodies are also seen and the platelet count is raised.

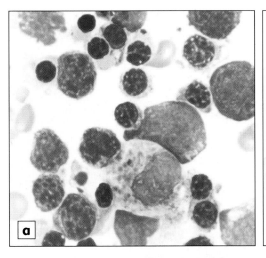

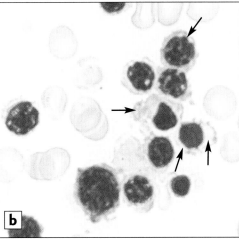

Fig. 5.23a and b β-Thalassaemia major: bone marrow aspirates showing (a) marked erythroid hyperplasia and erythroblasts with vacuolated cytoplasm; degenerate forms and a macrophage that contains pigment are present. (b) Erythroblasts with pink-staining cytoplasmic inclusions ('haemoglobin lakes', arrowed), precipitates of excess α-globin chains.

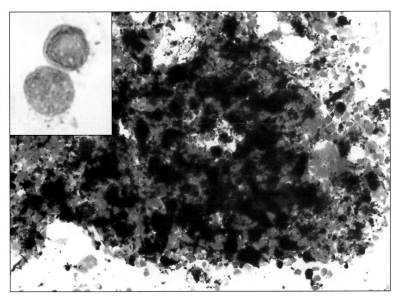

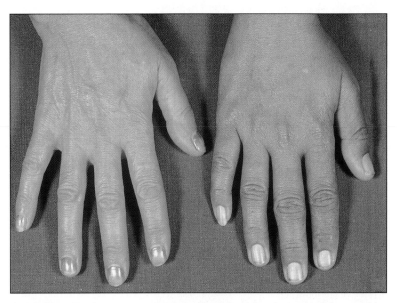

Fig. 5.24 β-Thalassaemia major: low power view of bone marrow fragment showing grossly increased iron stores, largely contained in macrophages as haemosiderin and (seen on electron microscopy) as ferritin. Bone marrow erythroblasts show prominent coarse iron granules (inset). (Perls' stain.)

Fig. 5.25 β-Thalassaemia major: the hand on the right is of a 16-year-old male patient and shows heavy melanin pigmentation; in contrast, his mother's hand (on the left) shows normal coloration. For comparison with the appearance of an adult male with genetic (primary) haemochromatosis *see Fig. 2.54.*

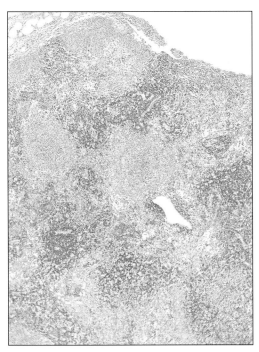

Fig. 5.26
β-Thalassaemia major: mesenteric adenitis caused by *Yersinia enterocolitica* infection. The lymph node contains large numbers of granulomas with central necrosis. In keeping with the severity of the disease the necrosis is more marked than that usually seen. The infection is particularly common in patients with iron overload. (Courtesy of Dr J Dyson.)

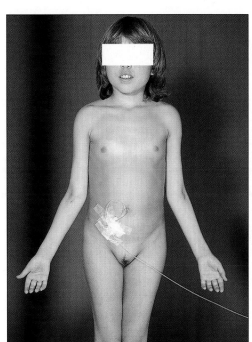

Fig. 5.27
β-Thalassaemia major: this 17-year-old girl shows reduced stature (height 134 cm) and delayed pubertal development. Since circulating growth hormone levels are usually normal, the lack of growth results from 'end-organ' failure. Subcutaneous infusion of desferrioxamine is in progress.

Bone development is delayed and abnormal (*Figs 5.28–5.30*). Damage and iron overloading occurs in the pancreas (*Figs 5.31 and 5.32*), often with diabetes mellitus, liver (*Figs 5.31, 5.33 and 5.34*) and myocardium (*Figs 5.35 and 5.36*), as well as damage to the other endocrine organs, particularly the hypothalamus, pituitary, thyroid and parathyroids (*Fig. 5.37*). Iron deposition may occur in bone (*Fig. 5.38*). Liver damage may also occur because of viral hepatitis from repeated transfusions (*Fig. 5.39*).

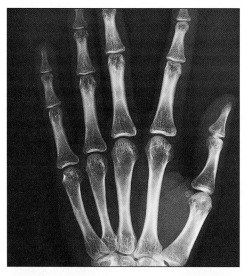

Fig. 5.28 β-Thalassaemia major: radiograph of the hand of a 19-year-old man. The estimated bone age is 14 years and there is failure of epiphyseal closure. Widening of the marrow cavity and thinning of trabeculae and cortex are also seen.

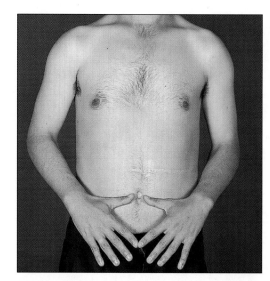

Fig. 5.29 β-Thalassaemia major: shortening of the upper arms because of premature epiphyseal closure of the humeral heads.

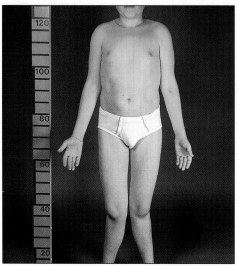

Fig. 5.30 β-Thalassaemia major: genu valgum deformity.

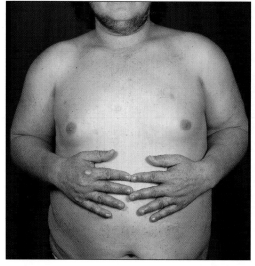

Fig. 5.31 β-Thalassaemia major: patient aged 37 years who had followed an intermedia course for 25 years but then required regular blood transfusions. Heavy melanin pigmentation, a spider naevus, gynaecomastia and a splenectomy scar are seen. He had diabetes mellitus, cirrhosis, hypothyroidism and hypoparathyroidism.

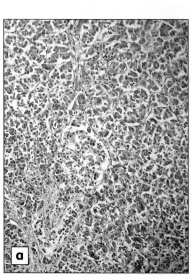
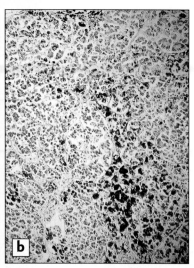

Fig. 5.32a and b β-Thalassaemia major: postmortem sections of pancreas showing (a) pigment (haemosiderin and lipofuscin) in acinar cells, macrophages and connective tissue, with less obvious pigment in the islet cells; and (b) gross iron (haemosiderin) deposits in all cell types, particularly marked in the acinar cells. [(a) H & E, and (b) Perls' stain.]

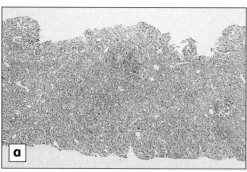
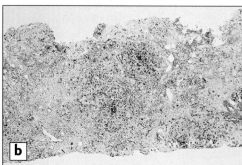

Fig. 5.33 a and b β-Thalassaemia major: needle biopsy of liver showing (a) disturbances of normal architecture with fibrosis in portal tracts and nodular regeneration of hepatic parenchymal cells; and (b) Grade IV siderosis with iron deposition in the hepatic parenchymal cells, bile duct epithelium, macrophages and fibroblasts. [(a) H & E, and (b) Perls' stain.]

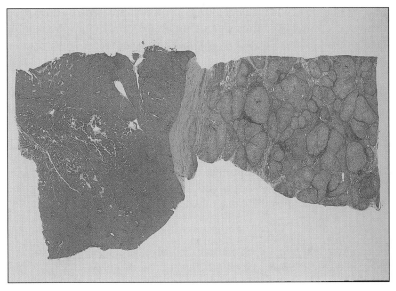

Fig. 5.34 β-Thalassaemia major: postmortem section taken from the liver of a 27-year-old male patient dying of hepatocellular carcinoma (on the left), with pre-existing hepatic cirrhosis (on the right) and hepatitis C infection. (Courtesy of Dr B Wonke.)

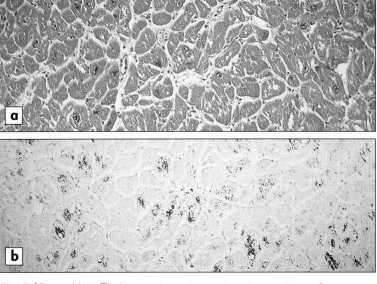

Fig. 5.35a and b β-Thalassaemia major: postmortem sections of myocardium seen by (a) H & E and (b) Perls' staining. The individual muscle fibres contain heavy deposits of iron pigment. In transfusional iron overload, iron deposition is most marked in the left ventricle (shown here) and interventricular septum.

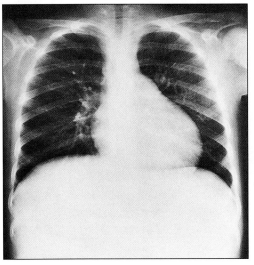

Fig. 5.36 β-Thalassaemia major: chest radiograph showing cardiomegaly caused by chronic anaemia and iron overload. Enlargement occurs mainly in the ventricles and interventricular septum.

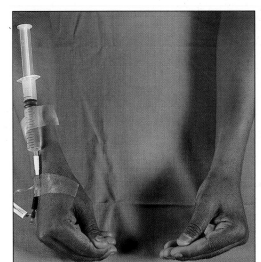

Fig. 5.37 β-Thalassaemia major: tetany (Trousseau's sign) caused by hypoparathyroidism caused by transfusional iron overload. An infusion of calcium is in progress. (Courtesy of Dr B Wonke.)

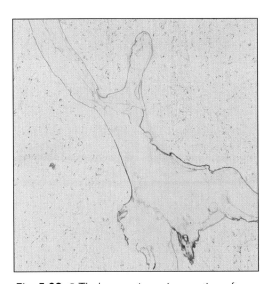

Fig. 5.38 β-Thalassaemia major: section of bone showing iron deposition in the cement lines of the trabecula and in macrophages (as haemosiderin) throughout the bone marrow. (Courtesy of Dr PG Bullough and Dr VJ Vigorita.)

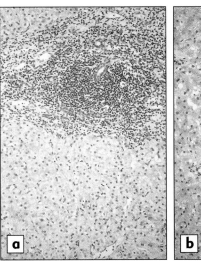
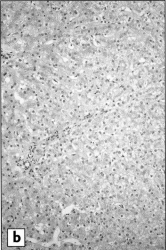
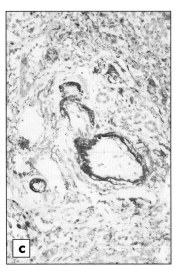

Fig. 5.39a–c β-Thalassaemia major: (a) liver biopsy showing heavy infiltration of portal tracts by lymphocytes. The serum was positive for hepatitis C RNA. Following 6 months' therapy with α-interferon there was considerable improvement in hepatic function and (b) liver biopsy showed clearing of the lymphocyte infiltration. (c) Liver biopsy showing heavy siderosis in parenchymal cells and in walls of vessels and sinuses (ferrocalcinosis). [(a, b) H & E, and (c) Perls' stain.]

Iron overload may, however, be substantially reduced by daily subcutaneous desferrioxamine infusions (*see Fig. 5.27*). The iron is then excreted as ferrioxamine in the urine, which appears red, and in bile.

Complications of desferrioxamine therapy may include ototoxicity with high tone deafness, retinal damage (*Fig. 5.40*) and, in children, 'pseudo' rickets changes in the bones (*Fig. 5.41*) or spinal platyspondylosis, in some cases with intervertebral calcification (*Fig. 5.42*), which may be accompanied by reduced growth. Alternative orally acting iron chelators are undergoing clinical trials. One of these, 1,2-dimethyl-3-hydroxypyrid-4-one (L_1, CP20, deferiprone) has been given to over 1000 patients for periods up to 10 years. It has proved effective at causing iron excretion (*Fig. 5.43*). Side effects that have occurred include agranulocytosis, joint pains or effusions, and (rarely) zinc deficiency (*Fig. 5.44*).

Splenectomy may be needed to reduce transfusion requirements. Other supportive measures include folic acid, hepatitis immunization and pneumococcal haemophilus and meningococcal immunization, plus regular prophylactic penicillin. Hormonal replacement therapy is needed in some cases, and calcium, vitamin D and biphosphonate for osteoporosis. Thalassaemia major may also be cured by bone marrow transplantation (*Fig. 5.45*).

β-Thalassaemia intermedia

The causes are listed in *Fig. 5.5*. One form results from homozygous haemoglobin Lepore (*Fig. 5.46*) or heterozygous Lepore in conjunction with another β chain abnormality. β-Thalassaemia intermedia is compatible with normal growth and development (*Fig. 5.47*), but is characterized by bone deformities (*Fig. 5.48*), extramedullary haemopoiesis (*Fig. 5.49*) and iron overload. Ankle ulcers (*Fig. 5.50*), probably the result of anoxia caused by anaemia and stasis of the local circulation, may arise as in thalassaemia major, sickle cell anaemia and other haemolytic anaemias.

Iron overload because of increased absorption and blood transfusion is treated by chelation and possible gentle venesections.

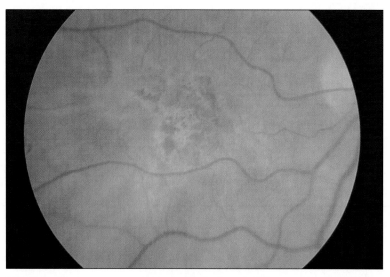

Fig. 5.40 Desferrioxamine toxicity: optic fundus of a 78-year-old man with primary acquired sideroblastic anaemia (myelodysplasia) and transfusional iron overload receiving desferrioxamine (2 g) subcutaneously daily and intravenously with blood transfusions. He complained of night blindness and loss of visual acuity. There is degeneration with hyperpigmentation of the macula.

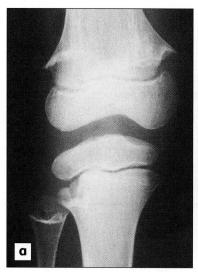
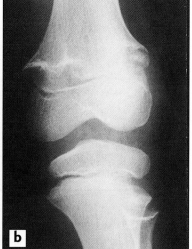

Fig. 5.41a and b Desferrioxamine toxicity: (a, b) pseudorickets in the knees of a child with β-thalassaemia major receiving desferrioxamine therapy. There is flaring of the metaphyses and poor mineralization of the distal metaphyses with normal epiphyses. (Courtesy of Dr V DeSanctis.)

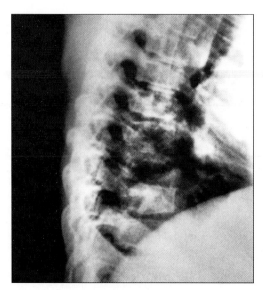

Fig. 5.42 Desferrioxamine toxicity: intervertebral calcification and platyspondylosis of the spine. (Courtesy of Dr B Wonke.)

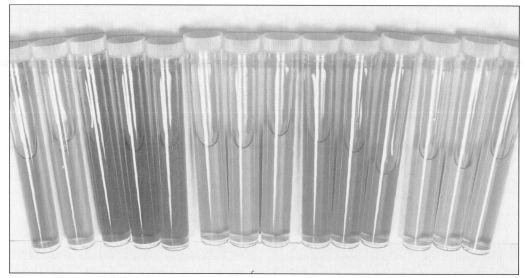

Fig. 5.43 Myelodysplastic syndrome: urine samples without (yellow) and with chelation therapy for transfusional iron overload. Subcutaneous desferrioxamine has resulted in orange urine, whereas oral 1,2-dimethyl-3-hydroxypyrid-4-one (deferiprone) has resulted in a darker, red urine. (Courtesy of Dr G Kontoghiorghes.)

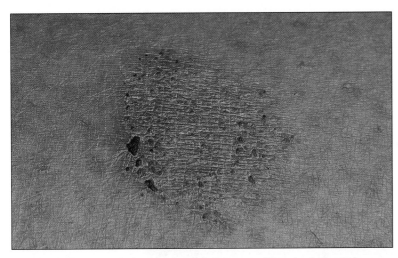

Fig. 5.44 Oral iron chelation: zinc deficiency causing raised, dry, itchy scaling patch in patient receiving deferiprone (L₁) long term.

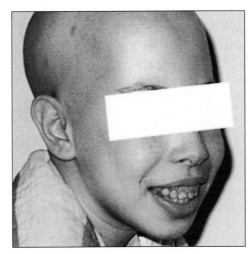

Fig. 5.45 β-Thalassaemia major: 14-year-old girl, after marrow transplantation from an HLA-matched sibling, shows hair loss as a result of chemotherapy, and bossing of the skull. (Courtesy of Prof. C Luccarelli.)

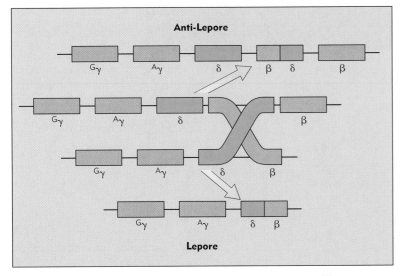

Fig. 5.46 Structure of haemoglobin-Lepore and anti-Lepore. These structural abnormalities are caused by crossing over of the δ- and β-globin genes at meiosis.

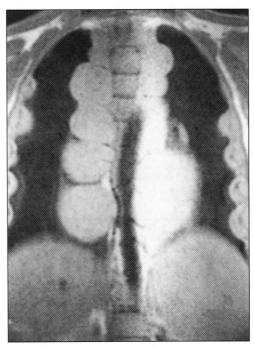

Fig. 5.47 β-Thalassaemia intermedia: this 29-year-old Cypriot patient had received occasional blood transfusions, with her haemoglobin ranging between 6.5 and 9.0 g/dl. She displays a thalassaemic facies with marked maxillary expansion, and had also developed pigment gallstones. She has normal sexual development and fertility, as shown by her 2-year-old son.

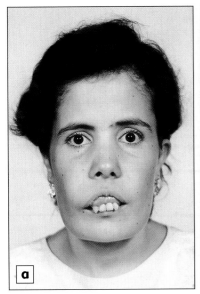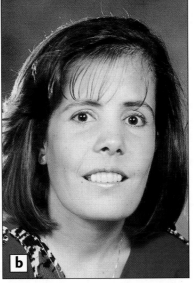

Fig. 5.48a and b β-Thalassaemia intermedia: facial bone deformities in a 20-year-old woman; (a) before surgery, (b) after surgical correction. [(a, b) Courtesy Dr B Wonke.]

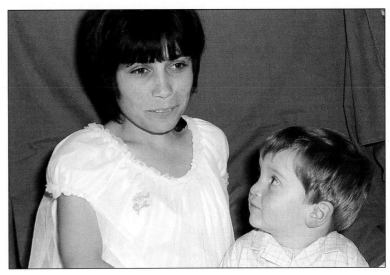

Fig. 5.49 β-Thalassaemia intermedia: magnetic resonance imaging (MRI) scan from a 42-year-old Turkish patient with bossing of the skull bones, maxillary expansion and splenomegaly (Hb, 9.7 g/dl; MCV, 78 fl; MCH, 23.5 pg; haemoglobin electrophoresis – Hb F, 98%; Hb A₂, 2.0%). The scan shows masses of extramedullary haemopoietic tissue arising from the ribs and in the paravertebral region without encroachment of the spinal cord.

β-Thalassaemia trait

In β-thalassaemia trait there is a hypochromic microcytic blood picture with a high red cell count (above 5.5×10^{12}/l; *Figs 5.51 and 5.52*) and raised haemoglobin A_2 percentage on haemoglobin electrophoresis.

β-Thalassaemia with a dominant phenotype

β-Thalassaemia with a dominant phenotype refers to a sub-group of β-thalassaemias that result in a thalassaemia intermedia phenotype in individuals who have inherited only a single copy of the abnormal β gene. Usually mutations affect exon 3 of the β-globin gene (*Fig. 5.53*). There is production of long unstable globin-gene protein, which, together with excess α chains, produces inclusions in normoblasts and red cells. The clinical features are those of a severe dyserythropoietic anaemia associated with splenomegaly. The inclusion bodies are seen in the bone marrow and in peripheral red cells after splenectomy (*Fig. 5.54*). These inclusion bodies could be visualized after methyl violet staining of fresh blood. A spectrum of different mutations underlying these dominantly inherited forms of β-thalassaemia have been identified and it is now clear that the phenotype of these disorders overlaps both the β-thalassaemias and the unstable haemoglobin variants. (*See* Thein SL. Dominantly inherited β-thalassaemia: molecular basis and pathophysiology. *Br J Haematol.* 1992;80:273–7.)

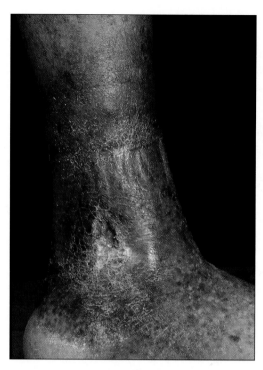

Fig. 5.50 β-Thalassaemia intermedia: ankle ulcer above the lateral malleolus.

Blood count in β-thalassaemia trait	
Haemoglobin	10.8 g/dl
Red blood cells	5.81×10^{12}/l
Packed cell volume	35%
Mean corpuscular volume	60.3 fl
Mean corpuscular haemoglobin	18.6 pg
Reticulocytes	1.8%
White blood cells	6.3×10^9/l
Platelets	288×10^9/l

Fig. 5.51 β-Thalassaemia trait: blood count in a woman (see *Fig. 5.52*).

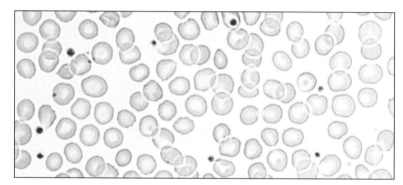

Fig. 5.52 β-Thalassaemia trait: peripheral blood film from a 20-year-old Cypriot woman shows microcytic hypochromic red cells with occasional target cells and poikilocytes. The red cell indices show a much reduced MCV (60.3 fl) and MCH (18.6 pg), despite the levels of the haemoglobin (10.8 g/dl) and packed cell volume (PCV, 35%) being only slightly below normal. The red cell count was raised to 5.81×10^{12}/l and haemoglobin electrophoresis showed a raised haemoglobin A_2 (4.5%) with a normal haemoglobin F (0.9%).

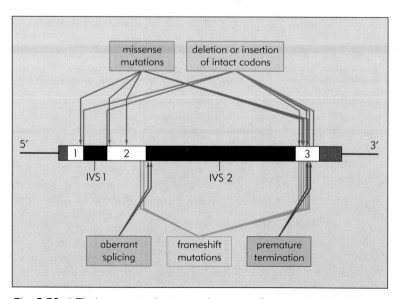

Fig. 5.53 β-Thalassaemia: dominant phenotype. Dominantly inherited β-thalassaemia. (Courtesy of Dr SL Thein.)

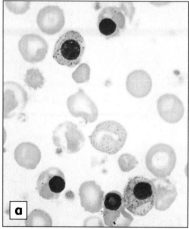
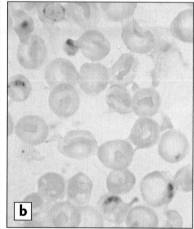

Fig. 5.54a and b β-Thalassaemia: dominant phenotype. Peripheral blood postsplenectomy: (a) May–Grünwald/Giemsa stain showing target cells, irregular contracted cells, punctate basophilia and numerous erythroblasts; (b) methyl violet stain showing inclusion bodies (pink) caused by precipitated α-globin chains. [(a, b) Courtesy of Dr SL Thein.]

Antenatal diagnosis

If both parents are carriers, fetal diagnosis is carried out, either using fetoscopy to obtain blood (*Fig. 5.55a*) and measuring the α/β chain synthesis ratio, or by amniocentesis or trophoblast biopsy (*Fig. 5.55b*) to obtain DNA for hybridization with relevant DNA probes (*Fig. 5.56*) or for analysis by one or other polymerase chain reaction (PCR) techniques (*Fig. 5.57*). These include analysis by direct restriction enzyme analysis, restriction fragment length polymorphism (RFLP) analysis (*Fig. 5.58*), use of oligonucleotide probes with radioactivity or horseradish peroxidase labelling, mismatched PCR amplification or other techniques. A homozygous fetus can then be aborted.

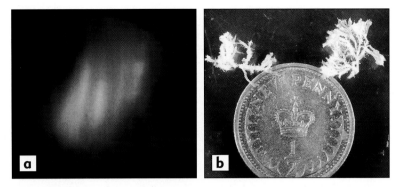

Fig. 5.55a and b Antenatal diagnosis: (a) fetal veins at 14 weeks, as seen through a fetoscope; (b) chorionic villus biopsy from a 12-week-old fetus. [Courtesy of (a) Mr C Rodeck and (b) Mr JW Keeling.]

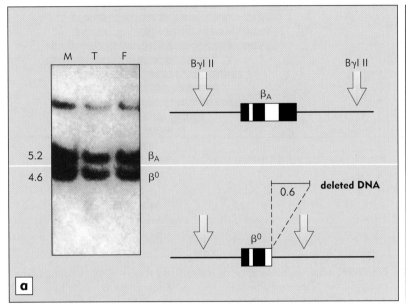

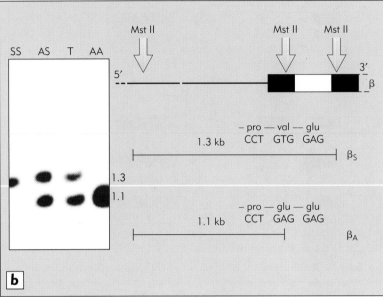

Fig. 5.56a and b Antenatal diagnosis: (a) restriction enzyme analysis of trophoblast DNA in Indian β⁰-thalassaemia. After digestion of DNA by the restriction enzyme Bgl II, the fragments are separated according to size by electrophoresis in agarose gel, transferred to nitrocellulose and a radioactive β-gene probe is added. Autoradiography shows hybridization to a 5.2 kb fragment when the chromosome contains a normal β_A gene, but to a 4.6 kb fragment on a chromosome carrying Indian β⁰ gene because of deletion of a 0.6 kb fragment. In this case, the fetus, like both parents, has β⁰ trait. (M, mother; T, trophoblast; F, father.) (b) In sickle cell anaemia DNA has been digested by Mst II. An adenine base in the normal β-globin gene is replaced by thymine in the sickle β-globin gene, removing a normal restriction site for Mst II and producing a 1.3 kb fragment which hybridizes with the β-globin gene probe. In this case, as the trophoblast DNA shows both normal (A) and sickle (S) restriction fragments, the fetus is AS (in other words, a sickle carrier). (Courtesy of Dr J Old and The Royal College of Obstetrics and Gynaecology.)

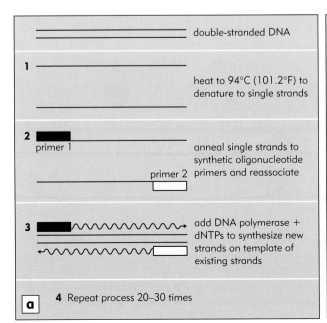

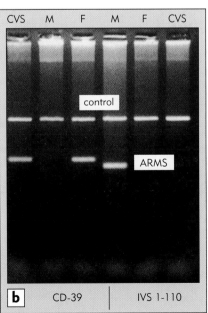

Fig. 5.57a and b α-Thalassaemia: antenatal diagnosis. (a) Polymerase chain reaction. Two primers are used, hybridizing to DNA on either side of the section of DNA to be amplified. Cycles of synthesis of new DNA using a heat-resistant DNA Taq polymerase and deoxynucleoside triphosphates (dNTPs), denaturation and synthesis of new DNA result in rapid amplification of the DNA over a million times. (b) The rapid prenatal diagnosis of β-thalassaemia by 'mismatched PCR' amplification refractory mutation system (ARMS). One parent has the common Mediterranean codon 39 (CD-39) mutation, the other the IVS1-110 G→A mutation. The fetus is heterozygous for the CD-39 mutation. (CVS, fetal DNA from chorionic villus sampling; F, father; M, mother; courtesy of Dr J Old and Prof. D Weatherall and modified from Hoffbrand AV, Pettit JE. *Essential Haematology*, 3rd edn. Oxford: Blackwell Scientific Publications; 1993.)

α-Thalassaemia

The gene deletions that produce α-thalassaemia are shown in *Fig. 5.59*. In its most severe form, in which all four genes are deleted, α-thalassaemia is incompatible with life and the fetus is stillborn or critically ill with hydrops fetalis (*Fig. 5.60*). The blood shows gross hypochromia and erythroblastosis (*Fig. 5.61*).

Deletion of three α-genes (haemoglobin H disease) presents as a moderately severe anaemia (Hb, 7.0–11.0 g/dl) with splenomegaly and a

hypochromic, microcytic blood film appearance (*Fig. 5.62*). Haemoglobin H (β_4) is demonstrable by special staining (*Fig. 5.63*) or haemoglobin electrophoresis.

α-Thalassaemia trait may be caused by deletion of two genes (α^0 trait). α^+ Trait may result from deletion of one of the pair of linked α-globin genes. In others both α genes are present, but one has a mutation or other genetic effect which partly or completely inactivates it. α-Thalassaemia trait shows a hypochromic, microcytic blood appearance

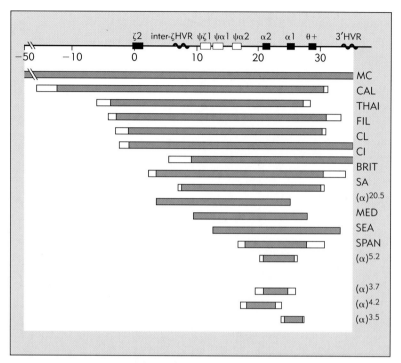

Fig. 5.58 α-Thalassaemia: restriction fragment length polymorphism analysis. A new restriction enzyme site, resulting from a polymorphic change in DNA close to a gene to be studied, reduces the size of the fragment of DNA produced by a restriction enzyme. The DNA is separated in a gel and the smaller size fragment is detected after using a probe for the gene. The size of fragment may also be different if the DNA close to the gene and between restriction sites contains a region that is hypervariable in size between individuals. The PCR technique can also be used instead of Southern blotting to detect RFLPs, providing primers on either side of the segment to be analyzed are available. (Modified from Hoffbrand AV, Pettit JE. *Essential Haematology*, 3rd edn. Oxford: Blackwell Scientific Publications; 1993.)

Fig. 5.59 α-Thalassaemia: the deletions that produce α-thalassaemia. The missing DNA is indicated by black lines. α^0-Thalassaemia results from deletion of both linked α-globin genes or mutations that completely inactivate both (not shown). α^+-Thalassaemia results from either deletion of one of the pair of linked α-globin genes or from a mutation that inactivates one of them partly or completely. One mutation affects the chain termination codon TAA and results in an elongated α chain (Haemoglobin Constant Spring) which is synthesized at a slower rate than normal. (Courtesy of Prof. DJ Weatherall.)

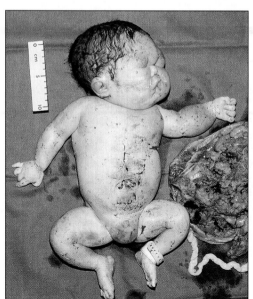

Fig. 5.60 α-Thalassaemia: hydrops fetalis, the result of deletion of all four α-globin genes (homozygous α^0-thalassaemia). The main haemoglobin present is Hb Bart's (γ_4). The condition is incompatible with life beyond the fetal stage. (Courtesy of Prof. D Todd.)

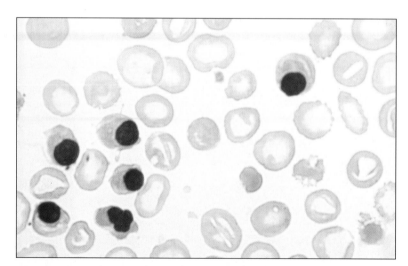

Fig. 5.61 α-Thalassaemia: peripheral blood film in homozygous α^0-thalassaemia (hydrops fetalis) at birth shows marked hypochromasia, polychromasia and many circulating erythroblasts.

of varying severity in adults. At birth, as much as 5–15% of Hb Bart's (γ_4) may be detected in α^0 trait, and up to 2% in α^+ trait. In α^0 trait an occasional cell in the adult blood film may show Hb H bodies after incubation with a dye such as brilliant cresyl blue.

X-Linked α-thalassaemia and mental retardation syndrome

The X-linked α-thalassaemia and mental retardation (ATR-X) syndrome is characterized by a severe form of mental retardation associated with characteristic dysmorphic facies (*Fig. 5.64*), genital abnormalities and an unusual, mild form of Hb H disease. In comparison with α-thalassaemia caused by deletions or point mutations in the α-globin cluster on chromosome 16p13.3, hypochromia and microcytosis are less prominent and, in some affected individuals, the red cell indices may fall in the normal range. Red cells with Hb

H inclusions can be demonstrated after incubation at room temperature in 1% brilliant cresyl blue solution. The frequency of such cells varies widely (0.001–40% red cells).

Carrier females are of normal appearance and intelligence. About 25% may exhibit very rare Hb H inclusions and this reflects the very skewed pattern of X inactivation present, with the disease-bearing X chromosome being preferentially inactive.

The disease gene responsible for the syndrome has been identified and maps to Xq13.3. It is called the ATR-X gene and is a member of a family of proteins (SWI/SNF) with ATPase and putative helicase activity. Members of this group have a wide range of functions, but it is thought they all act by interaction with chromatin. It seems likely that ATR-X acts on its target genes (including α-globin) as a transcriptional regulator (*Fig. 5.65*).

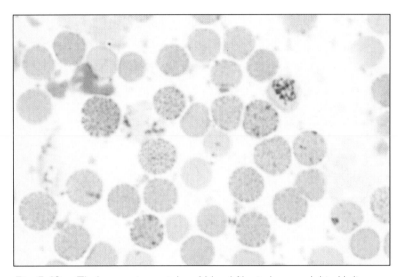

Fig. 5.62 α-Thalassaemia: peripheral blood film in haemoglobin H disease (three α-globin gene deletion or α^0/α^+-thalassaemia) shows marked hypochromic and microcytic cells with target cells and poikilocytes. The patient was a normally developed 23-year-old man with a spleen enlarged to 6 cm below the costal margin, moderate anaemia (Hb, 9.9 g/dl) and grossly reduced red cell indices. (MCV, 59 fl; MCH, 19 pg). Electrophoresis showed Hb A, 76.6%; Hb A$_2$, 2.5%; Hb F, 0.9%; Hb H (β_4), 20%.

Fig. 5.63 α-Thalassaemia: peripheral blood film in haemoglobin H disease stained supravitally with brilliant cresyl blue. Some of the cells show multiple, fine, deeply staining deposits which are precipitated aggregates of α-globin chains ('golf-ball' cells). Reticulocytes are also stained.

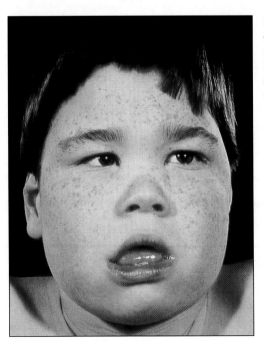

Fig. 5.64
α-Thalassaemia/mental retardation syndrome: boy with characteristic dysmorphic facies. (Courtesy of Dr DR Higgs.)

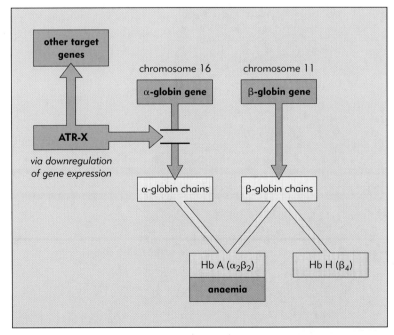

Fig. 5.65 α-Thalassaemia/mental retardation syndrome: action of ATR-X on expression of α-globin and other genes. (Courtesy of Dr DR Higgs.)

THE STRUCTURAL HAEMOGLOBIN VARIANTS

Sickle cell anaemia

Sickle cell anaemia is the most common of the severe structural haemo-globin variants (*Fig. 5.66*). It is the result of substitution of valine for glutamic acid in the sixth position of the β chain, caused by a single base change in the corresponding portion of DNA (*see Fig. 5.56b*). Sickle haemoglobin (Hb S) is insoluble at low oxygen partial pressures and tends to crystallize, which causes the red cells to assume a sickle-like appearance. The oxygen is given up to tissues relatively easily.

The patient has few symptoms of anaemia, despite a haemoglobin level in the steady state of 6–8 g/dl, and has a chronic haemolytic anaemia punctuated by sickle crises. Typically, the patient is of asthenic build (*Figs 5.67*) and is mildly jaundiced. Ulcers around the ankle are common (*Fig. 5.68*).

Bone deformities may be present (*Figs 5.69–5.71*). If the small bones of the hands and feet are affected, there may be unequal growth of the digits ('hand–foot' syndrome; *Figs 5.72–5.75*).

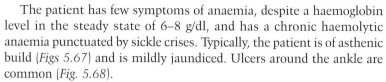

Diseases caused by structural haemoglobin variants
Sickle syndromes
Sickle cell (SS) anaemia
Sickle cell/haemoglobin C (SC)
Sickle cell/haemoglobin D (SD)
Sickle cell/β-thalassaemia
Haemolytic anaemia
Unstable haemoglobin
Polycythaemia
High oxygen affinity haemoglobin
Methaemoglobinaemia
Haemoglobin M
Thalassaemia syndromes
Haemoglobin Lepore
Chain-termination haemoglobins
Some unstable haemoglobins

Fig. 5.66 Structural haemoglobin variants: diseases.

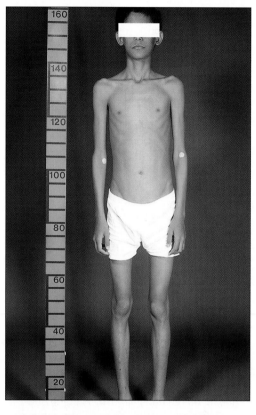

Fig. 5.67 Sickle cell anaemia: this patient of Middle Eastern origin is tall with long thin limbs, a large arm span and narrow pectoral and pelvic girdles. Sexual development is normal.

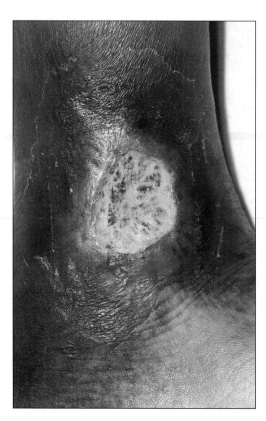

Fig. 5.68 Sickle cell anaemia: ulcer above ankle.

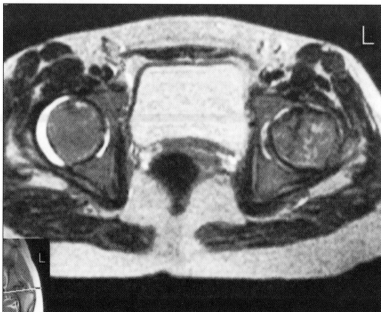

Fig. 5.69 Sickle cell/β-thalassaemia: axial T2-weighted MRI scan of the hips of a 17-year-old female, showing a small area of high signal in the anterior portion of the right hip with a low intensity rim. This is typical of early avascular necrosis. The irregular outline and signal in the left hip is results from more advanced avascular necrosis.

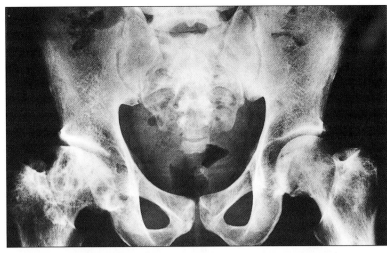

Fig. 5.70 Sickle cell anaemia: radiograph of the pelvis shows avascular necrosis with flattening of the femoral heads, more marked on the right, coarsening of the bone architecture and cystic areas in the right femoral neck caused by previous infarcts.

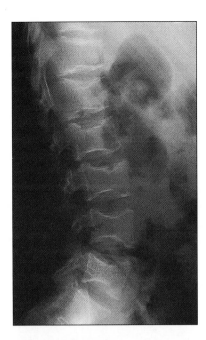

Fig. 5.71 Sickle cell anaemia: radiograph of spine showing 'fish bone' deformity as a result of indentation of vertebral bodies by intervertebral discs.

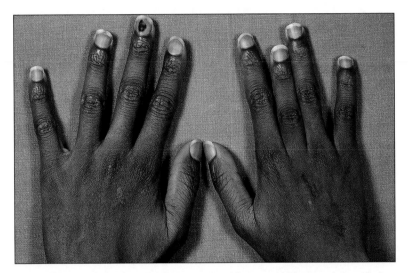

Fig. 5.72 Sickle cell anaemia: hands of an 18-year-old Nigerian boy with the 'hand–foot' syndrome. There is marked shortening of the right middle finger because the dactylitis in childhood affected the growth of the epiphysis.

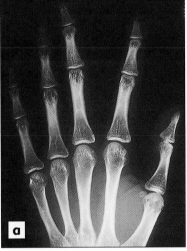

Fig. 5.73a and b Sickle cell anaemia: (a, b) radiographs of the hands shown in *Fig. 5.72*. The right middle metacarpal bone is shortened because of infarction of the growing epiphysis during childhood. The patient was receiving intravenous rehydration during a painful crisis.

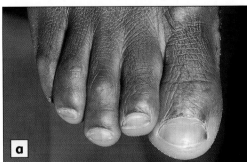

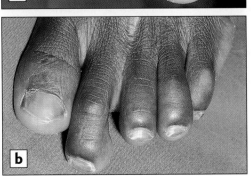

Fig. 5.74a and b Sickle cell anaemia: (a, b) the toes of the patient in *Fig. 5.72* show irregularities in length.

Fig. 5.75 Sickle cell anaemia: hand of an 18-month-old child with painful, swollen fingers (dactylitis) caused by infarction of the metacarpal bones of the index and ring fingers. This acute syndrome rarely occurs after 2 years of age.

As a result of infections together with infarcts, pneumonia (*Fig. 5.76*) may occur; it may be difficult to distinguish from the chest syndrome caused by blockage of small vessels and fat embolism from infarcted bones, especially the ribs (*Figs 5.77 and 5.78*). The central nervous system may be damaged by infarction. Transcranial Doppler studies may help to determine the risk of a stroke (*Fig. 5.79*). Osteomyelitis may also occur, usually from *Salmonella* spp. (*Fig. 5.780*), but sometimes from other organisms (*Fig. 5.81*). Parvovirus infection may cause

an 'aplastic' crisis. Infarcts may also occur in the kidney – papillary necrosis is particularly common (*Fig. 5.82*).

Following occlusion of small vessels in the retina during sickle cell crises, there may be characteristic regrowth of blood vessels at the affected sites (*Fig. 5.83*). Infarction and atrophy of the spleen are usual after childhood (*Fig. 5.84*).

The blood film shows the presence of sickle cells and target cells (*Fig. 5.85*), as well as, in most adult cases, features of splenic atrophy

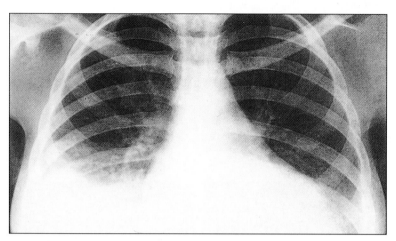

Fig. 5.76 Sickle cell anaemia: chest radiograph of an 18-year old female admitted in crisis with a pulmonary syndrome. There is generalized cardiomegaly and increased vascularity of the lungs, typical of a chronic haemolytic anaemia. In addition, there is shadowing, particularly in the right lower and middle lobes, which resolved slowly on antibiotic therapy and was considered to result from infection and small vessel obstruction.

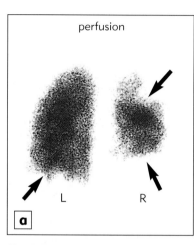
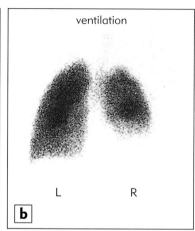

Fig. 5.77a and b Sickle cell anaemia: ventilation–perfusion lung scan of the patient in *Fig. 5.76* shows (a) perfusion measured with technetium 99^m-aggregated albumin (50 μm particles); (b) ventilation using krypton 81^m. The ventilation defect at the base of the right lung (R) suggests infection only, but the multiple perfusion defects apparent in other areas of both lungs (arrowed) suggest blockage of segmental and subsegmental arteries. [(a, b) Courtesy of Dr A Hilson.]

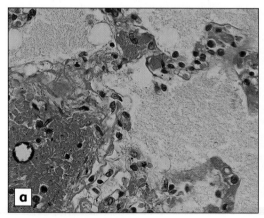
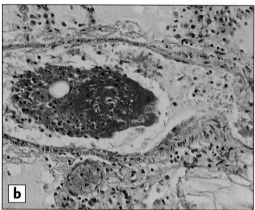

Fig. 5.78a and b Sickle cell anaemia: chest syndrome. (a) High-power view of lung showing alveolar oedema, fat embolism within an arteriole surrounded by sickle cells and microthrombi in the alveolar capillaries. Fat embolism is the white non-staining hole (from which fat has dissolved out in processing). (b) High-power view of an arteriole showing fat embolism with associated thrombus. [(a) H & E; (b) Martius scarlet blue with fibrin staining red; (a, b) courtesy of Prof. S Lucas.]

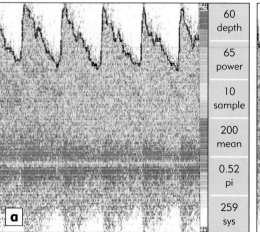
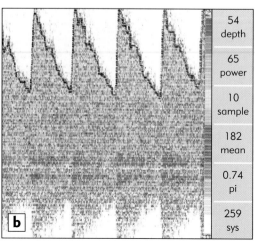

60 depth	54 depth
65 power	65 power
10 sample	10 sample
200 mean	182 mean
0.52 pi	0.74 pi
259 sys	259 sys

Fig. 5.79a and b Sickle cell anaemia: sonograms obtained using a pulsed transcranial Doppler instrument from (a) right and (b) left middle cerebral arteries (MCAs) in an 11-year-old-boy with sickle cell disease who presented with severe headaches, but no neurological signs. Maximum mean velocities in the right and left MCAs are 200 and 182 cm/s at depths of 6.0 and 5.4 cm, respectively. Although MRI was normal, MR angiography showed bilateral turbulence, suggestive of stenosis, in both MCAs. For patients with an MCA velocity >200 cm/s, the risk of stroke within 40 months is 40%; this child was therefore commenced on regular transfusions with resolution of his headaches. [(a, b) Courtesy of Dr JPM Evans and Dr F Kirkham.]

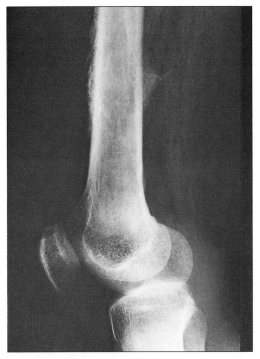

Fig. 5.80 Sickle cell anaemia: lateral radiograph of the lower limb and knee in salmonellal osteomyelitis. The periosteum is irregularly raised in the lower third of the femur.

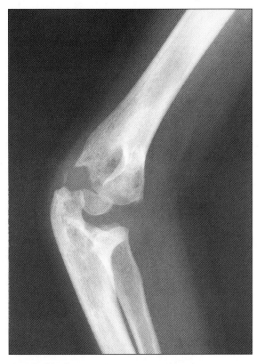

Fig. 5.81 Sickle cell anaemia: lateral radiograph of the elbow joint in staphylococcal osteomyelitis shows destructive changes in the humerus and ulna.

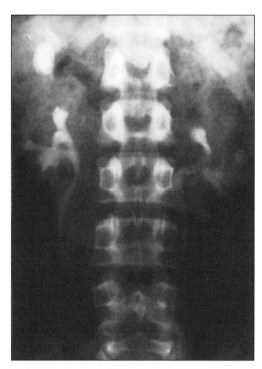

Fig. 5.82 Sickle cell anaemia: intravenous pyelogram. There is clubbing of the calyceal outline in the left kidney. The patient, a 24-year-old man, also shows two large opaque pigment gallstones. The bone trabeculae in the ribs and vertebrae are fine because of expanded erythropoiesis.

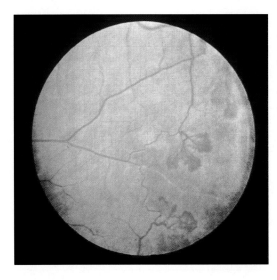

Fig. 5.83 Sickle cell anaemia: retina showing peripheral vascular fronds resulting from formation of arteriovenous anastomoses.

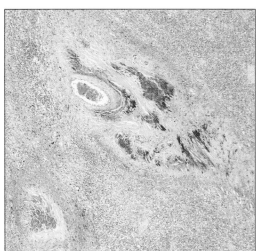

Fig. 5.84 Sickle cell anaemia: section of atrophied spleen showing deposits of haemosiderin in nests of macrophages (Gamna–Gandy bodies) around the vessels. There is severe reduction of both red and white pulp. (H & E stain.)

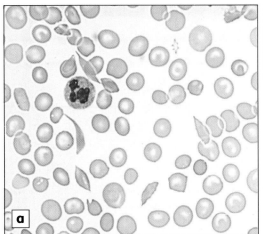

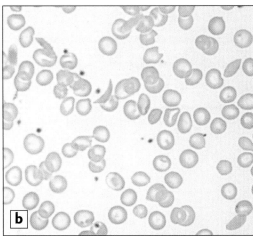

Fig. 5.85a and b Sickle cell anaemia: peripheral blood films showing (a) deeply staining sickle cells with target cells and polychromasia; (b) sickle, hypochromic and target cells.

(*Fig. 5.86*). The haemopoietic marrow expands down the long bones (*Fig. 5.87*) and the myeloid:erythroid ratio is reversed.

The different types of haemoglobin may be separated and quantitated by electrophoresis in cellulose acetate (*Fig. 5.88*) or agar gel.

Sickle cell trait gives a normal blood appearance, possibly with an occasional sickle cell present, unless a crisis is induced, for example by anoxia or severe infection. Recurrent haematuria because of renal papillary necrosis is an occasional problem. Usually combinations of sickle trait with other haemoglobin defects, such as β-thalassaemia

trait (*Fig. 5.89*) or C trait (*Fig. 5.90*), give rise clinically to mild forms of sickle cell disease.

The main clinical problem in sickle cell anaemia, recurring crises, is managed by rehydration, pain relief, antibiotic therapy as appropriate and, in severe cases, exchange transfusion (*see Fig. 19.15*). Blood transfusions may also be needed in aplastic crises, during pregnancy and pre-operatively to reduce the haemoglobin S content of the blood, and are sometimes used long-term to 'switch off' recurring crises. Patients with sickle cell disease, especially those with SC disease, tend

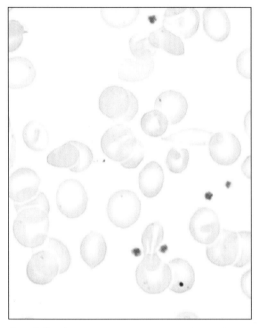

Fig. 5.86 Sickle cell anaemia: peripheral blood film in a patient with splenic atrophy. Howell–Jolly and Pappenheimer bodies are seen in addition to the sickle and target cells.

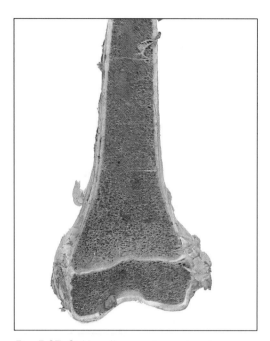

Fig. 5.87 Sickle cell anaemia: postmortem longitudinal section of femur showing expansion of red (haemopoietic) marrow down the shaft towards the knee, with thinning of cortical bone. (Courtesy of Dr JE McLaughlin.)

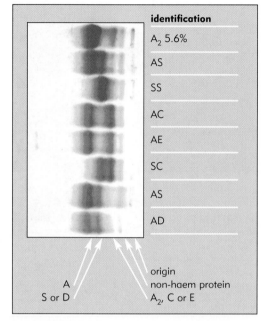

identification

A$_2$ 5.6%

AS

SS

AC

AE

SC

AS

AD

origin
A — non-haem protein
S or D — A$_2$, C or E

Fig. 5.88 Sickle cell anaemia: haemoglobin electrophoresis in cellulose acetate, Ponceau S stain. S and D, and A$_2$, C and E, run together. Agar gel separation is usually used to distinguish these. The uppermost lane shows the raised Hb A$_2$ level of β-thalassaemia trait.

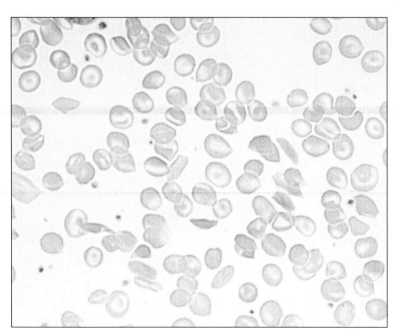

Fig. 5.89 Sickle cell/β-thalassaemia: peripheral blood film showing sickle cells, target cells and microcytic hypochromic cells.

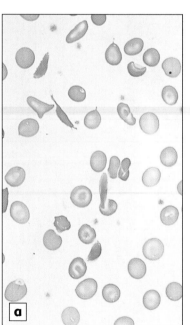 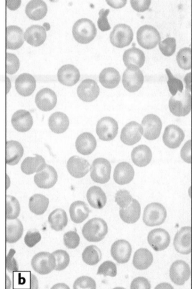

Fig. 5.90a and b Sickle cell/haemoglobin C disease: (a, b) peripheral blood films in which sickle cells and target cells are prominent. (b) Peripheral blood film showing typical irregularly contracted cells. [(b) Courtesy of Dr BA Bain.]

to suffer thromboembolic problems and may require antiplatelet or anticoagulant therapy. Hydroxyurea therapy results in amelioration of sickle cell disease in many patients.

Other structural haemoglobin defects

Other common haemoglobin abnormalities include haemoglobin C (*Fig. 5.91*) which may be combined with β^0-thalassaemia (*Fig. 5.92*), haemoglobin D and haemoglobin E diseases (*Figs 5.93 and 5.94*). Rare syndromes produced by haemoglobin abnormalities include haemolytic

anaemia because of an unstable haemoglobin (*Fig. 5.95*), hereditary poly-cythaemia, hereditary methaemoglobinaemia and thalassaemia syndromes caused by structural variants.

F-cells

In normal adults the synthesis of fetal Hb (Hb F) is reduced to very low levels (<0.6%) and the Hb F is restricted to a subpopulation of erythrocytes termed 'F-cells' which contain, in addition, adult haemoglobin (Hb A $\alpha_2\beta_2$). Increased levels of Hb F in adult life are characteristic

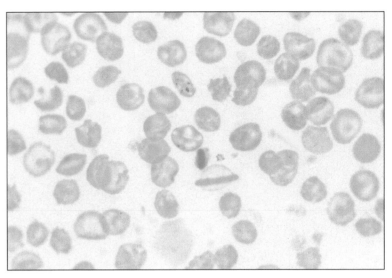

Fig. 5.91 Homozygous haemoglobin C disease: peripheral blood film showing many target cells and irregularly contracted cells. The patient showed a mild haemolytic anaemia with low MCV and MCH, splenomegaly and gallstones.

Fig. 5.92 Haemoglobin C/β^0-thalassaemia: peripheral blood film showing crystals of haemoglobin C in cells otherwise empty of haemoglobin. (Courtesy of Dr BA Bain.)

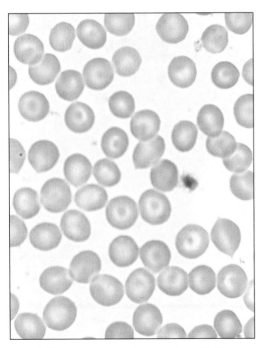

Fig. 5.93 Homozygous haemoglobin E disease: peripheral blood film showing target cells and deeply staining contracted cells. The patient was not anaemic. Red cell indices (MCV, MCH) were reduced.

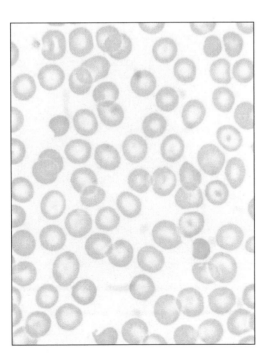

Fig. 5.94 Homozygous haemoglobin E: blood film showing hypochromia, microcytosis, target cells and irregularly contracted cells. (Hb, 11.9 g/dl; RBC, 6.84 × 10⁹/l; MCV, 54 fl; MCH, 17.4 pg; courtesy of Dr BA Bain.)

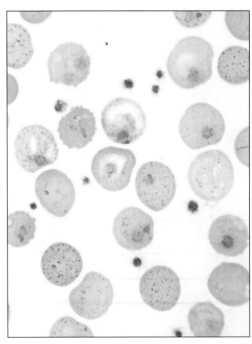

Fig. 5.95 Unstable haemoglobin (Hb-Hammersmith): postsplenectomy peripheral blood film shows many cells with punctate basophilia, or containing single or multiple inclusion bodies composed of precipitated, denatured haemoglobin (seen as Heinz bodies on special staining). The underlying lesion is substitution of the amino acid phenylalanine by serine at position 42 in the β chain.

of a heterogeneous group of genetic disorders termed Hereditary Persistence of Fetal Hb (HPFH) and δβ-thalassaemias. The distribution of Hb F could be heterocellular or pancellular and this has been a criterion for differentiating the δβ-thalassaemias from the HPFHs (*Fig. 5.96*). Presently, it is not clear if this picture may simply be a reflection of the sensitivity of the technique.

There is a slight increase of fetal haemoglobin in adult blood in a variety of acquired disorders, such as megaloblastic anaemia, acute myeloid leukaemia and paroxysmal nocturnal haemoglobinuria.

Circulating fetal red cells may be found in mothers in the immediate postpartum period, following mixing of fetal and maternal blood at delivery; such cells may be detected by the Kleihauer technique (*Fig. 5.97*).

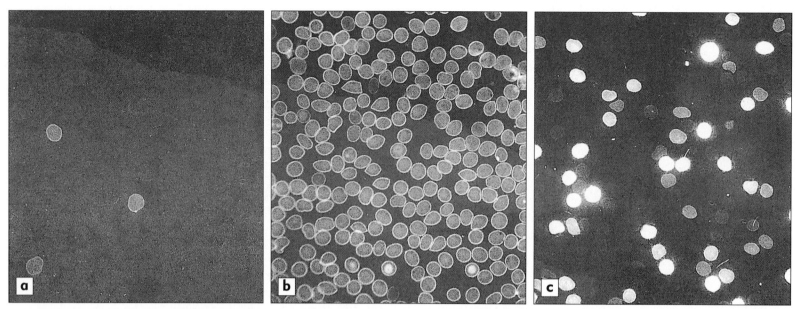

Fig. 5.96a–c Fetal haemoglobin in peripheral blood anti γ-immunofluorescence stain: (a) normal blood heterocellular distribution (Hb F, 0.4%; F cells, 2.5%). (b) Indian hereditary persistence of fetal haemoglobin (Hb F, 22%; F cells, 100%). (c) Heterocellular HPFH (Hb F, 2.5%; F cells, 30%). (Courtesy of Dr SL Thein.)

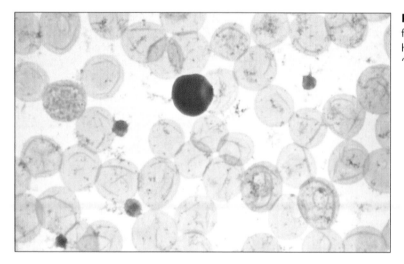

Fig. 5.97 Fetal haemoglobin: acid elution (Kleihauer) technique showing a fetal red cell in maternal blood. The darkly staining fetal cell contains fetal haemoglobin which has resisted elution at low pH. The adult cells appear as 'ghosts' because the adult haemoglobin has been leached out of the cells.

chapter

6

Aplastic, Dyserythropoietic and Secondary Anaemias

APLASTIC ANAEMIA

Aplastic (hypoplastic) anaemia comprises pancytopenia caused by hypoplasia of the marrow. It may be transient, as following cytotoxic therapy, but the term is usually used to denote the chronic forms of the condition. The condition may be congenital or acquired (*Fig. 6.1*).

In about half the acquired cases no cause can be found. The response to antilymphocyte globulin (ALG) or cyclosporin in a substantial proportion of these idiopathic cases, however, suggests that an immune mechanism may be involved. The success of bone marrow transplantation implies that the haemopoietic microenvironment of the marrow is intact, at least in the majority of cases.

The cause of the anaemia in about a third of the patients appears to be damage by a drug or toxin to the haemopoietic stem cells, which are then reduced in number as they lose their ability to self-renew and proliferate. The drugs most frequently associated with aplastic anaemia are the sulphonamides, chloramphenicol and gold; but a wide range of drugs has been implicated. In some patients these drugs give rise to only a selective neutropenia or thrombocytopenia. Aplastic anaemia may also be caused by radiation or infection, particularly viral hepatitis (non-A, non-B, non-C).

A typical blood count for a patient with severe aplastic anaemia is given in *Fig. 6.2*. The anaemia is mildly macrocytic or normocytic. The clinical features are those of anaemia, haemorrhage caused by thrombocytopenia or infections because of neutropenia. Bleeding is usually into the skin as petechiae or ecchymoses, or into or from interior surfaces (*Fig. 6.3*), but may also occur into internal organs (*Fig. 6.4*), cerebral haemorrhage being the major risk. Infections are usually bacterial

(*Fig. 6.5*), but viral (*Fig. 6.6*), fungal (*Fig. 6.7*), and protozoal infections may also occur, particularly later in the disease.

Congenital aplastic anaemia

The congenital forms of aplastic anaemia may be associated with other congenital defects, as in the Fanconi syndrome, an autosomal recessive inherited disease that is genetically and phenotypically heterogeneous. It is defined by cellular hypersensitivity to DNA cross-linking agents, for example diepoxybutane and mitomycin C, and is one of

Blood count in severe aplastic anaemia	
Haemoglobin	6.2 g/dl
Red blood cells	2.0×10^{12}/l
Packed cell volume	22%
Mean corpuscular volume	110 fl
Mean corpuscular haemoglobin	31 pg
Reticulocytes	0.1%
White blood cells	0.9×10^9/l
neutrophils	13%
eosinophils	0%
basophils	0%
monocytes	21%
lymphocytes	66%
Platelets	5×10^9/l

Fig. 6.2 Aplastic anaemia: typical blood count in severe aplastic anaemia.

Causes of aplastic anaemia
Congenital
Fanconi
Non-Fanconi
Associated with dyskeratosis congenita
Acquired
Idiopathic
Secondary:
Drugs – hypersensitivity (e.g. chloramphenicol, gold, sulphonamides)
Drugs – cytotoxics (e.g. busulfan, cyclophosphamide)
Irradiation
Infection: postviral hepatitis
Toxins: e.g. insecticides, benzene

Fig. 6.1 Aplastic anaemia: causes.

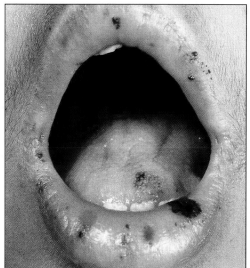

Fig. 6.3 Aplastic anaemia: spontaneous mucosal haemorrhages in a 10-year-old boy with severe congenital (Fanconi) anaemia. [Hb, 7.3 g/dl; WBC, 1.1 × 10^9/l (neutrophils, 21%; lymphocytes, 77%); platelets, <5.0 × 10^9/l.]

several congenital diseases associated with genomic instability (*Fig. 6.8*). There are random chromosomal breaks with endoreduplication and chromatid exchange can be demonstrated in peripheral lymphocytes. Patients may be mildly or severely affected with many congenital anomalies; the disease often progresses to myelodysplasia and acute myeloid leukaemia. Skeletal, renal and other defects may be present, as well as hyperpigmentation, small stature from birth and hypogonadism (*Figs 6.9–6.14*). Fanconi anaemia patients fall into at least five complementation groups as defined by cell fusion experiments (*Fig. 6.15*). The genes for the two most frequent subtype, FAA and FAC, have been cloned and sequenced, but the functions of the FAA and FAC proteins are unknown. No evidence indicates that specific complementation groups are associated with particular clinical syndromes, except that the IVS4+4A→T mutation in the FAC genes, common in the Askenazi Jewish population is associated with a severe clinical phenotype.

A less common association of the congenital form of aplastic anaemia is dyskeratosis congenita, in which there is skin pigmentation, nail dystrophy and mucosal leucoplakia (*Figs 6.16 and 6.17*). The gene DKC is located at chromosome Xq28. Girls may be affected and both autosomal dominant and recessive forms may occur. There may also be epiphora, telangiectasia and alopecia, as well as mental retardation, growth failure, pulmonary disease, hypogonadism, dental caries and/or loss and skeletal abnormalities; in contrast to Fanconi anaemia, the chromosomal pattern is normal.

Bone marrow appearances

Bone marrow fragments show reduced cellularity (*Fig. 6.18*), with fat spaces occupying >75% of the marrow. The trails are also reduced in cellularity, with particularly low numbers of megakaryocytes and often a predominance of lymphocytes and plasma cells. The hypoplasia is

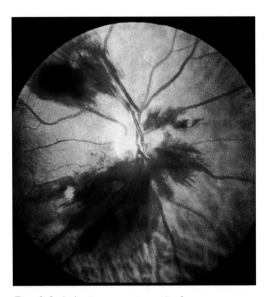

Fig. 6.4 Aplastic anaemia: retinal haemorrhages in a patient with acquired disease and profound thrombocytopenia.

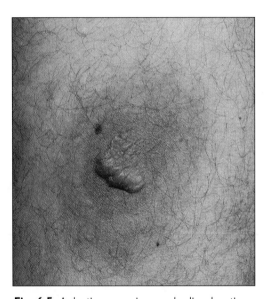

Fig. 6.5 Aplastic anaemia: purple discoloration and blistering of the skin caused by infection with *Pseudomonas aeruginosa*.

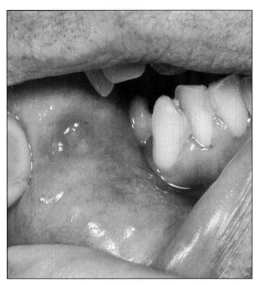

Fig. 6.6 Aplastic anaemia: ulceration of the buccal mucosa associated with severe neutropenia. Herpes simplex virus was grown from the ulcers. (Total leucocyte count, 0.8 × 10^9/l; neutrophils, 20%.)

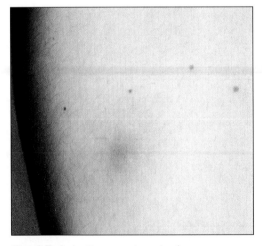

Fig. 6.7 Aplastic anaemia: raised, erythematous skin nodule from infection with *Candida albicans*, which was also present in the bloodstream. The patient, a 27-year-old woman, had previously been treated with antibacterial agents for prolonged periods of fever caused by bacterial infections.

Diseases of genomic instability			
Disease	**Damaging agent**	**Neoplasm**	**Function**
Fanconi anaemia	Cross-linking agents	Acute myeloid leukaemia, hepatic, gastrointestinal and gynaecological tumours	Unknown
Xeroderma pigmentosa	UV light	Squamous cell carcinomas	Excision repair
Ataxia telangiectasia	Ionizing radiation	Lymphoma, ?chronic lymphocytic leukaemia	Afferent pathway to p53
Bloom's syndrome	Alkylating agents	Acute lymphoblastic leukaemia	Cell-cycle regulation
Cockayne's syndrome	UV light	Basal cell carcinoma	Transcription coupled repair
Hereditary nonpolyposis colon cancer	Unknown	Adenocarcinoma of colon, ovarian cancer	DNA mismatch pair

Fig. 6.8 Aplastic anaemia: diseases of genomic instability. (UV, ultraviolet; adapted from D'Andrea AD, Grompe, M. Molecular biology of Fanconi anemia; implications for diagnosis and therapy. *Blood*. 1997;90:1725–36.)

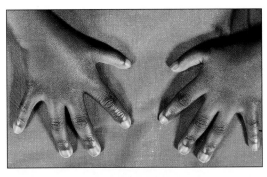

Fig. 6.9 Fanconi anaemia: the hands of the child shown in *Fig. 6.13* show symmetrical abnormalities of the thumbs, resulting in their resemblance to fingers. (Courtesy of Dr B Wonke.)

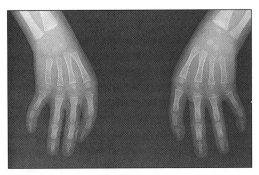

Fig. 6.10 Fanconi anaemia: radiograph shows absent thumbs.

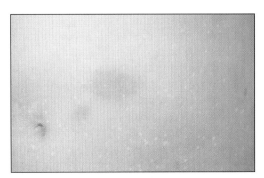

Fig. 6.11 Fanconi anaemia: café-au-lait spot, pigmentation and punctate areas of depigmentation over the abdominal wall. (Courtesy of Prof. EC Gordon-Smith.)

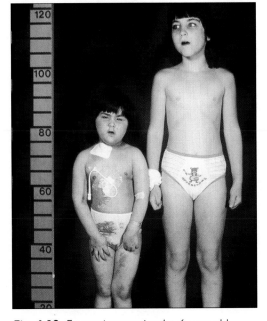

Fig. 6.12 Fanconi anaemia: the 6-year-old patient shows short stature and a minor degree of microcephaly compared with her normal older sister, who was HLA-identical and the donor for bone marrow transplantation.

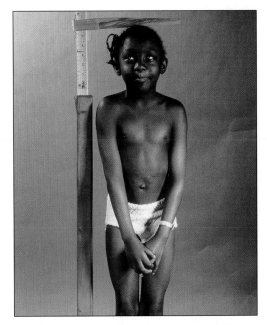

Fig. 6.13 Fanconi anaemia: this 9-year-old child shows typical short stature of 1.06 m (42 inches). (Courtesy of Dr B Wonke.)

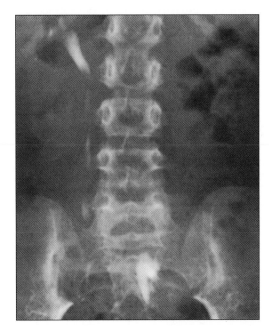

Fig. 6.14 Fanconi anaemia: intravenous pyelogram of the child shown in *Fig. 6.13* shows a normal right kidney, but a left kidney that is abnormally placed in the pelvis.

Complementation groups of Fanconi anaemia		
Subtype	Percentage of Fanconi anaemia patients	Chromosome location
A	66.0	16q24.3
B	4.3	?
C	12.7	9q22.3
D	4.3	3p22–26
E	6.4	?
F	2.1	?
G	2.1	?
H	2.1	?

Fig. 6.15 Fanconi anaemia: complementation groups. (Courtesy of Dr C Mathew.)

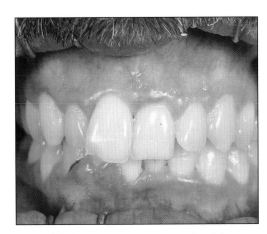

Fig. 6.16 Dyskeratosis congenita: this 24-year-old man with long-standing aplastic anaemia has irregularities of tooth size and shape, and of the gum margins.

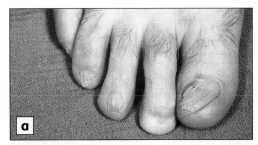
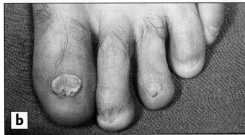

Fig. 6.17a and b Dyskeratosis congenita: (a, b) the feet of the patient shown in *Fig. 6.16* show grossly abnormal nails and excessive hair in an abnormal distribution.

best shown by trephine biopsy (*Fig. 6.19*). There may be areas of normal cellularity despite the overall hypocellularity (*Fig. 6.20*) and lymphoid follicles may be prominent (*Fig. 6.21*).

As therapy differs according to the degree of aplasia, a standard classification of severity has been adopted. Criteria for severe disease are:

- $<50 \times 10^5$/l reticulocytes;
- $<10 \times 10^9$/l platelets;
- $<0.5 \times 10^9$/l granulocytes in peripheral blood;
- $>80\%$ of the remaining cells in the marrow are non-myeloid.

When any three of these four conditions persists for more than 2 weeks the patient is categorized as having severe aplastic anaemia.

During the recovery phase, cellularity increases to normal (*Fig. 6.22*); the platelet count is usually the last of the blood cell counts to recover completely. Overt paroxysmal nocturnal haemoglobinuria (PNH) or a subclinical PNH defect may develop transiently or chronically, and some of these patients may have aplasia of the marrow.

Ferrokinetics

Ferrokinetic studies show a slow clearance of transferrin-bound radio-iron, with predominant uptake in the liver and reduced incorporation

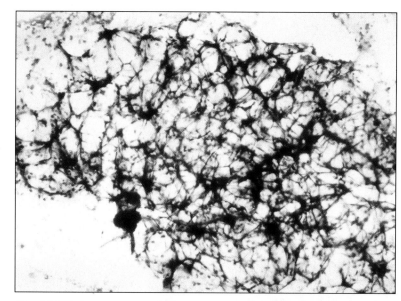

Fig. 6.18 Aplastic anaemia: low-power view of bone marrow fragment showing severe reduction of haemopoietic cells and an increase in fat spaces.

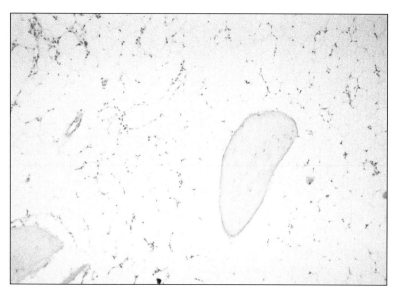

Fig. 6.19 Aplastic anaemia: trephine biopsy of posterior iliac crest shows gross hypocellularity with replacement by fat.

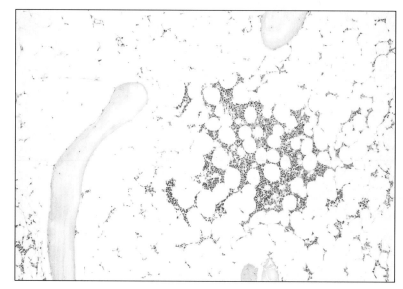

Fig. 6.20 Aplastic anaemia: trephine biopsy shows some haemopoietic cellular foci in an otherwise grossly hypocellular marrow.

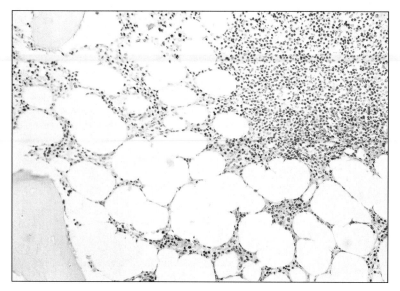

Fig. 6.21 Aplastic anaemia: higher power view of the biopsy shown in *Fig. 6.20*, showing grossly hypocellular marrow with a remaining lymphoid follicle in the upper right field.

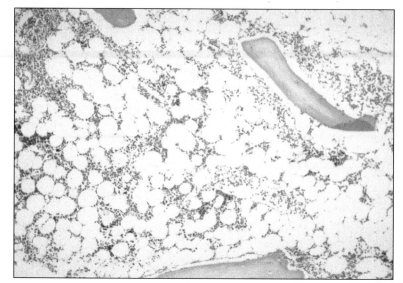

Fig. 6.22 Aplastic anaemia: trephine biopsy (same case as shown in *Fig. 6.20*), showing partial recovery of cellularity 4 weeks after treatment with antilymphocyte globulin. Peripheral blood cell counts also rose moderately.

into circulating red cells. Scanning studies show absence of iron uptake by the bone marrow, with accumulation of iron in the liver (*Fig. 6.23*).

Treatment

Once diagnosed, the cause of severe aplastic anaemia must be eliminated if possible. The patient is managed with support care (e.g. platelets, antibiotics, blood transfusions). If an HLA-matching sibling is available, allogeneic bone marrow transplantation is considered. A haematological recovery is promoted by ALG in 40–50% of cases; cyclosporin may also be of benefit and the combination of ALG and cyclosporin with corticosteroids is moderately more effective than these drugs used alone. Androgens are used in some cases.

RED CELL APLASIA

The causes of pure red cell aplasia are listed in *Fig. 6.24*. Like aplastic anaemia, it may be congenital, familial or acquired. In the congenital Diamond–Blackfan syndrome (*Figs 6.25 and 6.26*), skeletal defects

Causes of red cell aplasia
Congential
Diamond–Blackfan syndrome
Acquired
Primary
Autoimmune: immunoglobulin inhibitors of erythroid precursors   or of erythropoietin T-cell inhibition of erythroid precursors transient erythroblastopenia of childhood
Secondary
Tumours: thymoma

lymphoma:
   Hodgkin
   non-Hodgkin
chronic lymphocytic leukaemia
large granular lymphocytic leukaemia
acute lymphoblastic leukaemia
other tumours

Infections: parvovirus (transient) human immunodeficiency virus viral hepatitis infectious mononucleosis others
Immune disorders: systemic lupus erythematosus rheumatoid arthritis
Drugs and chemicals (e.g. benzene,   diphenylhydantoin, isoniazid)
Nutritional deficiencies: riboflavin vitamin B_{12} or folate deficiency

Fig. 6.24 Red cell aplasia: causes.

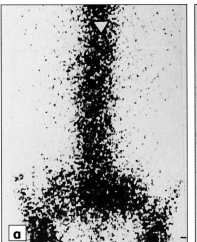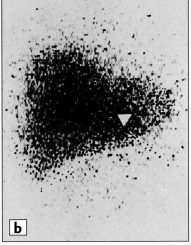

Fig. 6.23a and b Aplastic anaemia: iron-52 (^{52}Fe) scans showing (a) normal concentration of isotope in the bones of the spine and pelvis, and (b) accumulation of iron isotope only in the liver in aplastic anaemia. The triangles mark the position of the xiphisternum.

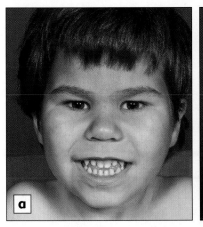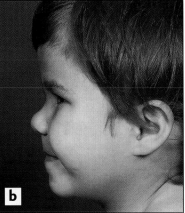

Fig. 6.25a and b Diamond–Blackfan syndrome: (a, b) 3-year-old boy with congenital red cell aplasia shows the typical facies, with a sunken bridge of the nose. He was treated with blood transfusions and subsequently corticosteroids to which he made a partial response and became transfusion independent. His mental development is normal but his growth has been partly retarded because of the corticosteroid therapy. [Hb, 6.1 g/dl; WBC, 7.2×10^9/l (neutrophils, 55%; lymphocytes, 41%); monocytes, 4%; platelets, 289×10^9/l.]

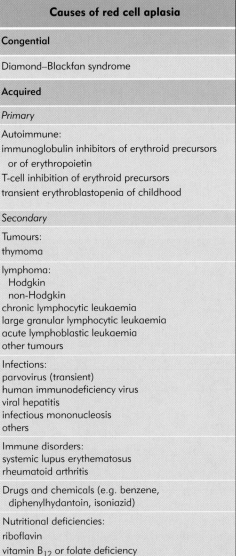

Fig. 6.26 Diamond–Blackfan syndrome: the 24-year-old woman on the right had received corticosteroid therapy as an infant and child to reduce the need for blood transfusions. This led to stunted growth (compare her normal mother). The patient had received over 100 units of blood and developed transfusional haemosiderosis with enlargement of the liver and spleen.

occur without renal and chromosomal abnormalities. The exact pattern of inheritance is unclear. Recently, the gene that encodes ribosomal protein S19 has been found mutated in patients with the Diamond–Blackfan syndrome. The acquired form may be idiopathic or may appear in conjunction with another disease, such as a thymoma (*Figs 6.27 and 6.28*).

A transient form of red cell aplasia occurs in the course of chronic and other haemolytic anaemias, but is best recognized in sickle cell anaemia. This form is the result of parvovirus B19 infection, with selective damage by the virus to bone marrow red cell progenitors. It is likely that a similar red cell aplasia occurs in normal subjects with this infection but is not clinically apparent because of the longer red cell lifespan. In all forms the bone marrow is of normal cellularity, but there is a relative absence of erythroid precursors (*Fig.*

6.29). In parvovirus B19 infection, giant proerythroblasts may be a feature (*Fig. 6.30*).

Pure red cell aplasia occasionally responds to thymectomy or other immunosuppressive therapy, corticosteroids or cyclosporin. If severe, it usually needs regular blood transfusions and iron chelation therapy.

CONGENITAL DYSERYTHROPOIETIC ANAEMIAS

The congenital dyserythropoietic anaemias (CDAs) are rare autosomal recessive diseases characterized clinically by anaemia, often with jaundice as a result of ineffective erythropoiesis and shortened red cell survival, and morphologically by abnormal red cell precursors in the bone marrow. The anaemia is usually macrocytic, and the reticulocyte count may be raised, but is low relative to the degree of anaemia.

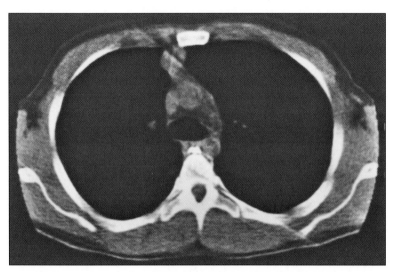

Fig. 6.27 Acquired red cell aplasia: upper mediastinal computed tomography scan shows a thymoma as a retrosternal mass of irregular outline. The patient, a 62-year-old man, had developed myasthenia gravis and pure red cell aplasia which required regular blood transfusions. (Courtesy of Dr R Dick.)

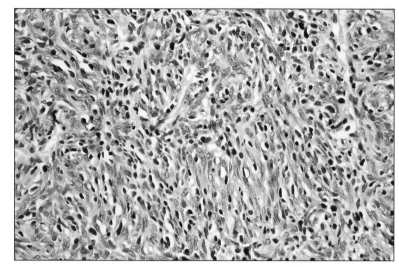

Fig. 6.28 Red cell aplasia: section of thymoma showing spindle cells and epithelial cells. The thymoma was removed surgically from a patient with severe red cell aplasia (Hb, 6.1 g/dl), neutropenia (WBC, 3.2×10^9/l; neutrophils, 0.4×10^9/l; platelets, 168×10^9/l). (H & E; courtesy of Dr JE McLaughlin.)

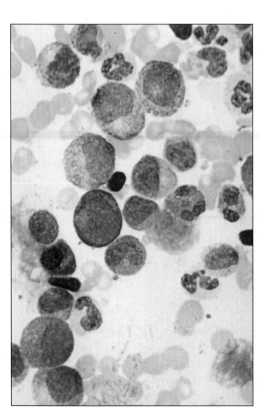

Fig. 6.29 Acquired red cell aplasia: bone marrow aspirate cell trail shows normal numbers of granulocytes and their precursors, but an absence of erythroblasts.

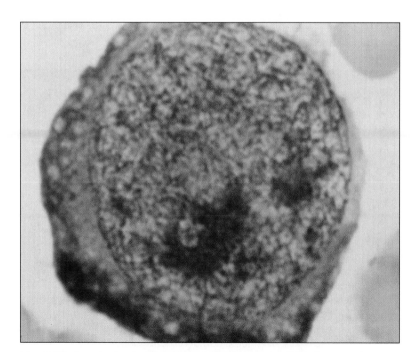

Fig. 6.30 Acquired red cell aplasia: bone marrow aspirate in parvovirus B19 infection showing a giant proerythroblast with cytoplasmic vacuolation and poorly defined intranuclear viral inclusions. (Courtesy of Prof. EC Larkin.)

The diseases are divided into three main groups according to the appearance of the bone marrow. In CDA I (*Figs 6.31 and 6.32*), megaloblastic changes and internuclear chromatin bridges are prominent. In the most frequent type, CDA II, also known as hereditary erythroblast multinuclearity with positive acidified serum test (HEMPAS), there are bi- and multinucleate erythroblasts (*Figs 6.33 and 6.34*). The cells lyse in acidified serum from about 30% of normal subjects, but not in the patient's serum (*Fig. 6.35*). This is because a naturally occurring IgM complement-binding antibody is present, but the antigen on HEMPAS red cells recognized by this antibody is not known. CDA III (*Figs 6.36 and 6.37*) is characterized by multinuclearity and gigantoblasts. The existence of a Type IV CDA, similar to a Type II CDA but with a negative acid lysis test, has been postulated.

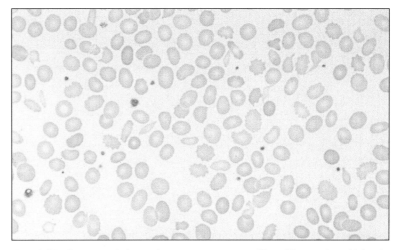

Fig. 6.31 Congenital dyserythropoietic anaemia (Type 1): peripheral blood film showing oval macrocytes, poikilocytes and small fragmented cells. The platelets and granulocytes are normal.

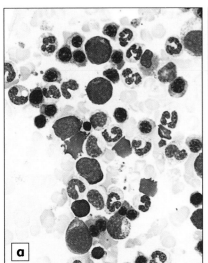

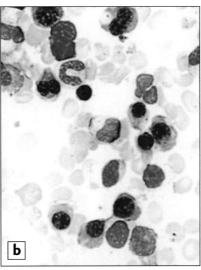

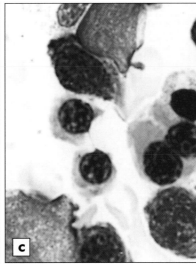

Fig. 6.32a–c Congenital dyserythropoietic anaemia (Type 1): bone marrow aspirate showing (a) erythroid hyperplasia, megaloblastic erythropoiesis and binucleate erythroblasts; (b, c) examples of cells with internuclear bridges.

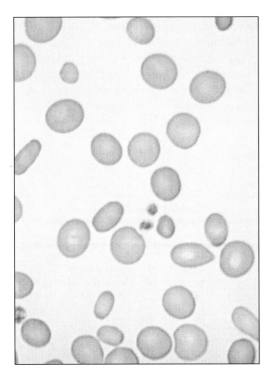

Fig. 6.33 Congenital dyserythropoietic anaemia (Type II): peripheral blood film showing marked red cell anisocytosis and poikilocytosis.

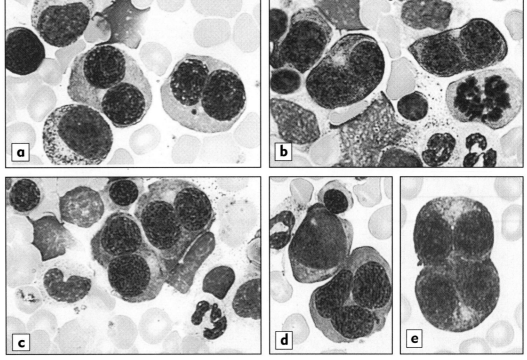

Fig. 6.34a–e Congenital dyserythropoietic anaemia (Type II): (a–e) selected high-power views of bone marrow aspirate showing multinucleate erythroblasts.

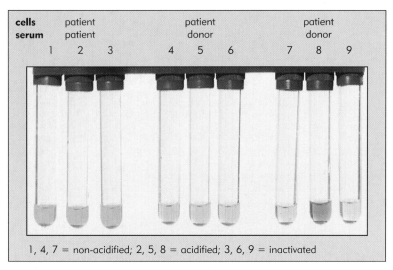

cells | patient | | | patient | | | patient | |
serum | patient | | | donor | | | donor | |
| 1 | 2 | 3 | 4 | 5 | 6 | 7 | 8 | 9

1, 4, 7 = non-acidified; 2, 5, 8 = acidified; 3, 6, 9 = inactivated

Fig. 6.35 Congenital dyserythropoietic anaemia (HEMPAS, Type II): in the samples from some normal donors the affected red cells show complement-dependent lysis in fresh acidified serum at 37°C, but not in the patient's own serum.

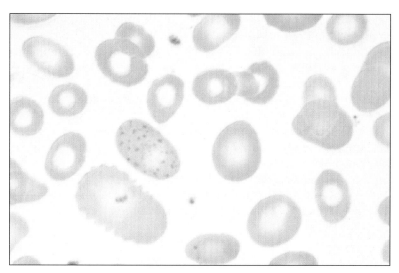

Fig. 6.36 Congenital dyserythropoietic anaemia (Type III): peripheral blood film shows gross macrocytosis, anisocytosis, poikilocytosis and punctate basophilia. (Courtesy of Dr IM Hann.)

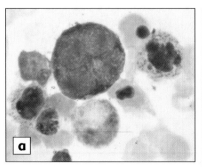 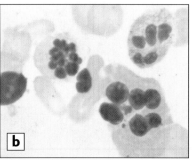 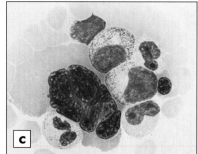 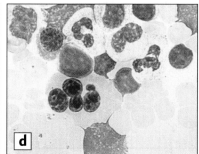

Fig. 6.37a–d Congenital dyserythropoietic anaemia (Type III): (a–d) selected high-power views of bone marrow aspirate showing multinucleate erythroblasts and karyorrhexis. (Courtesy of Dr IM Hann.)

SECONDARY ANAEMIAS

Many anaemias are not part of a primary blood disorder, but occur in patients with other systemic disease. In these anaemias there are often a number of contributing factors, such as iron and folate deficiencies, haemolysis, marrow infiltration or marrow suppression by therapy.

In chronic inflammatory or malignant conditions, usually with a raised erythrocyte sedimentation rate, there is also a mild normochromic or hypochromic anaemia (Hb, >9.0 g/dl) associated with low serum iron, reduced total iron-binding capacity and normal or raised serum ferritin. The severity of this anaemia is related to the severity of the underlying disease. Bone marrow iron stores are normal or increased, but siderotic granules are not seen in developing erythroblasts (*Fig. 6.38*). This 'anaemia of chronic disorders' is thought to arise as a result of a combination of failure of iron release from reticuloendothelial cells, reduced red cell survival and an inadequate erythropoietin response, caused by release of cytokines [e.g. tumour necrosis factor, interleukin-1 (IL-1) and IL-6] from inflammatory cells.

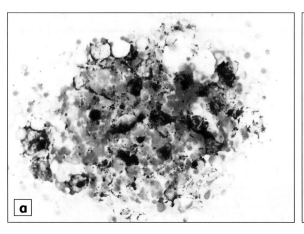 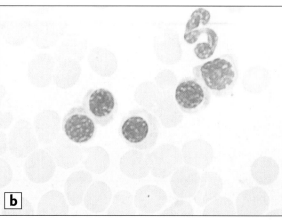

Fig. 6.38a and b Secondary anaemia: bone marrow aspirate showing (a) fragments containing adequate iron in the reticuloendothelial cells and (b) no siderotic granules in the developing erythroblasts. (Perls' stain.)

In the majority of patients with systemic disease and anaemia, no particular morphological features are seen in the blood other than mild hypochromasia. In liver disease, however, red cell macrocytosis, acanthocytosis and target cell formation (*Fig. 6.39*) are frequent. The mean cell volume is particularly raised when alcohol is the underlying cause. Bleeding caused by oesophageal or gastric varices, peptic ulceration, folate deficiency or haemolysis, especially in Zieve's syndrome (jaundice, hyperlipidaemia, hypercholesterolaemia and haemolytic anaemia with excess alcohol intake), may complicate the picture. In chronic renal failure, 'burr' cells and other bizarre poikilocytes are characteristic (*Fig.*

6.40; *see also Fig. 4.32*). In disseminated adenocarcinoma, microangiopathic haemolytic anaemia (*Fig. 6.41*; *see also Fig. 4.48*) may occur. Small acanthocytic forms occur in some patients with hypothyroidism (*Fig. 6.42*). Infections cause a wide variety of changes (*Fig. 6.43*; *see also Fig. 4.57*).

Connective tissue diseases are also important causes of anaemia in which haemolysis, renal failure and anaemia of chronic disorders may all play a part. The lupus erythematosus cell test, used to diagnose systemic lupus erythematosus, has now been replaced by tests for antinuclear factor (*Fig. 6.44*) and DNA binding.

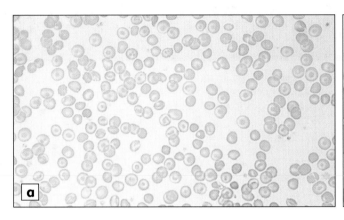

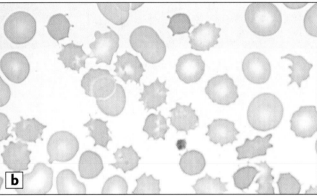

Fig. 6.39a and b Liver disease: peripheral blood films showing (a) marked target cell formation and (b), at higher magnification, marked red cell acanthocytosis.

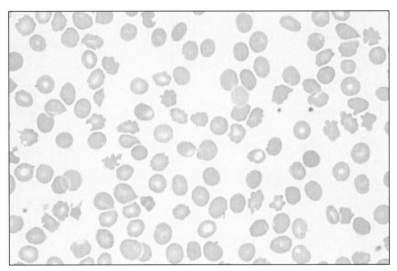

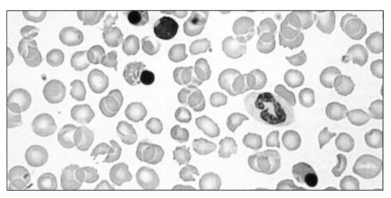

Fig. 6.41 Carcinomatosis: peripheral blood film of microangiopathic haemolytic and leucoerythroblastic anaemia in a 52-year-old man who presented with severe anaemia (Hb, 4.1 g/dl; reticulocytes, 18%) associated with widespread adenocarcinoma in the bone marrow. The primary site was unknown. There are deeply staining fragmented red cells, polychromasia and circulating erythroblasts. Platelets were severely reduced (32×10^9/l) and fibrin degradation products were present in serum.

Fig. 6.40 Renal failure: peripheral blood film showing coarse acanthocytes and 'burr' cells.

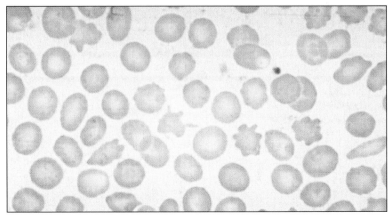

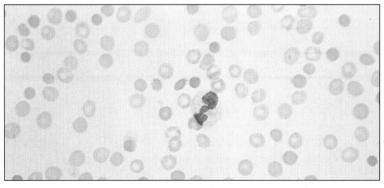

Fig. 6.43 Haemolytic anaemia: peripheral blood film in patient with haemolytic anaemia in clostridial septicaemia showing red cell contraction and spherocytosis. (From Hoffbrand AV, Pettit JE. *Essential Haematology*, 3rd edn. Oxford: Blackwell Scientific Publications; 1993.)

Fig. 6.42 Hypothyroidism: peripheral blood film showing mild macrocytosis, poikilocytosis and irregular acanthocytosis.

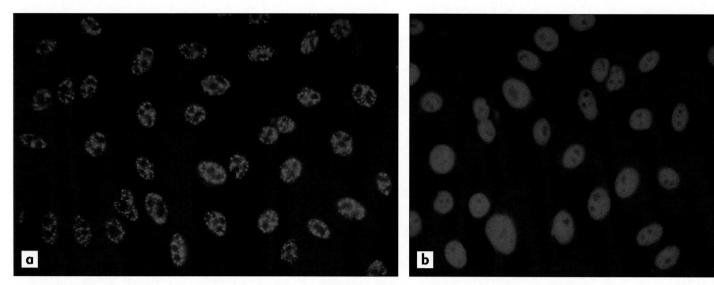

Fig. 6.44 Connective tissue disease: antinuclear factor test by indirect immunofluorescence on human epithelial carcinoma cell line HEP-2. (a) Mixed connective tissue disease showing a positive speckled pattern; (b) systemic lupus erythematosus showing a homogeneous pattern. [(a, b) Courtesy of the Department of Immunology, Royal Free School of Medicine; from Hoffbrand AV, Pettit JE. *Essential Haematology*, 3rd edn. Oxford: Blackwell Scientific Publications; 1993.]

7 Benign Disorders of Leucocytes

Normal white cell appearances and production were discussed in Chapter 1 and the present chapter is concerned with conditions which may be associated with abnormal white cell morphology or numbers, only some of which are associated with clinical problems. The primary immunodeficiency syndromes and the acquired immune deficiency syndrome (AIDS) are dealt with in this chapter. The acute and chronic leukaemias, myelodysplasia, lymphomas and myeloma are discussed in Chapters 8–12.

HEREDITARY VARIATION IN WHITE CELL MORPHOLOGY

Pelger–Huët anomaly

In the Pelger–Huët anomaly, characteristic bilobed neutrophils are found in the peripheral blood. Occasional unsegmented neutrophils with round nuclei are also seen, particularly during infection (*Fig. 7.1*). The inheritance is dominant. The condition appears to be of no clinical significance and the affected cells have not been shown to be functionally abnormal. 'Pseudo-Pelger' cells occur in acute myeloid leukaemia and the myelodysplastic syndromes.

May–Hegglin anomaly

In the May–Hegglin anomaly, a rare condition that has a dominant inheritance pattern, abnormal condensations of RNA appear as mildly basophilic inclusions in the neutrophil cytoplasm (*Fig. 7.2*). The majority of patients also have thrombocytopenia and giant platelets. Although most affected individuals have no clinical abnormality, in some there are haemorrhagic manifestations. Similar cytoplasmic inclusions, which are termed Döhle bodies, may be seen in neutrophils during severe infections (*see Fig. 7.12*) and occasionally in normal pregnancy.

Chédiak–Higashi syndrome

Chédiak–Higashi syndrome is a severe anomaly associated with giant neutrophil granules. A similar granular abnormality is seen in granulopoietic cells in the marrow and in eosinophils, monocytes and lymphocytes (*Fig. 7.3*). The inheritance is autosomal recessive. Affected children usually have neutropenia and thrombocytopenia, and suffer from recurrent severe infections. Clinical examination frequently reveals partial albinism and marked hepatosplenomegaly. The majority die in childhood from infection or haemorrhage.

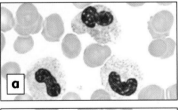
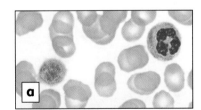
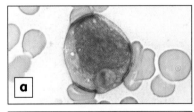
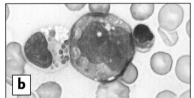

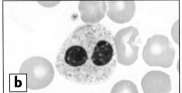
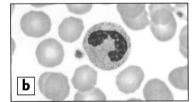
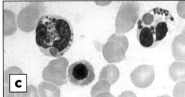
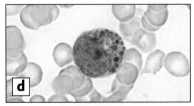

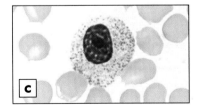
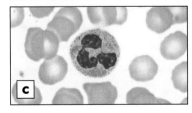
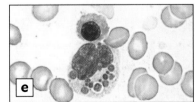
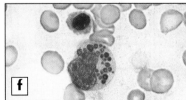

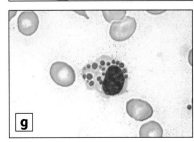

Fig. 7.1a–c Pelger–Huët anomaly: coarse clumping of the chromatin in (a) neutrophils and (b) 'pince-nez' configurations; (c) a single rounded nucleus seen mostly in rare homozygous patients. 'Pseudo-Pelger' neutrophils can be seen in myeloid leukaemias and the myelodysplastic syndromes.

Fig. 7.2a–c May–Hegglin anomaly: (a–c) the neutrophils contain basophilic inclusions 2–5 μm in diameter. These inclusions are similar to Döhle bodies (*see Fig. 7.12*), but are not related to infection. There is an associated mild thrombocytopenia with giant platelets (a).

Fig. 7.3a–g Chédiak–Higashi syndrome: bizarre giant granules are found in the cytoplasm of all types of leucocytes and their precursors: (a) promyelocyte; (b) promonocyte and lymphocyte; (c) neutrophils; (d) early eosinophil; (e, f) monocytes; and (g) lymphocyte.

Alder's (Alder–Reilly) anomaly

Alder's (Alder–Reilly) anomaly gives rise to deep purple granules in neutrophils (*Fig. 7.4*). Similar abnormal granules are found in other granulocytes, monocytes and lymphocytes. The inheritance is autosomal recessive and the majority of affected individuals have no clinical problems. Similar leucocyte abnormalities are seen in patients with mucopolysaccharide storage disorders, such as Hurler's and Maroteaux–Lamy syndromes, and occasionally in amaurotic family idiocy (for instance, Spielmeyer–Vogt syndrome; see below).

Mucopolysaccharidoses VI and VII

Abnormal granulation of blood granulocytes and monocytes, together with lymphocyte vacuolation, is found in the Maroteaux–Lamy syndrome, which is also known as mucopolysaccharidosis VI (*Fig. 7.5*). The striking white cell abnormality may also be seen in patients with mucopolysaccharidosis VII. These lysosomal storage disorders are caused by an inherited deficiency of enzymes concerned in the breakdown of acid mucopolysaccharides. Storage-related abnormalities of connective tissue, the heart, the bony skeleton and the central nervous system (CNS) produce clinical disabilities similar to, but milder than, those found in classic Hurler's syndrome (mucopolysaccharidosis I).

Other causes of lymphocyte vacuolation

Similar lymphocyte vacuoles may be found (rarely) in patients with inherited defects of enzymes that are involved in the catabolism of oligosaccharide components of glycoproteins (e.g. mannosidosis), and in the rare Spielmeyer–Vogt syndrome (*Fig. 7.6*).

Disorders of phagocytic function

Disorders of phagocytic function may be inherited or acquired. Inherited disorders involve adherence, mobility and migration (e.g. leucocyte adhesion deficiency), or phagocytosis and killing. Chronic granulomatous disease (CGD) is a rare disease of killing; 60% of cases are X-linked, the others are autosomal recessive (*Fig. 7.7*). Neutrophils, eosinophils and monocytes are affected. The patient presents with recurrent infections, usually with catalase-positive organisms (*Fig. 7.8*), Gram-negative bacilli or *Aspergillus* spp., often in the first year of life. Inability of the neutrophils to reduce nitroblue tetrazolium dye suggests the diagnosis.

LEUCOCYTOSIS

The term leucocytosis refers to an increase in white blood cells (usually to above 12×10^9/l). The most frequent cause is an increase in blood neutrophils. Other leucocytoses involve a predominance of one of the other white cell types found in the blood.

Neutrophil leucocytosis (neutrophilia)

An increase in neutrophils in the blood of more than 7.5×10^9/l is one of the most frequent abnormalities found in blood counts and blood films (*Fig. 7.9*). Clinically, fever often results from the release of leucocyte pyrogen. In most neutrophilias the number of band forms increases; occasionally, more primitive cells such as metamyelocytes and myelocytes appear in the peripheral blood (the so-called left shift). In most causes of reactive neutrophil leucocytosis (*Fig. 7.10*), toxic changes appear in the neutrophil cytoplasm and on occasion Döhle bodies are present (*Figs 7.11 and 7.12*). The neutrophil alkaline phosphatase score (*Fig. 7.13*) is characteristically elevated.

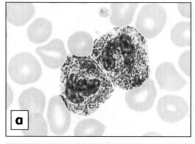
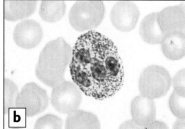

Fig. 7.4a and b Alder's anomaly: (a, b) coarse red-violet granules in neutrophils. In this case there was no associated clinical abnormality.

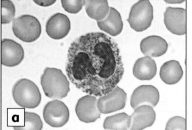
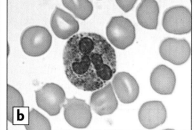
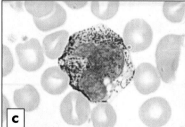
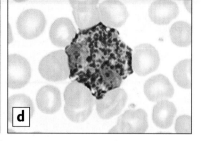
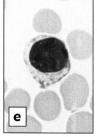
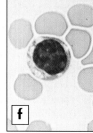

Fig. 7.5a–f Maroteaux–Lamy syndrome: (a, b) coarse red–violet granules in neutrophils, (c) monocyte and (d) basophil, and (e, f) prominent vacuolation of lymphocytes. In this variant of Hurler's syndrome, there are severe skeletal abnormalities and clouding of the cornea.

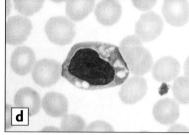
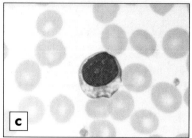
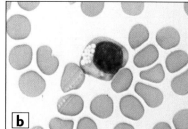
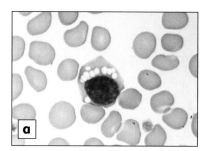

Fig. 7.6a–d Lymphocyte vacuolation: further examples of prominent cytoplasmic vacuolation in lymphocytes in (a, b) mannosidosis and in (c, d) the Spielmeyer–Vogt syndrome (juvenile onset amaurotic idiocy).

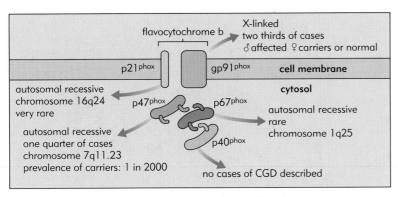

Fig. 7.7 Chronic granulomatous disease: NADPH oxidase components shown to be defective in CGD. The NADPH oxidase is composed of a flavocytochrome b in the membrane of the phagocytic vacuole. This is made up of a protein, gp91^{phox}, which is the flavocytochrome itself and has the NADPH FAD and two haem binding sites. Its gene, located on the X-chromosome, is abnormal in about two thirds of cases of CGD. The gene of the other subunit (p21^{phox}) of this molecule is located on chromosome 16; very occasional defects of this can cause CGD. The genes of the cytosolic proteins p47^{phox} and p67^{phox} are located on chromosome 7 and 1, respectively. Activation of the oxidase is associated with translocation of these two proteins from the cytosol to the membrane, where they bind to the flavocytochrome b. Autosomal recessive CGD is normally associated with the lesion p47^{phox} in about one quarter of cases, and occasionally with p67^{phox} (Courtesy of Prof. AW Segal.)

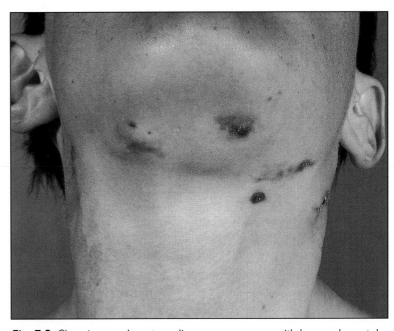

Fig. 7.8 Chronic granulomatous disease: young man with large submental and cervical nodes with poorly healed sinuses as a result of staphylococcal infection. Cervical lymphadenitis, poor healing and sinus formation are characteristic and can be confused with tuberculosis because of the granulomatous tissue reaction. (Courtesy of Prof. AW Segal.)

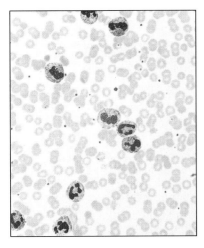

Fig. 7.9 Neutrophil leucocytosis: large numbers of band-form and segmented neutrophils in the peripheral blood. The patient had abdominal sepsis. (WBC, 45 × 10^9/l; neutrophils, 41 × 10^9/l.)

Causes of neutrophil leucocytosis	
Bacterial infections Pyogenic – localized or generalized	**Corticosteroid therapy**
	Acute haemorrhage and haemolysis
Inflammation, necrosis Cardiac infarct, ischaemia, trauma, vasculitis	**Myeloproliferative disorders** Polycythaemia vera, myelofibrosis, chronic myeloid leukaemia
Metabolic disorders Uraemia, acidosis, gout, poisoning, eclampsia	**Chronic myelomonocytic leukaemia**
	Malignant neoplasms

Fig. 7.10 Neutrophil leucocytosis: causes.

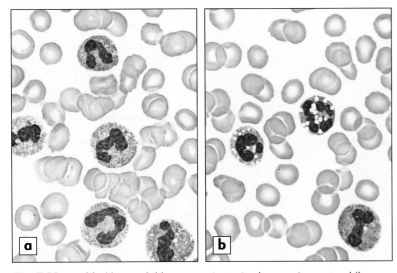

Fig. 7.11a and b Neutrophil leucocytosis: toxic changes in neutrophils include (a) the presence of red–purple granules in the band-form neutrophils and (b) cytoplasmic vacuolation.

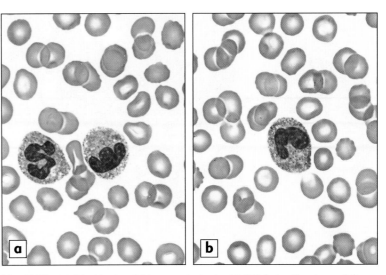

Fig. 7.12a and b Neutrophil leucocytosis: (a, b) Döhle bodies, basophilic inclusions of denatured RNA, can be seen in the cytoplasm of these neutrophils.

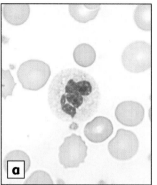
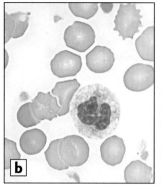
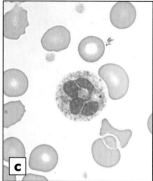
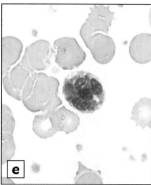
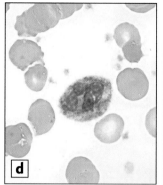

Fig. 7.13a–e Neutrophil alkaline phosphatase score: after cytochemical staining for alkaline phosphatase activity, 100 neutrophils are assessed for intensity of staining. From (a) to (e), the cells score 0, 1, 2, 3 and 4, respectively. High scores are found typically in reactive neutrophil leucocytoses, polycythaemia vera and myelofibrosis. Very low scores are found in chronic myeloid leukaemia.

Eosinophil leucocytosis (eosinophilia)

Eosinophilia is the term applied to an increase in blood eosinophils above 0.4×10^9/l (*Fig. 7.14*); the causes of eosinophilia are listed in *Fig. 7.15*.

There are a number of pulmonary eosinophilic syndromes of varying severity; they are characterized by transient pulmonary infiltrates (*Fig. 7.16a*) cough, fever and peripheral eosinophilia. Corticosteroid treatment usually results in the resolution of symptoms and the prompt clearance of infiltrates (*Fig. 7.16b*). Similar changes may occur in some parasitic infestations when migrating parasites lodge in the lungs.

Monocytosis and basophil leucocytosis

Conditions associated with monocytosis (*Fig. 7.17*) are listed in *Fig. 7.18*. A basophil leucocytosis is seen most frequently in patients with chronic myeloid leukaemia (*Fig. 7.19*) or polycythaemia vera. Moderate increases in blood basophils also occur in myxoedema, chickenpox, smallpox and ulcerative colitis.

LEUKAEMOID REACTION

The leukaemoid reaction is a benign but excessive leucocytosis that is characterized by the presence of immature cells (blasts, promye-

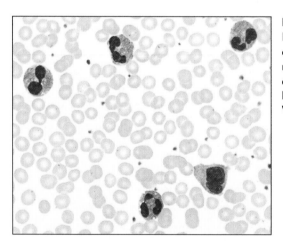

Fig. 7.14 Eosinophilia: four eosinophils and a monocyte in dermatitis herpetiformis. (Total WBC, 20×10^9/l.)

Causes of eosinophilia	
Allergies Asthma, hayfever, urticaria, drugs (e.g. gold, allopurinol)	**Eosinophilic leukaemia**
Parasites Ancylostomiasis, ascariasis, filariasis, trichinosis, toxocariasis	**Miscellaneous** Eosinophilic granuloma, erythema multiforme, polyarteritis nodosa, sarcoidosis, hypereosinophilic syndrome, post-irradiation, pulmonary eosinophilia (including Löffler's syndrome), tropical eosinophilia
Skin diseases Eczema, psoriasis, dermatitis herpetiformis	
Neoplastic disease Hodgkin lymphoma and others	

Fig. 7.15 Eosinophilia: causes.

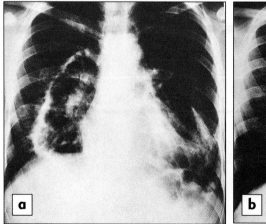
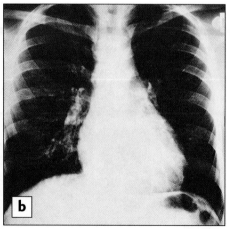
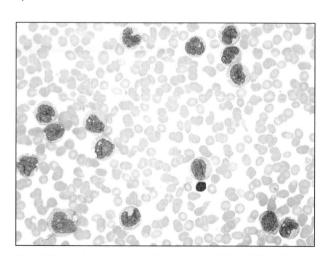

Fig. 7.16a and b Pulmonary eosinophilia: chest radiographs showing (a) diffuse infiltrates in the right middle and lower, and left lower zones. Prominent band shadows suggest areas of collapse. The patient had been taking sulfasalazine for ulcerative colitis. This drug was stopped and prednisolone commenced. (b) The radiograph shows the same patient 3 weeks later; there is almost complete resolution of the pulmonary changes.

Fig. 7.17 Monocytosis: in this peripheral blood film of chronic myelomonocytic leukaemia (myelodysplasia), with the exception of a single lymphocyte (centre), all the nucleated cells shown are monocytes. (Total WBC, 36×10^9/l; monocytes, 30×10^9/l.)

locytes and myelocytes) in the peripheral blood. Whereas most leukaemoid reactions involve blood granulocytes (*Fig. 7.20*), lymphocytic reactions also occur in some. The majority of these reactions are found in association with severe or chronic infections, and sometimes they are also a feature of widespread metastatic cancer or severe haemolysis. Leukaemoid reactions occur more frequently in children.

From the diagnostic point of view, the main problem is to distinguish these reactions from chronic myeloid leukaemia. Changes such as toxic granulation, Döhle bodies and a high neutrophil alkaline phosphatase (NAP) score are characteristically found in leukaemoid reactions, while large numbers of myelocytes, a low NAP score and the presence of the Philadelphia chromosome indicate chronic myeloid leukaemia.

LEUCOERYTHROBLASTIC REACTION

Another blood cell variation is leucoerythroblastic reaction, in which erythroblasts as well as primitive white cells are found in the peripheral blood (*Figs 7.21 and 7.22*). This reaction is most frequently found when a distortion of marrow architecture is present, because of either proliferative disorders of the marrow or marrow infiltrations, or extramedullary erythropoiesis. The principal causes of the leucoerythroblastic reaction are listed in *Fig. 7.23*.

NEUTROPENIA

Neutropenia is defined by a blood neutrophil count of less than 2.5×10^9/l. Note, however, that many African and Middle Eastern popula-

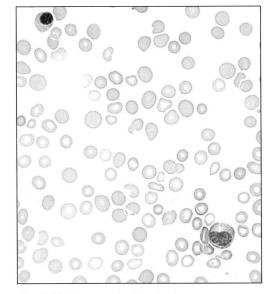

Fig. 7.18 Monocytosis: causes.

Causes of monocytosis
Infections Tuberculosis, brucellosis, bacterial endocarditis, malaria, kala-azar, trypanosomiasis, typhus
Other inflammatory diseases Sarcoidosis, ulcerative colitis, Crohn's disease, rheumatoid arthritis, systemic lupus erythematosus
Hodgkin's disease and other malignant neoplasms
Acute myelomonocytic and monocytic leukaemias, FAB classification AML – M₄ and M₅
Myelodysplastic syndrome, FAB classification chronic myelomonocytic leukaemia

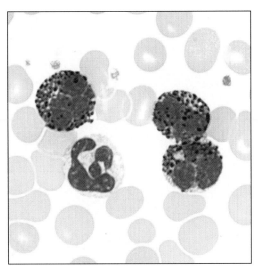

Fig. 7.19 Basophilia: high power view of three basophils and a neutrophil in a peripheral blood film of chronic myeloid leukaemia. (Total WBC, 73×10^9/l; basophils, 7.3×10^9/l.)

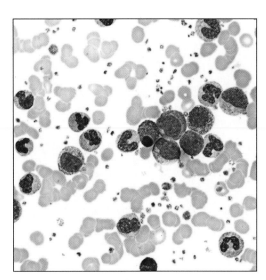

Fig. 7.20 Leukaemoid reaction: neutrophils, stab forms, metamyelocytes, myelocytes and a single necrobiotic neutrophil (centre) in staphylococcal pneumonia. (WBC, 94×10^9/l.)

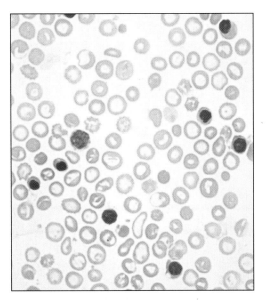

Fig. 7.21 Leucoerythroblastic change: an erythroblast, a myelocyte, red cell polychromasia, anisocytosis and poikilocytosis, including 'teardrop' forms, in myelofibrosis. (Hb, 9.5 g/dl; WBC, 5×10^9/l; 6 erythroblasts per 100 WBC; platelets, 45×10^9/l.)

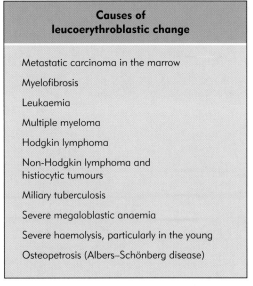

Fig. 7.22 Leucoerythroblastic change: erythroblasts, two lymphocytes, red cell polychromasia, hypochromia, poikilocytosis, acanthocytosis and spherocytosis. The differential white cell count included metamyelocytes and myelocytes. This is a case of homozygous α-thalassaemia (Hb Bart's disease).

Causes of leucoerythroblastic change
Metastatic carcinoma in the marrow
Myelofibrosis
Leukaemia
Multiple myeloma
Hodgkin lymphoma
Non-Hodgkin lymphoma and histiocytic tumours
Miliary tuberculosis
Severe megaloblastic anaemia
Severe haemolysis, particularly in the young
Osteopetrosis (Albers–Schönberg disease)

Fig. 7.23 Leucoerythroblastic change: causes.

tions have normal ranges with significantly lower limits than this. Clinical problems related to recurrent infections are associated with absolute levels below $0.5 \times 10^9/l$, and neutrophil counts of less than $0.2 \times 10^9/l$ carry grave risks. Neutropenia may be selective or part of a general pancytopenia (*Fig. 7.24*). The majority of neutropenias are caused by reduced granulopoiesis; but, in some patients, the reduced neutrophil counts are caused by increased removal of neutrophils by the reticuloendothelial system or by other tissues. Significant shifts of neutrophils from the circulating population to the marginal pool attached to the vascular endothelium may also be responsible.

Kostmann's syndrome

A severe congenital neutropenia, Kostmann's syndrome, is autosomal recessive. It presents as bacterial infections early in life. The neutrophil count is usually $<0.2 \times 10^9/l$. Bone marrow shows reduced or absent myeloid precursors. Point mutations in the gene coding for the G-CSF receptor have been detected in patients whose condition transforms into acute myeloid leukaemia (*Fig. 7.25*). Treatment is to give G-CSF and antibiotics.

Shwachman–Diamond syndrome

The Shwachman–Diamond syndrome consists of exocrine pancreatic deficiency with neutropenia and, like Kostmann's syndrome, it is autosomal recessive. It may be accompanied by anaemia, thrombocytopenia, short stature, metaphyseal chondrodysplasia and mental retardation. It may progress to myelodysplasia and acute myeloid leukaemia (*Fig. 7.26*).

Clinical and bone marrow findings

In severe neutropenia, painful and intractable infections of the buccal mucosa (*Figs 7.27 and 7.28*), throat, skin (*Fig. 7.29*) and the anal region often occur (*see also* Chapter 8).

Bone marrow examination is essential in all patients who present with severe neutropenia. Evidence of leukaemia or other infiltrations is

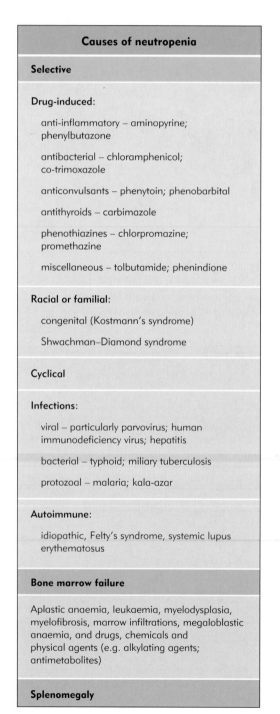

Fig. 7.24 Neutropenia: causes.

Causes of neutropenia
Selective
Drug-induced:
anti-inflammatory – aminopyrine; phenylbutazone
antibacterial – chloramphenicol; co-trimoxazole
anticonvulsants – phenytoin; phenobarbital
antithyroids – carbimazole
phenothiazines – chlorpromazine; promethazine
miscellaneous – tolbutamide; phenindione
Racial or familial:
congenital (Kostmann's syndrome)
Shwachman–Diamond syndrome
Cyclical
Infections:
viral – particularly parvovirus; human immunodeficiency virus; hepatitis
bacterial – typhoid; miliary tuberculosis
protozoal – malaria; kala-azar
Autoimmune:
idiopathic, Felty's syndrome, systemic lupus erythematosus
Bone marrow failure
Aplastic anaemia, leukaemia, myelodysplasia, myelofibrosis, marrow infiltrations, megaloblastic anaemia, and drugs, chemicals and physical agents (e.g. alkylating agents; antimetabolites)
Splenomegaly

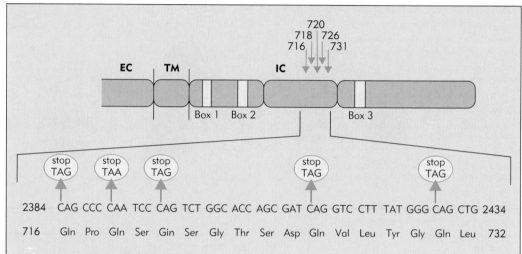

Fig. 7.25 Severe congenital neutropenia (Kostmann's syndrome): mutations in the gene coding for the G-CSF receptor have been described in different cases. (EC, IC, extra- and intracellular parts of the receptor; TM, transmembrane; Boxes 1–3, segments with homology to structures in other haemopoietic growth factor receptor genes; courtesy of Dr IP Touw and Prof. B Lowenberg.)

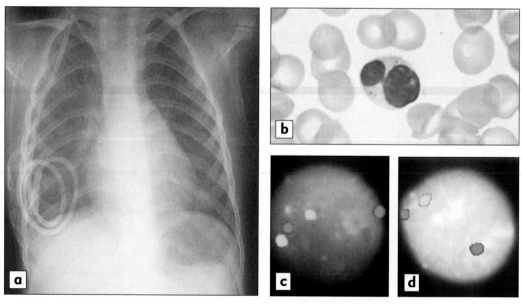

Fig. 7.26a–d Shwachman–Diamond syndrome transformed to myelodysplasia: (a) chest radiograph showing characteristic 'cupping' deformity of the ribs; (b) peripheral blood showing Pelger neutrophil. (c, d) fluorescence *in situ* hybridization technique showing (c) control and (d) patient with monosomy 7 (red, internal control; yellow, chromosome 7 centromeric probe). [(a–d) Courtesy of Dr OP Smith.]

found in many. In patients with selective depression of granulopoiesis, a reduction in all granulocyte precursors occurs (*Fig. 7.30*). In some cases, granulopoietic cells are absent (*Fig. 7.31*), but in others promyelocytes and myelocytes are present with no evidence of mature neutrophils.

Felty's syndrome

About 1% of patients with rheumatoid arthritis have associated splenomegaly (*Fig. 7.32*) and neutropenia. Some of these patients also show skin ulceration over the anterior surface of the tibia (*Fig. 7.33*).

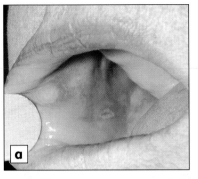 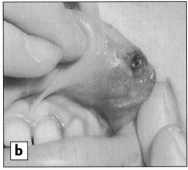

Fig. 7.27a and b Neutropenia: (a, b) ulceration of the buccal mucosa and upper lip in two patients with severe neutropenia.

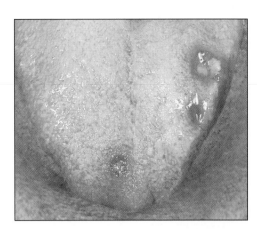

Fig. 7.28 Neutropenia: ulceration of the tongue in severe neutropenia.

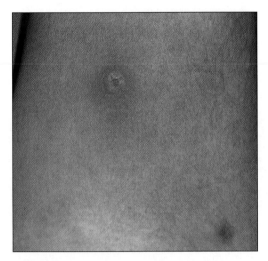

Fig. 7.29 Neutropenia: infected skin lesion with extensive surrounding subcutaneous cellulitis in severe neutropenia. Cultures grew *Staphylococcus aureus* and *Pseudomonas pyocyanea*.

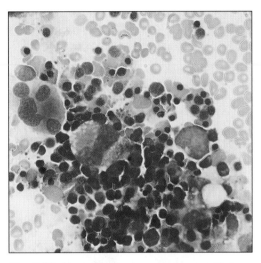

Fig. 7.30 Neutropenia: bone marrow aspirate showing an absence of granulopoietic cells. The small fragment and cell trail contain mainly erythroblasts and megakaryocytes.

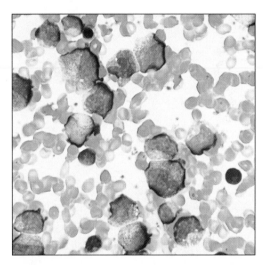

Fig. 7.31 Agranulocytosis: bone marrow aspirate showing numerous promyelocytes and myelocytes with mature neutrophils absent. (Courtesy of Prof. RD Brunning and the AFIP.)

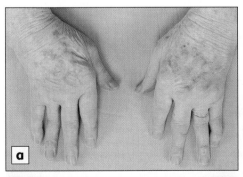
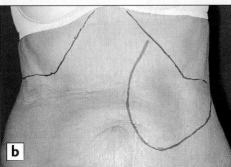

Fig. 7.32a and b Felty's syndrome: (a) the deformities of rheumatoid arthritis include prominent ulnar styloids, ulnar deviation of the hands, swan-neck deformities (best seen in the right fourth finger and left fourth and fifth fingers) and wasting of the intrinsic muscles; (b) splenic enlargement.

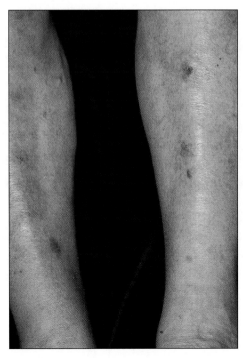

Fig. 7.33 Felty's syndrome: skin ulceration on the anterior surface of the leg (same patient as shown in *Fig. 7.32*).

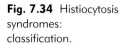

Classification of the histiocytosis syndromes

Dendritic cell related

Langerhan cell hystiocytosis
Juvenile xanthogranuloma
Solitary dendritic cell histiocytomas

Macrophage related

Haemophagocytic lymphohistiocytosis:
    primary (genetic)
    secondary
Sinus histiocytosis with massive lymphadenopathy
Solitary macrophage histiocytomas

Malignancies

AML FAB types M_4 and M_5
Extramedullary monocytic tumours
Chronic myelomonocytic leukaemia
Dendritic cell sarcomas
Macrophage-related sarcomas

Fig. 7.34 Histiocytosis syndromes: classification.

The neutropenia in Felty's syndrome is thought to result from anti-neutrophil autoantibodies; the bone marrow characteristically shows increased granulopoiesis. In patients with recurrent infections, splenectomy often results in a return to normal of blood neutrophil numbers.

HISTIOCYTIC PROLIFERATIONS

These are characterized by infiltration of tissues with cells of the macrophage–monocyte lineage and are divided into three classes (*Fig. 7.34*):
- benign abnormalities of dendritic cells;
- benign disorders of macrophages; and
- malignancies.

The malignant diseases are described in Chapter 11. The benign disorders are described and illustrated here.

Langerhan cell histiocytosis

Langerhan cell histiocytosis (LCH) comprises the diseases previously known as histiocytosis X – Letterer–Siwe disease, Hand–Schüller–Christian disease and eosinophilic granuloma of bone. Langerhan cells, distinguished on electron microscopy by the presence of Birbeck granules (*Fig. 7.35*), eosinophils, lymphocytes, neutrophils and macrophages, infiltrate a wide variety of organs, especially skin (*Fig. 7.36*), bone, lymph nodes, liver, spleen and bone marrow. The disease may be 'single' or multisystem. The lungs, CNS and gastrointestinal tract may also be involved. Multisystem LCH

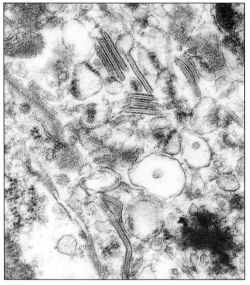

Fig. 7.35 Langerhan cell histiocytosis: Birbeck granules in the cytoplasm. These are rod-shaped structures with a central striated line that terminates in some cases in a vesicular dilatation, which gives a tennis racquet appearance. They may arise secondary to receptor-mediated endocytosis and are not present in normal monocytes and non-Langerhan macrophages. (courtesy of Prof. P Lanzkowsky.)

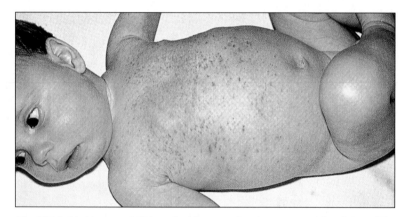

Fig. 7.36 Multisystem LCH: typical haemorrhagic eczematoid rash in a 10-month-old child. (Courtesy of Dr MD Holdaway.)

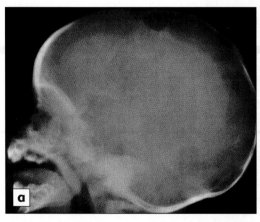
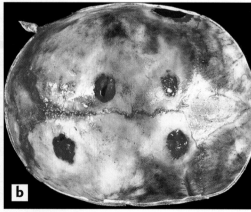

Fig. 7.37a and b Multisystem LCH: skull of an infant seen (a) radiographically and (b) at necropsy shows the typical osteolytic deposits in the vault.

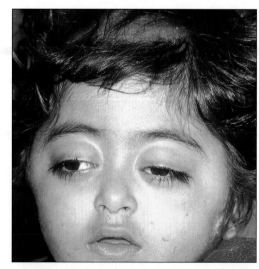

Fig. 7.38 Multisystem LCH: prominent bossing of the frontal bone and proptosis in a child with multiple skull deposits. (Courtesy of Dr U O'Callaghan.)

affects children initially in the first 3 years of life, with hepatosplenomegaly, lymphadenopathy and eczematoid skin eruptions. Localized lesions occur frequently in the skull (*Fig. 7.37 and 7.38*), ribs and long bones. Diabetes insipidus, caused by involvement of the hypothalamus and pituitary stalk (*Fig. 7.39*), occurs in both single and multisystem disease. The bone marrow is sometimes involved, later lesions being characterized by accumulation of lipid-laden macrophages (*Fig. 7.40*). In localized disease in bone a high proportion of eosinophils may be present (*Fig. 7.41*).

Haemophagocytic lymphohistiocytosis

Haemophagocytic lymphohistiocytosis (HLH) occurs in a familial primary form with a recessive inheritance pattern that affects infants and young children and an acquired secondary form precipitated by viral, bacterial, fungal or protozoan infections, which occurs particularly in immunocompromised patients. HLH presents with fever, splenomegaly, pancytopenia, liver dysfunction and coagulation changes. Histiocytic hyperplasia and haemophagocytosis occur in bone marrow (*Fig. 7.42*),

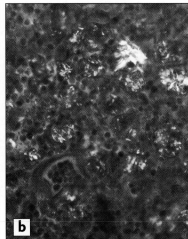

Fig. 7.39 Multisystem LCH: magnetic resonance imaging showing thickened pituitary stalk with absent posterior pituitary signal on T1 weighted images. (Courtesy of Dr DKH Webb.)

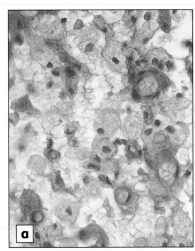

Fig. 7.40a and b Multisystem LCH: frozen sections of a skeletal lesion stained using the Sudan IV technique and viewed under (a) normal and (b) polarized light. The staining reaction indicated accumulation in the cytoplasm of neutral fat and cholesterol.

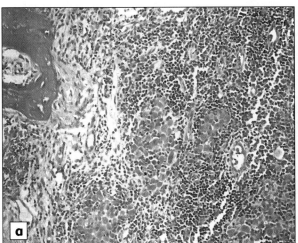
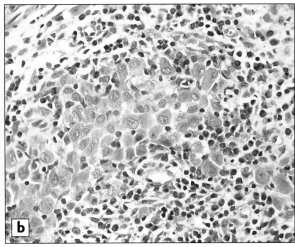

Fig. 7.41a and b Single system LCH: trephine biopsy of a 28-year-old-man with skeletal lesions shows (a) replacement of normal haemopoietic tissue by sheets of histiocytes and eosinophils; (b) higher power view of the abnormal histiocytes and eosinophils.

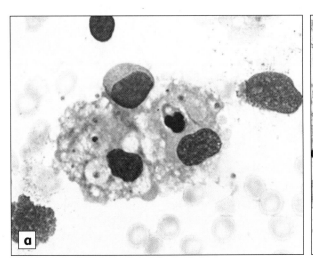
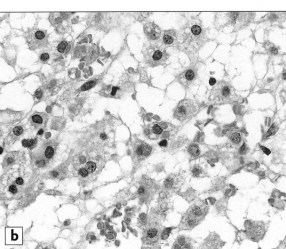

Fig. 7.42a and b Virus-associated haemophagocytic lymphohistiocytosis: (a) bone marrow aspirate showing a group of histiocytes that have engulfed red cells and erythroblasts. (b) Bone marrow trephine biopsy showing replacement of normal architecture by erythrophagocytic histiocytes. This reactive condition associated with viral infection may be confused with malignant histiocytosis. [(a) Courtesy of Dr S Knowles; (b) courtesy of Prof. KA MacLennan.]

liver, spleen or lymph nodes and other tissues, and in the familial form there is often CNS involvement (*Fig. 7.43*).

Sinus histiocytosis with massive lymphadenopathy

Sinus histiocytosis with massive lymphadenopathy is a rare condition seen most frequently in young blacks and is characterized by lymphadenopathy, fever, leucocytosis and hypergammaglobulinaemia. It is thought to be the result of an abnormal reaction to viral infection. The cervical nodes are usually involved (*Fig. 7.44*). Histologically, the nodes show marked sinusoidal dilatation by macrophages with foamy cytoplasm (*Fig. 7.45*) and plasma cells. Although the disease may follow a protracted course, recovery is usually spontaneous and total.

LYMPHOCYTOSIS

The main causes of an increase in the absolute lymphocyte count are listed in *Fig. 7.46*. Greatly raised levels are usually seen in adults with chronic lymphocytic leukaemia. Infants with pertussis and children with acute infectious lymphocytosis, an unusual viral disease, may also have very high lymphocyte counts. Lymphocytoses with large numbers of atypical or 'reactive' cells are most often seen in

infectious mononucleosis, in other viral illnesses (including infectious hepatitis) and in toxoplasmosis. Unusually heavy smoking is probably, although this is unclear, associated with a benign polyclonal lymphocytosis (*Fig. 7.47*).

Infectious mononucleosis

Infectious mononucleosis (glandular fever) is a disorder characterized by sore throat, fever, lymphadenopathy and atypical lymphocytes in the blood. The disease appears to be the result of infection with Epstein–Barr (EB) virus. In affected patients, heterophil antibodies against sheep red cells are found in the serum at high titres (Paul–Bunnell test).

Most patients present with lethargy, malaise and fever. On examination the majority show lymphadenopathy (*Fig. 7.48*).

Generalized inflammation of the oral and pharyngeal surfaces with follicular tonsillitis (*Fig. 7.49*) is usual, and some patients show palatal petechiae (*Fig. 7.50*). Periorbital and facial oedema (*Fig. 7.51*) or a morbilliform rash (*Fig. 7.52*) may be present.

Palpable splenomegaly occurs in over half the patients. Occasionally subcapsular haematomas of the spleen (*Fig. 7.53*) are present, and have a tendency to rupture. Jaundice as a result of liver involvement occurs in a minority of patients.

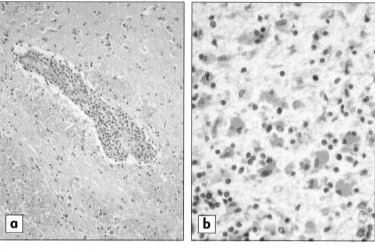

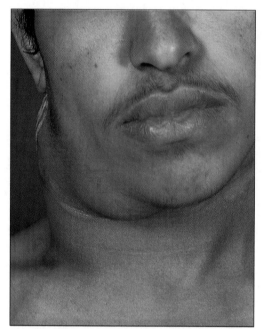

Fig. 7.44 Sinus histiocytosis with massive lymphadenopathy: massive painless cervical lymphadenopathy in a teenager from the Middle East. This resolved spontaneously over a 2-year period.

Fig. 7.43a and b Familial haemophagocytic lymphohistiocytosis: (a) section of brain at necropsy showing a collection of lymphocytes in the perivascular (Virchow–Robin) space; (b) higher magnification shows histiocytes that contain both red cells (erythrophagocytosis) and lymphocytes (lymphophagocytosis) in the parenchyma. [(a, b) Courtesy of Dr JE McLaughlin.]

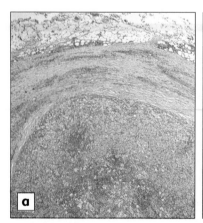
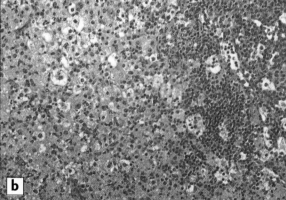
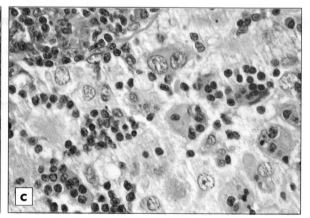

Fig. 7.45a–c Sinus histiocytosis with massive lymphadenopathy: (a) lymph node biopsy showing marked capsular and pericapsular fibrosis The sinuses are distended by a proliferation of histiocytes. This condition may occasionally be confused with a histiocytic lymphoma. (b) Higher power shows a confluent mass of histiocytes with abundant vacuolated cytoplasm can be seen. There is a focal collection of lymphocytes and residual medullary cords. (c) Higher power view showing characteristic histiocytes with engulfment of lymphocytes. [(c) Courtesy of Prof. KA MacLennan.]

Causes of lymphocytosis

Acute infections
   rubella, pertussis, mumps, infectious mononucleosis, acute infectious lymphocytosis

Chronic infections
   tuberculosis, brucellosis, infective hepatitis, syphilis

Thyrotoxicosis

Smoking

Chronic lymphocytic leukaemia (see Chapter 10)

Other lymphoid leukaemias and lymphomas (see Chapters 10 and 11)

Large granular lymphocytosis

Fig. 7.46 Lymphocytosis: causes.

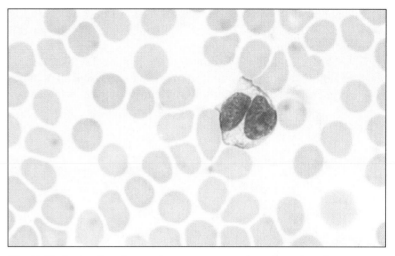

Fig. 7.47 Benign lymphocytosis: representative binucleate lymphocyte in the peripheral blood of a heavy smoker with polyclonal lymphocytosis. (Courtesy of Dr BA Bain.)

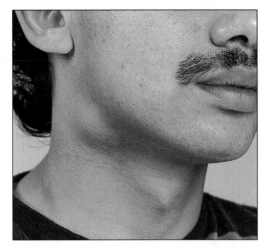

Fig. 7.48 Infectious mononucleosis: cervical lymphadenopathy in a 19-year-old man who presented with fever and pharyngitis.

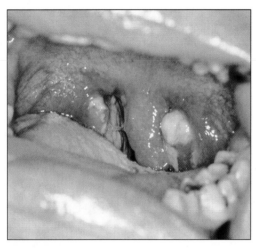

Fig. 7.49 Infectious mononucleosis: gross swelling and haemorrhagic erythema of the oropharynx. The tonsils are covered by a purulent exudate.

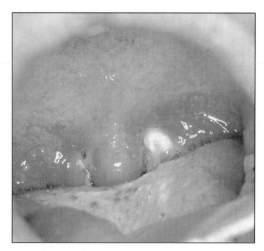

Fig. 7.50 Infectious mononucleosis: oropharynx (same case as shown in *Fig. 7.49*) showing marked swelling of the uvula and tonsils, and palatal petechial haemorrhage.

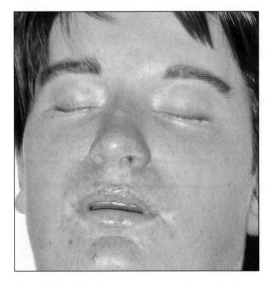

Fig. 7.51 Infectious mononucleosis: marked facial and periorbital oedema.

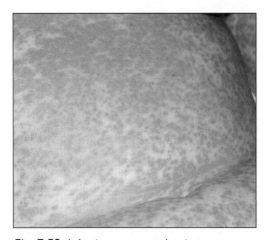

Fig. 7.52 Infectious mononucleosis: morbilliform erythematous skin eruption. There was generalized lymphadenopathy and the spleen was enlarged to 3 cm below the left costal margin.

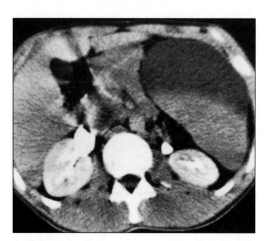

Fig. 7.53 Infectious mononucleosis: abdominal computed tomography (CT) scan showing massive enlargement of the spleen with a large anterior subcapsular haematoma (area of decreased density).

The diagnosis is suspected by finding a moderate lymphocytosis ($10-20 \times 10^9$/l) and large numbers of atypical lymphocytes in the peripheral blood film (*Fig. 7.54*).

A number of conditions, including acute leukaemia, toxoplasmosis, infectious hepatitis, human immunodeficiency virus (HIV) infection and follicular tonsillitis, are likely to create initial problems of diagnosis. Lymph node biopsy or fine-needle aspiration cytology of the affected nodes may be helpful (*Figs 7.55–7.65*). In infectious

mononucleosis the cytology is dominated by reactive lymphocytic changes (*Fig. 7.57*), while in toxoplasmosis characteristic small groups of histiocytes may be found (*Fig. 7.58*). Also, CT scans may be helpful in distinguishing benign lymphadenopathy from lymphoma (*Fig. 7.59*).

Lymph node biopsy may be needed to distinguish benign conditions (e.g. infectious, immune reactions, vasculitides) from malignant conditions (*Figs 7.60–7.65*).

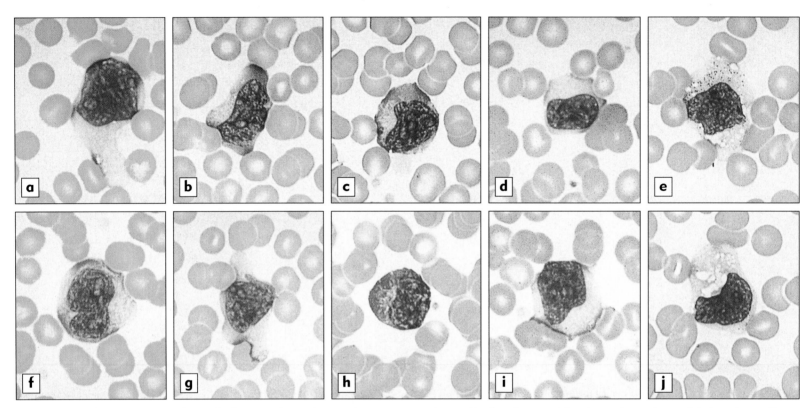

Fig. 7.54a–j Infectious mononucleosis: (a-j) representative 'reactive' lymphocytes in the peripheral blood film of a 21-year-old man. These are T lymphocytes reacting to B cells infected by the Epstein–Barr virus. The cells are large with abundant vacuolated cytoplasm; the nuclei often show a fine blast-like chromatin pattern. The edges of the lymphocytes are often indented by adjacent red cells.

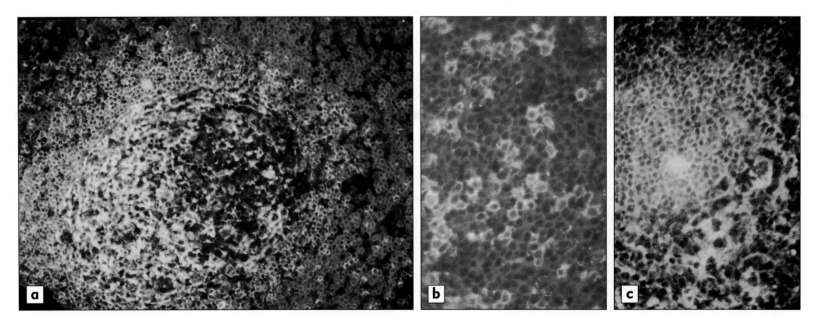

Fig. 7.55a–c Reactive lymphadenopathy: T cells (red rhodamine labelling) occupy the paracortical area surrounding the mainly B lymphocyte corona that expresses IgM (green fluorescein labelling). A number of T cells are scattered within the germinal centre, where immune complexes are also stained strongly by the IgM antisera. (b) The T cells within the paracortical area are a mixture of CD4$^+$ helper (red) and CD8$^+$ suppressor/cytotoxic (green) cells. (c) At the edge of a germinal centre is a mixture of B lymphocytes expressing χ (red) or λ (green) light chains. [(a–c) Courtesy of Dr M Chilosi, Prof. G Janossy and Dr C Pizzolo.]

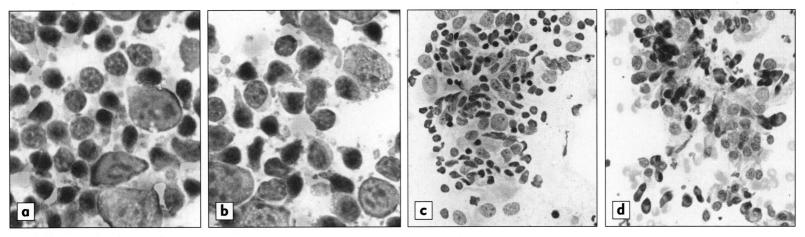

Fig. 7.56a–d Reactive lymphadenopathy: fine-needle aspirate of cervical lymph node showing (a, b) a pleomorphic lymphoid population with large immunoblasts, centroblasts, paler centrocytes and small lymphocytes; (c) small and medium sized lymphoid cells and histiocytes; (d) plasma cells, histiocytes and lymphocytes.

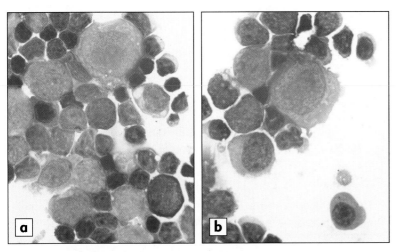

Fig. 7.57a and b Infectious mononucleosis: (a, b) fine-needle aspirate of cervical lymph node showing a pleomorphic lymphoid population including immunoblasts, centroblasts, centrocytes and small lymphocytes.

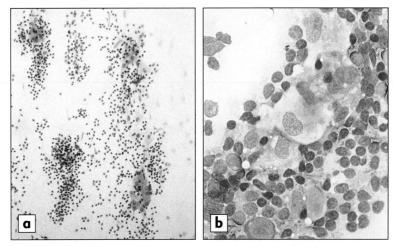

Fig. 7.58a and b Toxoplasmosis: fine-needle aspirate of cervical lymph node showing (a) groups of histiocytic cells in the cell trails; (b) at higher magnification predominantly small lymphocytes that surround these histiocytes are seen. [(a) Papanicolaou's stain; (b) May–Grünwald/Giemsa stain.]

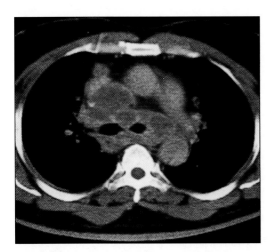

Fig. 7.59 Tuberculosis: CT scan showing tuberculous lymph nodes in the mediastinum. This is typical of tuberculosis. Lymphoma can occasionally produce this appearance. (Courtesy of Dr L Berger.)

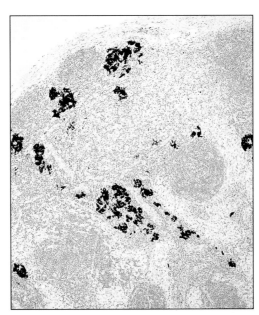

Fig. 7.60 Tattoo pigment in the sinus areas of a lymph node. (Courtesy of Dr JE McLaughlin.)

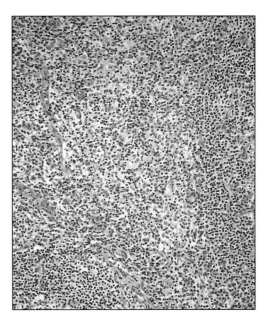

Fig. 7.61 Dermatopathic lymphadenopathy: clear cytoplasm of interdigitating reticulum cells gives an area of pallor above a follicle. Occasional phagocytic cells that contain melanin are visible. (Courtesy of Dr JE McLaughlin.)

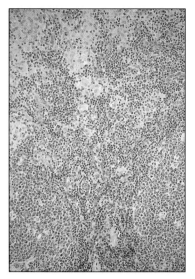

Fig. 7.62 Toxoplasmosis: small clusters of epithelial histiocytes above two hyperplastic follicles. (Courtesy of Dr JE McLaughlin.)

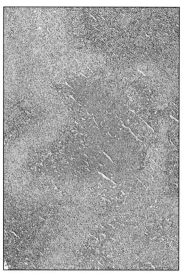

Fig. 7.63 Cat scratch disease: a geographical area of necrosis within a granuloma is visible. (Courtesy of Dr JE McLaughlin.)

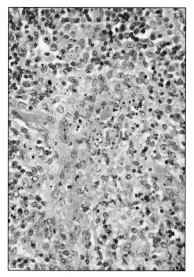

Fig. 7.64 Kawasaki's disease: vasculitic reaction in a lymph node. (Courtesy of Dr JE McLaughlin.)

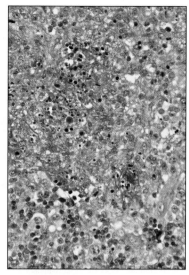

Fig. 7.65 Kawasaki's disease: fibrin (red) deposition in the wall of a small blood vessel. (Courtesy of Dr JE McLaughlin.)

Kikuchi's disease

Kikuchi's disease (also called Kikuchi–Fujimoto and histiocytic necrotizing lymphadenitis) was first recognized in Japan, but is now known to have world-wide distribution. It is more common in young women, presenting with persistent tender or non-tender lymphadenopathy; fever and a viral-like prodromal syndrome are frequent, and mild leukopenia may be present. Cervical nodes are involved most often, but any group of nodes may be affected. No associated virus has been found, and systemic lupus erythematosus (SLE) is suggested by the histopathology, but Kikuchi patients rarely develop SLE (*Fig. 7.66*).

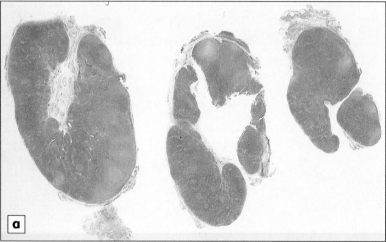

Fig. 7.66a–e Kikuchi disease: (a) whole mount of lymph node 'bread-sliced' into three parts showing pale circumscribed areas of necrosis; (b) low-power view of cortical area of necrosis; (c) high-power view of necrosis with karyorrhectic debris (note the absence of neutrophils); (d) adjacent 'cuff' of lymphoblasts, including T-cell blasts and macrophages; (e) characteristic 'crescentic' or 'signet cell' macrophages adjacent to areas of necrosis. [(a–e) Courtesy of Dr T Levine.]

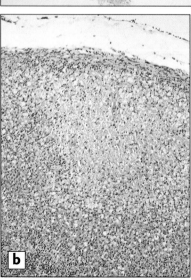

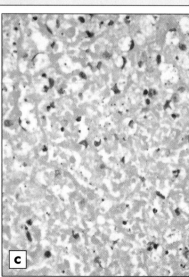

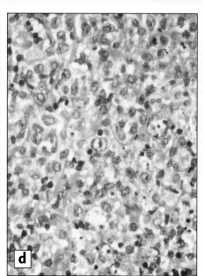

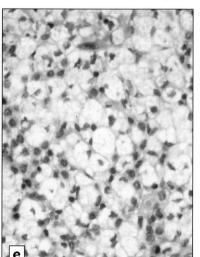

PRIMARY IMMUNODEFICIENCY DISORDERS

The main types of primary and secondary immunodeficiency disease are listed in *Fig. 7.67*. A detailed map of the site of the defect in the congenital immune deficiencies is given in *Fig. 7.68*. In severe combined immunodeficiency disease, the T- and B-lymphocyte systems fail to develop. There is severe lymphopenia and hypogammaglobulinaemia. Affected infants fail to thrive (*Fig. 7.69*) and die early in life from recurrent infections, such as by *Pneumocystis carinii*, cytomegalovirus, other viruses, fungi and bacteria. Atrophy of the thymus occurs (*Fig. 7.70*); the lymph nodes and spleen are small and devoid of lymphoid cells. The most common cause is deficiency of the enzyme adenosine deaminase

Fig. 7.67 Immunodeficiency disorders: letters A–H refer to *Fig. 7.68*.

Immunodeficiency disorders	
Primary	**Secondary**
B cell	**B cell**
F – X-linked hypogammaglobulinaemia (Bruton-type immunodeficiency)	Myeloma
E – μ chain defects	Nephrotic syndrome
G – Immunodeficiency with hyper IgM	Protein-losing enteropathy
H – Selective deficiency of IgA or IgM	**T cell**
H – Common variable immunodeficiency disease	HIV infection
	Hodgkin lymphoma
T cell	Non-Hodgkin lymphoma
C – Thymic hypoplasia (DiGeorge syndrome)	Drugs (e.g. corticosteroids, cyclosporine, azathioprine)
Mixed B and T cell	**Mixed B and T cell**
B, C, D – Severe combined immunodeficiency disease	Chronic lymphocytic leukaemia
Bloom's syndrome	Chemotherapy, radiotherapy, stem cell transplantation
Ataxia telangiectasia	
Wiskott–Aldrich syndrome	
A – Reticular dysgenesis	

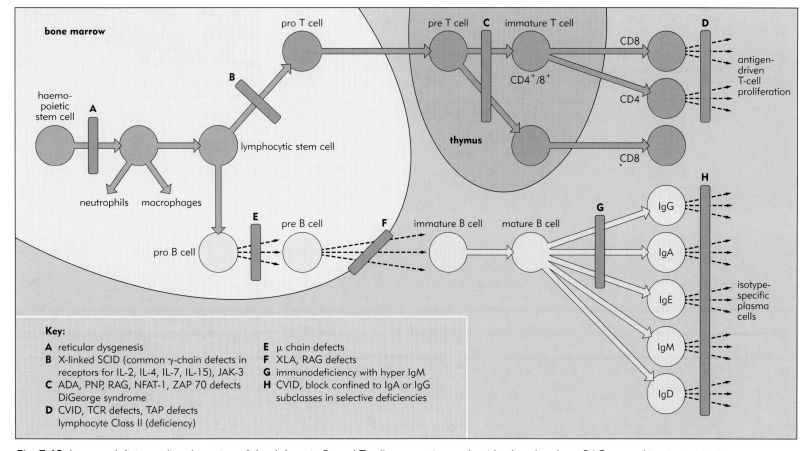

Key:
A reticular dysgenesis
B X-linked SCID (common γ-chain defects in receptors for IL-2, IL-4, IL-7, IL-15), JAK-3
C ADA, PNP, RAG, NFAT-1, ZAP 70 defects DiGeorge syndrome
D CVID, TCR defects, TAP defects lymphocyte Class II (deficiency)
E μ chain defects
F XLA, RAG defects
G immunodeficiency with hyper IgM
H CVID, block confined to IgA or IgG subclasses in selective deficiencies

Fig. 7.68 Immunodeficiency disorders: sites of the defects in B- and T-cell development in different types of congenital immune deficiency. (ADA, adenosine deaminase; CVID, common variable immunodeficiency; JAK-3, Janus associated kinase; NFAT-1, nuclear factor of activated T cells; PNP, purine nucleoside phosphorylase; RAG, recombination activation genes; SCID, severe combined immunodeficiency; TAP, transporter associated with antigen presentation; XLA, X-linked agammaglobulinaemia; ZAP-70, zeta associated protein; courtesy of Dr ADB Webster.)

(ADA; *Fig. 7.71*). Deficiency of another enzyme, purine nucleoside phosphorylase, causes a more selective lack of T cells. Deficiency of ADA has been treated successfully by bone marrow transplantation and most recently by 'gene therapy' in which the ADA gene is introduced into the patient's lymphocytes *in vitro*, and are then reinfused.

In the very rare syndrome of lymphoreticular dysgenesis, development of both the reticuloendothelial and lymphoid systems fails. Affected infants die soon after birth from overwhelming infection. Lymphopenia is marked, and stigmata of splenic atrophy may be found in the peripheral blood (*Fig. 7.72*).

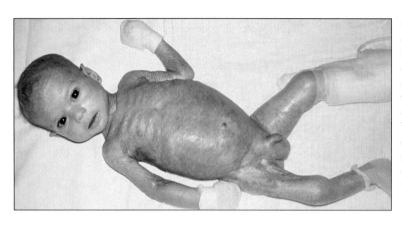

Fig. 7.69 Severe combined immunodeficiency disease caused by ADA deficiency: severely wasted infant with distended abdomen. There was widespread candidal infection of the mouth and chronic diarrhoea. (Courtesy of Prof. RI Levinsky.)

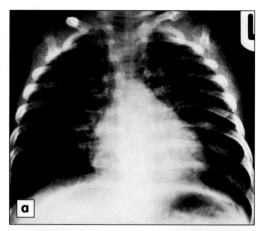

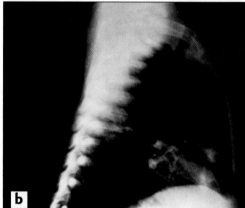

Fig. 7.70a and b Severe combined immunodeficiency disease: chest radiographs of the infant in *Fig. 7.69*. (a) The posteroanterior view shows absence of thymic shadow in the superior mediastinum; (b) the lateral view confirms the lack of thymus tissue deep in the sternum. [(a, b) Courtesy of Prof. RI Levinsky.]

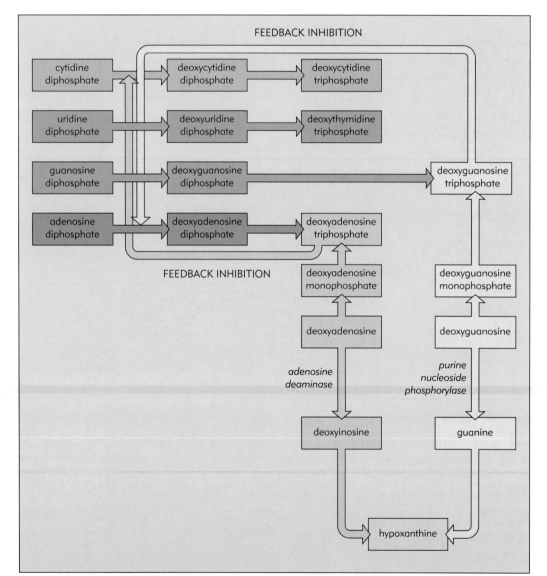

Fig. 7.71 Role of adenosine deaminase (ADA) and purine nucleoside phosphorylase (PNP) in purine degradation. ADA deficiency causes death of cortical thymocytes by accumulation of deoxyadenosine triphosphate (which inhibits DNA synthesis). PNP deficiency produces toxicity to T cells by accumulation of deoxyguanosine triphosphate. ADA and PNP are also involved in adenosine and guanosine degradation, respectively. In both types of deficiency, other biochemical mechanisms of toxicity to proliferating and non-proliferating lymphoid cells may occur.

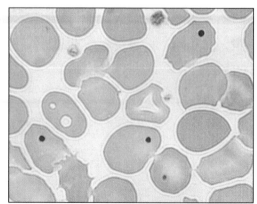

Fig. 7.72 Lymphoreticular dysgenesis: peripheral blood film of a 1-week-old infant. The large numbers of Howell–Jolly bodies (small granular remnants of DNA) are the result of splenic agenesis. There was severe lymphopenia. (Absolute lymphocyte count, 0.1×10^9/l.)

ACQUIRED IMMUNE DEFICIENCY SYNDROME

Acquired immune deficiency syndrome (AIDS) is caused by infection with HIV, a retrovirus of the lentivirus subgroup.

The predominant effects of HIV are produced through infection of T helper (CD4+) cells (*Fig. 7.73*). Some CD4+ cells are lysed directly

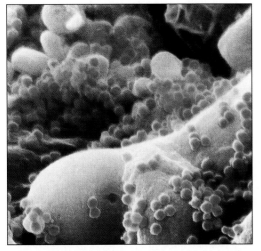

Fig. 7.73 AIDS: scanning electron micrograph of a T lymphocyte infected by the HIV virus. This close-up view shows the hexagonal outline of the virus particles. The virus subgroups (clades) differ in viral sequence. (Courtesy of Lennart Nilsson; © Boehringer Ingelheim International GmbH.)

by replicating HIV, but the virus remains latent in most host cells, unrecognized by the patient's immune system. When such latently infected T cells are activated, the virus replicates and cell death follows. The CD4 antigen appears to be the main receptor for HIV, and CD4+ antigen-presenting cells are also an important site for viral replication. A chemokine receptor, CCR-5 or CCR-4, is also required for cell entry.

Transmission of the virus is usually by sexual contact, or by blood or blood products, or by breast milk. Particularly common in homosexual men, AIDS is also seen frequently in intravenous drug abusers, haemophiliacs and other patients who require multiple blood transfusions, as well as in heterosexual contacts of AIDS cases.

The clinical outcome of infection has been classified into four stages or groups (*Fig. 7.74*). The viral load may be as high as 10^7 RNA copies/ml during acute infection. A prodromal period of about 6 weeks follows the initial infection, after which symptoms that resemble infectious mononucleosis may occur. A proportion of patients pass through the asymptomatic and persistent lymphadenopathy stages to the AIDS-related complex (ARC) and fully developed AIDS.

Examination of involved lymph nodes reveals characteristic abnormalities (*Figs 7.75 and 7.76*). Depletion of CD4 cells is progressive, and the peripheral blood shows lymphopenia and an alteration in the T-lymphocyte subsets, with a fall in the CD4+:CD8+ (helper:suppressor)

Clinical stages of human immunodeficiency virus disease
Group 1
Acute infection
Infectious mononucleosis-type illness, fever, lymphadenopathy, arthralgia, myalgia, mild meningoencephalitis, myelopathy
Diagnosis confirmed by seroconversion
Group 2
Asymptomatic infection with positive serology
Anaemia, neutropenia, thrombocytopenia, low CD4 counts, hypergammaglobulinaemia
Group 3
Persistent generalized lymphadenopathy
Group 4
Acquired immune deficiency syndrome (AIDS)
Constitutional symptoms – fever, malaise, weight loss, diarrhoea
Neurological symptoms – peripheral neuropathy, myelopathy, AIDS dementia, complex progressive multifocal leucoencephalopathy
Secondary infections:
pulmonary – *Pneumocystis carinii*, cytomegalovirus (CMV), *Cryptococcus* spp., atypical mycobacteria (e.g. *Mycobacterium avium*), toxoplasmosis, histoplasmosis
gastrointestinal – *Candida* spp., mycobacteria, *Salmonella* spp., cryptosporidiosis, herpes simplex virus (HSV), CMV
skin – HSV, herpes zoster, *Candida* spp., hairy leukoplakia
central nervous system – *Cryptococcus* spp., CMV, *Toxoplasma* spp.
Malignant tumours – Kaposi's sarcoma, non-Hodgkin lymphoma, primary lymphoma of the brain, squamous carcinoma of oral and rectal mucosae

Fig. 7.74 HIV virus: clinical stages of infection. Group 4 is subdivided into the AIDS-related complex (ARC – generalized lymphadenopathy with persistent fever; weight loss; unexplained diarrhoea; haematological abnormalities; CNS manifestations) and full-blown AIDS with severe opportunistic infections and/or neoplasms.

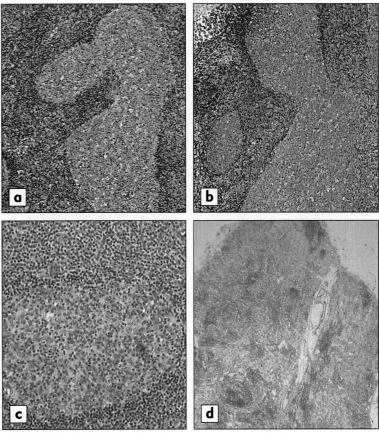

Fig. 7.75a–d AIDS: sections of lymph nodes infected by HIV show a spectrum of histological changes. (a, b) Type I includes follicular and paracortical hyperplasia. Mitotically active germinal centres are numerous in the medulla as well as the cortex and present a 'geographical outline'. Mitotic figures are abundant and there is extensive cytolyis and phagocytosis of cell remnants by tingible body histiocytes. The mantle zones are attenuated and (in places) absent, and the follicles appear confluent. The interfollicular tissue shows an increase in small vessels. (c) In the Type II pattern, there is loss of germinal centres but diffuse lymphoid hyperplasia. (d) In Type III, an end-stage in fatal cases, lymphocyte depletion predominates. [(a, b) Courtesy of Dr JE McLaughlin; (c) reproduced with permission from Ioachim HL. *Pathology of AIDS*. New York: Gower Medical Publishing; 1989.]

ratio from the normal value of 1.5–2.5:1 to <1:1 (*Fig. 7.77*). A polyclonal rise in serum immunoglobulins is often found, in some cases with a paraprotein present. The diagnosis is confirmed by detection of antibodies to one or other HIV surface antigens, or by detection of the antigens themselves (*Fig. 7.78*). Haematological abnormalities may include anaemia, neutropenia or thrombocytopenia (*Fig. 7.79*); these are often autoimmune in origin, but sometimes result from direct infection of haemopoietic stem and progenitor cells in the bone marrow. The cytopenias may also be caused by dysplastic changes (*Figs 7.80–7.83*) marrow lymphoma or fibrosis (*Fig. 7.84*).

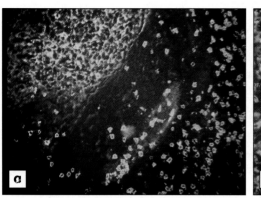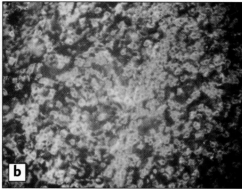

Fig. 7.76a and b AIDS: indirect immunofluorescence of sections of lymph nodes. (a) In the normal nodes the CD8$^+$ lymphocytes (orange) are mainly in the paracortex. The germinal centre consists of B lymphocytes and dendritic reticular cells (green). (b) In lymphadenopathy caused by HIV infection, the germinal centre is disrupted and invaded by CD8$^+$ cells. [(a, b) Courtesy of Prof. G Janossy.)]

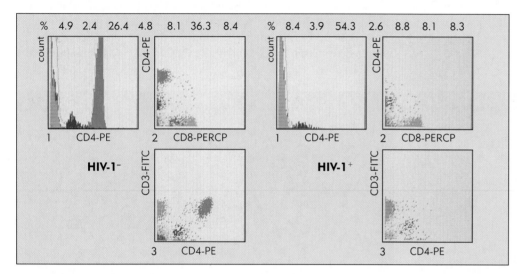

Fig. 7.77 The depletion of CD4$^+$ T lymphocytes in HIV-1 infection. T lymphocytes co-express CD3 and CD4 antigens on 'helper'-type cells and CD3 and CD8 antigens on 'suppressor/cytotoxic'-type cells. These three markers (CD3, CD4 and CD8) can be analyzed together in the same sample using monoclonal antibodies labelled by different dyes and then counted on flow cytometers as a precise measure of CD4 depletion. In normals (HIV-1$^-$) the ratio between CD3$^+$, CD4$^+$ (PE, light blue) and CD3$^+$, CD8$^+$ (PERCP, orange) T cells is about 1.3–1.8; in HIV-1 infection (HIV-1$^+$) the CD3$^+$, CD4$^+$ cells are depleted and the CD3$^+$, CD8$^+$ T cells predominate (CD4/CD8 ratio: <1.0). In this figure the various displays show triple-colour analysis. Modern flow cytometers perform this routine test with absolute T-cell counting and define the absolute CD4 count in whole blood samples. (Courtesy of Prof. G Janossy.)

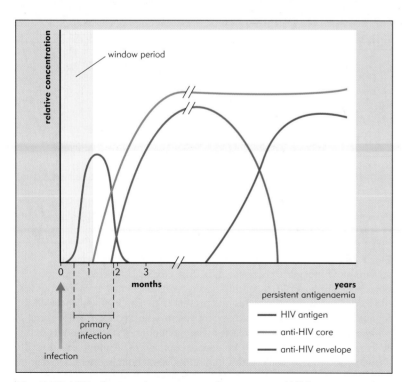

Fig. 7.78 HIV infection: the sequence of expression of HIV antigens and different antibodies following primary infection. (Courtesy of Prof. MC Contreras and the North London Blood Transfusion Centre.)

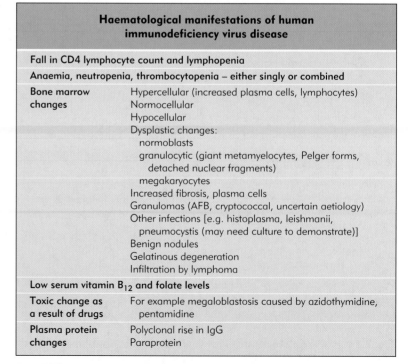

Haematological manifestations of human immunodeficiency virus disease	
Fall in CD4 lymphocyte count and lymphopenia	
Anaemia, neutropenia, thrombocytopenia – either singly or combined	
Bone marrow changes	Hypercellular (increased plasma cells, lymphocytes)
	Normocellular
	Hypocellular
	Dysplastic changes:
	normoblasts
	granulocytic (giant metamyelocytes, Pelger forms, detached nuclear fragments)
	megakaryocytes
	Increased fibrosis, plasma cells
	Granulomas (AFB, cryptococcal, uncertain aetiology)
	Other infections [e.g. histoplasma, leishmanii, pneumocystis (may need culture to demonstrate)]
	Benign nodules
	Gelatinous degeneration
	Infiltration by lymphoma
Low serum vitamin B$_{12}$ and folate levels	
Toxic change as a result of drugs	For example megaloblastosis caused by azidothymidine, pentamidine
Plasma protein changes	Polyclonal rise in IgG
	Paraprotein

Fig. 7.79 HIV infection: haematological manifestations.

134

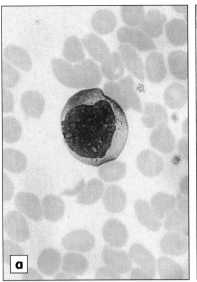

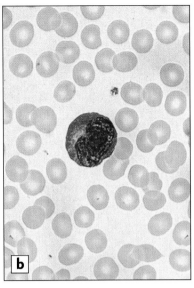

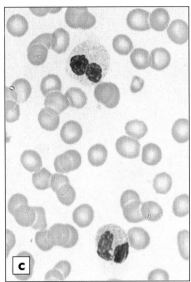

Fig. 7.80a–c HIV infection: peripheral blood showing (a, b) immunoblasts and (c) pseudo-Pelger cells. [(c) Courtesy of Dr D Swirsky.]

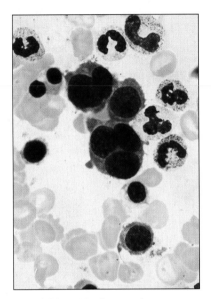

Fig. 7.81 HIV infection: bone marrow aspirate showing dyserythropoietic changes.

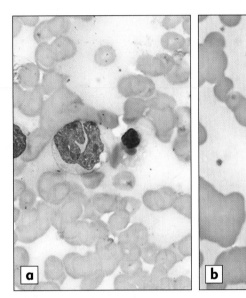

Fig. 7.82a and b HIV infection: dysmyelopoiesis with (a) giant metamyelocyte and (b) detached nuclear fragment. [(b) Courtesy of Dr BA Bain.]

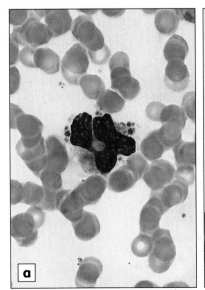

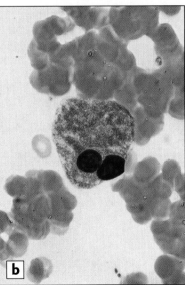

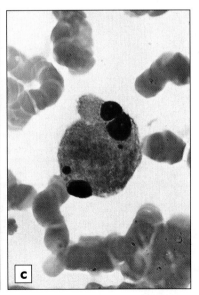

Fig. 7.83a–c HIV infection: (a–c) bone marrow aspirate showing dysplastic megakaryoctes.

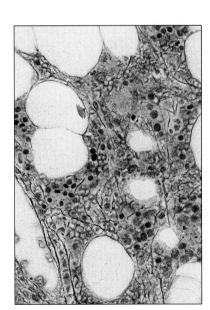

Fig. 7.84 HIV infection: bone marrow trephine biopsy showing dense reticulin network. Silver stain. (Courtesy of Dr C Costello.)

A wide spectrum of opportunistic organisms cause infections in AIDS patients, including atypical mycobacteria (*Fig. 7.85*), *Pneumocystis carinii* (*Fig. 7.86*), cytomegalovirus (*see Figs 14.12 and 14.13*), and *Cryptococcus, Histoplasma* (*Fig. 7.87*) and *Leishmania* (*Fig. 7.88*). Often non-specific granuloma are found (*Fig. 7.89*). A proportion of the patients develop Kaposi's sarcoma, a vascular skin tumour of endothelial cell origin (*Figs 7.90 and 7.91*), while other patients may develop non-Hodgkin lymphoma, which is likely to be high grade, and they have a 20% incidence of lymphoma in the CNS (*Figs 7.92–7.94*).

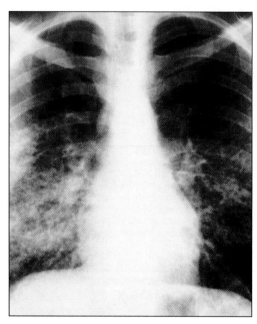

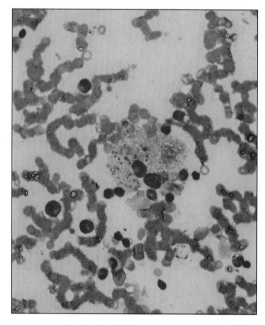

Fig. 7.85a and b AIDS: bone marrow trephine biopsy. (a) Granuloma showing strong positivity with Ziehl–Nielsen stain. (b) Higher power shows large numbers of acid-fast bacilli. [(a, b) Courtesy of Dr BW Baker and Dr EB Knottenbelt.]

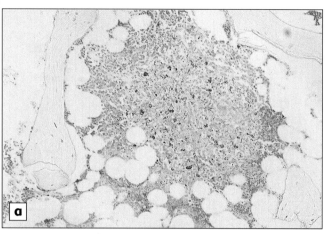

Fig. 7.86 AIDS: chest radiograph in *Pneumocystis carinii* infection, showing extensive, predominantly central interstitial opacities.

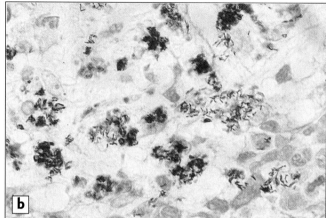

Fig. 7.87 AIDS: bone marrow aspirate showing histoplasmosis, visible as faintly staining fine fungal organisms in macrophages. (Courtesy of Dr C Costello.)

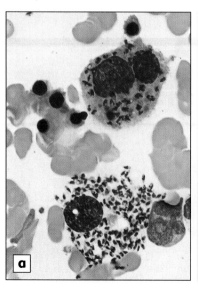

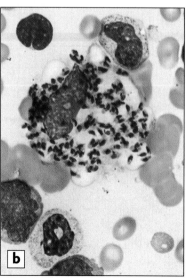

Fig. 7.88a and b AIDS: bone marrow aspirate showing Leishman–Donovan bodies. [(a, b) Courtesy of Dr D Swirsky.]

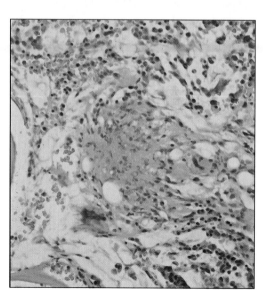

Fig. 7.89 AIDS: bone marrow trephine biopsy showing granuloma of uncertain aetiology. (Courtesy of Dr C Costello.)

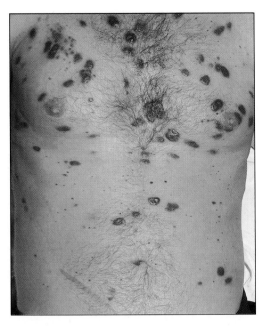

Fig. 7.90 AIDS, Kaposi's sarcoma: multiple vascular tumours of endothelial origin on the chest of an HIV antigen-positive homosexual male. (Courtesy of Dr IVD Weller.)

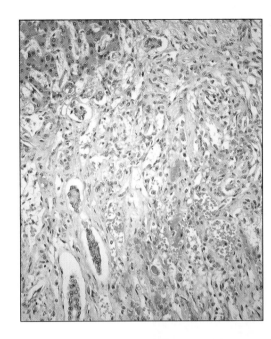

Fig. 7.91 AIDS, Kaposi's sarcoma: infiltration of the portal areas of the liver.

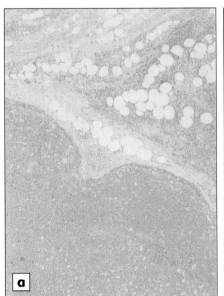

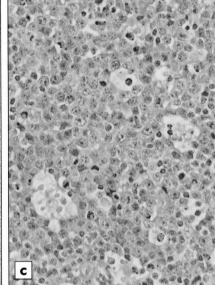

Fig. 7.92a–c AIDS, non-Hodgkin lymphoma: (a) lymph node showing replacement of normal architecture by tumour, which is extending into surrounding fat; (b, c) higher magnifications show the tumour to comprise lymphoblasts and 'starry sky' tingible body macrophages.

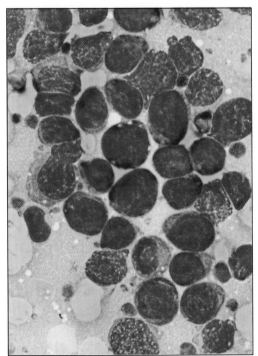

Fig. 7.93 AIDS, non-Hodgkin lymphoma: fine-needle aspirate of cervical lymph node showing lymphoblasts with cytoplasm that is strongly basophilic. Some of the cells show prominent cytoplasmic vacuoles (same case as shown in *Fig. 7.92*).

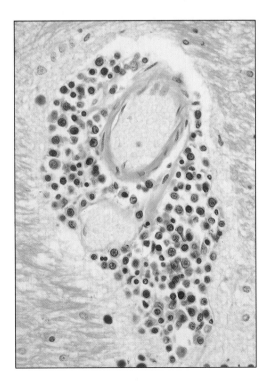

Fig. 7.94 AIDS, non-Hodgkin lymphoma: invasion of perivascular space of the brain by a high-grade systemic lymphoma. (Courtesy of Dr JE McLaughlin.)

AUTOIMMUNE LYMPHOPROLIFERATIVE SYNDROME

Autoimmune lymphoproliferative syndrome is characterized by lymphadenopathy (*Fig. 7.95*), hepatosplenomegaly, autoimmune haemolytic anaemia, neutropenia, thrombocytopenia and hypergammaglobulinaemia with a high proportion of circulating $CD3^+$, $CD4^-$ and $CD8^+$ T cells. The lymph nodes show loss of normal architecture with reduction of B cells (*Fig. 7.96*). The disease is associated with mutations in the FAS gene with defective apoptosis in response to anti-FAS antibody and presumably failure of normal apoptosis by lymphoid cells *in vivo*.

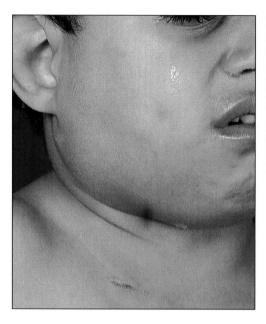

Fig. 7.95 Autoimmune lymphoproliferative syndrome: 8-year-old girl with marked generalized lymphadenopathy and hepatosplenomegaly. Her brother had similar clinical findings. (Courtesy of Prof. HG Prentice.)

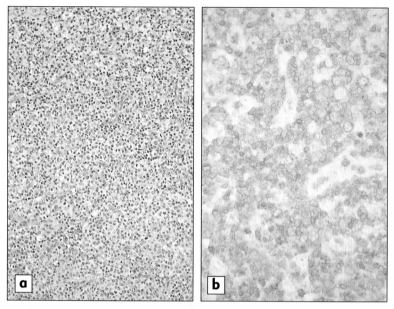

Fig. 7.96a and b Autoimmune lymphoproliferative syndrome: (a) lymph node biopsy at low power showing replacement of normal architecture by a uniform population of T lymphocytes with effacement of cortical structures. (b) Immunoperoxidase stain at higher power showing that the majority of lymphocytes express CD3 antigens. [(a, b) Courtesy of Dr JE McLaughlin and Prof. HG Prentice.]

8

Acute Leukaemias

The acute leukaemias are the result of accumulation of early myeloid or lymphoid precursors in the bone marrow, blood and other tissues, and are thought to arise by somatic mutation(s) of a single cell within a minor population of stem or early progenitor cells in the bone marrow or thymus (*Fig. 8.1*). Acute leukaemia may arise *de novo* or be the terminal event in a number of pre-existing blood disorders, for instance polycythaemia rubra vera, chronic myeloid leukaemia or one of the myelodysplastic syndromes. At presentation at least 30% and usually more than 80% of marrow cells are 'blasts'.

The diseases are divided into two main subgroups, acute myeloid (myeloblastic) leukaemia (AML) and acute lymphoblastic leukaemia (ALL), and further subdivided on morphological grounds into various

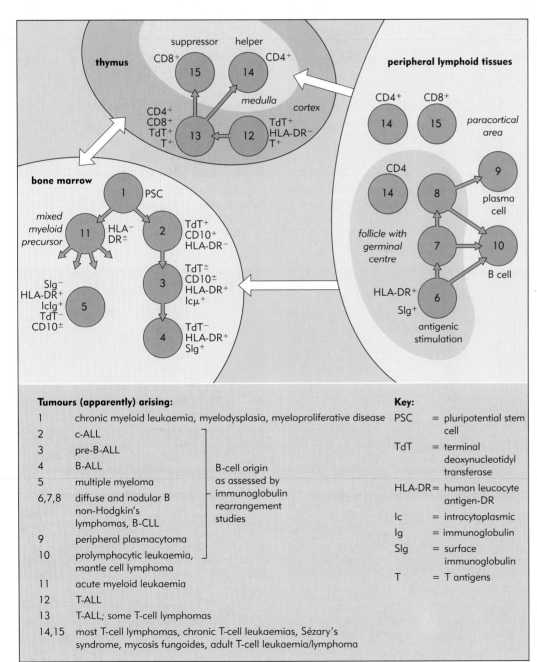

Fig. 8.1 Tumour cells: similarities between the tumour cells of acute and chronic leukaemias, malignant lymphomas and myeloma and early bone marrow, thymic or peripheral lymphoid cells. Although the malignant cells may resemble these progenitor or more mature cells, it is possible that the cell of origin of the hamatological malignancy is an earlier (more primitive) cell. (Modified from Hoffbrand AV, Pettit JE. *Essential Haematology*, 2nd edn. Oxford: Blackwell Scientific Publications; 1984.)

Tumours (apparently) arising:

1	chronic myeloid leukaemia, myelodysplasia, myeloproliferative disease
2	c-ALL
3	pre-B-ALL
4	B-ALL
5	multiple myeloma
6,7,8	diffuse and nodular B non-Hodgkin's lymphomas, B-CLL
9	peripheral plasmacytoma
10	prolymphocytic leukaemia, mantle cell lymphoma
11	acute myeloid leukaemia
12	T-ALL
13	T-ALL; some T-cell lymphomas
14,15	most T-cell lymphomas, chronic T-cell leukaemias, Sézary's syndrome, mycosis fungoides, adult T-cell leukaemia/lymphoma

2, 3, 4, 6, 7, 8, 9, 10: B-cell origin as assessed by immunoglobulin rearrangement studies

Key:

PSC = pluripotential stem cell

TdT = terminal deoxynucleotidyl transferase

HLA-DR = human leucocyte antigen-DR

Ic = intracytoplasmic

Ig = immunoglobulin

SIg = surface immunoglobulin

T = T antigens

subcategories (*Fig. 8.2*). The French–American–British (FAB) scheme divides AML into subtypes M_0 to M_7 and ALL into subtypes L_1, L_2 and L_3. There are additional unusual types [see also the World Health Organization (WHO) classification in Appendix 2].

CLINICAL FEATURES

Acute leukaemia presents with features of bone marrow failure (anaemia, infections, easy bruising or haemorrhage) and may or may not include features of organ infiltration by leukaemic cells. The organs usually involved are the lymph nodes, spleen and liver, meninges and central nervous system (CNS), testes (particularly in ALL) and skin (particularly in the M_3 type of AML). Rarely, a visible deposit of leukaemic blasts is seen in the eye (*Fig. 8.3*) or in other tissues (*Figs 8.4 and 8.5*). Occasionally patients show Sweet's syndrome (acute febrile neutrophilic dermatitis), which occurs in other malignant diseases (*Fig. 8.6*).

Infections are often bacterial in the early stages and particularly affect the skin (*Figs 8.7 and 8.8*), pharynx, perianal (*Fig. 8.9*) and perineal (*Fig. 8.10*) regions. Bacterial infections may lead to the adult respiratory distress syndrome (*Fig. 8.11*). Fungal infections are particularly common in patients with prolonged periods of neutropenia (*Figs 8.12–8.14*) who have undergone multiple courses of chemotherapy and antibiotic therapy.

Acute leukaemia: morphological classification
Myeloid (AML)
M_0: minimally differentiated
M_1: without maturation
M_2: with maturation
M_3: hypergranular promyelocytic
M_4: myelomonocytic
M_5: (a) monoblastic, (b) monocytic
M_6: erythroleukaemia
M_7: megakaryoblastic
Rare types (e.g. eosinophilic, natural killer)
Lymphoblastic (ALL)
L_1: small, monomorphic
L_2: large, heterogeneous
L_3: Burkitt-cell type

Fig. 8.2 French–American–British (FAB) classification of acute leukaemias: the myeloid leukaemias are divided into eight types (M_{0-7}) and lymphoblastic leukaemias into three (L_{1-3}).

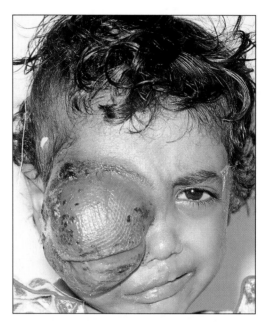

Fig. 8.3 Acute myeloid leukaemia: chloroma of the eye in a 12-year-old girl with AML M_2.

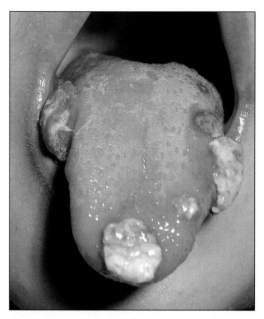

Fig. 8.4 Acute myeloid leukaemia: raised lesions on the tongue caused by deposits of leukaemic blasts in a 41-year-old man with AML M_4.

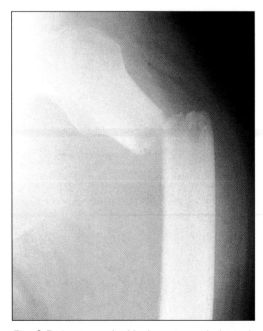

Fig. 8.5 Acute myeloid leukaemia: pathological fracture of left upper femur in an 82-year-old woman.

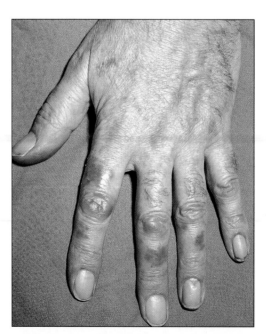

Fig. 8.6 Acute myeloid leukaemia: Sweet's syndrome (acute febrile neutrophilic dermatosis) in a 62-year-old man with AML M_4: bullous pyoderma. (Courtesy of Prof. HG Prentice.)

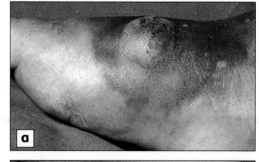
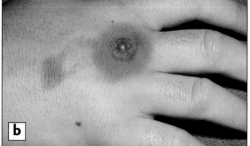

Fig. 8.7a and b Acute myeloid leukaemia: (a) a purplish black bullous lesion with surrounding erythema caused by infection from *Pseudomonas pyocyanea* on the foot; (b) similar but less marked infection on the back of the hand.

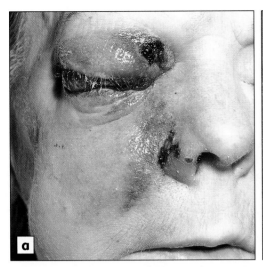

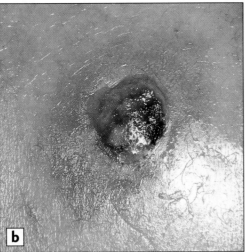

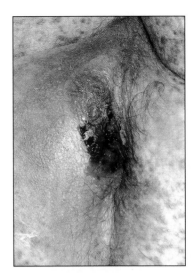

Fig. 8.9 Acute myeloid leukaemia: this perianal lesion was found to be the result of a mixed infection by *Escherichia coli* and *Streptococcus faecalis*.

Fig. 8.8a and b Acute myeloid leukaemia: *Staphylococcus aureus* was isolated from (a) infection of the right orbit and surrounding tissue and (b) a necrotic erythematous skin ulcer.

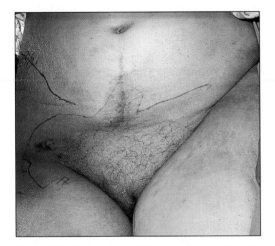

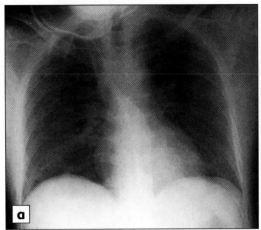

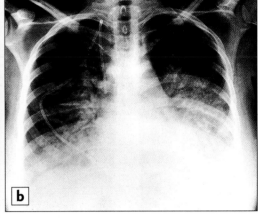

Fig. 8.10 Acute myeloid leukaemia: cellulitis of the perineum, lower abdomen and upper thighs caused by *Pseudomonas pyocyanea*.

Fig. 8.11a and b Acute myeloid leukaemia: (a) chest radiograph of 22-year-old man showing widespread interstitial shadowing resulting from adult acute respiratory distress syndrome associated with *Streptococcus mitis* infection during induction therapy; (b) interstitial shadowing in lower and mid-zones bilaterally in a 23-year-old woman with septicaemia from *Pseudomonas pyocyanea* following chemotherapy. She developed a fatal adult respiratory distress syndrome.

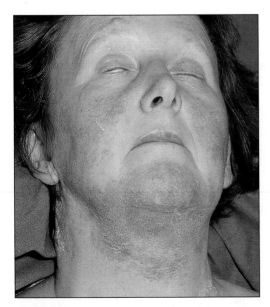

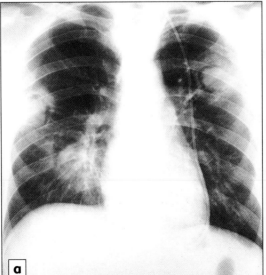

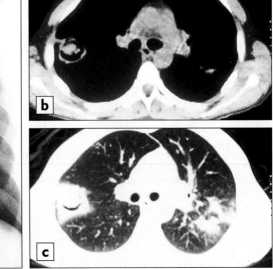

Fig. 8.12 Acute myeloid leukaemia: spreading cellulitis of the neck and chin resulting from mixed streptococcal and candidal infection, previous chemotherapy and prolonged periods of neutropenia.

Fig. 8.13a–c Acute myeloid leukaemia: this 32-year-old-man had received repeated chemotherapy for refractory disease. Three pulmonary mycotic cavities are visible: (a) radiograph; (b, c) computed tomography (CT) scans. [(b, c) Courtesy of Dr AR Valentine.]

Other viral (especially herpetic), protozoal or fungal infections are frequent, particularly in the mouth, and may become generalized and life-threatening (*Figs 8.15–8.18*). Haemorrhage of the skin or mucous membranes is usually petechial (*Figs 8.19 and 8.20*).

Infiltration of the skin that presents as a widespread, raised, non-itchy haemorrhagic rash and swelling of the gums (*Fig. 8.21*) are characteristic of the M₅ type of AML; nodular and localized skin infiltrates may also occur (*Fig. 8.22*).

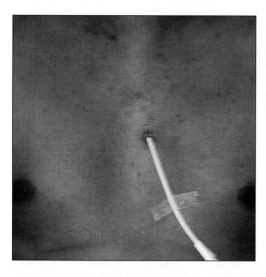

Fig. 8.14 Acute myeloid leukaemia: candidal septicaemia. Typical skin rash in a 22-year-old Sri-Lankan man with severe neutropenia caused by intensive chemotherapy.

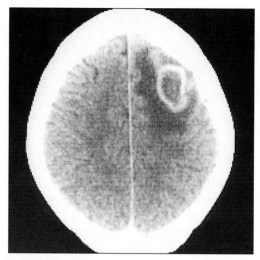

Fig. 8.15 Acute myeloid leukaemia: CT scan showing encapsulated brain lesion in right frontal zone caused by aspergillosis infection with surrounding hypodense area caused by inflammation.

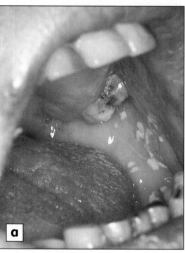
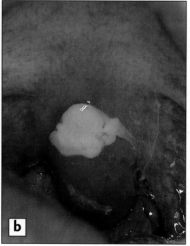

Fig. 8.16a and b Acute myeloid leukaemia: (a) plaques of *Candida albicans* in the mouth, with a lesion of herpes simplex on the upper lip; (b) candidal plaque on the soft palate.

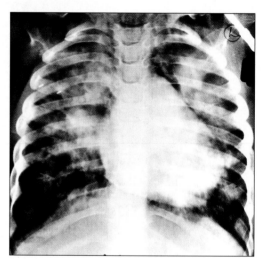

Fig. 8.17 Acute myeloid leukaemia: chest radiograph showing patchy consolidation bilaterally caused by measles infection in a child. (Courtesy of Prof. JM Chessells.)

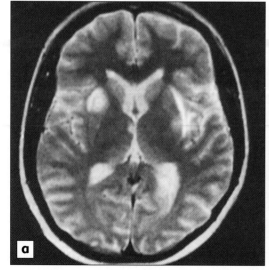
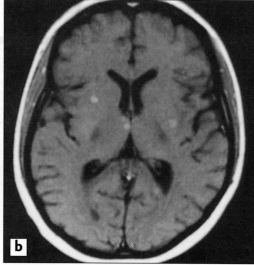
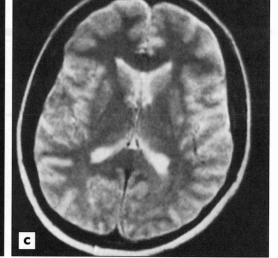

Fig. 8.18a–c Acute myeloid leukaemia: (a, b) magnetic resonance imaging (MRI) scans showing multiple small opacities. The patient, a 23-year-old woman, complained of headaches and diplopia. The diagnosis of toxoplasmosis was made and (c) she responded rapidly to anti-toxoplasmosis therapy. [(a–c) Courtesy of Dr AR Valentine.]

In ALL, lymphadenopathy is more common (*Fig. 8.23*). In the T-cell variant (T-ALL), there is often upper mediastinal enlargement, caused by a thymic mass, which responds rapidly to therapy (*Fig. 8.24*). Although meningeal involvement is more frequent in children and younger subjects with ALL, it may occur at all ages, presenting with nausea, vomiting, headaches, visual disturbances, photophobia

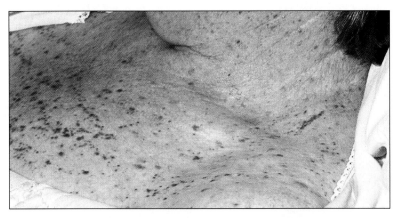

Fig. 8.19 Acute myeloid leukaemia: petechial haemorrhages covering the upper chest and face in severe thrombocytopenia.

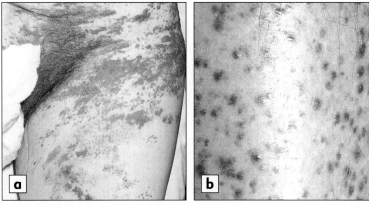

Fig. 8.20a and b Acute myeloid leukaemia: (a) marked ecchymoses, petechial haemorrhages and bruises over the groin and thigh; (b) close-up view of petechial haemorrhages over the leg.

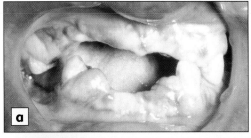
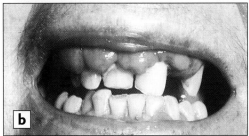

Fig. 8.21a and b Acute myeloid leukaemia, M₅ subtype: (a, b) leukaemic infiltration of the gums results in their expansion and thickening, and partial covering of the teeth.

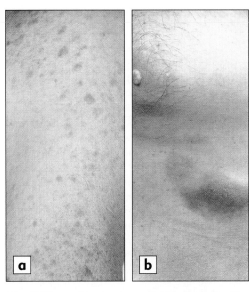

Fig. 8.22a and b Acute myeloid leukaemia, M₅ subtype: (a) multiple, raised, erythematous skin lesions caused by leukaemic infiltration; (b) close-up view of nodular skin lesion.

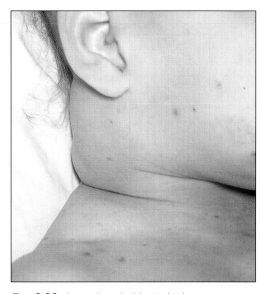

Fig. 8.23 Acute lymphoblastic leukaemia: marked cervical lymphadenopathy in a 4-year-old boy. (Courtesy of Prof. JM Chessells.)

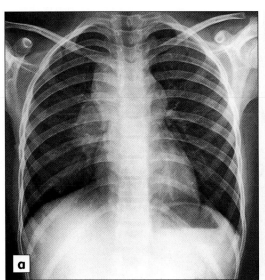
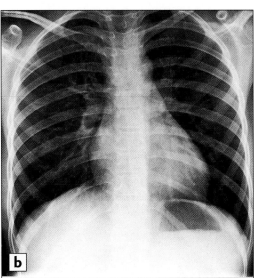

Fig. 8.24a and b Acute lymphoblastic leukaemia, T-cell subtype: chest radiographs of a 4-year-old boy showing (a) upper mediastinal widening caused by thymic enlargement; (b) disappearance of thymic mass following 1 week of therapy with vincristine and prednisolone.

and features of the cranial nerve palsies (*Fig. 8.25*). Papilloedema may be found on examination (*Fig. 8.26*) and infiltration may occur at any site (*Figs 8.27 and 8.28*). Testicular relapse is common, although it is only rarely detectable clinically on presentation (*Fig. 8.29*). Bone involvement may produce characteristic radiographic findings (*Fig. 8.30*).

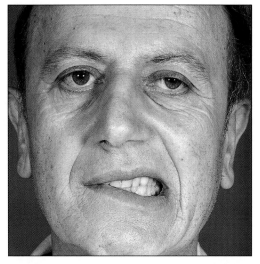

Fig. 8.25 Acute lymphoblastic leukaemia: this 59-year-old man has facial asymmetry because of a right lower motor neuron seventh nerve palsy resulting from meningeal leukaemic infiltration. (Courtesy of Prof. HG Prentice.)

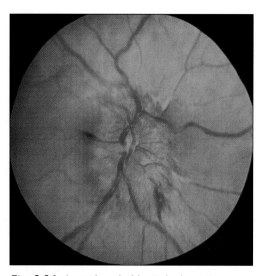

Fig. 8.26 Acute lymphoblastic leukaemia: papilloedema caused by meningeal disease. There is blurring of the disk margin with venous enlargement and retinal haemorrhages.

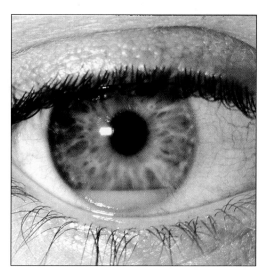

Fig. 8.27 Acute lymphoblastic leukaemia: leukaemic infiltration in the anterior chamber of the eye obscures the lower rim of the iris.

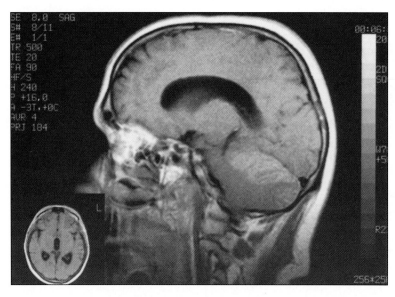

Fig. 8.28 Acute lymphoblastic leukaemia: MRI scan showing dilated cerebral ventricles with expansion of the cerebellum and blockage of the viaduct between the third and fourth ventricles. The patient, a 33-year-old man, presented with headache, diplopia and blast cells in the cerebrospinal fluid. (Courtesy of Dr AR Valentine.)

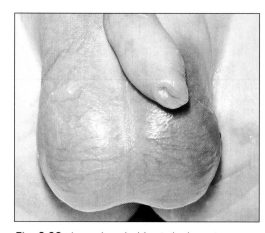

Fig. 8.29 Acute lymphoblastic leukaemia: testicular swelling and erythema of the left side of the scrotum caused by testicular infiltration. (Courtesy of Prof. JM Chessells.)

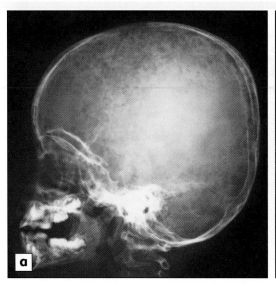

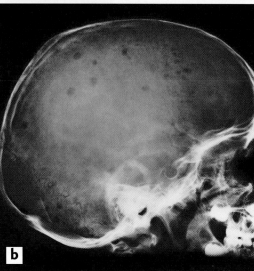

Fig. 8.30a and b Acute lymphoblastic leukaemia: radiographs of childrens' skulls showing (a) mottled appearance caused by widespread leukaemic infiltration of bone and (b) multiple punched-out lesions caused by leukaemic deposits. (Courtesy of Prof. JM Chessells.)

Revised criteria for the classification of acute myeloid leukaemia

M₀

Large, agranular blasts (resemble ALL L₂, rarely L₁). Myeloperoxidase negative or <3% positive; B-, T-lineage markers negative; CD13 and/or CD33 positive; myeloperoxidase positive by immunochemistry or electron microscopy; TdT may be positive.

M₁

Blast cells, agranular and granular types (Types I and II) >90% of non-erythroid cells. At least 3% of these are peroxidase or Sudan black positive.

Remaining 10% (or less) of cells are maturing granulocytic cells.

M₂

Sum of agranular and granular blasts (Types I and II) is from 30 to 89% of non-erythroid cells.

Monocytic cells, <20%.

Granulocytes from promyelocytes to mature polymorphs, >10%.

M₃

Majority of cells are abnormal promyelocytes with heavy granulation.

Characteristic cells that contain bundles of Auer rods ('faggots') invariably present.

Note: Microgranular variant also occurs (Fig. 8.40)

M₄

In the marrow, blasts >30% of non-erythroid cells.

Sum of myeloblasts, promyelocytes, myelocytes and later granulocytes is between 30 and 80% of non-erythroid cells.

>20% of non-erythroid cells are monocyte lineage.

If monocytic cells exceed 80%, diagnosis is M₅.

Notes: If marrow findings as above and peripheral blood monocytes (all types) are >5.0 × 10⁹/l, diagnosis is M₄.

If monocyte count <5.0 × 10⁹/l, M₄ can be confirmed on basis of serum lysozyme, combined esterase, etc.

Diagnosis of M₄ confirmed if >20% of marrow precursors are monocytes (confirmed by special stains).

M₄ with eosinophilia

Eosinophils >5% of non-erythroid cells in marrow.

Eosinophils are abnormal.

Eosinophils are chloroacetate and periodic acid–Schiff positive.

M₅

80% of marrow non-erythroid cells are monoblasts, promonocytes or monocytes.

M₅ₐ, 80% of monocytic cells are monoblasts.

M₅ᵦ, <80% of monocytic cells are monoblasts, remainder are predominantly promonocytes and monocytes.

M₆

The erythroid component of the marrow exceeds 50% of all nucleated cells.

30% of the remaining non-erythroid cells are agranular or granular blasts (Types I and II).

Note: If >50% erythroid cells but <30% blasts, diagnosis becomes myelodysplastic syndrome.

M₇

30% at least of nucleated cells are blasts.

Blasts identified by platelet peroxidase on electron microscopy, or by monoclonal antibodies.

Increased reticulin is common.

Fig. 8.31 FAB classification for acute myeloid leukaemia. (Modified from Bennett JM, Catovsky D, Daniel MT, *et al.* Proposed revised criteria for classification of acute myeloid leukemia. A report of the French–American–British Cooperative Group. *Ann Intern Med.* 1985;103:620–5.)

MICROSCOPICAL APPEARANCES

Acute myeloid leukaemia

The FAB classification criteria are given in *Fig. 8.31*. On May–Grünwald/Giemsa staining the M₀ subclass is the least differentiated (*Fig. 8.32*) and can only be diagnosed with certainty after immunophenotyping and immunocytochemistry and/or electron microscopy. The M₁ subclass shows agranular and granular blasts (*Fig.*

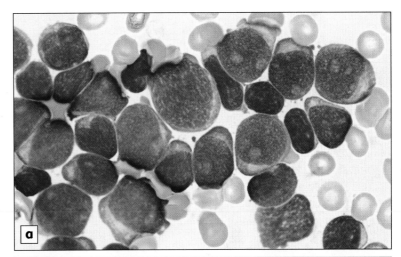

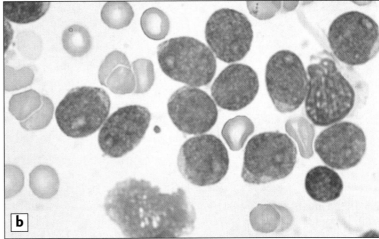

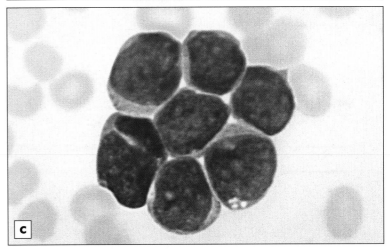

Fig. 8.32a–c Acute myeloid leukaemia, M₀ subtype: (a–c) bone marrow aspirates showing large blasts resembling ALL L₂ subtype. Granules are absent (Type I blasts), myeloperoxidase and Sudan black staining negative, CD13 and/or CD33 positive; myeloperoxidase is positive by electron microscopy or immunocytochemistry. TdT may be positive. (Courtesy of Dr MT Daniel, Prof. JM Bennett and Dr AB Mehta.)

8.33), the blasts showing less than 20 granules (type I and II). The M₂ subclass shows definite differentiation to promyelocytes (*Fig. 8.34*). Rare

subtypes show abnormal metachromatic granules (*Fig. 8.35*) with or without basophilic granules (*Figs 8.36–8.38*).

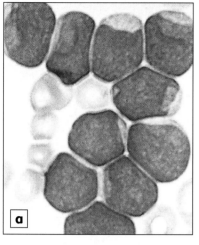
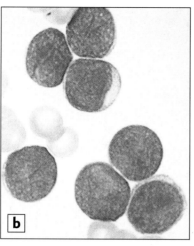
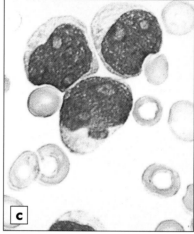
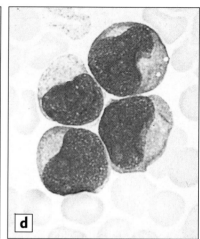

Fig. 8.33a–d Acute myeloid leukaemia, M₁ subtype: (a–d) bone marrow aspirates showing blasts with large, often irregular, nuclei with one or more nucleoli, and with varying amounts of eccentrically placed cytoplasm. Either no definite granulation (Type I blasts) is present or a few azurophilic granules and occasional Auer rods can be seen. At least 3% of cells stain with Sudan black or myeloperoxidase.

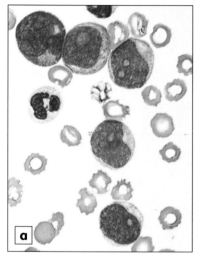
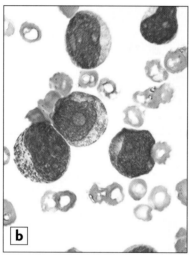
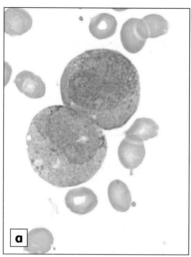
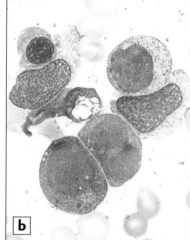

Fig. 8.34a and b Acute myeloid leukaemia, M₂ subtype: bone marrow aspirates showing (a) blasts similar to those in *Fig. 8.33*, but promyelocytes with azurophilic granules are also present; (b) blast cells with folded nuclei, one or two nucleoli, <20 azurophilic granules (Type II blasts) or >20 azurophilic granules (Type III blasts) per cell and occasional Auer rods.

Fig. 8.35a and b Acute myeloid leukaemia, M₂ subtype: (a, b) unusual large, vacuolated inclusions (pseudo-Chédiak–Higashi) are present in blast cells. (Courtesy of Dr D Swirsky.)

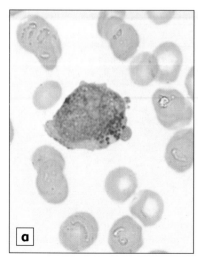
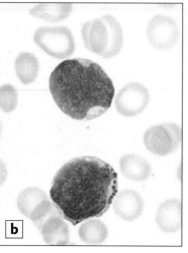
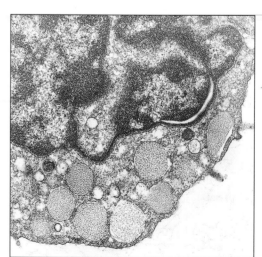

Fig. 8.37 Acute myeloid leukaemia, M₂ subtype: ultrastructure of the blasts shown in *Fig. 8.36*. Cytoplasmic granules show stippled pattern. (Courtesy of Prof. D Catovsky.)

Fig. 8.36a and b Acute myeloid leukaemia, M₂ subtype: (a, b) rare basophilic differentiation (peripheral blood). [(a, b) Courtesy of Prof. D Catovsky.]

The typical form of M_3 (acute promyelocytic leukaemia) shows bundles of rod-like structures ('faggots' or Sultan bodies), which are aggregates of granules and can be seen with special stains (*Fig. 8.39*). These cells contain procoagulant material which, when released into the circulation, causes disseminated intravascular coagulation; this type also has a microgranular variant (*Fig. 8.40*). In AML M_3, treatment with all-*trans* retinoic acid (ATRA) produces differentiation of the blasts (*Fig. 8.41*) often with full remission being obtained.

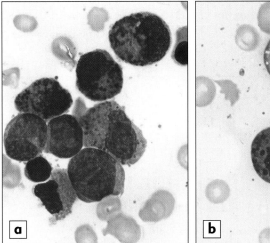

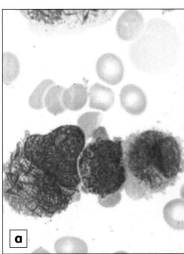 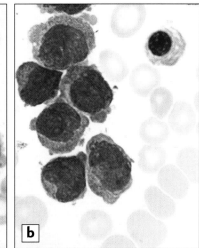

Fig. 8.38a and b Acute myeloid leukaemia, $M_2 E_0$ subtype: (a) three myeloblasts and four abnormal eosinophils with metachromatic granules; (b) neoplastic myelocyte with coarse basophilic and eosinophilic granulation. [(a, b) Courtesy of Dr K van Poucke and Prof. M Peetermans.]

Fig. 8.39a and b Acute myeloid leukaemia, M_3 subtype: (a, b) promyelocytes containing coarse azurophilic granules, and bundles of Auer rods ('faggots') in (a). The nuclei contain one or two nucleoli. The subtype is associated with the 15:17 chromosome translocation (see *Fig. 8.100*).

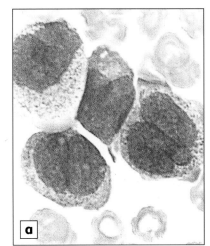 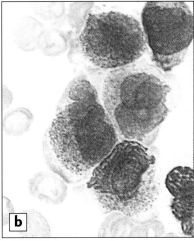 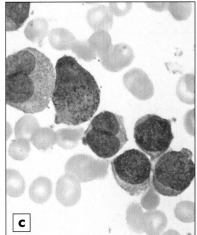 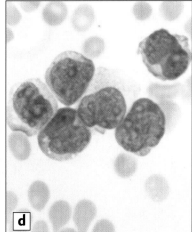

Fig. 8.40a–d Acute myeloid leukaemia, M_3 subtype: (a–d) microgranular variant. The usually bilobed cells contain numerous small azurophilic granules. [(a, b) Courtesy of Prof. JM Bennett.]

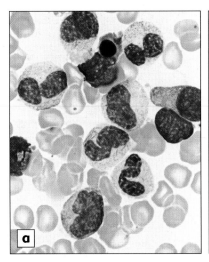 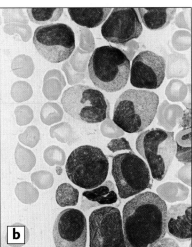 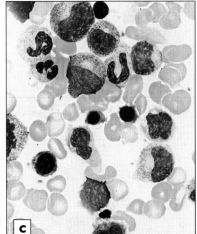 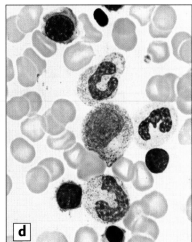

Fig. 8.41a–d Acute myeloid leukaemia, M_3 subtype: (a–d) differentiation of myeloblasts into myelocytes and neutrophils during treatment with ATRA. Abnormal myelocytes and neutrophils containing Auer rods are seen. [(a–d) Courtesy of Prof. MT Daniel.]

147

M$_4$ (myelomonocytic leukaemia) shows a mixture of blasts with promyelocytic and monocytic differentiation, the latter consisting of less than 20% of the total (*Fig. 8.42*). In one subtype, there are abnormal eosinophils as well as inversion (inv) of chromosome 16 (*Fig. 8.43*).

M$_{5a}$ (monoblastic leukaemia; *Fig. 8.44*) shows over 20% monoblasts. M$_{5b}$ shows more differentiated 'promonocytes' or monocytic cells. Serum and urinary lysozyme are high.

An unusual subtype with M$_4$ or M$_5$ features shows erythrophagocytosis (*Fig. 8.45*). In subclass M$_6$ (erythroleukaemia) over 50% of cells are erythroid precursors with bizarre dyserythropoietic forms (*Figs 8.46 and 8.47*). Features of myelodysplasia are also present in other cell lines.

Acute megakaryoblastic leukaemia (M$_7$) is rare. It is often associated with fibrosis of the marrow (*Fig. 8.48*) and is recognized by the appearance of the blasts, special staining for platelet peroxidase, electron microscopy and/or monoclonal antibodies to cell surface antigens (*Fig. 8.49*).

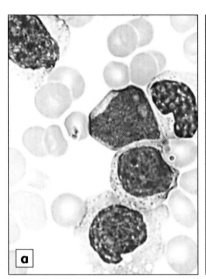
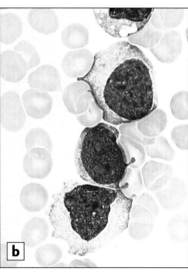
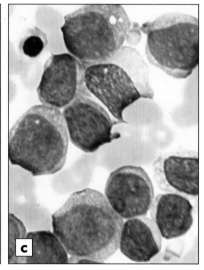
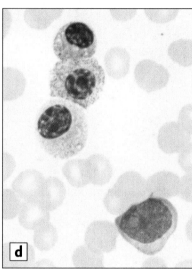

Fig. 8.42a–d Acute myeloid leukaemia, M$_4$ subtype: (a–c) blast cells contain cytoplasmic granules (myeloblasts and promyelocytes) or pale cytoplasm with occasional vacuoles and granules, and folded or rounded nuclei (monoblasts). (d) Abnormal pseudo-Pelger forms may occur.

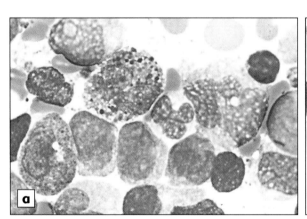
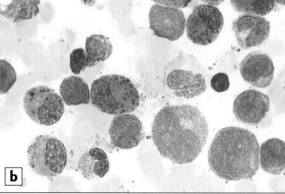

Fig. 8.43a and b Acute myeloid leukaemia, M$_4$ subtype: (a, b) blast cells, abnormal myelomonocytic cells and eosinophils with basophilic granules. Cytogenetic analysis showed inv(16) (p13;q22). [(a) Courtesy of Dr M Bilter and Prof. J Rowley; (b) courtesy of Prof. D Catovsky.]

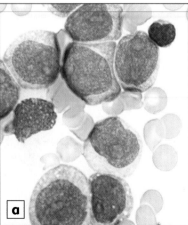
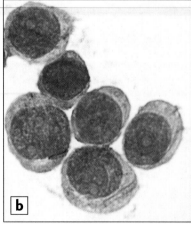
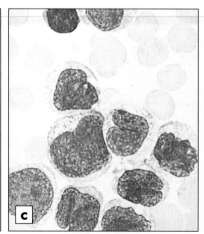
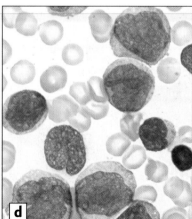

Fig. 8.44a–d Acute myeloid leukaemia, M$_5$ subtype: blast cells with pale cytoplasm or perinuclear 'haloes' and cytoplasmic vacuoles but only occasional granules. Their usually centrally placed nuclei are folded, rounded or kidney-shaped. (a, b) M$_{5a}$ subtype: 80% of the cells are monoblasts; (c, d) M$_{5b}$ subtype: less than 80% of the cells are monoblasts. The remaining cells are promonocytes and monocytes. The cells in (b) show ribosome lamellar complexes. [(b, d) Courtesy of Prof. D Catovsky.]

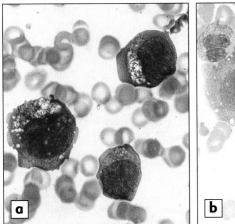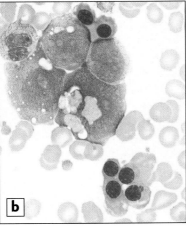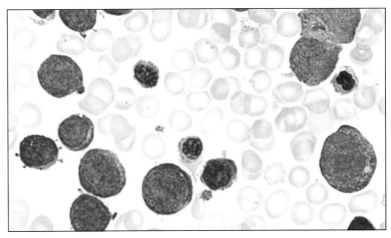

Fig. 8.45a and b Acute myeloid leukaemia: M_4/M_5 subtype with erythrophagocytosis and t(8;16). (a) In this case the blasts were M_5 subtype; other similar cases are M_4 subtype. A bleeding diathesis with features of fibrinolysis (not disseminated intravascular coagulation as in M_3) is often present. (b) Child with M_4/M_5 subtype with t(8;16) showing erythrophagocytosis. [(a) Courtesy of Prof. D Catovsky; (b) Courtesy of Dr D Swirsky.]

Fig. 8.46 Acute myeloid leukaemia, M_6 subtype: there is a preponderance of erythroid cells at all stages of development.

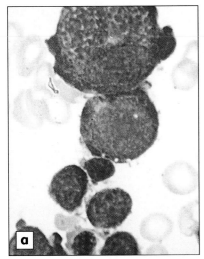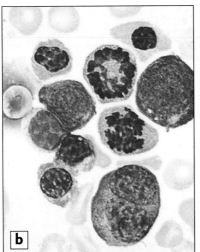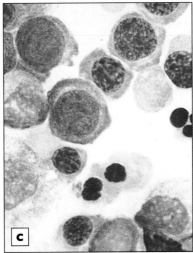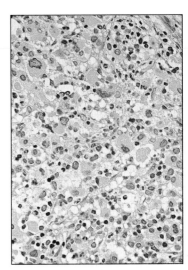

Fig. 8.47a–c Acute myeloid leukaemia, M_6 subtype: (a–c) high-power views of bone marrow aspirate showing erythroid predominance with many dyserythropoietic features, such as multinucleate cells (gigantoblasts), vacuolated cytoplasm, abnormal mitoses and megaloblastic nuclei.

Fig. 8.48 Acute myeloid leukaemia, M_7 subtype: bone marrow trephine biopsy showing large blasts with amorphous pink cytoplasm interspersed with residual small haemopoietic cells.

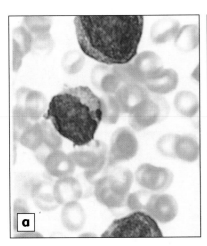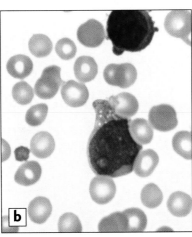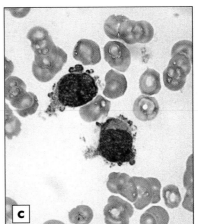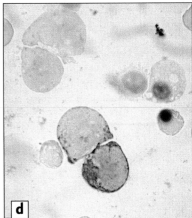

Fig. 8.49a–d Acute myeloid leukaemia, M_7 subtype: (a–d) the megakaryoblasts are large primitive cells with basophilic cytoplasm. Some show abortive platelet budding. (d) The cells are positive for platelet peroxidase; immunoperoxidase stain. [(b–d) Courtesy of Prof. D Catovsky.]

Rare types of acute myeloid leukaemia

Rare types of AML include eosinophilic leukaemia (*Fig. 8.50*), acute natural killer (NK) cell leukaemia (*Fig. 8.51*) and mast cell leukaemia (*Fig. 8.52*). A rare appearance of the marrow in AML, partial necrosis, is shown in *Fig. 8.53*.

Acute lymphoblastic leukaemia

Lymphoblasts show little evidence of differentiation. Cases with smaller, more uniform cells with scanty cytoplasm are classified as L₁ (*Fig. 8.54*), whereas those with blasts differing widely in size, with prominent nucle-oli and greater amounts of cytoplasm, are classified as L₂ (*Fig. 8.55*). L₂ tends to include more of the adult cases and also most of those immunologically typed as T-ALL. Rare subtypes show coarse granules (*Fig. 8.56a*) or a reactive eosinophilia (*Fig. 8.56b*).

The L₃ variant shows multiple small vacuoles throughout a basophilic cell cytoplasm and often overlying the nucleus (*Fig. 8.57*); this appearance corresponds usually to the rare B-cell or Burkitt type. The bone marrow in all variants is hypercellular, with leukaemic blasts comprising at least 80% of the marrow cell total (*Fig. 8.58*). In ALL, blasts may be seen in the cerebrospinal fluid (*Fig. 8.59*) or testes (*Fig. 8.60*).

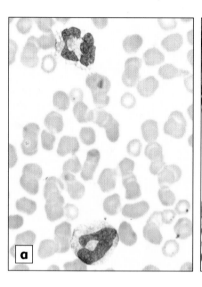
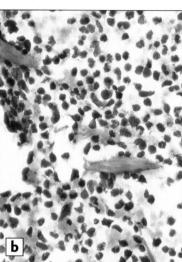
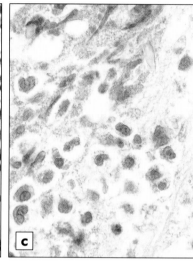

Fig. 8.50a–c Acute myeloid leukaemia, rare eosinophilic subtype: 55-year-old male patient treated with chemotherapy for carcinoma of the bladder 10 years previously. (a) peripheral blood showing abnormal eosinophils; (b) bone marrow aspirate showing eosinophilic blasts, necrotic cells and Charcot–Leyden crystals; (c) bone marrow trephine showing necrotic cells and Charcot–Leyden crystals. (Hb, 11.0 g/dl; WBC, 23.2 × 10⁹/l; platelets, 24 × 10⁹/l; courtesy of Dr AG Smith.)

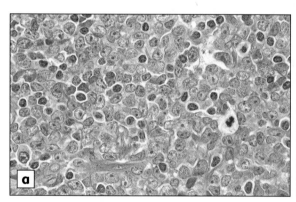
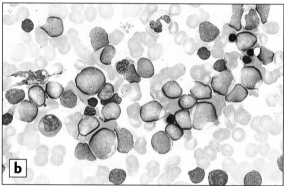

Fig. 8.51a and b Acute myeloid leukaemia, NK cell subtype: 54-year-old man with cervical lymphadenopathy. (a) Biopsy showed diffusive infiltration of cells with round and irregular small nucleoli and scanty cytoplasm. (b) The bone marrow shows an infiltrate of immature blasts with L₂ morphology. The cells were myeloperoxidase negative but CD2⁺, CD7⁺, CD33⁺, CD56⁺, and HLA-DR⁺. [(a, b) Courtesy of Dr R Suzuki.]

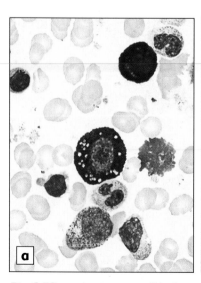
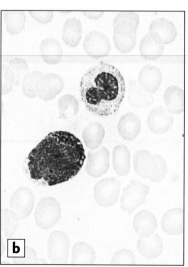
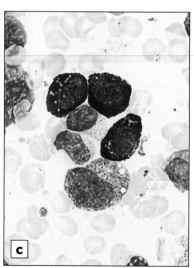
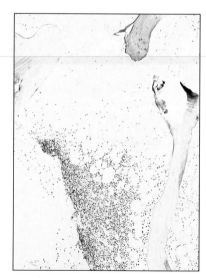

Fig. 8.52a–c Acute mast cell leukaemia: (a–c) bone marrow showing typical blasts with basophilic and vacuolated cytoplasm. In this case the leukaemia arose *de novo*; other cases follow systemic mastocytosis (although usually other forms of AML complicate this disease) or occur as transformation of chronic myeloid leukaemia.

Fig. 8.53 Acute myeloid leukaemia: trephine biopsy showing partial necrosis of bone marrow. (Courtesy of Dr R Kumar.)

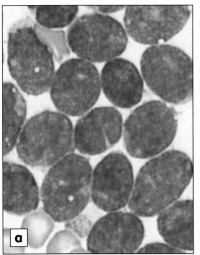 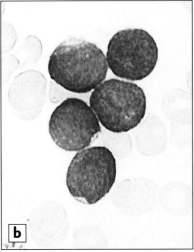 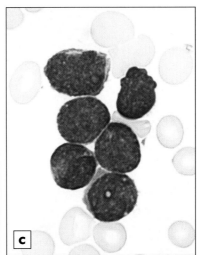 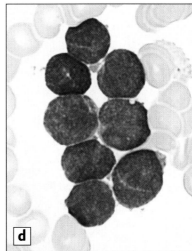

Fig. 8.54a–d Acute lymphoblastic leukaemia, L₁ subtype: (a–d) rather small, uniform blast cells with scanty cytoplasm, and rounded or cleft nuclei with usually a single nucleolus.

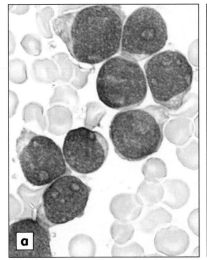 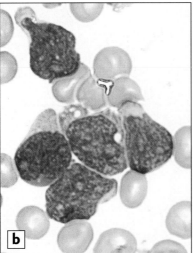 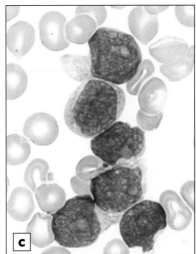 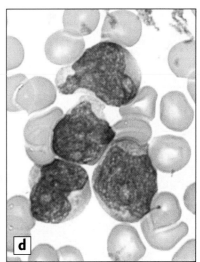

Fig. 8.55a–d Acute lymphoblastic leukaemia, L₂ subtype: (a–d) blast cells that vary considerably in size and amount of cytoplasm; the nuclear:cytoplasmic ratio is rarely as high as in L₁. The nuclei are variable in shape and often contain many nucleoli.

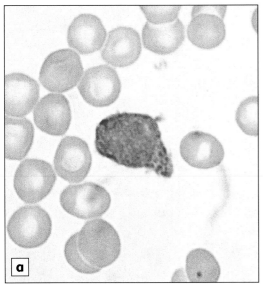 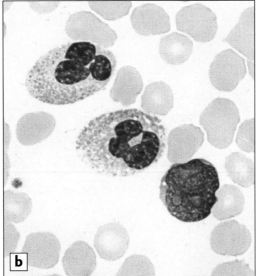 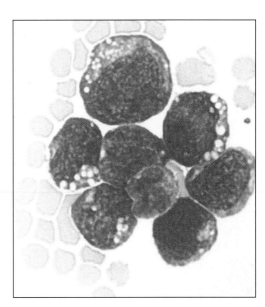

Fig. 8.56a and b Acute lymphoblastic leukaemia: (a) rare subtype with granules; (b) rare subtype with eosinophilia – peripheral blood film showing a lymphoblast and two eosinophils. [WBC, 36 × 10⁹/l; lymphoblasts, 14 × 10⁹/l; eosinophils, 20 × 10⁹/l; (a) courtesy of Dr Cantu-Reynoldi; see also Cantu-Reynoldi A, Invenizzi R, Biondi A, *et al*. Biological and clinical features of acute lymphoblastic leukaemia with cytoplasmic granules or inclusions: description of eight cases. *Br J Haematol*. 1989;73:309–14.]

Fig. 8.57 Acute lymphoblastic leukaemia, L₃ subtype: blast cells with deeply staining blue cytoplasm containing numerous small perinuclear vacuoles. This appearance is usually associated with the B-cell type.

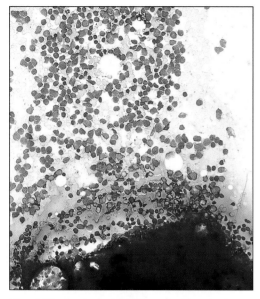

Fig. 8.58 Acute lymphoblastic leukaemia: low-power view with bone marrow fragment showing hypercellularity of cellular trails of which over 80% are blast cells.

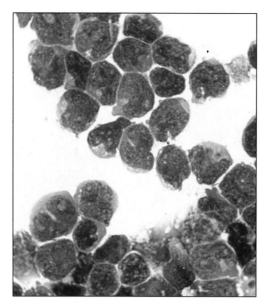

Fig. 8.59 Acute lymphoblastic leukaemia: high-power view of cytospin of cerebrospinal fluid, showing a deposit of blast cells of varying morphology. The patient presented with the features of meningeal leukaemia.

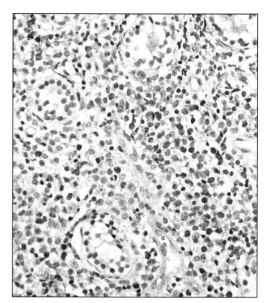

Fig. 8.60 Acute lymphoblastic leukaemia: low-power view of testicular infiltrate, showing leukaemic blast cells in the interstitial tissues and in the seminiferous tubular epithelium.

Cytochemistry in acute leukaemia					
	precursor B-ALL	T-ALL	AML		
			M_1–M_3	M_4–M_5	M_6–M_7
Myeloperoxidase	–	–	+/++	+	–
Sudan black	–	–	+/++	+	–
Non-specific esterase	–	–	–	++	+ (focal)
periodic acid–Schiff	+ (coarse)	–	–	+	+ (fine)
acid phosphatase	–	+ (focal)	–	+ (diffuse)	+ (focal)

Fig. 8.61 Acute leukaemia: cytochemistry.

CYTOCHEMISTRY

Cytochemical stains may aid the identification of the different subtypes of acute leukaemia (*Fig. 8.61*). In AML, special stains such as myeloperoxidase or Sudan black are used to confirm the presence of granules in the myeloid cells. The dual esterase stain may also be used (*Fig. 8.62*). Monocytic differentiation is demonstrated by non-specific esterase staining which may be combined with chloracetate staining to differentiate monoblasts and myeloblasts in the same case (*Fig. 8.63*). The periodic acid–Schiff (PAS) reagent may show block positivity in the M_6 variant (*Fig. 8.64*). The presence of monoblasts may also be shown by measuring serum lysozyme or by demonstrating microscopically lysozyme secretion by the monoblasts (*Fig. 8.65*).

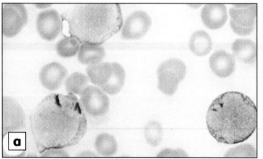

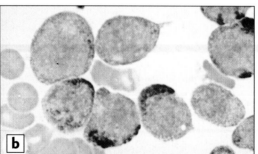

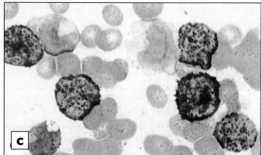

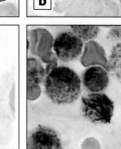

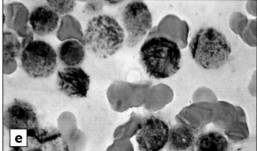

Fig. 8.62a–e Acute myeloid leukaemia: bone marrow aspirates of (a, b) M_2 subtypes show black-staining cytoplasmic granules and Auer rods; (c) M_4 subtype myeloblasts with black cytoplasmic granules (the monoblasts show only background staining); (d) M_2 subtype shows multiple, blue-staining cytoplasmic granules; (e) M_3 subtype shows multiple Auer rods ('faggots'). [(a–c) Sudan black; (d) myeloperoxidase; (e) dual esterase stains; (e) courtesy of Prof. JM Bennett.]

In ALL, the special stains of value are:
- PAS, which shows block positivity in non-B, non-T-ALL, usually showing the c-ALL (CD10) antigen (*Fig. 8.66*);
- acid phosphatase, which shows eccentric Golgi body staining in T-ALL (*Fig. 8.67*); and
- oil red O, which stains lipid material in L_3 ALL (*Fig. 8.68*) that appears as vacuoles on conventional May–Grünwald/Giemsa staining.

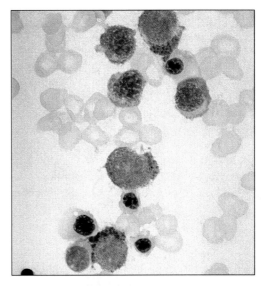

Fig. 8.64 Acute myeloid leukaemia, M_6 subtype: bone marrow aspirate in which the cytoplasm of some of the erythroblasts shows block positive red staining by PAS.

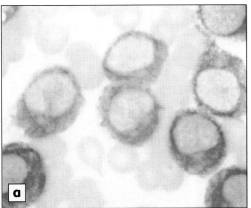

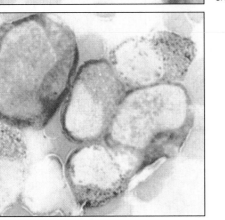

Fig. 8.63a and b Acute myeloid leukaemia: bone marrow aspirates of (a) M_5 subtype shows deep orange staining by non-specific esterase, and of (b) M_4 subtype shows deep orange staining of the monoblast cytoplasm by non-specific esterase and blue staining of myeloblast cytoplasm by chloracetate.

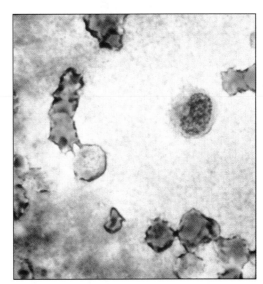

Fig. 8.65 Acute myeloid leukaemia, M_5 subtype: the bone marrow aspirate plate has been layered with the organism *Micrococcus lysodeikticus*. There is clearing of the organism around a monoblast because of secretion of lysozyme (muramidase) by the cell. (Courtesy of Prof. D Catovsky.)

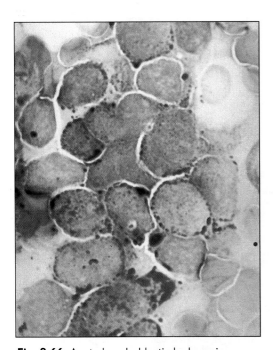

Fig. 8.66 Acute lymphoblastic leukaemia, precursor B: bone marrow aspirate showing cells with one or more coarse granules in the cytoplasm. PAS stain.

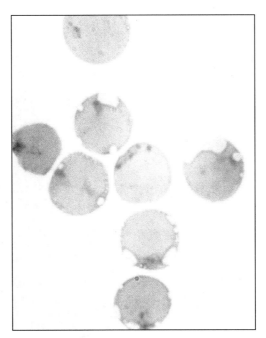

Fig. 8.67 Acute lymphoblastic leukaemia, T-cell subtype: bone marrow aspirate shows red cytoplasmic staining with marked coloration of the Golgi zone adjacent to or indented into the nucleus. Acid phosphatase stain.

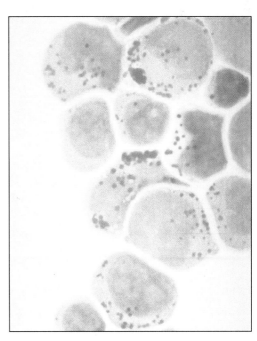

Fig. 8.68 Acute lymphoblastic leukaemia, L_3 subtype: bone marrow aspirate stained with oil red O shows prominent cytoplasmic lipid collections corresponding to some of the vacuoles shown by Romanowsky staining (*see Fig. 8.57*).

IMMUNOLOGICAL MARKERS

Immunofluorescence, immunoperoxidase and alkaline phosphatase–anti-alkaline phosphatase (AP–AAP) techniques are particularly useful in the determination of the leukaemia and lymphoma subtypes. A typical panel of (monoclonal) antibodies used in acute leukaemia diagnosis is shown in *Fig. 8.69*.

The sequence of expression for some markers is given in *Figs 1.96 and 1.101*. In ALL, blasts are usually positive for the nuclear enzyme terminal deoxynucleotidyl transferase (TdT). Tests for this may be combined with membrane staining for HLA-DR and for the common ALL antigen CD10 (c-ALLA), which are both usually positive in precursor B-ALL (*Figs 8.70 and 8.71*). In pro-B (null) ALL, CD10 is negative. For the T-cell antigens that are positive in T-ALL (*Fig. 8.72*), pre-T-ALL is distinguished by absence of CD2. Cytoplasmic (c)CD22 is a relatively specific marker for B-lineage ALL and cCD3 for T-lineage ALL. Testing for TdT is particularly valuable for the detection of blasts at extramedullary sites, since no TdT⁺ cells occur normally outside the marrow or thymus (*Figs 8.73 and 8.74*), and for detecting populations of lymphoblasts in cases of mixed ALL/AML arising *de novo* or during transformation of chronic myeloid leukaemia (*Figs 8.75 and 8.76*).

In pre-B-ALL, intracytoplasmic immunoglobulin is expressed and may be detected by indirect immunofluorescence (*Fig. 8.77*). The cells usually show some degree of vacuolization and the cytogenic abnormality t(1;19) is often present. In B-ALL, surface immunoglobulin is present but TdT is negative (*Fig. 8.78*). Fluorescence-activated cell sorting (FACS) analysis may be used instead of microscopy for immunological analysis of the cell population (*Fig. 8.79*). Characteristic antigens may also be demonstrated by enzyme-linked cytochemistry instead of immunofluorescence (*Fig. 8.80*). Immunoglobulin gene probes (*Fig. 8.81*) and poly-

Immunological markers and gene rearrangements in acute leukaemia				
	B-lineage ALL	**B-ALL**	**T-ALL**	**AML**
'Stem cell'				
Terminal deoxynucleotidyl transferase (TdT)	+	–	+	–
HLA-DR	+	+	–	±
CD34	±	–	–	±
B-cell associated				
CD10	+ (in pro-B)	±	–	–
CD19 (m)	+	+	–	–
CD20	+	+	–	–
cCD22	+	+	–	–
CD79a (cyt)	+	+	–	–
μ chain (cyt)	+ (pre-B)	+	–	–
SmIg	–	+	–	–
T-cell associated				
CD2	–	–	+ (– in met)	-
cCD3	–	–	+	–
CD5	–	–	+	–
CD7	–	–	+	–
Myeloid/monocytic associated				
Anti-MPO	–	–	–	+
CD11	–	–	–	+
CD13	–	–	–	+
CD14	–	–	–	+ (especially M_4, M_5)
CD33	–	–	–	+
Megakaryoblastic (platelet gpIIb/IIIa)	–	–	–	+ (M_7)
CD41				
CD42		–		
CD61	–	–	–	+ (M_6)
Glycophorin A (gp41)		–		
Immunoglobulin genes	Rearranged	Rearranged	Germ line (or rearranged)	Germ line
T-cell receptor genes	Germ line (or rearranged)	Germ line	Rearranged	Germ line

Fig. 8.69 Acute leukaemia: immunological markers and gene rearrangements. A substantial minority of cases show a mixed phenotype with, for example, lymphoid markers (TdT, CD7) positive in AML or myeloid markers (e.g. CD11, CD13) positive in ALL. Some of these mixed cases show a mixed phenotype in individual cells (biphenogenic), whereas others show a dual population of myeloid and lymphoid cells (bilineal) (*see Fig. 8.76*). Rare types include NK cell leukaemia. (cyt, intracytoplasmic; m, membrane; MPO, myeloperoxidase.)

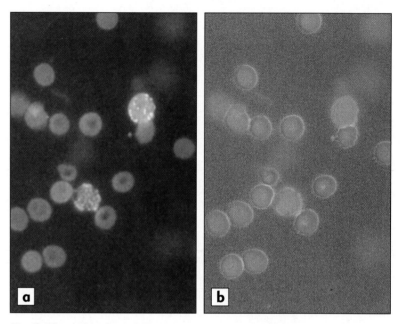

Fig. 8.70a and b Acute lymphoblastic leukaemia, c-ALL subtype: (a) bone marrow aspirates seen by indirect immunofluorescent staining for TdT using fluorescein labelling (green), and for CD10 antigen using avidin labelling (orange); one of the cells is double stained. (b) The same cells as seen by phase-contrast microscopy. [(a, b) Courtesy of Prof. G Janossy.]

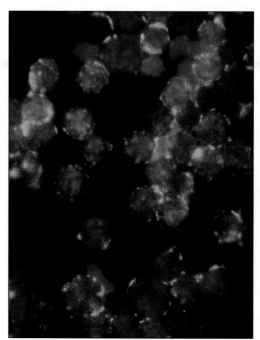

Fig. 8.71 Acute lymphoblastic leukaemia, c-ALL subtype: bone marrow aspirate seen by indirect immunofluorescence shows nuclear TdT (green) and membrane HLA-DR antigen (orange). Most cells are double stained but some cells show only one of the antigens. (Courtesy of Prof. G Janossy.)

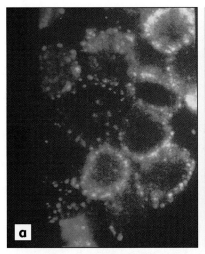

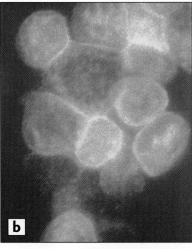

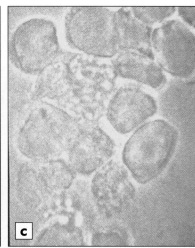

Fig. 8.72a–c Acute lymphoblastic leukaemia, T-ALL subtype: bone marrow aspirates seen by indirect immunofluorescence show (a) red cell membrane T antigen; (b) green-staining nuclear TdT. (c) The same cells as seen by phase-contrast microscopy. [(a–c) Courtesy of Prof. G Janossy.]

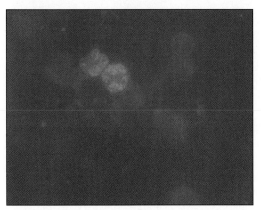

Fig. 8.73 Acute lymphoblastic leukaemia: indirect immunofluorescent staining of cerebrospinal fluid for TdT. These few cells, difficult to recognize morphologically, show nuclear TdT staining typical of lymphoblasts. (Courtesy of Dr KF Bradstock.)

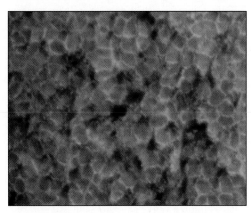

Fig. 8.74 Acute lymphoblastic leukaemia, c-ALL subtype: testicular infiltrate seen by indirect immunofluorescence shows nuclear TdT as green and membrane HLA-DR antigen as orange. (Courtesy of Prof. G Janossy.)

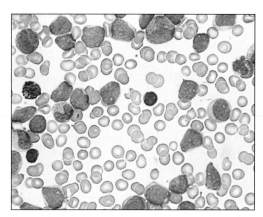

Fig. 8.75 Acute leukaemias, mixed cell (myeloid/lymphoblastic) type: bone marrow aspirate showing blasts of varying size and morphology. Some have scanty cytoplasm without granules, while others, usually larger, have eccentric nuclei, substantial cytoplasm and granules.

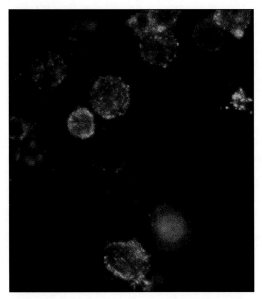

Fig. 8.76 Acute leukaemia, mixed cell type: bone marrow aspirate seen by indirect immunofluorescence shows one population of cells (lymphoblastic) to have nuclear TdT (green) while another population (myeloid) has myeloid surface antigen (yellow/orange). (Courtesy of Prof. G Janossy.)

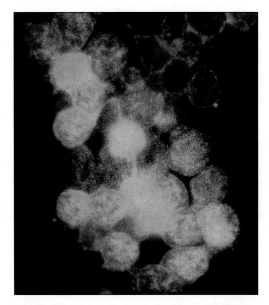

Fig. 8.77 Acute lymphoblastic leukaemia, pre-B subtype: bone marrow aspirate seen by indirect immunofluorescence. The blast cells show nuclear TdT as green and intracytoplasmic immunoglobulin as orange. (Courtesy of Prof. G Janossy.)

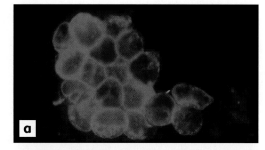

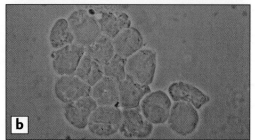

Fig. 8.78a and b Acute lymphoblastic leukaemia, B subtype: bone marrow aspirate seen by indirect immunofluorescence. (a) The cells are invariably negative for nuclear TdT but show the presence of surface immunoglobulin; (b) as seen by phase-contrast microscopy. [(a, b) Courtesy of Prof. G Janossy.]

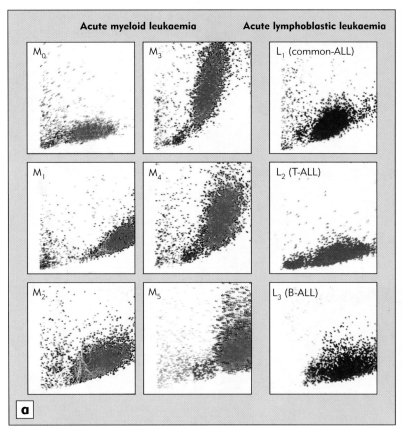

Acute myeloid leukaemia

M₀ M₃

M₁ M₄

M₂ M₅

Acute lymphoblastic leukaemia

L₁ (common-ALL)

L₂ (T-ALL)

L₃ (B-ALL)

a

Triple I
CD13–33/CD19/CD7

forward scatter 1

A

c
b
a

side scatter 2

CD7
b
c
a

CD13–33

c
a

b

CD13-FITC
+CD33-FITC 3
CD19-PE 4
CD7-biotin
+SAperCPO 5

B

Triple II
CD34/CD10/Class II

forward scatter 1

C

a

side scatter 2

Class II
a

CD34

a

CD34-FITC 3
CD10-PE 4
Class 11-
perCP 5

D

b

Fig. 8.79a and b (a) Acute leukaemia: five-parameter analysis with flow cytometry. The five parameters are two scatters and three antibodies (see below). The side scatter (granularity) and forward scatter (cell size) are depicted in the figures. These scatter characteristics can be correlated with the haematological morphology such as the FAB classification of leukaemias as shown. The colour coding in the various cases of leukaemias derives from the immunological phenotype. In all cases the same triple markers are used, including myeloid antibodies (CD13 and CD33, green), anti-B lineage reagent (CD19, blue) and anti-T lineage reagent (CD7, red). It is clear that the M₁–M₅ cases are labelled with the myeloid antibodies. In addition, the case with the relatively undifferentiated myeloid leukaemia (M₀) also reacts with the CD7 antibody and therefore yields a superimposed orange colour (green and red). The small lymphocytes in all myeloid cases are residual T cells (CD7⁺, red). The common ALL (L₁) and the Burkitt-like (L₃) B-ALL are of B lineage and therefore are labelled blue (CD19). The case with L₂ morphology is T-ALL labelled red (CD7). Such an investigation gives not only the morphological, but also the immunological features of the different populations in acute leukaemia.

(b) Immunodiagnosis of leukaemia – the concept of multiparameter analysis using flow cytometry in a case of ALL of B-lineage. The blast cells show lymphoblastic scatter (a in **A**) and reactivity with CD19 B lineage (painted red). The five parameters simultaneously studied are: forward scatter (1; granularity) and side scatter (2; size) plus staining with three monoclonal antibodies. These are labelled with different fluorochromes such as fluorescein (3; FITC), phycoerythrin (4; PE) and a third dye (5; perCP). The first triple (**A**, **B**) not only shows that this is a case of B-lineage ALL (CD19⁺), but also that a few residual small normal T lymphocytes (CD7⁺, blue) and granular myeloid cells (CD13⁺, CD33⁺) are present. The second triple staining reveals that the blast cells express CD10 (ALL antigen, PE), Class II antigen (perCP) and a marker of immaturity (CD34, FITC). These triple stained cells give a black colour (in **C** and **D**), but a few double stained blasts (pink and orange dots in **D**) are discernible. The diagnosis is common ALL (positive for CD19, CD10, CD34 and Class II). The programme is Paint-a-Gate on a FACScan flow cytometer (Becton Dickinson). (Courtesy of Prof. G Janossy and Dr R Peters.)

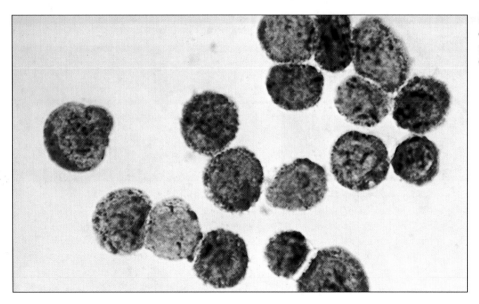

Fig. 8.80 Acute lymphoblastic leukaemia: bone marrow aspirate stained by the AP–AAP technique to demonstrate the presence of the HLA-DR antigen. (Courtesy of Dr D Campana.)

merase chain reaction (PCR) analysis (*Fig. 8.82*) show that the cells in precursor B-ALL and B-ALL show clonal rearrangements of their immunoglobulin genes, thus confirming their B-cell origin. This is also the case for B-cell chronic lymphocytic leukaemia, B-cell non-Hodgkin lymphoma, myeloma and hairy cell leukaemia (*Fig. 8.83*). The T-cell receptor genes (δ, γ, β and α) show clonal rearrangement in the T-cell tumours (e.g. T-ALL, T-CLL, T-cell lymphoma and Sézary's disease). Cross-lineage rearrangements may also occur, for instance the T-cell receptor δ gene is rearranged or deleted in 70–80% of B-lineage ALL cases (*Figs 1.94, 1.95 and 8.84*).

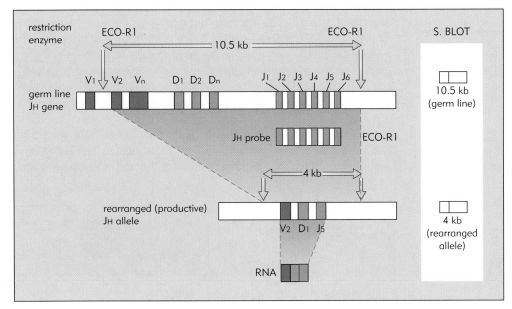

Fig. 8.81 Southern blot: clonal rearrangement of immunoglobulin genes in B-lineage ALL.

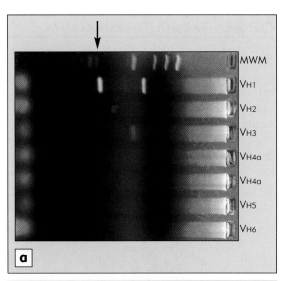

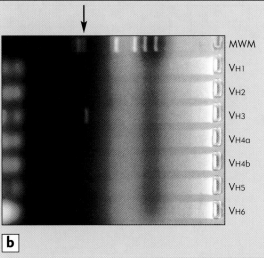

Fig. 8.82a and b Leukaemia analysis: representative ethidium bromide gel analysis by the IgH chain gene fingerprinting technique of leukaemic samples at presentation. DNA (1 μg) from two patients with ALL was tested with seven different VH primers specific for each of the VH families (VH1–6) in combination with the JH consensus primer. One third of each PCR reaction was then loaded and subjected to electrophoresis on a 1.5% agarose gel and visualized by ethidium bromide staining. A discrete visible band is seen only in one of the patients' DNA samples, indicating the presence (a) of a VH1 family rearrangement in patient A and (b) of a VH3 family rearrangement in patient B. The molecular weight marker (MWM) used is the Hae III digest of the ΦX174 DNA. The size of the individual MW fragments are (in kb) as follows: 1.3, 1.0, 0.87, 0.6, 0.31, 0.28, 0.27, 0.23, 0.19. The arrow indicates a MW of 0.31 kb corresponding to the correct size of the amplified rearranged VH gene. Primer–dimer complex is visible at the bottom of the figure. (Courtesy of Dr L Foroni.)

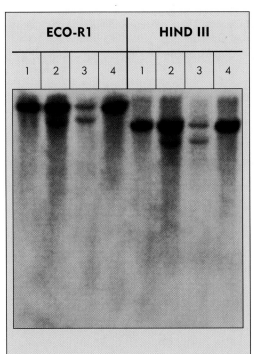

Fig. 8.83 Autoradiograph of Southern blot DNA analysis in ALL: DNA extracted from the peripheral blood of a patient with c-ALL has been digested by restriction enzymes ECO-RI and HIND III. Track 1 is of normal leucocytes; tracks 2 and 3 are of leukaemic blasts; and track 4 is of the promyelocytic cell line HL60. In all tracks except 3 the cells have been concentrated before DNA extraction. The DNA digests have been subjected to electrophoresis in agarose and transferred to nitrocellulose. A ³²P-labelled genomic DNA probe to the JH region of the IgM heavy chain gene has been added to hybridize with complementary DNA in the DNA digests.

All the tracks show a band of similar MW corresponding to the JH region in the germ line configuration. Tracks 2 and 3 show an additional band of lower MW caused by clonal rearrangement of the heavy chain gene in the c-ALL DNA. (Courtesy of Dr R Taheri and Dr JD Norton.)

Scoring system for biphenotypic acute lymphoblastic leukaemia			
Points	**B lineage**	**T lineage**	**Myeloid lineage**
2	CD79a cCD22	cCD3	MPO (any method including anti-MPO)
1	cμ chain CD10 CD19	CD2 CD5	CD33 CD13 CD117 (ckit-receptor)
0.5	TdT	TdT CD7	CD11b/11c CD14/15

Fig. 8.84 Biphenotypic acute leukaemia: suggested scoring system. Score >2 in two lineages is biphenotypic. If CD79a is not used, gene rearrange-ment analysis can be added. IgH rearrangement scores 0.5 for B lineage, and TCR β or δ rearrangement 1.0 for T lineage. (Modified from Catovsky D, Hoffbrand AV. Acute leukaemia. In: Hoffbrand AV, Lewis SM, Tuddenham ECD (eds). *Postgraduate Haematology*. Oxford: Butterworth–Heinemann; 1998:373–404.)

ELECTRON MICROSCOPY

The identification of different types of blast cell is possible using electron microscopy, combined with cytochemical or immunological markers. The electron microscopic appearances of a megakaryoblast are shown in *Fig. 8.85*.

CONGENITAL ACUTE LEUKAEMIA

Fig. 8.86 illustrates a rare type of acute leukaemia, congenital acute leukaemia. This is usually myeloid and characterized by extensive extramedullary infiltration, including in the skin.

Acute leukaemia and Down syndrome
An increased incidence of both ALL and AML occurs in Down syndrome. In the first year of life, AML is the more usual (*Fig. 8.87*). A transient myeloproliferative syndrome also occurs more frequently in Down syndrome than in normal infants. The blood and bone marrow appearances are morphologically similar to those in AML, with usually over 30% of blasts in the blood (*Figs 8.88–8.90*).

CYTOGENETICS

The human somatic cell contains 23 pairs of chromosomes. These are numbered 1 to 22 plus one pair, the sex chromosomes, being XX in females and XY in males (*see Fig. 1.30*). The term 'karyotype' is used to describe the chromosomal make-up of a cell. The letters p and q are used to refer to the short and long arms of the chromosomes (*Fig. 8.91*), respectively; translocations are indicated by t, followed by the chromosomes involved in a first set of parentheses and the chromosome bands involved in a second set of parentheses. *Fig. 8.92* gives examples of translocations found in acute leukaemia. The dark or lighter staining bands are detected by the Giemsa (G) or quinacrine (Q) techniques and are numbered from the centromere outward. Inv indicates an inversion,

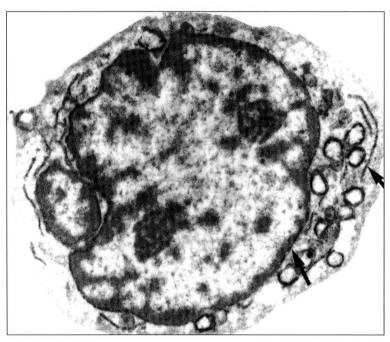

Fig. 8.85 Megakaryoblast: morphologically, this cell resembles a lymphoblast but is identified by the reactivity with the platelet–peroxidase reaction (linear black areas) in the endoplasmic reticulum and nuclear membrane (arrows). Mitochondria are non-specifically positive (× 9250). (Courtesy of Dr E Matutes and Prof. D Catovsky.)

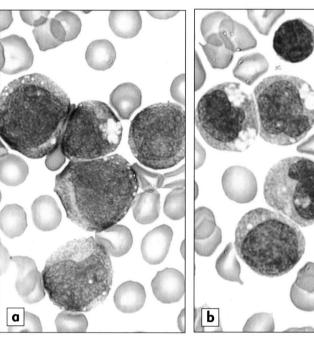

Fig. 8.86a and b Congenital acute myeloid leukaemia: (a, b) peripheral blood films of a male infant who presented at birth with anaemia, hepatosplenomegaly and skin lesions. There are large numbers of myeloblasts with prominent cytoplasmic vacuolation. [Hb, 10.1 g/dl; WBC, 92 × 10^9/l; blasts, 85%; platelets, 15 × 10^9/l; (a, b) courtesy of Prof. JM Chessels.]

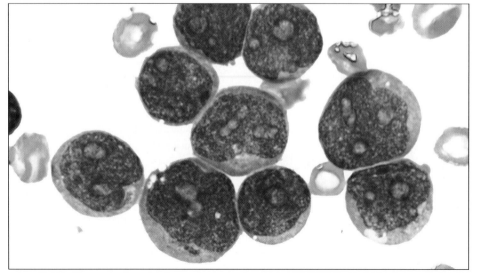

Fig. 8.87 Acute myeloid leukaemia: Down syndrome. Peripheral blood showing numerous myeloblasts in a child aged <1 year. (Courtesy of Prof. RD Brunning and the AFIP.)

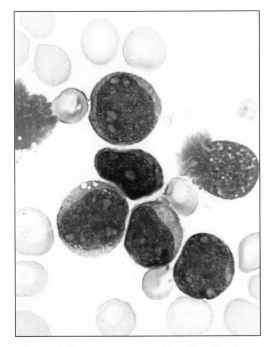

Fig. 8.88 Transient myeloproliferative disorder: Down syndrome. Peripheral blood film from a 3-day-old girl with Down syndrome [Hb, 16.2 g/dl; WBC, 62 × 10⁹/l (blasts, 50–55%); platelets, 28 × 10⁹/l]. The blasts have basophilic cytoplasm, dispersed nuclear chromatin and several nucleoli. Azurophilic granules are present in one of the blasts. The WBC increased to 77 × 10⁹/l on day 5, but then resolved spontaneously by 8 weeks, when the blood film was normal. There was no recurrence within a 5-year follow-up. (Courtesy of Prof. RD Brunning and the AFIP.)

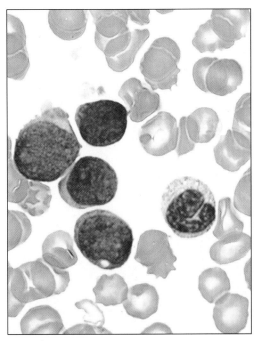

Fig. 8.89 Transient myeloproliferative disorder: Down syndrome. Peripheral blood film from a 20-day-old girl (Hb, 16.4 g/dl; WBC, 54 × 10⁹/l, platelet count normal). Approximately 50% of the white blood cells are blasts. The platelets are large; occasional platelets are poorly granulated. The white cell count returned to normal after 3 weeks, but increased 3 months later following a bacterial infection when blast cells were again numerous. This resolved but relapsed 2 months later, upon which the child was treated for acute leukaemia. (Courtesy of Prof. RD Brunning and the AFIP.)

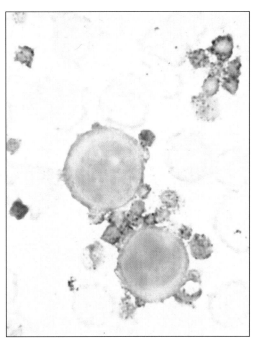

Fig. 8.90 Transient myeloproliferative disorder: Down syndrome. Peripheral blood from the child described in *Fig. 8.89* reacted with monoclonal antibody to CD61 (platelet glycoprotein IIIa; AP–AAP technique). The megakaryocytes, promegakaryocytes and platelets are positive; the blasts (not shown) were non-reactive. (Courtesy of Prof. RD Brunning and the AFIP.)

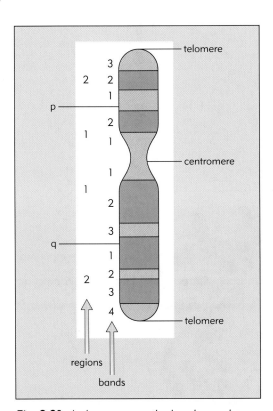

Fig. 8.91 A chromosome: the bands may be divided into sub-bands according to staining pattern. (Modified from Hoffbrand AV, Pettit JE. *Essential Haematology*, 3rd edn. Oxford: Blackwell Scientific; 1993.)

Fig. 8.92 Acute leukaemia: cytogenetic abnormalities.

Cytogenetic abnormalities in acute leukaemias	
Acute myeloid leukaemia	**Acute lymphoblastic leukaemia**
Relatively specific	**Precursor B-ALL**
M₁ t(3;v)*	t(12;21) (p13;q22)¶
M₂ t(8;21) (q22;q22)	t(9;22) (q34;q11)
M₃ t(15;17) (q22;q21)	t(4;11) (q21;q23)
M₄ inv(16) (p13;q22) or del(16) (q22)†	t(1;19) (q23;p13)
M₄(M₅) t(8;16) (p11;p13)	del(6q)
M₅ₐ t(11;v) (q23;v)	t(11;14) (q13;q32)
M₅ᵦ t(8;16)(p11;p13)	t or del 12p12
M₆ del(20)(q11)	6q–
	9p–
Others	+21
t(9;22) (q34;q11) M₁, biphenotypic	Hyperdiploidy 50–65 chromosomes
t(6;9) (p23;q34)‡ M₂, M₄	Near haploidy 26–34 chromosomes
t(3;3) (q21;q29) inv(3) (q21;q26)§	
+9 M₆	**B-ALL**
+11, +13 M₀, M₁	t(8;14) (q24;q32)
+22 M₄ Eo	t(8;22) (q24;q11)
+4 M₂, M₄ with MDS	t(2;8) (p11–13;q24)
+8 M₁, M₄, M₅	
+21	**T-ALL**
5q–/–5 secondary AML, MDS	t or del 14q11
	t(11;14) (p13;q11)
7q–/–7 secondary AML, MDS	t(10;14) (q24;q11)
	t(1;14) (p34;q11)
t or del secondary AML	6q–
ˊ12p11–p13‡	9p–
*v = various other chromosomes	§associated with thrombocytosis
†associated with abnormal eosinophils	¶detectable only by molecular methods
‡with increased basophils	

ins an insertion and del a deletion; + or – in front of a number indicates gain or loss of the whole chromosome, while + or – after a number means a gain or loss of part of the chromosome.

Cytogenetic analysis of acute leukaemia cells may help to confirm the diagnosis and indicate the subtype in which characteristic abnormalities may occur (*Figs 8.92 and 8.93*).

A normal male karyotype is illustrated in *Fig. 8.94*. The cytogenetic abnormality hyperdiploidy (*Fig. 8.95*) is found in 35% of children with ALL and is associated with a good prognosis. The translocations shown in *Figs 8.96 and 8.97*, with the exception of derived [der(19)], are associated with a poor prognosis. Translocations t(9;22) (*see Fig. 9.1*), t(1;19) and the variant der(19), and t(4;11) are characteristic for early B-lineage

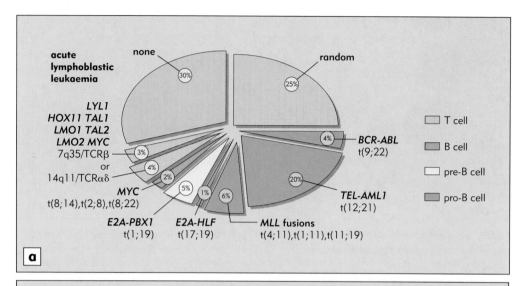

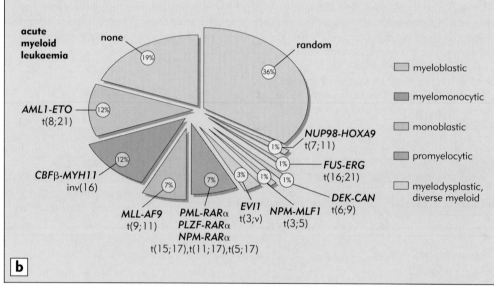

Fig. 8.93a and b Acute leukaemia: Cytogenetic abnormalities. Distribution of translocation-generated oncogenes in (a) AML and (b) ALL. (Modified from Look AT. Oncogenic transcription factors in the human acute leukaemias. *Science*. 1997;278:1059–64.)

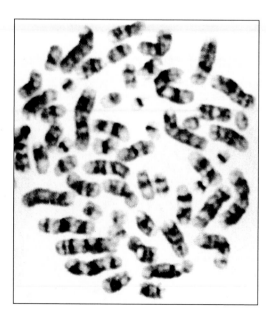

Fig. 8.94 Chromosomes (adult male): normal 46 chromosomes in metaphase from a G-banded marrow cell. (Courtesy of Prof. LM Secker-Walker.)

Fig. 8.95 Acute lymphoblastic leukaemia, L₁ subtype: 58 chromosomes in a hyperdiploid metaphase from a marrow cell. (Courtesy of Prof. LM Secker-Walker.)

ALL and t(8;14) for B-ALL (*Figs 8.96 and 8.97*). Abnormalities found in AML are t(6;9) (p23;q34) associated with basophilia, t(8;21) (q22;q22) in M$_2$, t(15;17) (q22;q21) in M$_3$ and inv(16) (p13;q22) in M$_4$ (*Figs 8.98–8.100*). The fluorescent *in situ* hybridization technique (FISH) may also be used to detect loss or gain of a chromosome or part of a chromosome or for chromosome translocation (*Figs 8.101 and 8.102*), in some cases where the translocated or lost material is not visible by light microscopy. A cryptic translocation t(12;21) (p13;q22) occurs in 30% of B-lineage ALL (*Fig. 8.103a*). Using the MLL probe, FISH can show rearrangements within the gene (*Fig. 8.103b*). Cryptic hemi- or homozygous loss of genes p16 INKa and p15 INKb situated at 9p21–22 occurs in up to 80% of childhood T-ALL.

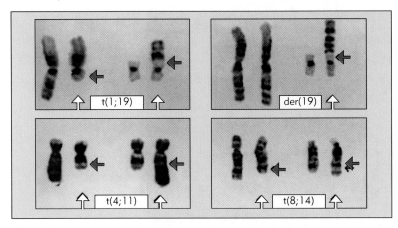

Fig. 8.96 Acute lymphoblastic leukaemia: partial karyograms showing common translocations in patients with ALL. The translocated chromosomes are on the right (arrowed) of each pair; the red arrows mark the regions of chromosome breakage and rejoining: t(1;19) (q21;p13); der(19)t(1;19) (q23;p13); t(4;11) (q21;q23); t(8;14) (q24;q32). (Courtesy of Prof. LM Secker-Walker.)

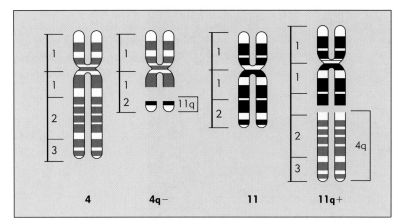

Fig. 8.97 Acute lymphoblastic leukaemia, L$_1$ subtype: from a patient with blasts of null phenotype (TdT$^+$, CD10$^-$). Systematized description of the structural aberration. The translocated chromosomes are on the right in each pair t(4;11). (Courtesy of Prof. LM Secker-Walker.)

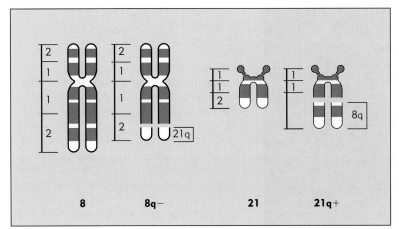

Fig. 8.98 Acute myeloid leukaemia, M$_2$ subtype: diagrammatic systematized description of the structural aberration t(8;21). (Courtesy of Prof. LM Secker-Walker.)

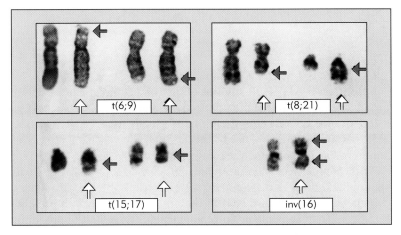

Fig. 8.99 Acute myeloid leukaemia: partial karyograms showing common rearrangements in AML. In each karyogram, the translocated chromosome is on the right (arrowed) in each pair; red arrows mark the regions of chromosome breakage and rejoining: t(6;9) (p22;q34); t(8;21) (q22;q22); t(15;17) (q22;q12); inv(16) (p13;q22). (Courtesy of Prof. LM Secker-Walker.)

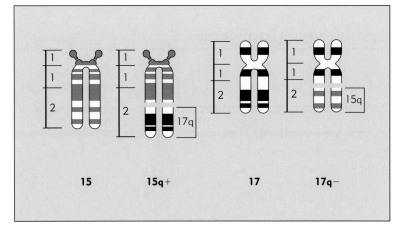

Fig. 8.100 Acute myeloid leukaemia, M$_3$ subtype (acute promyelocytic leukaemia, APL): systematized description of the structural aberration t(15;17). (Courtesy of Prof. LM Secker-Walker.)

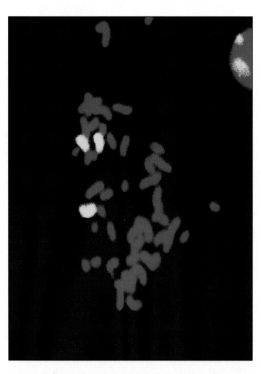

Fig. 8.101 Acute myeloid leukaemia: M₆ subtype. Fluorescent *in situ* hybridization (FISH) technique using a chromosome 8 painting probe. The probe was visualized indirectly using the biotin–avidin system. Three copies of chromosome 8 (trisomy 8) are present. (Courtesy of Dr A Kasprzyk.)

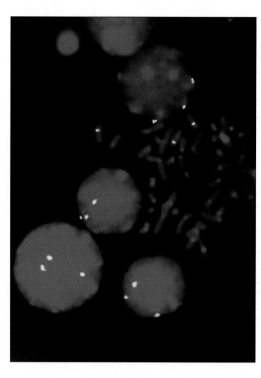

Fig. 8.102 Acute myeloid leukaemia: M₆ subtype. FISH technique using a chromosome 8 centromere probe. Three copies of chromosome 8 (trisomy 8) are present. (Courtesy of Dr CJ Harrison.)

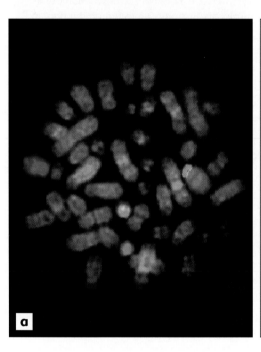

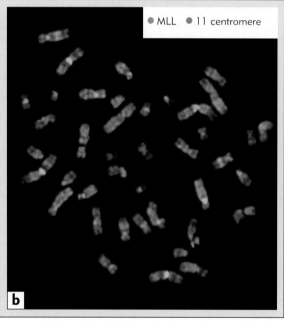

● MLL   ● 11 centromere

Fig. 8.103a and b Acute lymphoblastic leukaemia: FISH analysis. (a) Metaphase from a childhood patient with ALL showing the translocation t(12;21) by chromosome 'painting'. Chromosomes 12 are painted red and chromosomes 21 green. This chromosome abnormality is not visible by conventional cytogenetic analysis. FISH elegantly reveals the exchange of material on the derived chromosomes 12 and 21. (b) FISH using probes for the centromere of chromosome 11 (green) and the *MLL* gene (red), normally on chromosome 11, reveals a reciprocal translocation between chromosomes 6 and 11 that results in the rearrangement of *MLL*, which is detected as a splitting of the *MLL* signal between the derived chromosomes 6 and 11. [(a, b) Courtesy of Dr CJ Harrison.]

MINIMAL RESIDUAL DISEASE

A number of different techniques may be used to search for residual leukaemia cells in the blood, bone marrow or other tissues of patients with acute leukaemia who have entered remission and have normal appearance of the blood film and bone marrow by conventional staining. These techniques include:

- cytogenetics;
- flow karyotyping;
- DNA analysis (e.g. of the immunoglobulin genes or T-cell receptor genes by Southern blotting);
- use of the FISH technique (see earlier);
- immunological analysis using double or triple marker analysis (*see* Fig. 8.79) to detect combinations of antigens that are infrequently or not present on normal bone marrow cells (*Fig. 8.104*); or

- use of one or other PCR technique.

For precursor B-ALL, PCR analysis of the third complementary determining region (CDR3) of the immunoglobulin heavy chain locus (*Fig. 8.105*) or of the T cell receptor δ gene is usually used. For T-ALL, the TCRγ or TCRδ genes are used. The original clone is characterized by Southern blotting or a PCR technique.

Primers are chosen so that the region rearranged in that clone will be amplified from remission marrow. Detection of the PCR product (which will be obtained if cells of the original clone are still present; *Fig. 8.106*) may be made by autoradiography. (*Fig. 8.107*) or ethidium bromide staining.

For AML, double immunological marker analysis may be useful if the cells show aberrant phenotypes, e.g. TdT⁺ and myeloid antigens. PCR

Immunological markers for minimal residual disease

Disease	Phenotype*	Frequency (%)†	Frequency in normal marrow (% positive cells ± SD)‡
B-lineage ALL	TdT/CD10/CD13	7	0.02 ± 0.01
	TdT/CD10/CD33	8	0.03 ± 0.02
	TdT/CD10/CDw65	7	0.02 ± 0.01
	TdT/CD10/CD21	10	0.02 ± 0.01
	TdT/CD10/CD56	9	<0.01
	TdT/cytoplasmic μ/CD34	14	0.03 ± 0.01
	KOR-SA3544	10	<0.01
	7.1	3	<0.01
T-lineage ALL	TdT/cytoplasmic CD3	90	<0.01
T-lineage AML	CD34/CD56	20	<0.01
	CDw65/CD34/TdT	15	<0.01

*TdT and CD10 can be replaced by CD19 and CD34.
†Greater than 10% positive leukaemic lymphoblasts
‡These positive cells had light-scattering properties typical of immature lymphoid or myeloid cells. The reduced expression of the indicated phenotypes by normal cells allows one leukaemic cell to be identified among 10,000 normal marrow cells.

Fig. 8.104 Acute leukaemia: immunophenotypic combinations used to study minimal residual disease. (Modified from Pui C-H, Campana D. In: *Haematology Education Programme of the 26th Congress of the International Society of Haematology*. Singapore; 1996:137–41.)

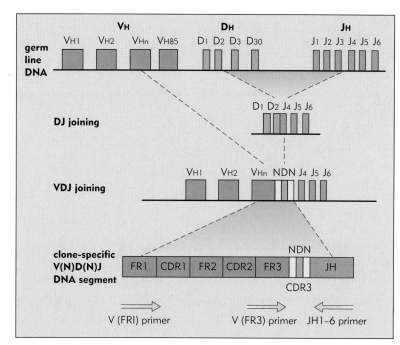

Fig. 8.105 IgH locus: the partial germ line locus is shown on top, followed by a hypothetical rearrangement event. Positions of primers which can be used for PCR gene amplification of the resulting rearrangement are shown by orange arrows. V, variable regions; D, diversity regions; J, joining regions; N, random regions inserted by TdT during gene rearrangement. (Courtesy of Dr L Foroni.)

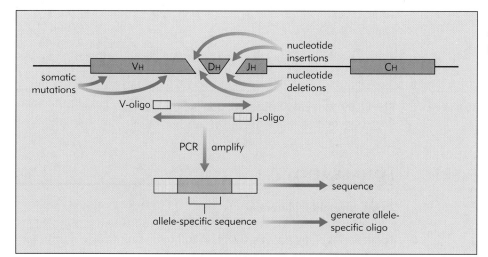

Fig. 8.106 Minimal residual disease: detection in precursor B-ALL using PCR amplification with clone-specific primers or probe.

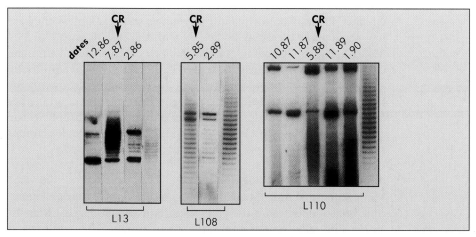

Fig. 8.107 Minimal residual disease: detection in precursor B-ALL using immunoglobulin fingerprinting technique. In each case the remission marrow (CR) shows a residual clone. (Courtesy of Dr M Deane and Dr JD Norton.)

Some of the translocations suitable for polymerase chain reaction analysis

Acute lymphoblastic leukaemia: B lineage

	Chromosomal translocation	Molecular target	DNA or RNA
Precursor B	t(9;22)	BCR-ABL	RNA
	t(1;19)	E2A-PBX1	RNA
	t(17;19)	HLF-E2A	RNA
	t(4;11)	AF4-MLL	RNA
	t(12;21)	TEL-AML1	RNA
	Hq23 translocations	MLL-AF	RNA
B-ALL	t(8;14)	MYC-Sμ	DNA

Acute lymphoblastic leukaemia: T lineage

	Chromosomal translocation	Molecular target	DNA or RNA
T-ALL	TAL interstitial deletion	TAL-SIL	DNA
	t(1;14)	TAL-1-TCRδ	DNA
	t(10;14)	HOX11-TCRδ	DNA
	t(11;14)	11p13-TCRδ	DNA

Acute myeloid leukaemia

FAB subtype	Chromosomal translocation	Molecular target	DNA or RNA
M₂	t(8;21)	CBFα-/MTGA*	RNA
M₂ or M₄	t(6;9)	DEK-CAN	RNA
M₃	t(15;17)	PML-RARα	RNA
M₄	inv 16	CBFβ-MCHII	RNA
Non-specific	t(9;22)	BCR-ABL	RNA
	t(9;11)	MLL-AF9	RNA

*CBFα = AMLI; MTGA = ETO

Fig. 8.108 Translocations suitable for PCR analysis: (upper) ALL, B lineage; (middle) ALL, T lineage; (lower) AML.

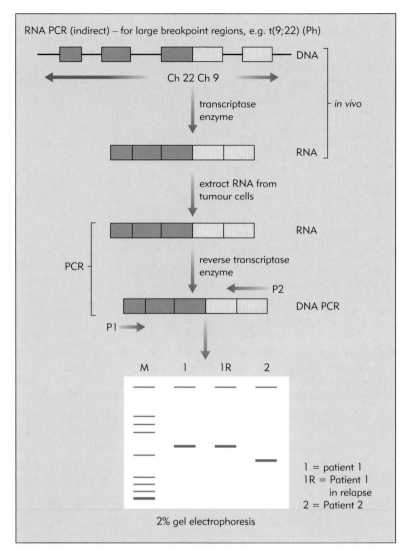

Fig. 8.109 Molecular cytogenetics: RNA PCR [indirect – for large breakpoint regions, e.g. t(9;22) (Ph)].

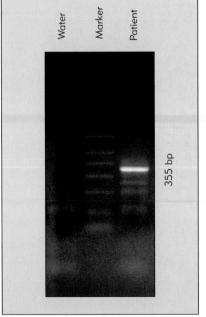

Fig. 8.110 Reverse transcriptase (RT): PCR analysis of an APL patient at diagnosis. The PML–RARA fusion product (cDNA) has been amplified using nested oligonucleotides from the *PML* and *RARA* genes. Lane 1, water control, Lane 2, low molecular weight (Cambio) DNA marker; Lane 3, patient sample. All APL patients with a t(15;17) translocation express either the 5' (a single 355 bp fusion message) or the 3' (a series of various fusion messages caused by alternate splicing) PML breakpoint. (Courtesy of Dr P Devaraj.)

techniques are valuable if there is a chromosome translocation (*Fig. 8.108*). These may use analysis of DNA if the breakpoints occur within a relatively small area of DNA (<1000 kb) or RNA with reverse transcriptase if the breakpoints occur over a larger area (*Figs 8.109 and 8.110*).

MANAGEMENT

Acute myeloid leukaemia

The principles of treatment of AML are outlined in *Fig. 8.111*. Induction therapy is given to obtain full remission which, if achieved, is consolidated with further courses of intensive combination chemotherapy, with a total of four or five courses. If an HLA-matching sibling is available, allogeneic stem cell transplantation (*see* Chapter 14) may be carried out in younger patients unless they are in a particularly good risk group [M₂ with t(8;21), M₃ with t(15;17), M₄ with inv(16) and complete remission has been achieved after one course]. For patients with M₃ with t(15;17) ATRA is given initially and usually continued throughout the first course of treatment. For those without a suitable donor, autologous transplantation or further consolidation is considered. For older patients, for example, those over 60 years of age with major general medical problems, less intensive chemotherapy or even support care only is often used.

Acute lymphoblastic leukaemia

Management of ALL involves therapy directed at remission induction, consolidation and the CNS, with late and 'late late' intensification and maintenance therapy. The drugs used for induction usually include vincristine, L-asparaginase, prednisolone or dexamethasone, and an anthracycline such as daunorubicin in adults (*Fig. 8.112*). Consolidation protocols often include cytosine arabinoside

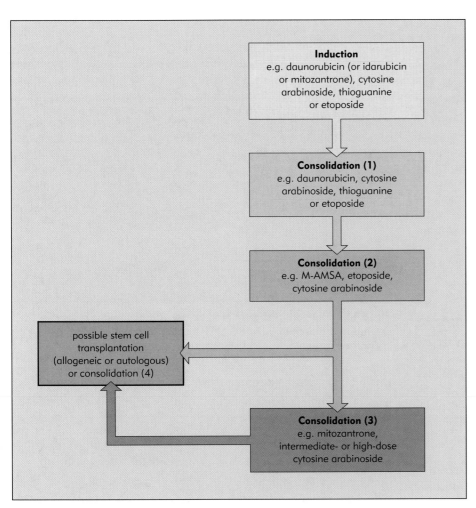

Fig. 8.111 Acute myeloid leukaemia: typical treatment regimen.

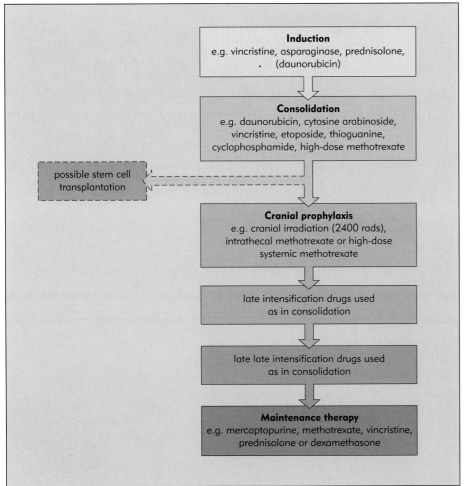

Fig. 8.112 Acute lymphoblastic leukaemia: typical treatment regimen.

(ara-C), etoposide, cyclophosphamide and 6-mercaptopurine or thioguanine, with the drugs used in induction. Cranial irradiation, intrathecal methotrexate or ara-C, and/or systemic high-dose methotrexate are used for CNS-directed therapy. The particular drugs used for late and 'late late' intensification and the number of cycles of therapy differ in different protocols. Maintenance therapy is given until 2 years from remission. Allogeneic stem cell transplantation is carried out in first remission, provided an HLA-matching sibling can act as a donor, in patients of relatively poor prognosis [e.g. male, adult, high white cell count at presentation, Philadelphia (Ph) chromosome positive, failure to enter remission in 4 weeks, persistence of minimal residual disease after 4 months]. Unrelated HLA-matched donors are used when the prognosis is particularly poor with chemotherapy alone (e.g. failure of remission, second remission or Ph-positive cases) and no HLA-matching sibling donors are available. Autologous stem cell transplantation for ALL in first remission is undergoing clinical trials.

DRUG RESISTANCE

Resistance to chemotherapy may have multiple causes. One is increased expression of a multi-drug resistance (MDR) gene which codes for a membrane glycoprotein PGP of molecular weight 170 kDa (p170) and which is responsible for efflux of a number of drugs, including anthracyclines, mitoxantrone, M-amasacrine, vinca alkaloids and epipodophyllotoxin from cells (*Figs 8.113 and 8.114*). Therapy to reverse MDR can be given with verapamil (but its action *in vivo* is too low), cyclosporin or one of its derivatives (e.g. PSC833), or other drugs specifically developed for MDR modulation [e.g. GG918 (amiodarone derivative)]. Drug resistance may also be associated with expression of other proteins including lung-resistance protein (LRP), which is the major component of vaults (ribonucleotide particles composed of four proteins and a small RNA particle), and the MDR-associated protein (MRP), a 190 kDa protein structurally related to PGP (15% homology).

Drug resistance may also result from overexpression of enzymes (of which the glutathione-S-transferases are the most studied) or from changes in the levels of the target molecules for an individual drug (e.g. dihydrofolate reductase, the target of methotrexate).

New drugs are currently under trial for treatment of relapsed or resistant disease including arsenic treatment for AML M$_3$, tyrosine kinase inhibitors and deacetylase inhibitors.

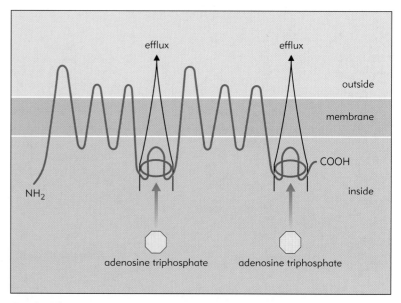

Fig. 8.113 Multi-drug resistant protein: the transmembrane protein belongs to a superfamily of ABG (ATP binding cassette) proteins, specialized for energy-dependent cellular transport.

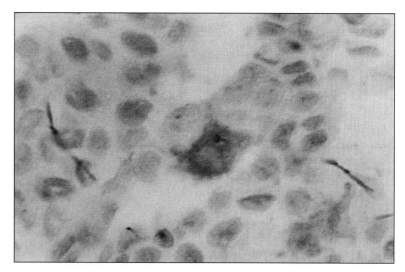

Fig. 8.114 Multi-drug resistant protein: detection by immunocytochemistry. (Courtesy of Dr M Lyttleton.)

Chronic Myeloid Leukaemias and Myelodysplasia

CHRONIC MYELOID LEUKAEMIA

Chronic myeloid leukaemia (CML) is most frequently seen in the middle-aged. In most patients there is replacement of normal marrow by cells with an abnormal G-group chromosome, the Philadelphia or Ph chromosome (*Fig. 9.1*). This abnormality is a result of reciprocal translocation involving chromosome 9 band q34 and chromosome 22 band q11. The cellular oncogene c-ABL, which codes for a tyrosine protein kinase (TPK), is translocated to a specific breakpoint cluster region (BCR) of chromosome 22. Part of the BCR (the 5' end) remains on chromosome 22, and the 3' end moves to chromosome 9 together with the oncogene c-SIS (which codes for a protein with close homology to one of the two subunits of platelet derived growth factor). As a result of the translocation onto chromosome 22, a chimeric BCR/c-ABL·mRNA is produced (*Fig. 9.2*),which results in the synthesis of a 210 kDa protein with considerably enhanced TPK activity compared to the normal 145 kDa c-ABL oncogene product (*Fig. 9.3*). The fusion gene may be detected by the fluorescent *in situ* hybridization (FISH) technique (*Fig. 9.4*).

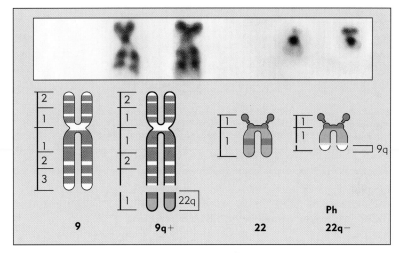

Fig. 9.1 Chronic myeloid leukaemia: partial karyotypes of G-banded chromosomes 9 and 22; the right-hand member of each pair shows the results of the reciprocal translocation. (Courtesy of Prof. LM Secker-Walker.)

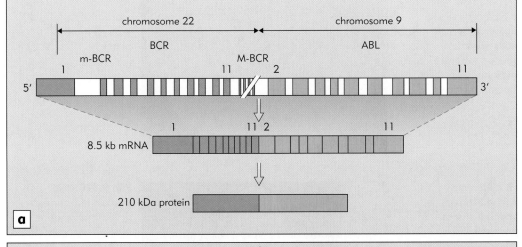

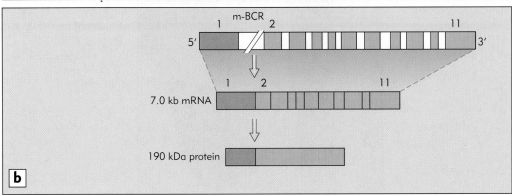

Fig. 9.2a and b Chronic myeloid leukaemia: (a) chimeric BCR/c-ABL mRNA encoded for partly by the BCR (breakpoint cluster region) of chromosome 22 and partly by the c-ABL oncogene translocated from chromosome 9 to 22. The breakpoint is almost always in the major BCR (M-BCR) region, a 5–6 kb region 3' to exon 11. Small exons numbered b_1, b_2, b_3, etc. occur in the M-BCR region, and the breakpoint is usually between b_3 and b_4 or b_2 and b_3, giving rise to fusion genes b_3a_2 or b_2a_2, respectively. The resultant 8.5 kb mRNA is expressed as a 210 kDa protein (p210). (b) In Ph$^+$ acute lymphoblastic leukaemia (ALL) the breakpoint may be in the M-BCR region, but may also occur in the first intron, the minor BCR (m-BCR) region. The fusion gene is termed e_1a_2. A 7.0 kb mRNA is formed which codes for a 190 kDa protein (p190).

Also, Ph⁻ CML may show translocation of c-ABL to chromosome 22, rearrangement of the BCR region and the presence of the 210 kDa kinase. Cases without this may be variants of myelodysplasia (*see Fig. 9.21*).

Cases of Ph⁺ ALL may show a similar molecular abnormality to that in typical Ph⁺ CML, but some show a breakpoint on chromosome 22 outside the major BCR region but in the first intron of the gene (minor or m-BCR breakpoint). In these, the product of the translocated c-ABL gene is a 190 kDa protein also of enhanced TPK activity (*Figs 9.3 and 9.4*).

Clinical features

The symptoms are related to hypermetabolism and include anorexia, lassitude, weight loss and night sweats. Splenomegaly is usual and frequently massive (*Fig. 9.5*). Features of anaemia, a bleeding disorder, visual disturbance because of retinal disease (*Figs 9.6 and 9.7*), neurological symptoms and occasionally gout (*Fig. 9.8*) may occur. As in chronic lymphocytic leukaemia (CLL), this condition is only discovered in some patients during routine blood counting. The white cell count is usually between 50×10^9 and 500×10^9/l (but may be over

Patterns of involvement of the Philadelphia chromosome	
Condition	**Pattern**
Normal	Ph⁻, BCR⁻ → 145 kDa TPK
Chronic myeloid leukaemia	Ph⁺, BCR⁺ → 210 kDa TPK
	Ph⁻, BCR⁺ → 210 kDa TPK
	Ph⁻, BCR⁻ → 145 kDa TPK (atypical cases; ?myelodysplasia)
Acute lymphoblastic leukaemia	Ph⁺, BCR⁺ → 210 kDa TPK (?blast transformation of CML)
	Ph⁺, BCR⁻ → 190 kDa TPK (?*de novo* ALL)
	Ph⁻, BCR⁻ → 145 kDa TPK (*de novo* ALL)

Fig. 9.3 Chronic myeloid leukaemia: patterns of involvement of the Ph chromosome, the BCR (5.8 kb) region and the c-ABL TPK in CML and ALL. (BCR⁺, rearrangement within the 5.8 kb BCR region.)

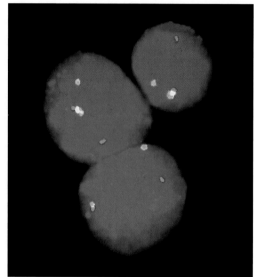

Fig. 9.4 Chronic myeloid leukaemia: three interphase cells from a patient with CML. The red signal indicates the presence of the ABL gene on the normal chromosome 9, the green signal represents the M-BCR on chromosome 22 and the co-localization of the green and red signals (which appears yellow in the region of the overlap) represents the fusion of BCR and ABL on the Ph chromosomes. All three cells are Ph⁺. (Courtesy of Dr CJ Harrison.)

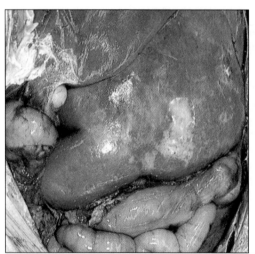

Fig. 9.5 Chronic myeloid leukaemia: abdominal contents of autopsy of a 54-year-old man. The grossly enlarged spleen extends towards the right iliac fossa. The central pale area covered by fibrinous exudate overlays an extensive splenic infarct. The liver is moderately enlarged.

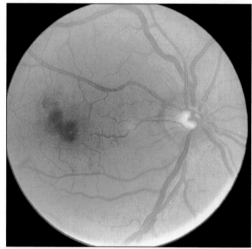

Fig. 9.6 Chronic myeloid leukaemia: ocular fundus in the hyperviscosity syndrome shows distended retinal veins and deep retinal haemorrhages at the macula. (Hb, 14 g/dl; WBC, 590 × 10⁹/l; platelets, 1050 × 10⁹/l.)

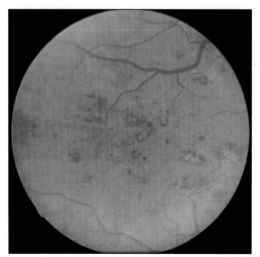

Fig. 9.7 Chronic myeloid leukaemia: ocular fundus (same case as shown in *Fig. 9.6*) showing prominent leukaemic infiltrates fringed by areas of retinal haemorrhage.

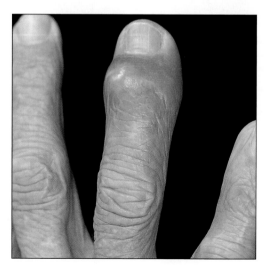

Fig. 9.8 Chronic myeloid leukaemia: acute inflammation and swelling of the fourth finger because of uric acid deposition. (Hb, 8.6 g/dl; WBC, 540 × 10⁹/l; platelets, 850 × 10⁹/l; serum uric acid, 0.85 mmol/l.

500 × 10⁹/l, *Fig. 9.9*), and a complete spectrum of granulocytic cells is seen in the blood film (*Figs 9.10–9.12*). Basophils are often prominent and the levels of myelocytes, metamyelocytes and neutrophils exceed those of the more primitive blast cells and promyelocytes. The bone marrow is hypercellular with a granulocytic predominance (*Fig. 9.13*).

Treatment

Previous treatments have now to be reconsidered with the introduction of STI-571, a specific inhibitor of the tyrosine kinase formed by the BCR-ABL fusion gene in CML. In early trials, this drug has been found to con-

trol the white cell count and result in the conversion of the marrow to partial or 100% Ph⁻ within a few months of therapy in patients resistant to α-interferon (α-IFN). Whether this results in cure of the disease and if so, in what proportion of patients, are the subjects of ongoing trials in newly diagnosed and previously treated patients. In those without an HLA-matching donor sibling, previous therapy has consisted of hydroxyurea initially to control the blood count, followed by α-IFN either alone or with hydroxyurea or cytosine arabinoside. α-IFN appears to prolong the chronic phase, particularly in those who respond well to it, 10–15% of patients becoming Ph⁻. For younger patients with an HLA-

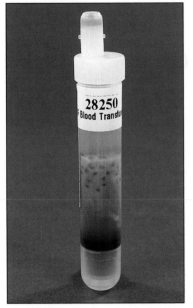

Fig. 9.9 Chronic myeloid leukaemia: peripheral blood, from a 22-year-old woman, showing vast increase in buffy coat. (Hb, 6.1 g/dl; WBC, 532 × 10⁹/l; platelets, 676 × 10⁹/l.)

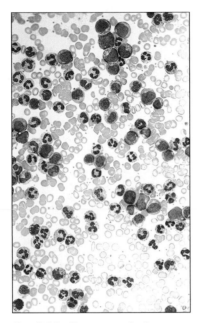

Fig. 9.10 Chronic myeloid leukaemia: peripheral blood film showing cells in all stages of granulocytic development. (Hb, 16.8 g/dl; WBC, 260 × 10⁹/l; platelets, 140 × 10⁹/l.)

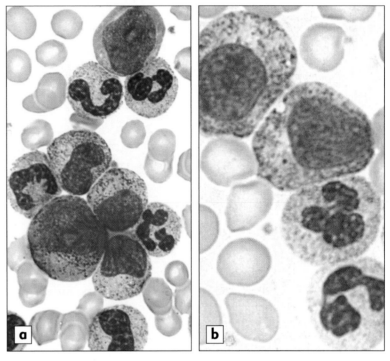

Fig. 9.11a and b Chronic myeloid leukaemia: (a, b) peripheral blood films showing a myeloblast, promyelocytes, myelocytes, metamyelocytes, and band and segmented neutrophils.

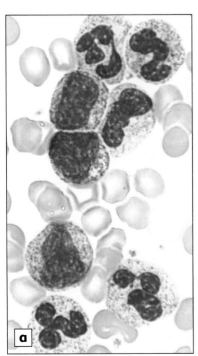

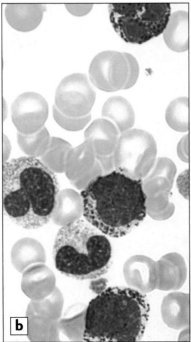

Fig. 9.12a and b Chronic myeloid leukaemia: peripheral blood films showing (a) myelocytes, a metamyelocyte, and band and segmented neutrophils and (b) basophils and metamyelocytes.

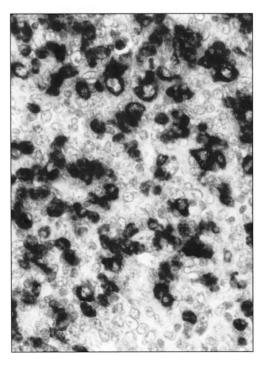

Fig. 9.13 Chronic myeloid leukaemia: Trephine bone marrow biopsy stained for neutrophil elastase (a myeloid-specific marker) with immunophosphatase. (Courtesy of Prof. DY Mason.)

matching sibling, stem cell transplantation has been recommended within the first year of treatment. Unrelated HLA-matched donors and autologous stem cell transplants have also been used early or, at later stages of the disease.

In about 70% of patients there is a terminal metamorphosis to an acute malignant form of leukaemia (*Figs 9.14–9.16*), which is associated with a rapid deterioration of the patient and progressive bone marrow failure. Infiltration of the skin (*Figs 9.17 and 9.18*) and other non-haemopoietic tissues may occur. The transformation may be myeloblastic, lymphoblastic (*Fig. 9.16*), mixed or (rarely) megakaryoblastic (*Figs 9.19 and 9.20*). It may be preceded by an accelerated phase when refractoriness to hydroxyurea or α-IFN, anaemia, thrombocytopenia, splenomegaly, marrow fibrosis and increasing basophilia may occur.

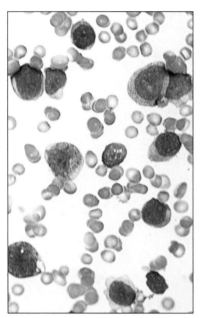

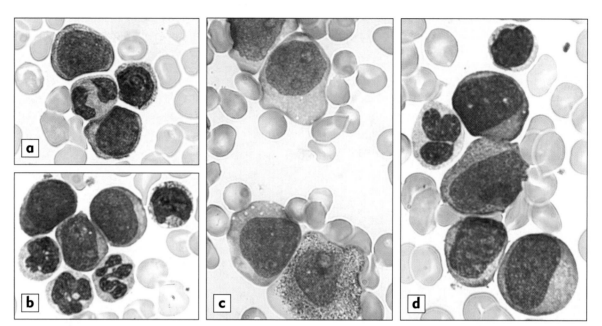

Fig. 9.14 Chronic myeloid leukaemia: peripheral blood film showing blast cell transformation. Over half the white cells seen are primitive blast forms. [Hb, 8.5 g/dl; WBC, 110 × 10⁹/l (blasts, 65 × 10⁹/l); platelets, 45 × 10⁹/l.]

Fig. 9.15a–d Chronic myeloid leukaemia: (a–d) peripheral blood films at high magnification showing myeloblastic transformation. Numerous myeloblasts, atypical neutrophils and abnormal promyelocytes are seen.

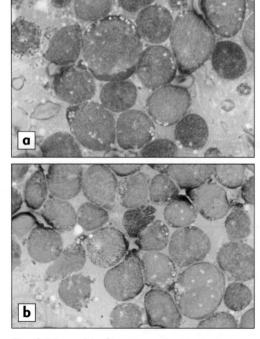

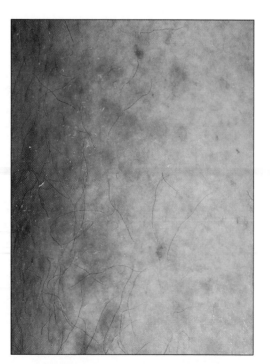

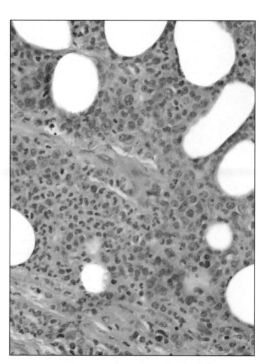

Fig. 9.16a and b Chronic myeloid leukaemia: (a, b) bone marrow aspirates showing lymphoblastic transformation. There are vacuolated lymphoblasts and residual basophil granulocytes or precursors. [(a) Courtesy of Dr K van Pouche and Prof. Z Berneman.]

Fig. 9.17 Chronic myeloid leukaemia: nodular leukaemic infiltrates in the skin over the anterior surface of the tibia in a 48-year-old woman with blast cell transformation

Fig. 9.18 Chronic myeloid leukaemia: histological section of the skin lesion shown in *Fig. 9.17*, illustrating extensive perivascular infiltration with mononuclear cells and polymorphs in the deeper layers of the dermis.

Philadelphia-negative chronic myeloid leukaemia
Some patients with typical disease are Ph⁻ but are found to have the BCR-ABL rearrangement on molecular analysis. Other patients with Ph⁻ and BCR-ABL rearrangement negative disease have a variant of CML that is usually associated with fewer myelocytes, more monocytoid cells and atypical neutrophils in the peripheral blood. Severe anaemia and thrombocytopenia are more frequent than in classic CML (*Fig. 9.21*).

The prognosis for Ph⁻ BCR-ABL⁻ is generally worse than that for Ph⁺ BCR-ABL⁺ or Ph⁻ BCR-ABL⁺ CML. A juvenile form of Ph⁻ CML occurs in children, often with marked lymphadenopathy and eczematoid rashes (*Fig. 9.22*). As with the adult Ph⁻ BCR-ABL⁻ form, morphological differences are found between this and classic CML (*Figs 9.23 and 9.24*).

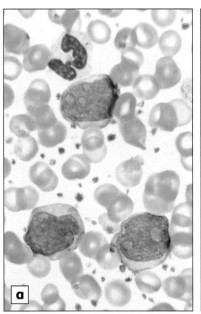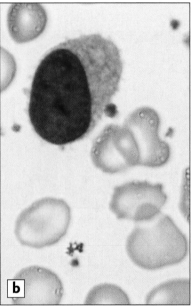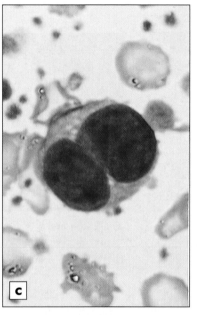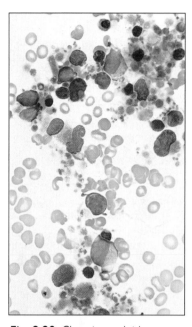

Fig. 9.19a–c Chronic myeloid leukaemia: megakaryoblastic transformation. (a–c) Peripheral blood films showing blast cells that stained positive for CD41. [(a) Courtesy of Dr RD Brunning and the US Armed Forces Institute of Pathology.]

Fig. 9.20 Chronic myeloid leukaemia: megakaryoblastic transformation. Bone marrow showing atypical megakaryocytes and megakaryoblasts. (Courtesy of Dr RD Brunning and the US Armed Forces Institute of Pathology.)

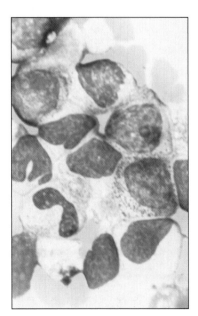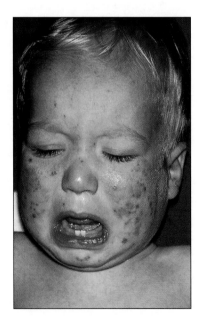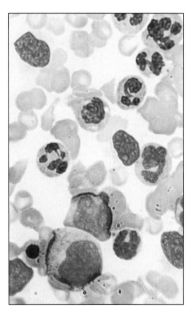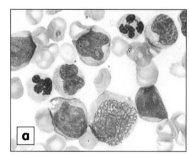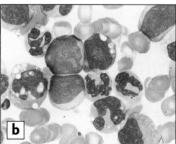

Fig. 9.21 Chronic myeloid leukaemia: Ph chromosome negative, BCR-ABL rearrangement negative. Bone marrow aspirate showing myelocytes, metamyelocytes and 'paramyeloid' cells, features of myelodysplasia.

Fig. 9.22 Juvenile CML: eczematoid facial rash and lip bleeding in an 8-month-old infant. There was moderate splenomegaly. Cytogenetic studies failed to demonstrate the presence of the Ph chromosome. (Hb, 10.5 g/dl; WBC, 120 × 10⁹/l; platelets, 85 × 10⁹/l; courtesy of Prof. JM Chessells.)

Fig. 9.23 Juvenile CML: peripheral blood film from the infant in *Fig. 9.22* shows a predominance of myelomonocytoid cells.

Fig. 9.24a and b Juvenile CML: (a, b) peripheral blood films at higher magnification showing occasional blast forms, myelomonocytic cells and atypical agranular band and segmented neutrophils.

MYELODYSPLASTIC SYNDROMES

The myelodysplastic syndromes usually occur in elderly subjects who present with an anaemia, persistent neutropenia and thrombocytopenia, or various combinations of these. Typically, the anaemia is macrocytic and there is no enlargement of the liver, spleen and lymph nodes.

Within this group of patients, some present with an absolute monocytosis of >1.0 × 10⁹/l, with or without splenomegaly. This is referred to as 'chronic myelomonocytic leukaemia' (CMML). Gum hypertrophy and skin deposits do not usually occur.

The myelodysplastic syndromes are classified into five subgroups (*Fig. 9.25*). (For a summary of blood and bone marrow findings in myelodysplastic syndromes, *see Fig. 9.41*.) Clinically, these patients have symptoms related to bone marrow failure with frequent infective episodes (*Figs 9.26 and 9.27*) and bleeding abnormalities (*Fig. 9.28*). As a consequence of these complications, many patients die of severe

French–American–British classification of the myelodysplastic syndromes
Refractory anaemia (RA)
RA with ring sideroblasts (RARS; ring sideroblasts >15%)
RA with excess blasts (RAEB; blasts 5–20%)
RAEB 'in transformation' (RAEB-T; blasts 20–30%)
Chronic myelomonocytic leukaemia (CMML)

Fig. 9.25 The myelodysplastic syndromes: the French–American–British classification. RARS is also known as primary acquired sideroblastic anaemia (see page 50).

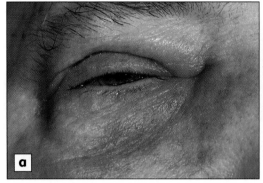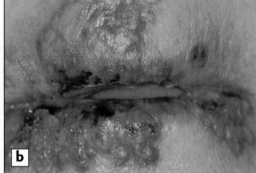

Fig. 9.26a and b Myelodysplastic syndrome: (a) skin infection spreading from the eyelids; (b) extensive herpes simplex eruptions spreading from the lip margins to adjacent skin. Both patients had refractory anaemia with excess blasts (RAEB).

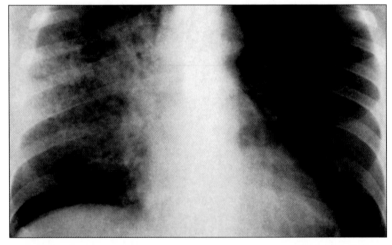

Fig. 9.27 Myelodysplastic syndrome: chest radiograph (portable film) of a 62-year-old man with legionnaires' disease. There is widespread patchy consolidation throughout the right lung.

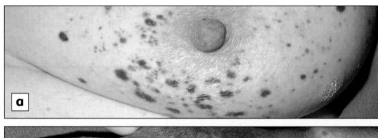

Fig. 9.28a and b Myelodysplastic syndrome: (a) extensive purpura of the skin of the breast in a 35-year-old woman with refractory anaemia (RA); (b) extensive ecchymoses and purpura of the skin over the back of the hand (same patient). (Hb, 8 g/dl; WBC, 4 × 10⁹/l; platelets, 20 × 10⁹/l.)

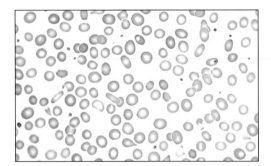

Fig. 9.29 Myelodysplastic syndrome: peripheral blood film in RA shows marked anisocytosis and poikilocytosis. [(Hb, 7.9 g/dl; WBC, 5.4 × 10⁹/l (neutrophils, 1.8 × 10⁹/l); platelets, 120 × 10⁹/l.]

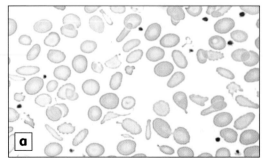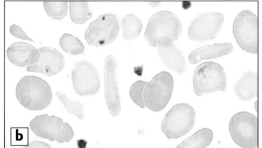

Fig. 9.30a and b Myelodysplastic syndrome: peripheral blood films in acquired sideroblastic anaemia (RARS) showing (a) marked red cell anisocytosis and poikilocytosis. Although the majority of cells are markedly hypochromic, there is a second population of normochromic cells. At higher magnification (b) a red cell shows two small basophilic inclusions (Pappenheimer bodies). Perls' staining demonstrated that similar inclusions were Prussian blue-positive (siderotic granules). These granules were far more numerous after splenectomy.

neutropenia or thrombocytopenia, but in others the disease progresses to frank acute myeloid leukaemia (AML). In the past these syndromes, particularly those with normal numbers of blasts (<5%) in the marrow, have been referred to as 'preleukaemia'.

The blood film abnormalities in each subgroup are highly variable. General features include macrocytic red cells, qualitative granulocytic and monocytic changes (see below), and giant platelets. In patients with RA gross morphological changes may not occur (*Fig. 9.29*). In RA with ring sideroblasts (RARS) a dimorphic red cell population frequently occurs (*Fig. 9.30*). Patients with RAEB often show leucoerythroblastic changes. The greatest number of blast cells is seen in RAEB 'in trans-

formation' (RAEB-T; *see Fig. 9.44*), and abnormal myelomonocytic cells and monocytosis (*Figs 9.31 and 9.32*) are characteristic of CMML. Thrombocytosis occurs typically in the 5q⁻ (an interstitial deletion, usually 5q11 or 5q13 to 5q33) syndrome variant of RA (*Fig. 9.33*).

The bone marrow in the myelodysplastic syndromes is typically hypercellular and shows morphological abnormalities, often in all three series of haemopoietic cells. There is usually evidence of dyserythropoiesis, with nuclear atypia, some megaloblastosis and ring sideroblasts (*Figs 9.34–9.39*). In about 20% of cases in all five subgroups an increase in reticulin occurs (*Fig. 9.40*), while in occasional cases the marrow is hypocellular.

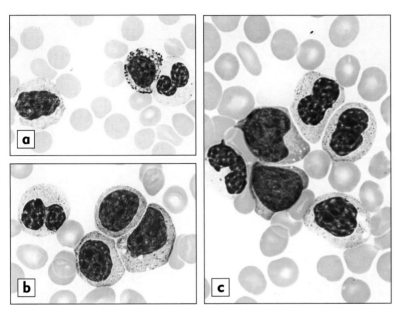

Fig. 9.31a–c Myelodysplastic syndrome: (a–c) peripheral blood films showing white cells in CMML. Many atypical myelomonocytic cells and pseudo-Pelger neutrophils, some agranular, are shown.

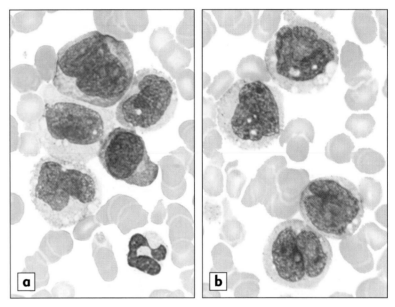

Fig. 9.32a and b Myelodysplastic syndrome: (a, b) peripheral blood films showing white cells in CMML. The majority of cells are more monocytoid than those in *Fig. 9.31* and the neutrophil shown is agranular.

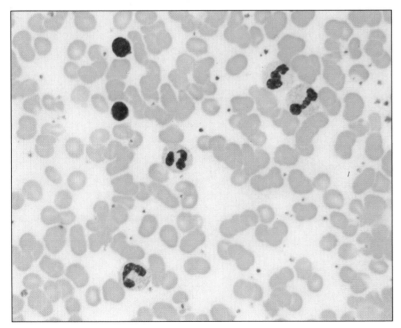

Fig. 9.33 Myelodysplastic syndrome: peripheral blood film from a 75-year-old woman with 5q⁻ syndrome showing macrocytes, hyposegmented neutrophils and thrombocytosis.

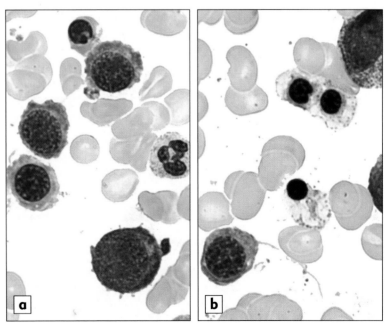

Fig. 9.34a and b Myelodysplastic syndrome: (a, b) bone marrow cell trails in RARS showing marked defective haemoglobinization and vacuolation in later-stage polychromatic and pyknotic erythroblasts.

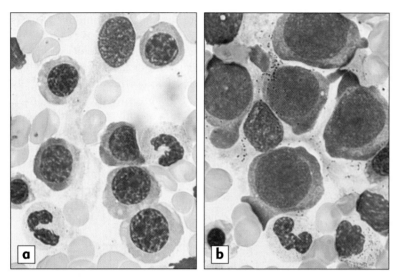

Fig. 9.35a and b Myelodysplastic syndrome: bone marrow cell trails in RARS showing (a) erythroblasts with vacuolation of cytoplasm in later cells and mild megaloblastic features; (b) a prominent group of proerythroblasts.

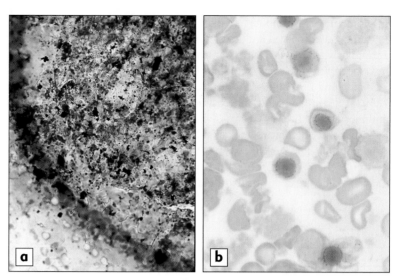

Fig. 9.36a and b Myelodysplastic syndrome: bone marrow fragment in RARS showing (a) increased iron stores and (b) pathological ring sideroblasts at higher magnification. (Perls' stain.)

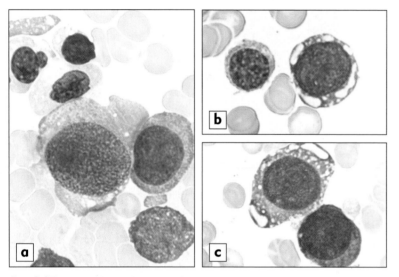

Fig. 9.37a–c Myelodysplastic syndrome: bone marrow aspirates in RAEB showing (a) abnormal proerythroblasts and megaloblast-like changes and (b, c) prominent cytoplasmic vacuolation in the basophilic erythroblasts, evidence of dyserythropoiesis.

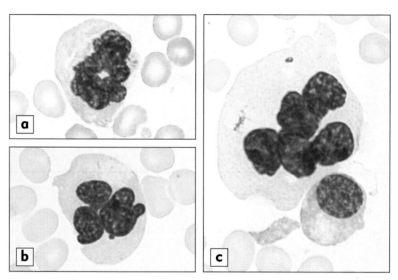

Fig. 9.38a–c Myelodysplastic syndrome: (a–c) bone marrow aspirates in RAEB showing three examples of polyploid multinucleate polychromatic erythroblasts, further evidence of gross dyserythropoiesis.

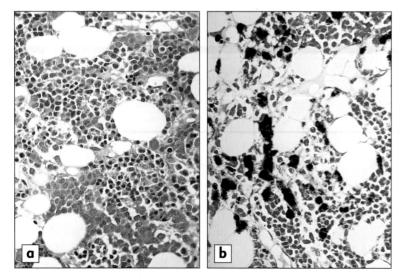

Fig. 9.39a and b Myelodysplastic syndrome: trephine biopsies in RAEB, showing (a) clusters of blast forms and prominent haemosiderin-laden macrophages. (b) The gross increase in reticuloendothelial iron stores is confirmed by Perls' staining.

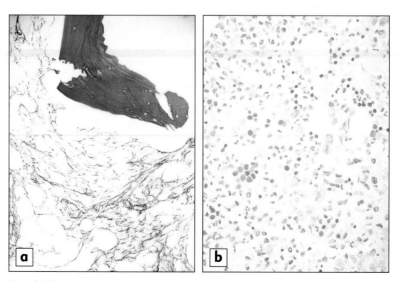

Fig. 9.40a and b Myelodysplastic syndrome: (a, b) trephine biopsy showing increased reticulin. (Silver impregnation stain.)

A summary of blood and bone marrow findings in myelodysplastic syndromes is given in *Fig. 9.41*.

Granulocytic abnormalities include hypogranular or agranular myelocytes, metamyelocytes and neutrophils, pseudo-Pelger cells and hypersegmented or polyploid neutrophils (*Fig. 9.42*).

Megakaryocytic abnormalities include small mononuclear or binucleate forms (*Fig. 9. 43*) or large megakaryocytes with multiple round nuclei and large granules in the cytoplasm.

In the more advanced myelodysplastic syndromes there is also an increase in the blast cell population but, by definition, these cells remain <30% of the marrow cell total (*Fig. 9.44*). When the level of blast cells exceeds this figure, it is assumed that an evolution to AML has occurred. Abnormal localization of immature precursors (ALIP) in the bone marrow in patients without excess blasts may be an independent prognostic factor (*Fig. 9.45*).

Blood and marrow findings in myelodysplastic syndromes					
Parameter	**RA**	**RARS**	**RAEB**	**RAEB-T**	**CMML**
Blood					
Haemoglobin	↓	↓	↓	↓	↓
Total WBC	N or ↓	N or ↓	↓	↓ or N or ↑	↑
Monocytes	N	N	N	↓ or N or ↑	↑
Blasts (%)	<1	<1	<5	>5	<5
Platelets	N or ↓	N or ↓	↓	↓	↓ or N or ↑
Marrow					
Sideroblasts (%)	<15	>15	<15	<15	<15
Myeloblasts (%)	<5	<5	5–20	20–30	0–20

Fig. 9.41 Myelodysplastic syndromes: blood and bone marrow findings.

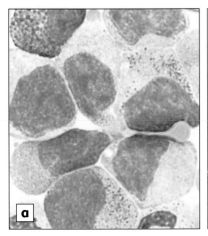
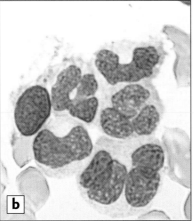
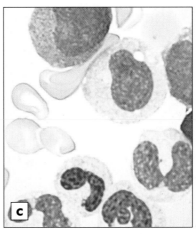

Fig. 9.42a–c Myelodysplastic syndrome: bone marrow aspirates in RAEB showing disturbed granulopoiesis with (a) agranular promyelocytes and (b, c) agranular neutrophils and abnormal myelomonocytic cells; some cells ('paramyeloid' cells) are difficult to classify as monocytic or granulocytic.

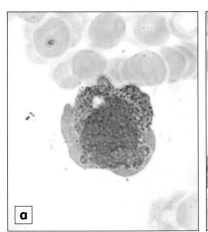
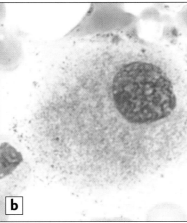
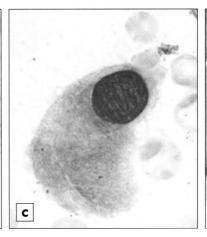
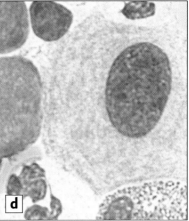

Fig. 9.43a–d Myelodysplastic syndrome: (a–d) bone marrow aspirates showing an atypical megakaryoblast and three atypical mononuclear megakaryocytes, all of which show evidence of cytoplasmic maturation and granulation.

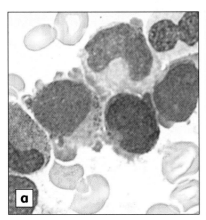
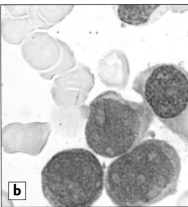
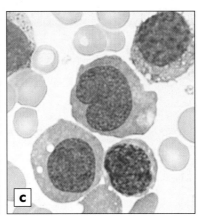

Fig. 9.44a–c Myelodysplastic syndrome: (a–c) bone marrow aspirates in RAEB-T showing increased numbers of blast cells, some of which have atypical features. The blast cells comprise 23% of the marrow cell total. Agranular neutrophils and myelomonocytic cells are also evident.

Cytogenetic abnormalities are common, occurring in 50% of primary and 90% of secondary myelodysplastic syndromes. They are more common in RAEB-T than in RA or RARS. Abnormalities include:

- chromosome deletion or loss [e.g. del 5q/monosomy 5 (*see Fig. 9.33*), del 7q/monosomy 7, del 11q, del 12p, del 13q, del 20q, monosomy 7 (*Fig. 9.46*), loss of Y];

- chromosome gain (e.g. trisomy 8, trisomy 11);
- chromosome rearrangement [e.g. t3q28 (3:3), t(1;7), 17p, iso 17q]; and
- complex karyotypes.

The management of these syndromes is unsatisfactory. Treatment is with supportive therapy alone or with mild chemotherapy (e.g. low-dose subcutaneous cytosine arabinoside). Trials of differentiating agents (e.g. retinoic acid) have shown occasional benefit. The haemopoietic growth factors G-CSF, GM-CSF, IL-3 and erythropoietin have been used in various trials and routine practice either alone or in combination with chemotherapy in an attempt to improve the blood count, but the number of patients who show clinically relevant responses and sustained responses is low. In younger patients intensive chemotherapy, as for AML, with or without stem cell transplantation, offers a possible cure.

Monosomy 7 syndrome of childhood

Monosomy 7 syndrome of childhood is a form of myelodysplasia that presents in children, usually boys, between the ages of 6 months and 8 years. Hepatosplenomegaly is normally marked. There is usually monocytosis and anaemia, as well as dysplastic changes in the marrow (*Fig. 9.46*). Transformation to AML is frequent.

MYELOKATHEXIS

A rare syndrome, myelokathexis may be related to myelodysplasia, but it occurs in young patients and is associated with chronic neutropenia and repeated infections. Marrow aspirates show many cells of the neutrophil series with hypersegmentation and longer than normal chromatin strands separating nuclear lobes (*Fig. 9.47*). Binucleate myelocytes, metamyelocytes and band forms are a feature. The mature neutrophils are functionally defective.

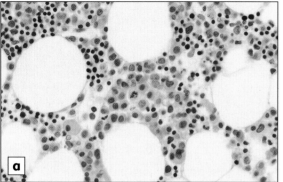
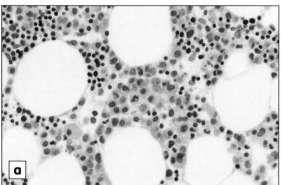

Fig. 9.45a and b Myelodysplastic syndrome: (a, b) trephine biopsy in CMML. Both views show abnormal intertrabecular localization of nests of immature myeloid cells (ALIPs).

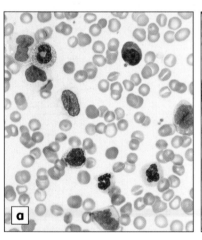
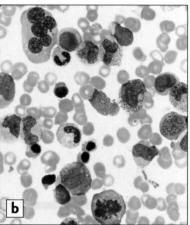
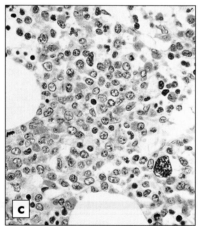

Fig. 9.46a–c Myelodysplastic syndrome, monosomy 7 of childhood: (a) peripheral blood film showing mature monocytes, neutrophils, occasional immature cells and a plasma cell. (b) Bone marrow aspirate showing increased numbers of monocytes and promonocytes and large multinucleated polychromatic erythroblasts (c) Trephine biopsy showing increased cellularity, a centrally placed ALIP and reduced megakaryocytes. [(a, b) Courtesy of Dr RD Brunning and the US Armed Forces Institute of Pathology.]

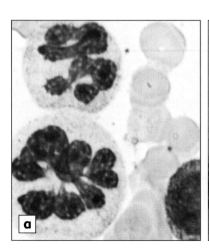
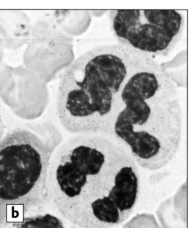
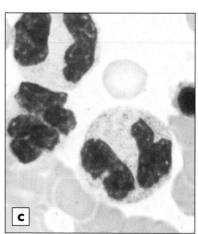

Fig. 9.47a–c Myelokathexis: (a–c) bone marrow aspirate showing large band and segmented neutrophils including hyperdiploid forms, with hypersegmentation and abnormal separation of nuclear lobes. Binucleate band forms are apparent.

10

Chronic Lymphoid Leukaemias

CHRONIC B-CELL LEUKAEMIAS

The chronic lymphoid leukaemias may be classified into B- and T-cell disorders (*Fig. 10.1*; see also the REAL and WHO classifications in Chapter 11).

CHRONIC LYMPHOCYTIC LEUKAEMIA

Chronic lymphocytic (lymphatic) leukaemia (CLL) is predominantly a disease of the elderly and is characterized by large numbers of lym-phocytes which accumulate in the blood, spleen, liver and lymph nodes. In the majority of cases, the cells are a monoclonal population of immature B lymphocytes with low-density surface immunoglobu-lin. Prolymphocytes (*see Fig. 10.30*) are also seen in variable propor-tions in the peripheral blood, the proportion increasing with more advanced disease in some cases.

Symmetrical enlargement of the superficial lymph nodes is found in most patients (*Figs 10.2 and 10.3*) and, rarely, there is also tonsil-lar involvement (*Fig. 10.4*). In advanced disease, there is both splenomegaly and hepatomegaly, and patients with thrombocytopenia

Classification of the chronic lymphoid leukaemias
B cell
B-Chronic lymphocytic leukaemia (CLL)
Common type CLL
B-CLL with >10%, but <55% prolymphocytes (CLL/PLL)
Richter's syndrome
B-Prolymphocytic leukaemia (B-PLL) with >55% prolymphocytes
Hairy cell leukaemia
Classic form
Variant form
Plasma cell leukaemia
Plasma cell and plasmablast
Leukaemia–lymphoma syndromes
Splenic lymphoma with villous lymphocytes
Waldenström's macroglobulinaemia (see Chapter 12)
Follicular lymphoma (see Chapter 11)
Mantle cell lymphoma (see Chapter 11)
Lymphoplasmacytic NHL (see Chapter 11)
Large cell (see Chapter 11)
T cell
Leukaemias
Large granular lymphocytic leukaemia
T-Prolymphocytic leukaemia
Leukaemia–lymphoma syndromes
Adult T-cell leukaemia–lymphoma (HTLV-1 positive)
Sézary syndrome
Peripheral T-cell lymphoma (HTLV-negative; see Chapter 11)

Fig. 10.1 Chronic lymphoid leukaemias: classification. (Modified from Bennett JM, Catovsky D, Daniel MT, *et al*. Proposals for the classification of chronic (mature) B and T lymphoid leukaemias. French–American–British (FAB) Cooperative Group. *J Clin Pathol*. 1989;42;567–84)

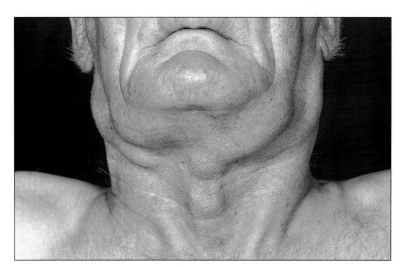

Fig. 10.2 Chronic lymphocytic leukaemia: bilateral cervical lymphadenopathy in a 65-year-old man. [Hb, 12.5 g/dl; WBC, 150 × 10⁹/l (lymphocytes, 140 × 10⁹/l); platelets, 120 × 10⁹/l.]

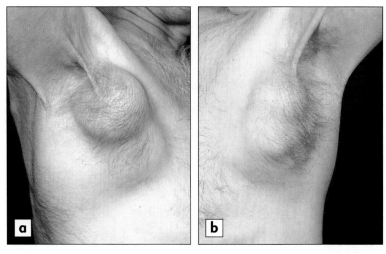

Fig. 10.3a and b Chronic lymphocytic leukaemia: (a, b) bilateral axillary lymphadenopathy (same patient as shown in *Fig. 10.2*).

may show bruising and extensive skin purpura (*Fig. 10.5*). Infections frequently result from immunoglobulin deficiency, neutropenia and lymphoid dysfunction. In many patients herpes zoster (*Figs 10.6 and 10.7*) or herpes simplex (*Fig. 10.8*) infections may be associated, and

oral candidiasis and other infections are also a frequent occurrence (*Fig. 10.9*).

The blood count in CLL reveals an absolute lymphocytosis (between 20×10^9 and 200×10^9/l is usual), and the peripheral blood has a

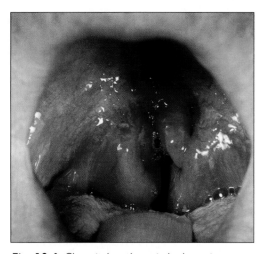

Fig. 10.4 Chronic lymphocytic leukaemia: massive enlargement of the pharyngeal tonsils (same patient as shown in *Fig. 10.2*).

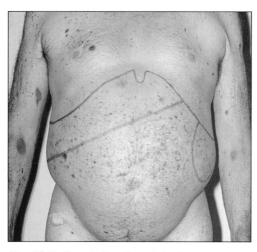

Fig. 10.5 Chronic lymphocytic leukaemia: purpuric haemorrhage and abdominal swelling in a 54-year-old man. The extent of liver and splenic enlargement is indicated. [Hb, 10.9 g/dl; WBC, 250×10^9/l (lymphocytes, 245×10^9/l); platelets, 35×10^9/l.]

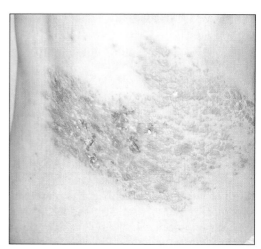

Fig. 10.6 Chronic lymphocytic leukaemia: herpes zoster infection in a 68-year-old woman.

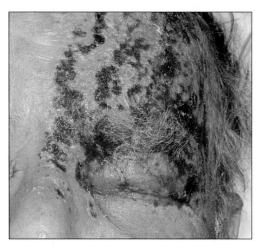

Fig. 10.7 Chronic lymphocytic leukaemia: herpes zoster infection in the territory of the ophthalmic division of the fifth cranial nerve.

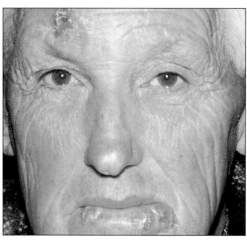

Fig. 10.8 Chronic lymphocytic leukaemia: herpes simplex eruptions of the lower lip and of the skin of the forehead.

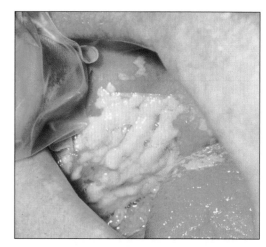

Fig. 10.9 Chronic lymphocytic leukaemia: extensive *Candida albicans* infection of the buccal mucosa of a 73-year-old woman.

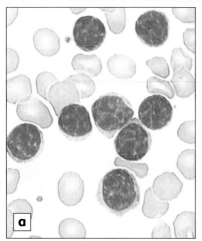 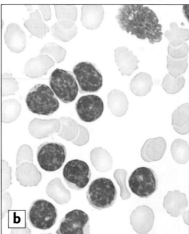 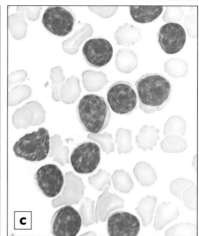 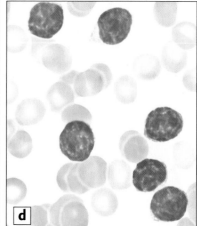

Fig. 10.10a–d Chronic lymphocytic leukaemia: (a–d) lymphocytes from the peripheral blood of four different patients show thin rims of cytoplasm, condensed coarse chromatin and only rare nucleoli.

characteristic lymphoid morphology (*Figs 10.10 and 10.11*). In advanced disease a normochromic anaemia and thrombocytopenia often occurs. About 10% of patients develop a secondary warm-type autoimmune haemolytic anaemia (*Fig. 10.12*) and in a smaller number of cases an autoimmune thrombocytopenia occurs. Approximately 20% of patients with CLL are asymptomatic and the diagnosis is made only when a routine blood test is performed. Rarely the lymphocytes show crystalline deposits of immunoglobulin (*Fig. 10.13*).

Bone marrow examination shows extensive replacement of normal marrow elements by lymphocytes, reaching 30–95% of the marrow cell total. Trephine biopsies (*Figs 10.14 and 10.15*) show nodular, interstitial or diffuse collections of abnormal cells. Patients with nodular or interstitial histology have a better prognosis. In patients with autoimmune haemolytic anaemia or thrombocytopenia the spleen is sometimes removed and shows a characteristic histology (*Fig. 10.16*).

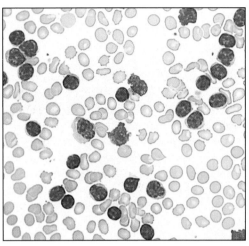

Fig. 10.11 Chronic lymphocytic leukaemia: peripheral blood film showing the increased numbers of lymphocytes and occasional characteristic 'smudge' cells. (Hb, 9.0 g/dl; WBC, 190 × 10⁹/l; platelets, 70 × 10⁹/l.)

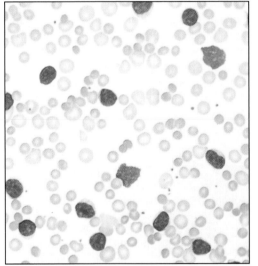

Fig. 10.12 Chronic lymphocytic leukaemia with autoimmune haemolytic anaemia: peripheral blood film shows increased numbers of lymphocytes, red cell spherocytosis and polychromasia. The direct antiglobulin test was strongly positive with IgG on the surface of the cells. [Hb, 8.3g/dl; reticulocytes, 150 × 10⁹/l; WBC, 110 × 10⁹/l (lymphocytes, 107 × 10⁹/l); platelets, 90 × 10⁹/l.]

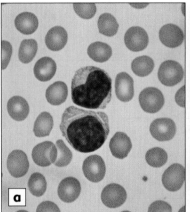
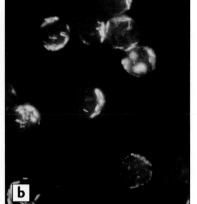

Fig. 10.13a and b Chronic lymphocytic leukaemia: the clonal B cells show crystalline deposits of immunoglobulin. (a) Jenner–Giemsa stain, (b) immunofluorescence. [(a, b) Courtesy of Prof. TJ Hamblin.]

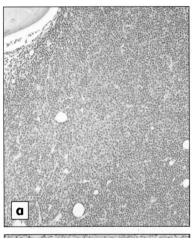
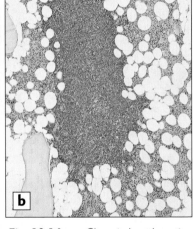
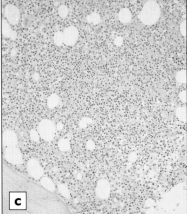

Fig. 10.14a–c Chronic lymphocytic leukaemia: trephine biopsies showing (a) a marked diffuse increase in marrow lymphocytes (closely packed cells with small dense nuclei); (b) a nodular pattern of lymphocyte accumulation (in a different patient); (c) interstitial infiltration.

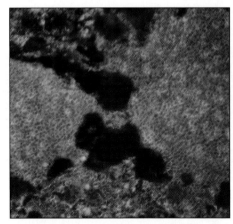

Fig. 10.15 Chronic lymphocytic leukaemia: trephine biopsy with two neoplastic lymphoid nodules containing predominantly B cells with positive reaction for IgM (green fluorescence). Numerous reactive T cells are identified by a monoclonal antibody to the CD3 antigen (red rhodamine staining). (Courtesy of Prof. G Pizzolo and Prof. Chilosi.)

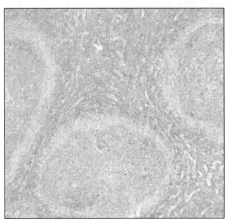

Fig. 10.16 Chronic lymphocytic leukaemia: histological section of spleen in a patient with secondary autoimmune haemolytic anaemia. There is expansion of lymphoid tissue in the periarterial sheaths of the white pulp and obvious red cell entrapment in the reticuloendothelial cords and splenic sinuses.

Cytogenetics

Frequent chromosomal changes in CLL are trisomy 12 (+12), deletions or translocations of the long arm of chromosome 13 at band q14, deletions of 6q21 or 27, deletions or translocations of 11q23 and, especially in patients in immunoblastic transformation, structural abnormalities of 17p (which involve the p53 gene). Mutations or deletions of the ataxia–telangiectasia (ATM) gene located at 11q22–23 are frequent, particularly in T-PLL. Some reports suggest that inherited mutations in the ATM gene may predispose to the development of CLL. Reciprocal translocations and interstitial deletions involving 13q14 are close to but usually separate from the retinoblastoma gene. Inv(14) (q11;q32) occurs in most cases of T-cell PLL, with reciprocal translocation [e.g. t(11,14)] in a minority. About 50% of the cases have trisomy 8. These abnormalities and (t1;14) (p13;q11) may occur in other T-cell diseases, as may other translocations that involve 14q11 and 14q32.

Apoptosis

In vivo, B-CLL cells have a long life, but they rapidly die in culture by apoptosis unless certain cytokines [e.g. interleukin-4 (IL-4) or γ- or α-interferon (IFN-γ or -α)] are added to the culture (*Figs 10.17–10.20*).

Membrane markers

The results of different membrane markers in chronic B-cell leukaemias are shown in *Fig. 10.21*. Characteristically, in CLL a score of 4 or 5 is obtained: weak expression of SmIg (score 1), negative staining for FMC7 (score 1) and CD79b (score 1), and positive staining for CD5 (score 1) and CD23 (score 1). B cell disorders other than CLL usually score 0–2.

VH gene status

The V heavy (VH) and V light (VL) chain genes undergo somatic hypermutations in the germinal centres. In CLL, the VH genes are mutated in approximately 50% of cases. Some reports suggest that non-mutated cases show more trisomy 12, p53 abnormalities, more expression of CD38, more atypical features and a poorer prognosis ("atypical CLL").

Staging and treatment

According to the extent of involvement of different lymphoid organs and the presence or absence of anaemia and thrombocytopenia from bone marrow failure, CLL may be divided into a number of clinical stages (*Fig. 10.22*).

Patients with early stages of CLL require no treatment. Those patients with advanced disease and increasing lymphadenopathy, systemic symptoms or marrow failure are usually treated with chlorambucil, and often with corticosteroids if there are autoimmune complications or bone marrow failure. Fludarabine is a useful purine analogue that is of value alone or in combination with cyclophosphamide or with mitozantrone and dexamethasone (FMD) in later stage disease. It is also being used for earlier stages. Local irradiation may be used in the treatment of massive lymphadenopathy, especially if this is compromising the function

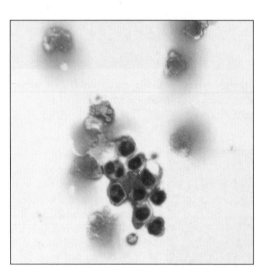

Fig. 10.17 Chronic lymphocytic leukaemia: death of cells *in vitro* by apoptosis after culture in medium and plasma. (Courtesy of Dr P Panayiotides.)

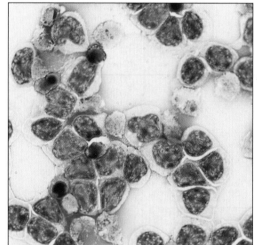

Fig. 10.18 Chronic lymphocytic leukaemia: death of some cells (small, darkly stained chromatin) by apoptosis after 30 hours culture in medium and plasma. (Courtesy of Dr P Panayiotides.)

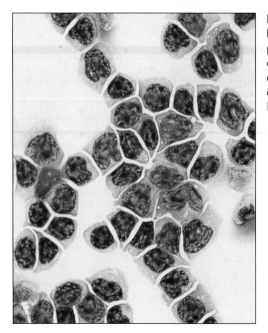

Fig. 10.19 Chronic lymphocytic leukaemia: prevention of apoptotic cell death by IL-4 addition to culture (10 days). (Courtesy of Dr P Panayiotides.)

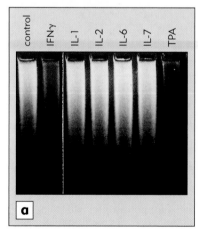
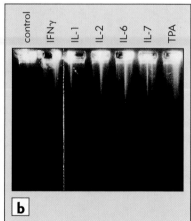

Fig. 10.20a and b Chronic lymphocytic leukaemia: (a) cells cultured at 37°C in medium and autologous plasma. DNA fragmentation shown (ladder pattern of 180 kb pieces) in control culture and in the presence of IL-1, IL-2, IL-6 and IL-7, but prevented by IFN-γ or TPA (phorbol ester). (b) As (a), but cells cultured at 4°C, at which temperature programmed cell death is inhibited. [(a, b) Courtesy of Dr P Panayiotides.]

of vital organs. In resistant cases, combination therapy [e.g. including with fludarabine (see above) or cyclophosphamide, doxorubicin, vincristine and prednisolone (CHOP)], is of benefit. Splenic irradiation or splenectomy is of value in selected patients.

Infections are often troublesome so active treatment with antibiotics or antiviral or antifungal agents may be needed. Concentrated immunoglobulin preparations, given intravenously, may be used in prophylaxis.

Chronic lymphocytic leukaemia: mixed cell types

Mixed cell cases include those showing a dimorphic population of small lymphocytes and prolymphocytes (>10% and <55%) (CLL/PLL) (*Figs 10.23 and 10.24*) and those showing a spectrum of small to large lymphocytes with <10% prolymphocytes. Some of the cases resemble typical CLL in clinical and laboratory features and in clinical course. Others show greater splenomegaly and markers more typical of PLL, are more refractory to therapy and follow a more aggressive

Membrane markers in chronic B-cell leukaemias								
	CLL	PLL	HCL	HCL-V	SLVL	FL	MZL	PCL
SIg	+/–	++	++	++	++	+	+	– (cyt Ig+)
CD5	+	–	–	–	–	–	+	–
CD19/CD20/37	+	+	+	+	+	+	+	–
FMC7/CD22	–/+	+	+	+	+	+	+	–
CD23	+	–/+	++	++	–/+	–/+	–/+	–
CD11c/25	–	–	++	+	+	?	?	–
CD25	–	–	++	–	–/+	–	–	–
CD38	–	–	–/+	–/+	–	–/+	–	++
CD103	–	–	+	+/–	–	–	–	–
HC2/CD103	–	–	+	–	–	–	–	–
HLA-DR	+	+	+	+	+	+	+	–
CD79b	–	++	–/+	?	++	++	++	?

SIg, surface immunoglobulin
CLL, B-cell chronic lymphocytic leukaemia
PLL, prolymphocytic leukaemia
HCL-V, hairy cell leukaemia variant
SLVL, splenic lymphoma with villous lymphocytes
FL, follicular lymphoma
MZL, mantle zone lymphoma
PCL, plasma cell leukaemia

Fig. 10.21 Membrane markers in chronic B-cell leukaemias.

Chronic lymphocytic leukaemia: clinical staging		
Rai classification of chronic lymphocytic leukaemia		
Stage 0	Lymphocytes >5 × 10⁹/1 and >40% of bone marrow cells	
Stage I	As Stage 0, with enlarged lymph nodes	
Stage II	As Stages 0 or I, with enlarged liver and/or spleen	
Stage III	As Stages 0, I or II, with Hb <10 g/dl	
Stage IV	As Stages 0, I, II or III, with platelets <100 × 10⁹/1	
Revised international classification of chronic lymphocytic leukaemia		
Group A (good prognosis)	Hb >10 g/dl	
	Platelets >100 × 10⁹/1	
	< three sites of palpable organ enlargement	
Group B (intermediate prognosis)	Hb >10 g/dl	
	platelets >100 × 10⁹/1	
	≥ three sites of palpable organ enlargement (one site = spleen or liver, or lymph nodes in the neck, axillae or groins)	
Group C (bad prognosis)	Hb <10 g/dl	
	platelets <100 × 10⁹/1	

Fig. 10.22 Chronic lymphocytic leukaemia: classifications of the clinical stages. (Rai classification, modified from Rai KR, Sawitsky A, Cronkite EP, *et al.* Clinical staging of chronic lymphocytic leukaemia. *Blood.* 1975;46:219–34.)

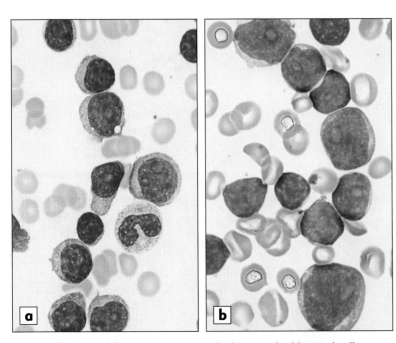

Fig. 10.23a and b Chronic lymphocytic leukaemia: (a, b) mixed cell type. The circulating lymphoid cells include >10%, but <55% prolymphocytes.

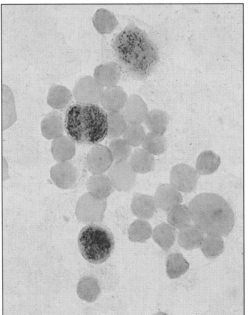

Fig. 10.24 Chronic lymphocytic leukaemia: mixed cell (CLL/PLL) type. Immunoperoxidase reaction using anti-Ki-1 (CD30) monoclonal antibody to detect proliferating cells. A positive reaction is seen in three cells. (Courtesy of Prof. D Catovsky.)

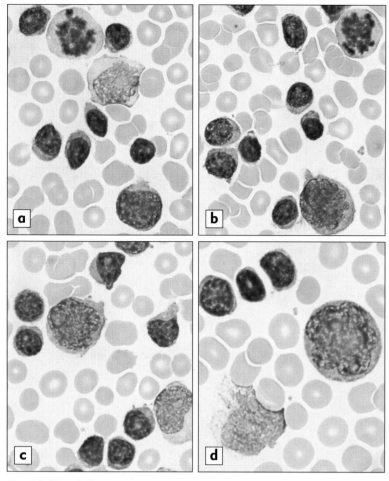

a b c d

Fig. 10.25a–d Chronic lymphocytic leukaemia: (a–d) Richter's syndrome (immunoblastic transformation). Peripheral blood films showing typical small lymphocytes, large blast cells and mitotic cells.

course than typical CLL. Some cases present with a mixed pattern that remains stable, but in others prolymphocytic transformation gradually progresses.

Richter's syndrome (immunoblastic transformation)

Some cases of CLL transform into a more aggressive stage, with the local formation of a mass of high-grade, large cell lymphoma (immunoblastic), which is often retroperitoneal, and sometimes with circulating immunoblastic cells if immunoblastic transformation is present in the marrow (*Figs 10.25–10.27*). Structural changes and mutations of p53, unusual in chronic-phase CLL, are frequent at this stage.

PROLYMPHOCYTIC LEUKAEMIA

Prolymphocytic leukaemia, a variant of CLL, usually occurs in the elderly and is associated with marked splenomegaly, absolute lymphocytosis (usually over $100 \times 10^9/l$) and minimal lymph node enlargement. Electron microscopy shows characteristic differences (*Figs 10.28 and 10.29*) and the blood film shows larger lymphocytes than are found in classic CLL (*Fig. 10.30*). In the majority of patients, surface marker studies indicate a B-cell origin of prolymphocytes, although the nature of the normal equivalent cell is unknown. Marker studies help to distinguish PLL from CLL by the stronger expression of surface Ig, FMC7 and cytoplasmic CD22, and weaker expression of CD5. In this mixed cell type more of the cells in the peripheral blood are proliferating (*see Fig. 10.24*). The prognosis is worse than in B-CLL. Treatment of PLL is unsatisfactory. It is usually resistant to chlorambucil or corticosteroids. Splenic irradiation, splenectomy, CHOP (see above) or fludarabine alone or in combination may be valuable in some cases.

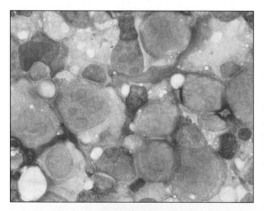

Fig. 10.26 Chronic lymphocyte leukaemia: Richter's syndrome. Imprint from enlarged lymph node showing large immunoblastic cells with multiple prominent nucleoli and a few residual small lymphocytes. (Courtesy of Prof. D Catovsky.)

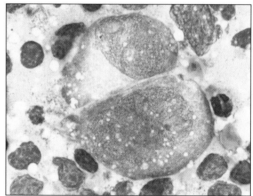

Fig. 10.27 Chronic lymphocytic leukaemia: Richter's syndrome. Imprint from lymph node showing two large immunoblasts surrounded by small lymphocytes.

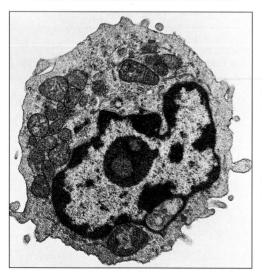

Fig. 10.28 B-cell prolymphocytic leukaemia: the B prolymphocyte is characterized by its relatively large size, moderately abundant cytoplasm, chromatin condensed in the periphery of the nucleus and a prominent nucleolus. (× 11,000; courtesy of Mrs D Robinson and Prof. D Catovsky.)

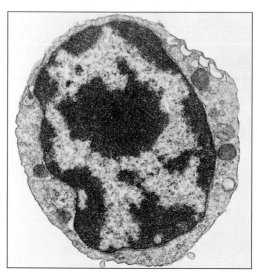

Fig. 10.29 B-cell chronic lymphocytic leukaemia: compared to *Fig. 10.28*, this cell is smaller, and has less cytoplasm [high nuclear/cytoplasmic (N/C) ratio)] and more marked nuclear chromatin with no visible nucleolus. (× 18,350; courtesy of Mrs D Robinson and Prof. D Catovsky.)

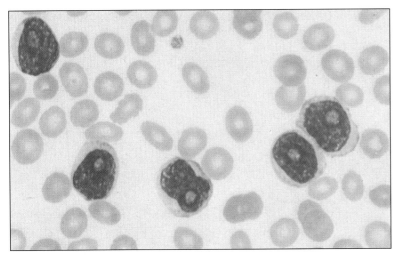

Fig. 10.30 B-cell prolymphocytic leukaemia: blood film showing prolymphocytes that have prominent central nucleoli and an abundance of pale cytoplasm. A high density of surface immunoglobulin confirmed their B-cell nature.

HAIRY CELL LEUKAEMIA

Patients with hairy cell leukaemia (HCL) usually present with pancytopenia and splenomegaly without lymphadenopathy. The characteristic cells, of B-lymphocyte origin, are seen in the peripheral blood (*Figs 10.31 and 10.32*) and may also be found in large numbers in marrow aspirates or from splenic imprints in patients who have undergone splenectomy (*Fig. 10.33*). Hairy cells also show characteristic cytochemical reactions (*Fig. 10.34*).

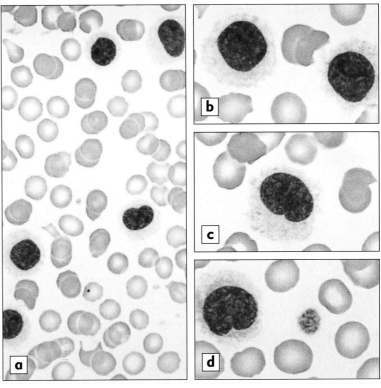

Fig. 10.31a–d Hairy cell leukaemia: peripheral blood films showing (a) typical 'hairy' cells, which have round or oval nuclei and a moderate amount of finely mottled, pale grey cytoplasm with irregular serrated ('hairy') edges; the chromatin is less dense than in typical small lymphocytes; (b–d) at higher magnification the nucleoli are clearly visible. [Hb, 9.4 g/dl: WBC, 25 × 10⁹/l (hairy cells, 23.5 × 10⁹/l); platelets, 90 × 10⁹/l.)

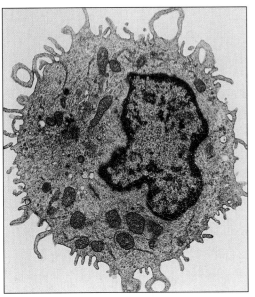

Fig. 10.32 Hairy cell leukaemia: hairy cell from the peripheral blood. Typical features are the abundant cytoplasm, low N/C ratio and cytoplasmic projections or villi that give the cell a 'hairy' appearance. (× 9200; courtesy of Mrs D Robinson and Prof. D Catovsky.)

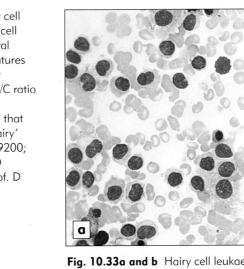

Fig. 10.33a and b Hairy cell leukaemia: (a) bone marrow aspirate showing a predominance of hairy cells in the cell trail; (b) splenic imprints showing typical nuclear and cytoplasmic features of the abnormal hairy cells.

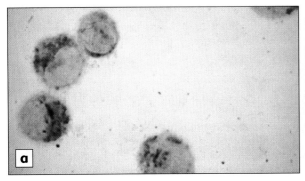

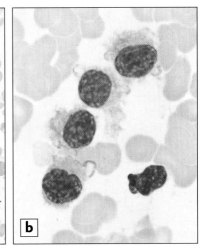

Fig. 10.34a and b Hairy cell leukaemia: typical cytochemical findings of hairy cells include (a) a strongly positive reaction to tartaric acid-resistant acid phosphatase (TRAP) and (b) a fine granular positivity with crescentic accumulation at one side of the nucleus following alpha-naphthyl butyrate esterase staining.

In many patients the marrow is difficult to aspirate and trephine biopsy is necessary for diagnosis. In these cases, diffuse infiltration by hairy cells (*Fig. 10.35*) and a dense reticulin fibre pattern (*Fig. 10.36*) are seen.

Histological sections of the spleen (*Figs 10.37 and 10.38*) and liver (*Figs 10.39 and 10.40*) may demonstrate unusual vascular 'lakes' caused by hairy cell infiltration of these organs.

Patients with HCL often respond well to splenectomy. In almost all cases, α-IFN, the adenosine deaminase inhibitor 2′-deoxycoformycin and 2-chlorodeoxyadenosine (2-CDA) produce substantial and prolonged improvement, and 2-CDA is now the usual drug of choice.

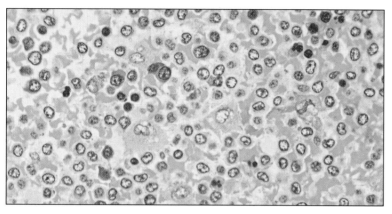

Fig. 10.35 Hairy cell leukaemia: bone marrow trephine biopsy showing extensive replacement of normal haemopoietic tissue by discrete mononuclear hairy cells. The nuclei are typically surrounded by a clear zone of cytoplasm. (Methacrylate section.)

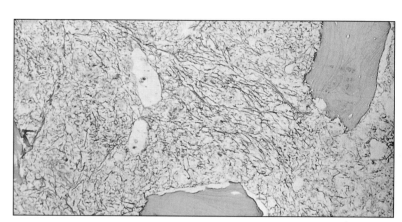

Fig. 10.36 Hairy cell leukaemia: bone marrow trephine biopsy showing increased fibre density and thickness in the reticulin fibre pattern. Silver impregnation technique.

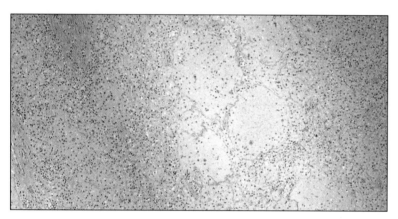

Fig. 10.37 Hairy cell leukaemia: histological section of spleen showing hairy cell infiltration of reticuloendothelial cords and sinuses. Numerous blood 'lakes' are seen in the centre of the field.

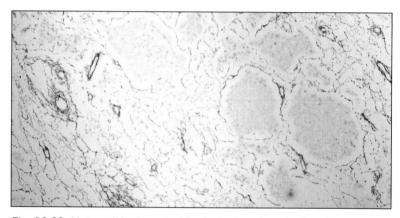

Fig. 10.38 Hairy cell leukaemia: histological section of spleen (same case as shown in *Fig. 10.37*) showing more clearly the reticulin fibre pattern outlining the abnormal venous 'lakes'. The presence of these structures may explain the extensive splenic red cell pooling that occurs in this disease. (Silver impregnation technique.)

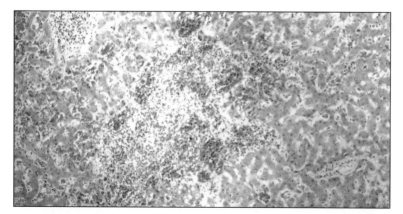

Fig. 10.39 Hairy cell leukaemia: histological section of liver shows hairy cell infiltration of sinusoids and portal tracts. There is sinusoidal ectasia and pseudoangiomatous transformation of hepatic blood vessels.

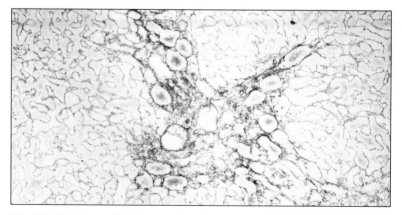

Fig. 10.40 Hairy cell leukaemia: histological section of liver (same case as shown in *Fig. 10.39*) showing the reticulin fibre pattern clearly, confirming the gross distortion of hepatic vascular architecture. It is thought that attachment of large numbers of hairy cells to the sinusoidal lining cells causes cell damage that results in these characteristic vascular abnormalities in the liver and spleen. (Silver impregnation technique.)

Hairy cell leukaemia variant

The rare cases of HCL variant usually present with a white cell count >40 × 10⁹/l and splenomegaly. The cells show a prominent nucleolus (*Fig. 10.41*) and are usually CD25 and TRAP (*Fig. 10.34*) negative. The response to treatment with IFN or 2-CDA is not as good as that for typical HCL.

PLASMA CELL LEUKAEMIA

Plasma cell leukaemia may occur as a primary disease or during the course of multiple myeloma (*see* page 238). There are >2 × 10⁹/l plasma cells in the peripheral blood and in some cases >100 × 10⁹/l. Usually features of myeloma are present – bone lesions, serum paraprotein and/or Bence–Jones proteinuria, often with hypercalcaemia and renal failure. The circulating cells may have the features of:

- lymphoplasmacytic cells;
- typical plasma cells (*Fig. 10.42a*); or
- plasmablasts (*Fig. 10.42b*).

Immunophenotyping shows that the cells are positive for the plasma cell marker CD38, are surface Ig⁻ but cytoplasmic Ig⁺; CD19, CD20, CD25 and HLA-DR are negative but in some cases CD10 is positive.

LEUKAEMIA–LYMPHOMA SYNDROMES

Splenic lymphoma with villous lymphocytes

Splenic lymphoma with villous lymphocytes is a primary splenic disease that occurs mainly in the elderly. The spleen may be massively enlarged but lymphadenopathy is rare. The peripheral blood shows a moderate lymphocytosis (usually up to 25 × 10⁹/l), the cells having an irregular plasma membrane with villi often confined to one pole of the cell (*Fig. 10.43a*). A monoclonal serum protein occurs in two-thirds of the cases. Cytogenic abnormalities include trisomy 3 in about 20% of cases and structural abnormalities that affect chromosome 7q in 20–30% of cases. In contrast to HCL, the bone marrow is usually easy to aspirate and typically shows an infiltrate of cells similar to those in the blood, but

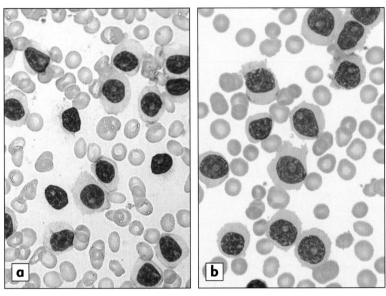

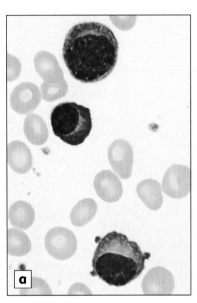 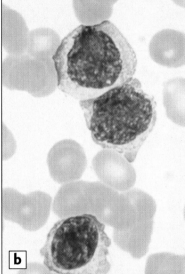

Fig. 10.41a and b Hairy cell leukaemia variant: (a, b) peripheral blood films showing cells with a prominent nucleolus, abundant pale cytoplasm and an irregular cytoplasmic border. (Courtesy of Prof. D Catovsky.)

Fig. 10.42a and b Plasma cell leukaemia: peripheral blood films showing (a) typical plasma cells; (b) plasmablasts.

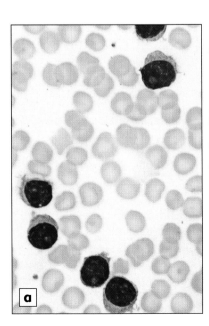 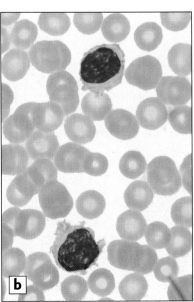 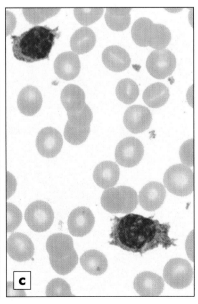

Fig. 10.43a–c Splenic lymphoma with villous lymphocytes: (a–c) peripheral blood films showing characteristic cells with irregular plasma membranes with short and thin villi often concentrated at one or two poles of the cells; the cells are larger than in typical CLL, the nucleus is round or ovoid and sometimes eccentric with a clumped chromatin pattern. [(a) Courtesy of Prof. D Catovsky; (b, c) courtesy of Prof. M Peetermans.]

it may reveal a nodular pattern (*Fig. 10.44*). Marker studies show strong expression of SIg, and positivity for B-cell antigens (CD19, CD20, CD22), as well as HLA-DR and FMC7. In some cases CD38 is positive, suggesting plasma cell differentiation. The spleen usually shows evidence of predominant white pulp involvement (*Figs 10.44 and 10.45*). Treatment, if needed, is by splenectomy, splenic irradiation or chlorambucil.

Lymphoplasmacytic lymphoma

Cases of lymphoplasmacytic lymphoma show monoclonal protein(s) in serum and circulating cells comprising small and large lymphocytes, including cells with eccentric nuclei and marked cytoplasmic basophilia (*Fig. 10.46*). The underlying condition may be Waldenström's macroglobulinaemia (*see* Chapter 12) or a low-grade lymphoma (*see* Chapter 11).

Follicular lymphoma in leukaemic phase

Many cases of follicular lymphoma show circulating follicular centre cells, ranging from 5×10^9 to 20×10^9/l (*Fig. 10.47*). The cells are small, they lack cytoplasm, the nuclear chromatin is featureless with no nucleoli and the nucleus of many cells is indented or clefted. In some cases, the lymphocyte count is higher and there may blast cells (centroblasts) present (*Fig. 10.48*).

Mantle cell lymphoma

In mantle cell lymphoma, in the leukaemic phase the circulating cells are medium-sized with nuclear indentations or clefts (*Fig. 10.49*). Nucleoli, if present, are ill-defined. The cells may resemble CLL of mixed cell type with few small cells. Nucleoli are inconspicuous. The cells are characteristically CD5$^+$, CD22$^-$ and show the chromosome abnormality t(11;14) (q13;q32) (*see* page 210).

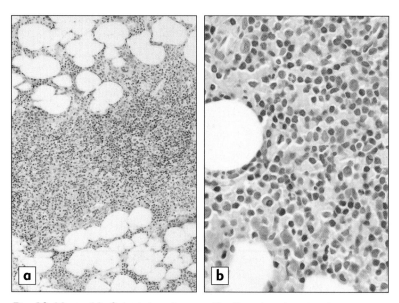

Fig. 10.44a and b Splenic lymphoma with villous lymphocytes: bone marrow trephine biopsies showing (a) nodular infiltrate; (b) diffuse interstitial infiltration by lymphocytes with lymphoplasmacytic forms. (Courtesy of Prof. KA MacLellan.)

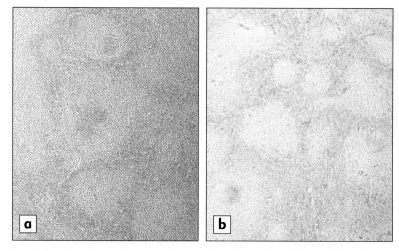

Fig. 10.45a and b Splenic lymphoma with villous lymphocytes: (a) splenic pulp showing predominant involvement of the white pulp areas by a uniform population of lymphoplasmacytic cells with clumped nuclear chromatin and a population of nucleolated cells, arranged in nodules with 'margination' (larger tumour cells at the periphery and smaller, germinal centre cells at the centre); (b) reticulin stain reveals the nodular distribution of the infiltrate. (Courtesy of Dr S Hamilton-Dutoit.)

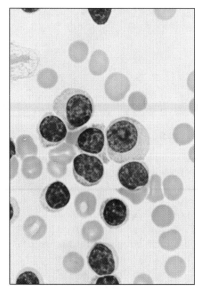

Fig. 10.46 Lymphoplasmacytic lymphoma in leukaemic phase: peripheral blood film.

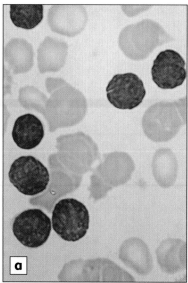

Fig. 10.47a and b Follicular lymphoma in leukaemic phase: (a, b) peripheral blood films showing small cells with scanty or absent cytoplasm, and deeply clefted nuclei with uniformly condensed chromatin.

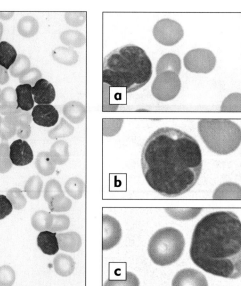

Fig 10.48a–c Non-Hodgkin lymphoma: (a–c) peripheral blood films showing abnormal large 'blast' forms or 'lymphosarcoma' cells in a patient with widely disseminated and terminal centroblastic lymphoma.

Large cell lymphoma

A leukaemic phase may occur in both B- and T-lineage large cell lymphomas and it is not possible to distinguish them by morphological criteria. The cells are large and pleomorphic, the cytoplasm is moderately or strongly basophilic and nucleoli may be inconspicuous or prominent (*Fig. 10.50*). The cells may show vacuolation, but appearance varies considerably from case to case, and immunological markers are needed to distinguish the cells from those of acute myeloid leukaemia. In some cases, large cell lymphoma supervenes on preceding low-grade small cell lymphoproliferative disease, and may also show circulating small cells.

LARGE GRANULAR LYMPHOCYTIC LEUKAEMIA (CHRONIC T-CELL LYMPHOCYTOSIS)

In large granular lymphocytic leukaemia (chronic T-cell lymphocytosis, T-CLL), patients usually have chronic neutropenia and anaemia and T-lymphocytosis, which persists for more than 3 months. Some patients show seropositive rheumatoid arthritis and splenomegaly. The T-cell receptor gene rearrangement analysis determines whether the cells are clonal, but the disease often runs a benign course. The cells may be large and have abundant cytoplasm and show multiple fine or coarse azurophil granules (*Figs 10.51 and 10.52*). Some of the cells are positive for tartrate resistant acid phosphatase. In the majority of cases the cells are positive for T-cell markers CD3$^+$ and CD8$^+$, but are usually CD4$^-$. Approximately 15% of cases have an immunophenotype of natural killer cells (CD3$^-$, CD56$^+$; *Fig. 10.53*).

T-CELL PROLYMPHOCYTIC LEUKAEMIA

T-Cell prolymphocytic leukaemia usually presents like B-cell PLL (B-PLL) with a high white cell count (>100 × 10^9/l), but is often associated with widespread lymphadenopathy, splenomegaly, serous effusions and skin lesions, and runs an aggressive course. The cells resemble those of B-PLL but may have a more irregular outline, a higher N/C ratio and an inconspicuous nucleolus. Two-thirds of the

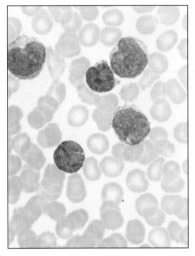

Fig. 10.49 Mantle zone lymphoma: peripheral blood film showing medium-sized cells with nuclear indentations and clefts. (Courtesy of Prof. D Catovsky.)

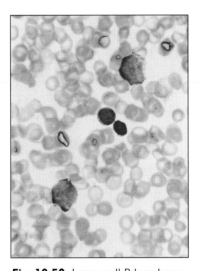

Fig. 10.50 Large cell B lymphoma in leukaemic phase: peripheral blood film showing large cells with irregular outline, nucleoli and scanty cytoplasm.

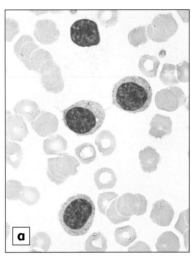
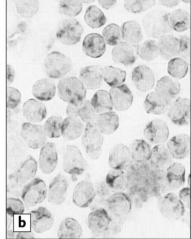

Fig. 10.51a and b Large granular lymphocytic leukaemia: peripheral blood films showing (a) abnormal lymphocytes and (b) characteristic 'clump' positivity in the Golgi zone using acid phosphatase staining.

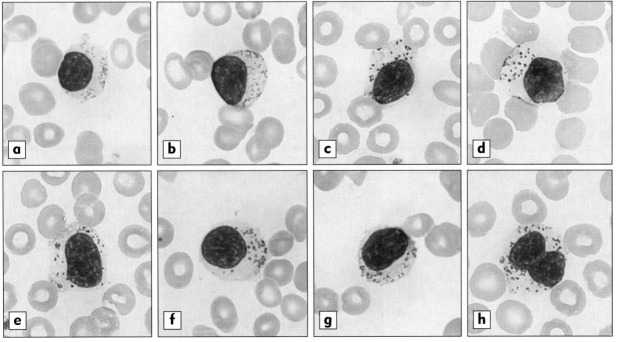

Fig. 10.52a–h Large granular lymphocytic leukaemia: (a–h) peripheral blood films showing representative large lymphocytes with multiple coarse, azurophilic, cytoplasmic granules. Immunological marker studies showed the cells to be CD8$^+$, CD3$^+$, CD16$^+$ and CD57$^+$. The patient had splenomegaly, chronic neutropenia and lymphocytosis. (Absolute lymphocyte count, 9.4 × 10^9/l.)

Membrane markers in the chronic T-cell leukaemias				
	LGLL*	T-PLL	ATLL	Sézary syndrome
CD2	+	+	+	+
CD3	+	+/–	+	+
CD5	–	+	+	+
CD7	–/+	++	–	–
CD4	–	+	+	+
CD8	+	+/–	–	–
CD25	–	–/+	++	–
CD56/57	+	–	–	–

LGLL, large granular lymphocyte leukaemia
T-PLL, T-cell prolymphocytic leukaemia
ATLL, adult T-cell leukaemia–lymphoma
*Approximately 15% of LGLL have an NK phenotype (CD3⁻, CD56⁺)

Fig. 10.53 Membrane markers in chronic T-cell leukaemias: these marker patterns are usual, but variant patterns also occur.

cases show inv(14) with similar breakpoints in 14q11 and 14q32. ATM mutations are frequent (*see* page 180). Most are CD4⁺, CD8⁻ (*Figs 10.54 and 10.55*).

ADULT T-CELL LEUKAEMIA–LYMPHOMA

Adult T-cell leukaemia–lymphoma is an unusual lymphoproliferative malignancy that occurs predominantly in Japan and in blacks of the West Indies and other Caribbean countries, and of the USA (*Figs 10.56 and 10.57*). Typically, the lymphoma evolves rapidly with early involvement of the lymph nodes, skin (*Fig. 10.56*), blood (*Fig. 10.57*) and bone marrow. The cells are CD4⁺, CD3⁺, TdT⁻.

The white cell count varies widely with between 10–80% of tumour cells. The neoplastic lymphoid cells vary in size and have an irregular nucleus, often with marked convolutions (*Figs 10.58 and 10.59*). Associated hypercalcaemia may lead to death in coma. The disease is caused by a C-type RNA retrovirus now designated as human T-cell lymphoma–leukaemia virus I (HTLV-I). The life cycle of a typical retrovirus is illustrated in *Fig. 10.60*. Invasion of the host cell causes cell proliferation, but there is no consistent integration site and no identified oncogene activation.

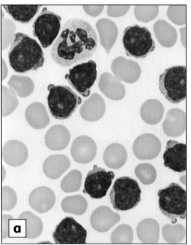
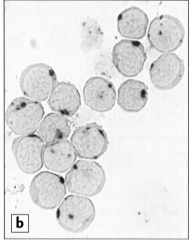

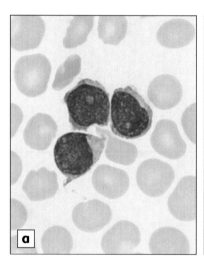
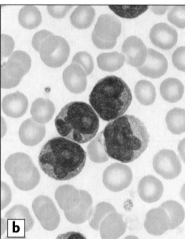

Fig. 10.54a and b Prolymphocytic leukaemia (T-cell type): blood films showing (a) prolymphocytes each with a prominent central nucleolus and a single neutrophil. Cell marker studies showed positive reactions with anti-T-cell antisera (CD2⁺, CD3⁺, CD4⁺, CD5⁺, CD7⁺, CD8⁻, CD25⁺) and an absence of surface immunoglobulin; (b) 'clump' positivity of these cells using acid phosphatase staining. (Hb, 10.5 g/dl; WBC, 240 × 10⁹/l; platelets, 60 × 109/l; courtesy of Prof. D Catovsky.)

Fig. 10.55a and b T-cell prolymphocytic leukaemia: (a, b) small cell type with scant cytoplasm and irregular nuclear outline.

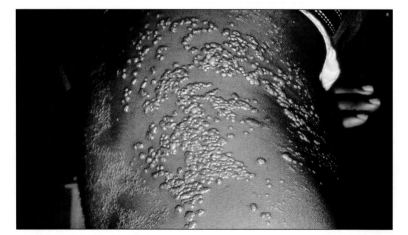

Fig. 10.56 Adult T-cell lymphoma–leukaemia syndrome: extensive involvement of the skin. (Courtesy of Dr JW Clark.)

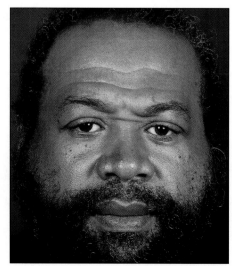

Fig. 10.57 Adult T-cell leukaemia–lymphoma in a 42-year-old male patient. He was diagnosed in Jamaica 5 years earlier to have paraplegia because of spinal disease. He presented with firm swelling of the salivary glands, but no superficial lymphadenopathy. (Hb, 12.3 g/dl; WBC, 28 × 10⁹/l; platelets, 134 × 10⁹/l; serum positive for anti-HTLV-I; serum calcium normal; no skin rash.)

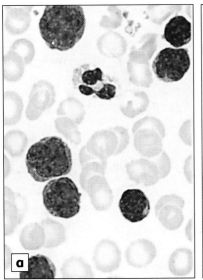
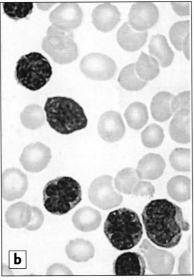
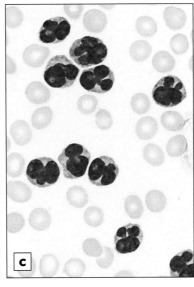

Fig. 10.58a–c Adult T-cell lymphoma–leukaemia syndrome: (a–c) peripheral blood films showing the characteristic abnormal lymphocytes with convoluted nuclei.

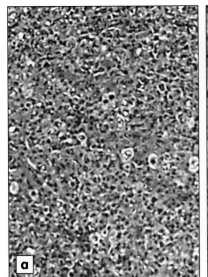
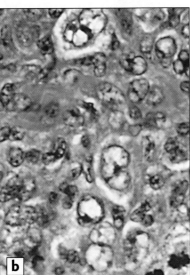
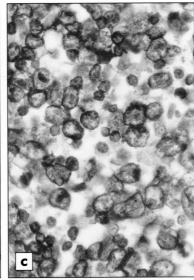

Fig. 10.59a–c Adult T-cell lymphoma–leukaemia syndrome: histological sections of lymph node showing (a) replacement of normal architecture by pleomorphic lymphoid cells; (b) occasional bizarre polylobulated giant cells and prominent mitotic figures at high magnification; (c) paraffin-stained (immunophosphatase) section for CD3. (Courtesy of Prof. DY Mason.)

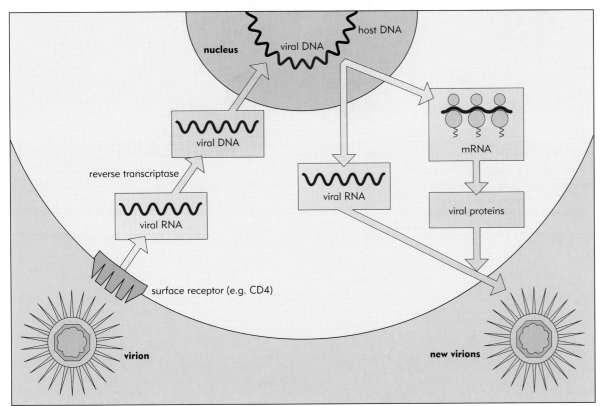

Fig. 10.60 Replication of retrovirus within a host cell.

SÉZARY SYNDROME

Sézary syndrome is closely related to mycosis fungoides (see page 000). It is characterized by a generalized exfoliative dermatitis. The epidermis is invaded by mononuclear T cells. The circulating abnormal Sézary cells show a grooved nuclear chromatin and are divided into large and small cell types (*Figs 10.61–10.64*). The larger cells are similar in size to neutrophils or monocytes and may have a tetraploid chromosome content. The nucleus is oval, round or reniform, with a cerebriform pattern on electron microscopy. In the more common small (Lutzner) cell type (*Fig. 10.63*), the cell is of a similar size to small lymphocytes, shows a similar grooved nuclear pattern with scant cytoplasm, sometimes with perinuclear cytoplasmic vacuoles, and stains positive with the periodic acid–Schiff (PAS) stain (*Fig. 10.64*). The Sézary cell is usually, but not necessarily, CD4$^+$, CD8$^-$.

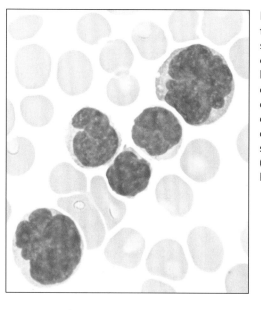

Fig. 10.61 Mycosis fungoides – Sézary syndrome: abnormal cells in the peripheral blood have characteristic, cerebriform, large and clefted nuclei with fine chromatin pattern and scanty cytoplasm. (Courtesy of Prof. D Catovsky.)

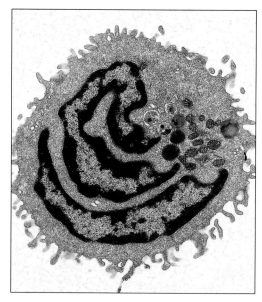

Fig. 10.62 Mycosis fungoides – Sézary syndrome: electronmicrograph of an abnormal T lymphocyte from the peripheral blood shows a deeply clefted nucleus. (× 8,000; courtesy of Dr E Matutes and Prof. D Catovsky.)

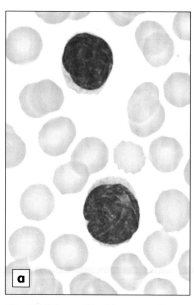
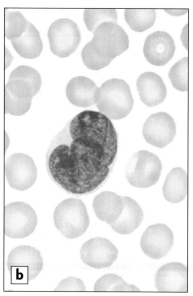

Fig. 10.63a and b Sézary syndrome: (a) small cell type (Lutzner cell) – the cells show grooved nuclear chromatin with a high N/C ratio; (b) large cell type with grooved nuclear pattern densely clumped chromatin and lower N/C ratio. (Courtesy of Prof. D Catovsky.)

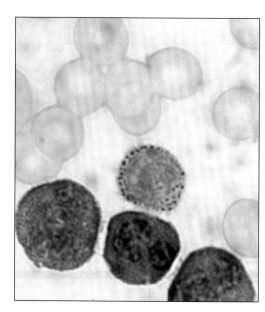

Fig. 10.64 Sézary syndrome: PAS-positive granules surrounding nucleus in a lymphocyte with convoluted nucleus. (Courtesy of Dr PM Canfield.)

Malignant Lymphomas
Written with KC Gatter, KA MacLennan and DY Mason

NON-HODGKIN LYMPHOMAS

Introduction

The term 'malignant lymphoma' embraces all neoplastic diseases that originate in the lymph nodes or extranodal lymphatic tissues. They comprise Hodgkin lymphoma (discussed later), which is relatively uniform in histology, and a large and heterogeneous category known as the non-Hodgkin lymphomas. The latter vary from highly proliferative and rapidly fatal disorders to indolent (although often incurable) malignancies which may be very well tolerated for 10–20 years or more.

It has been known for many years that non-Hodgkin lymphomas represent monoclonal expansions of B, T or natural killer (NK) cells. Evidence for this comes both from the expression of a single type of Ig on the cell surface and/or within the cytoplasm, and also from studies of Ig or T-cell receptor gene rearrangement. It is possible to find a 'normal counterpart' for many types of non-Hodgkin lymphoma, and the number of these diseases (more than 40 distinct entities) reflects the rich diversity of maturation stages and subpopulations of reactive human lymphoid cells. Recently, evidence has accumulated, based on analysis of microdissected single cells, that the Reed–Sternberg cells characteristic of Hodgkin lymphoma are also clonal in origin, deriving from B cells.

In the past, following the terminology of Rappaport from the 1960s, many large cell non-Hodgkin lymphomas were referred to as 'histiocytic', but it is now evident that the vast majority of neoplasms arising from the monocyte–phagocyte system present as leukaemias, and that true 'histiocytic lymphomas' are exceedingly rare. The latter are summarized at the end of the section on non-Hodgkin lymphoma.

Sometimes the difference between lymphomas and lymphoid leukaemias (acute and chronic) is unclear. Since lymphomas can be leukaemic, and leukaemias can be lymphomatous (e.g. they can present as solid tumour deposits), the obvious question is why there appear to be two categories of disease. The answer is that an artificial distinction has arisen from the traditions of medical practice: the diseases known as lymphomas are diagnosed by histopathologists and treated by oncologists or haematologists; whereas neoplasms that present as leukaemias are diagnosed and treated by haematologists. Apart from causing confusion for the beginner, this arbitrary distinction can result in a single lymphoproliferative disease entity being categorized as two diseases. Little evidence, for example, shows that small lymphocytic lymphoma differs from chronic lymphocytic leukaemia, or that lymphoblastic neoplasms that arise from precursor B cells should be subdivided into leukaemias and lymphomas, but such distinctions are often made, and patient management may suffer.

Geographic variation, viruses, chromosomes and oncogenes

Given the role of the immune system in responding to stimuli in the environment, it is not surprising that the frequencies of some types of non-Hodgkin lymphoma vary markedly between different parts of the world. For example, two lymphoma categories that are common in Western countries, Hodgkin lymphoma and follicular lymphoma, are much rarer in Eastern and less developed countries, whereas large B cell lymphomas and T cell neoplasms are more frequent in the latter areas. Conversely, some subtypes of non-Hodgkin lymphoma which are only rarely seen in Western countries can be found at much higher frequency elsewhere. This may be partly accounted for by local patterns of exposure to viruses or other pathogens, as summarized in *Fig. 11.1*. In each of these instances the infectious agent presumably provides a stimulating effect on lymphoid cell growth, but how this interacts with other cellular mechanisms to induce neoplastic transformation remains unclear. However, some clues to the molecular aetiology of lymphomas have been provided by the study of

Geographic distribution of lymphoma and infectious agents			
Lymphoma type	**Infectious agent**	**Geographic distribution**	**Evidence for aetiological role**
Burkitt's lymphoma	Epstein–Barr virus (EBV) and malaria	Endemic form essentially restricted to areas of holoendemic malaria	Correlation with malaria prevalence Constant presence of EBV in tumour cells
Nasal-type (angiocentric) lymphoma	EBV	Areas of South-East Asia and South America	Presence of virus in tumour cells Serological evidence of active infection
Gastric mucosa-associated lymphoid tissue lymphoma (MALT)	Helicobacter pylori	Associated with poor socioeconomic conditions	Lymphoma associated with *H. pylori* gastritis May respond to antibiotic treatment
Adult T cell leukaemia/lymphoma	HTLV-1	Southwest Japan and Caribbean	Neoplasm only found in carriers of virus

Fig. 11.1 Lymphoma and infectious agents: geographical distribution.

chromosomal alterations (*Fig. 11.2*), and in many instances the consequences of these alterations have been identified at the DNA level (*Figs 11.3 and 11.4*).

Clinical features and diagnosis
Symptomatology
The clinical presentation of non-Hodgkin lymphoma is more variable than that of Hodgkin lymphoma, and the pattern of tumour spread is not as regular. Furthermore, a greater proportion of patients present with disease in organs other than lymph nodes, or with leukaemic manifestations.

Clinical examination
Patients may present with asymmetrical painless enlargement of lymph nodes in one or more peripheral lymph node regions (*Fig. 11.5*). This presentation is often associated with widespread involvement of lymph nodes (e.g. mesenteric and retroperitoneal nodes) that is not detectable on routine clinical examination (*Fig. 11.6*). The liver and spleen (*Figs 11.7 and 11.8*) may also be enlarged.

Of those patients with non-Hodgkin lymphoma, 10–15% present with extranodal disease at sites of involvement, which include the skin (*Fig. 11.9*) and soft tissue (*Fig. 11.10*). When the gastrointestinal

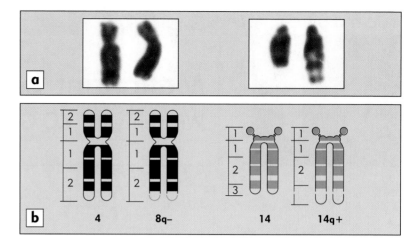

Fig. 11.2a and b Burkitt's lymphoma: (a) partial karyotypes of G-banded chromosomes 8 and 14 from a child. The translocated chromosomes are on the right in each pair. The cellular oncogene c-MYC moves with the translocated portion of chromosome 8 and is juxtaposed to the Ig heavy-chain locus. (b) A systematized description of the structural aberration (see also *Fig. 11.4*). More rarely, cases of Burkitt's lymphoma show (8;22) or (2;8) translocations, involving, respectively, the κ and λ light chain genes. [(a, b) Courtesy of Prof. LM Secker-Walker.]

Fig. 11.3 Non-Hodgkin lymphoma: chromosome translocations and their genetic consequences.

Chromosomal translocations in non-Hodgkin lymphomas and their genetic consequences			
Neoplasm	**Translocation**	**Genes involved**	**Consequences**
B cell neoplasms			
Burkitt's	t(8;14)(q24;q32)*	c-MYC and IgH	Activation of c-MYC (DNA-binding protein)
MALT	t(11;18)(q21;q21)	AP12 and MLT	Reduced apoptosis
	t(1;14)(p24;q32)	BCL-10	More aggressive disease
Follicular	t(14;18)(q32;q21)	IgH and BCL-2	Activation of BCL-2 (apoptosis inhibitor)
Mantle cell	t(11;14)(q13;q32)	BCL-1 and IgH	Activation of BCL-1 (cyclin D1)
Diffuse large B cell	t(3;14)(q27;q32)	BCL-6	Extranodal disease; better prognosis
T cell neoplasms			
Acute lymphoblastic	t(1;14)(p32;q11)	TAL-1/SCL and α-TCR	Activation of TAL-1/SCL (haemopoietic transcription factor)†
Anaplastic large cell	t(2;5)(p23;q35)	ALK and NPM	Creation of hybrid NPM–ALK tyrosine kinase

*Rare variant translocations involve the κ or λ Ig genes instead of the Ig heavy chain gene.
†An interstitial deletion at chromosome 1q32 can also activate the TAL-1/SCL gene.

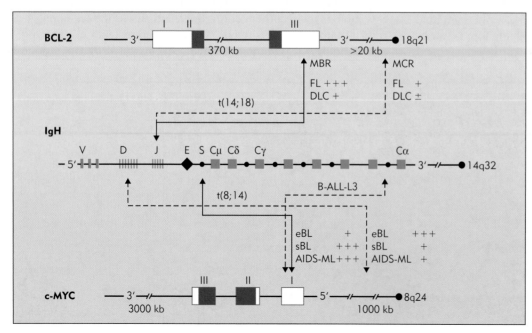

Fig. 11.4 Non-Hodgkin lymphoma: molecular analysis of common breakpoints found in reciprocal translocations involving IgH and BCL-2 (follicular lymphoma) or IgH and c-MYC (in Burkitt's lymphoma). Exons of BCL-2 and c-MYC are represented by rectangles with roman numeral designation above. Coding regions of BCL-2 and c-MYC are solid red rectangles. (MBR, major breakpoint cluster region; MCR, minor breakpoint cluster region; V, variable region; D, diversity region; J, joining region; E, enhancer; S, switch region; C, constant regions of IgH genes; FL, follicular lymphoma; DLC, diffuse large B cell lymphoma type; ALL, acute lymphoblastic leukaemia; eBL, endemic Burkitt's lymphoma; sBL, sporadic Burkitt's lymphoma, AIDS-ML, AIDS-related malignant lymphoma; +++, majority of cases; +, minority of cases; ±, some cases.)

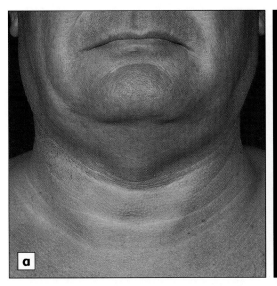
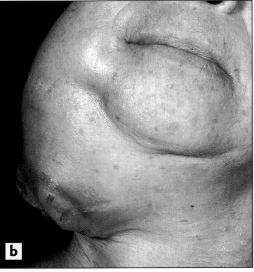
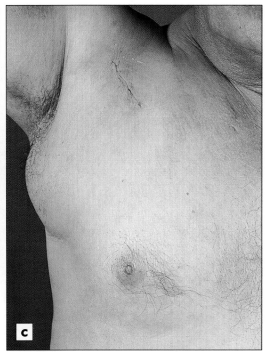

Fig. 11.5a–c Non-Hodgkin lymphoma: (a) bilateral cervical lymphadenopathy in a patient with diffuse lymphocytic lymphoma; (b) massive enlargement of lymph nodes in the left submandibular area, with extensive ulceration of the overlying skin in a patient with diffuse large B cell lymphoma; (c) massive enlargement of axillary nodes with mass extending subcutaneously and also intramuscularly in the right infraclavicular and supraclavicular regions in a patient with diffuse large B cell lymphoma.

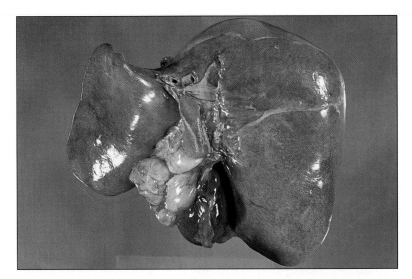

Fig. 11.6 Large B cell lymphoma: enlarged porta hepatis lymph nodes seen at autopsy.

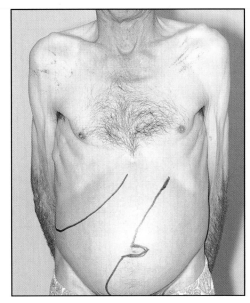

Fig. 11.7 Non-Hodgkin lymphoma: massive enlargement of the spleen and hepatomegaly in diffuse lymphocytic lymphoma. (Hb, 9.5 g/dl; WBC, 6.0×10^9/l; lymphocytes, 2.7×10^9/l; platelets, 80×10^9/l.)

Fig. 11.8 Large B cell lymphoma: macroscopic appearance of spleen removed at laparotomy, showing widespread replacement of splenic tissue by pale tumour and extensive areas of necrosis.

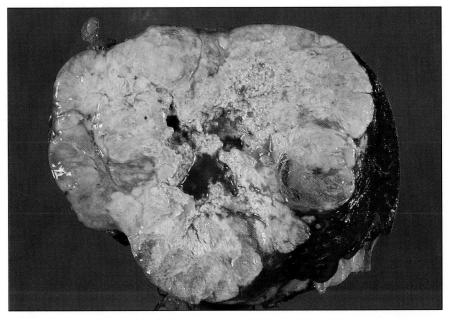

tract is involved patients may present with acute abdominal symptoms. However, in some instances extranodal involvement represents a tumour that arises in lymphoid tissue at sites such as the gastrointestinal tract or jaw, and/or locally spreads from these sites (*Fig.* 11.11). Some lymphoma subtypes show a predilection for certain tissues (*Fig. 11.12*), which sometimes reflects the distribution of the normal counterpart from which they derive (*Fig. 11.13*).

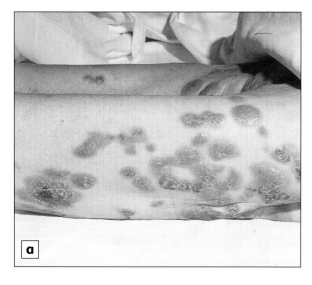

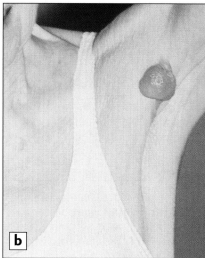

Fig. 11.9a and b Non-Hodgkin lymphoma: cutaneous deposits in (a) advance large B cell lymphoma and (b) follicular lymphoma.

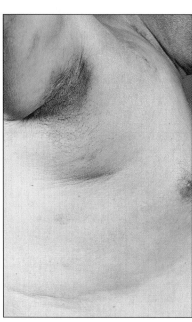

Fig. 11.10 Non-Hodgkin lymphoma: high grade invasion of anterior and lateral chest wall by direct spread into muscle from the axillary lymph nodes (same patient as shown in *Fig. 11.5c*).

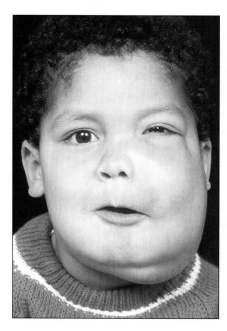

Fig. 11.11 Burkitt's lymphoma: characteristic facial swelling caused by extensive tumour involvement of the mandible and surrounding soft tissues. (Courtesy of Prof. JM Chessells.)

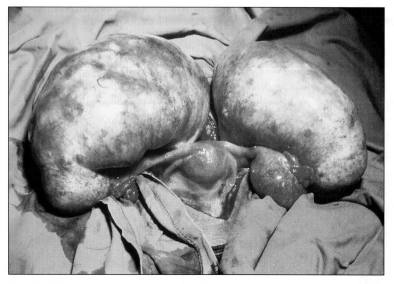

Fig. 11.12 Burkitt's lymphoma: gross bilateral involvement of the ovaries.

Distribution of lymphoid neoplasms and their cells of origin	
Neoplasm	**Cell of origin and its localization**
Mycosis fungoides and/or Sézary syndrome	Epidermal associated T cell
MALT lymphoma	Mucosa and/or epithelium associated T cell
Follicular lymphoma	Germinal centre
Myeloma	Bone marrow plasma cell
Nasal (angiocentric) lymphoma	Nasopharyngeal T/NK cell
Enteropathy-associated T cell lymphoma	Small intestinal intraepithelial T cell
Hepatosplenic lymphoma	γ/δ T cell in splenic red pulp and liver

Fig. 11.13 Lymphoid neoplasms: distribution and cells of origin.

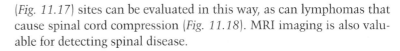
Imaging

Imaging may play an important part in diagnosis and in assessing the distribution of non-Hodgkin lymphoma ('staging'). For example, involvement of intrathoracic (*Figs 11.14–11.16*) and intra-abdominal (*Fig. 11.17*) sites can be evaluated in this way, as can lymphomas that cause spinal cord compression (*Fig. 11.18*). MRI imaging is also valuable for detecting spinal disease.

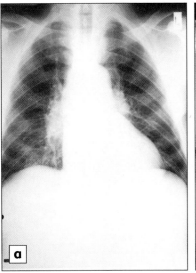
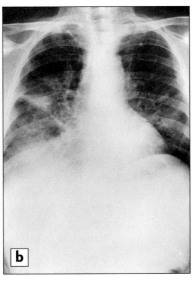

Fig. 11.14a and b Small lymphocytic lymphoma: chest radiographs showing (a) bilateral hilar lymph node enlargement and (b) interstitial and confluent shadowing particularly in the lower and mid-zones caused by lymphomatous infiltration (as shown by biopsy).

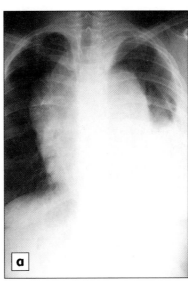
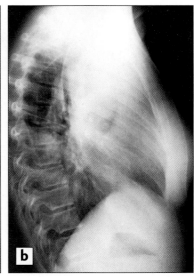

Fig. 11.15a and b T cell lymphoblastic lymphoma: (a) chest radiograph showing gross enlargement of the mediastinal lymph nodes and a pleural effusion on the left; (b) the lateral view confirms anterior mediastinal disease with posterior displacement of the trachea.

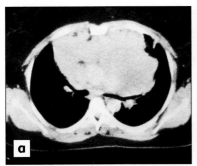
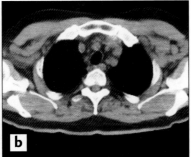

Fig. 11.16a and b Non-Hodgkin lymphoma: CT scans through the mid-thorax show (a) gross enlargement of anterior mediastinal, paratracheal and hilar nodes in T lymphoblastic lymphoma; (b) anterior mediastinal and paratracheal lymph node enlargement in follicular lymphoma.

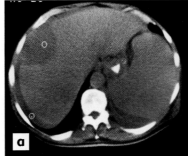
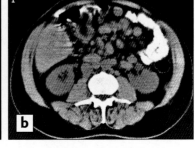

Fig. 11.17a and b Non-Hodgkin lymphoma: CT scans through the abdomen show (a) hepatic and splenic enlargement and a prominent radiolucent focus in the right lobe of the liver (ascitic fluid is present and contrast medium is present in the gut) and (b) mesenteric and some para-aortic lymph node enlargement.

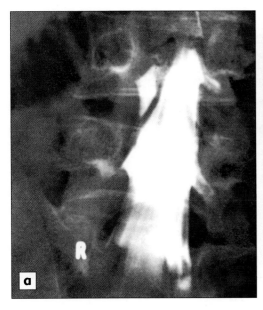
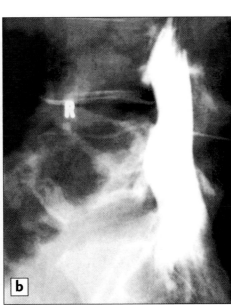

Fig. 11.18a and b Non-Hodgkin lymphoma in the anterior lumbar canal: (a) anteroposterior and (b) lateral myelograms demonstrate an extradural deposit in the anterior lumbar canal, commencing at L4.
[(a, b) Courtesy of Dr D Nag.]

Morphological diagnosis

Microscopic tissue examination is of importance for two purposes. First, it may be used to show involvement in tissues for which clinical examination and imaging are not informative, such as the skin (*Fig. 11.19*) or bone marrow. The latter tissue shows focal or diffuse involvement in about 20% of patients (*Figs 11.20–11.22*). Other sites at which tumour infiltration may be evident on microscopic examination include the central nervous system (CNS; *Figs 11.23 and*

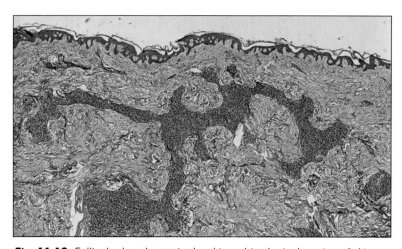

Fig. 11.19 Follicular lymphoma in the skin: a histological section of skin with follicular lymphoma shows sheets of tumour cells in the dermis.

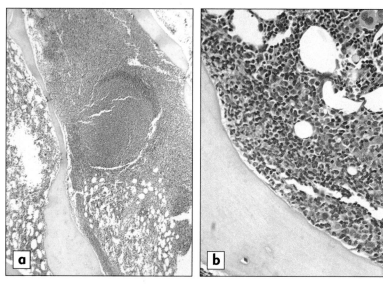

Fig. 11.20a and b Non-Hodgkin lymphoma in the bone marrow: (a) trephine biopsy in follicular lymphoma shows almost complete replacement of normal haemopoietic tissue in the upper field and a paratrabecular collection of neoplastic lymphoid cells below; (b) higher power shows the demarcation between the paratrabecular centrocytes and centroblasts and the normal haemopoietic cells and fat.

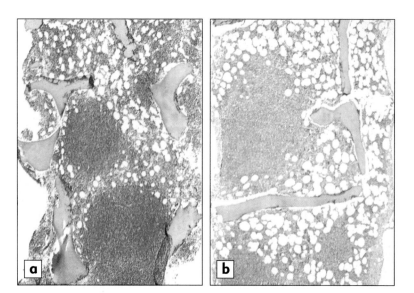

Fig. 11.21a and b Non-Hodgkin lymphoma in the bone marrow: (a, b) trephine biopsies from two patients, showing extensive focal deposits of lymphoma cells.

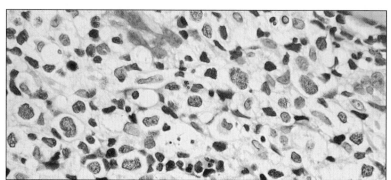

Fig. 11.22 Non-Hodgkin lymphoma in the bone marrow: a trephine biopsy shows a large cell lymphoma infiltrating haemopoietic marrow.

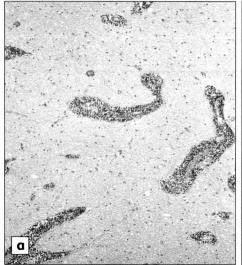
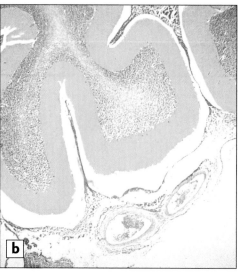

Fig. 11.23a and b Lymphoblastic lymphoma in the brain: sections of brain in CNS relapse showing (a) nodular invasion along perivascular spaces and (b) extensive involvement of the meninges. A similar pattern of involvement occurs in primary lymphoma of the brain. In the past these primary tumours may have been categorized as microgliomas. [(a, b) Courtesy of Dr BB Berkeley.]

11.24), lung (*Fig. 11.25*) and thyroid (*Fig. 11.26*). Also, many types of lymphoid neoplasms that are initially tissue-based may spread to the blood, particularly in an advanced or terminal stage (*Fig. 11.27*). Haematological examination of bone marrow aspirates may also detect involvement by lymphoma (*Fig. 11.28*), although trephine biopsies should also be examined.

The other purpose for which microscopic examination is essential is in establishing that a lymphoid proliferation is neoplastic and in

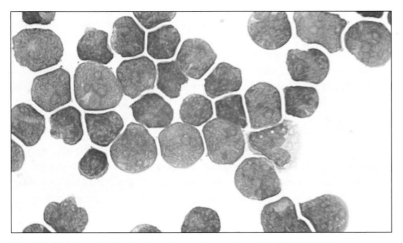

Fig. 11.24 Lymphoblastic lymphoma in cerebrospinal fluid: high-power view of a cytospin preparation of cerebrospinal fluid in CNS relapse shows typical lymphoblasts.

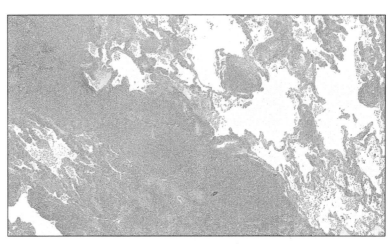

Fig. 11.25 Primary small lymphocytic lymphoma in the lung: low-power view of a histological section shows sheets of neoplastic lymphocytes at the edge of the tumour infiltrating the surrounding lung along bronchovascular bundles and alveolar septae.

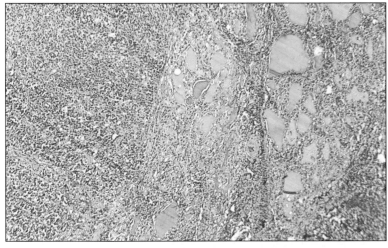

Fig. 11.26 Primary large B cell lymphoma of the thyroid: a histological section shows sheets of neoplastic cells (left) and remaining colloid-filled acini (right). Immunoperoxidase staining for light chains confirmed the monoclonality of the tumour cells.

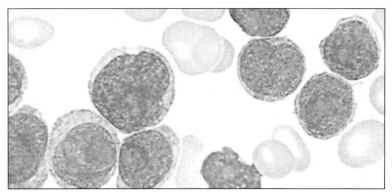

Fig. 11.27 Peripheral blood involvement in terminal large B cell lymphoma: a film showing abnormal large blast cells in a patient with widely disseminated disease.

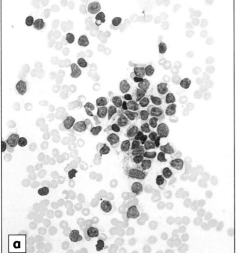

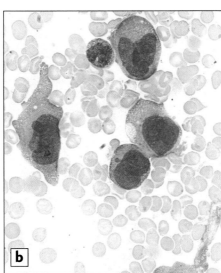

Fig. 11.28a and b Bone marrow aspirates in non-Hodgkin lymphoma: (a) dominance of neoplastic lymphocytes in the cell trail in small lymphocytic lymphoma; (b) higher power view of large neoplastic cells in large B cell lymphoma – the smaller cell is a monocyte.

deciding on the lymphoma subtype. By convention this is carried out by histopathological examination of a lymph node or tissue biopsy, but also given below are details of the use of cell smears prepared from aspirated material by the 'fine needle' technique.

Tissue sample processing

Biopsies are processed as for other histological samples although the great importance in diagnosis of cell morphological detail means that adequate and rapid fixation is essential. Fixatives do not penetrate rapidly through a large lymph node so that biopsies should be taken without delay to the laboratory. It is an unfortunate fact that the main obstacle to lymphoma diagnosis is no longer lack of knowledge of lymphoma subtypes or the inexperience of pathologists, but the poor quality of many biopsy specimens.

Ideally fresh tissue should also be given to the laboratory for freezing, and it can be kept if necessary prior to this in saline or culture medium for at least 24 hours without deterioration. This tissue can then be examined if necessary by techniques that are not applicable to routinely fixed samples (e.g. immunostaining of cryostat sections for denaturation-sensitive markers or molecular biological analysis).

Fine needle aspiration cytology

Fine needle aspiration of enlarged lymph nodes is a useful screening procedure in cases of suspected malignant lymphoma. The principal causes of lymphadenopathy are given in *Fig. 11.29*. It is also particularly useful in establishing supplemental information on regional or extra-regional involvement during staging of the disease and it may avoid the trauma of additional surgery when disease recurrence is suspected clinically. Aspirates are stained by Romanovsky or Papanicolaou techniques, but information may also be obtained by immunocytochemical staining of the cell smears or by flow cytometric analysis of suspended cells. Histological confirmation of an initial suspected diagnosis of malignancy is essential.

Figs 11.30–11.32 show aspirates from cases of lymphoma, while *Figs 11.33–11.44* show examples of metastatic carcinoma and malignant melanoma diagnosed by aspiration cytology. Although the majority of these conditions are easily distinguished cytologically from malignant lymphoma, metastatic small cell or undifferentiated tumours, such as small cell carcinoma of the lung (*Fig. 11.45*), metastatic or primary

Causes of lymphadenopathy	
Localized	**Generalized**
Local infection	**Infections**
Pyogenic infection (e.g. pharyngitis, dental abscess, otitis media), actinomyces	Viral (e.g. infectious mononucleosis, measles, rubella, viral hepatitis), human immunodeficiency virus
Viral infection (e.g. cat scratch fever, lymphogranuloma venereum)	Bacterial (e.g. brucellosis, syphilis, tuberculosis, salmonella, bacterial endocarditis)
Tuberculosis	Fungal (e.g. histoplasmosis)
Lymphoma	Protozoal (e.g. toxoplasmosis)
Hodgkin lymphoma	**Non-infectious inflammatory diseases**
Non-Hodgkin lymphoma	For example sarcoidosis, rheumatoid arthritis, systemic lupus erythematosus, other connective tissue diseases, Kikuchi's disease, serum sickness
Metastatic tumours	
Carcinoma	**Leukaemia, especially CLL, ALL**
Malignant melanoma	**Lymphoma**
	Non-Hodgkin lymphoma
	Hodgkin lymphoma
	Waldenström's macroglobulinaemia
	Rarely, metastatic tumours
	Angioimmunoblastic lymphadenopathy
	Sinus histiocytosis with massive lymphadenopathy
	Autoimmune lymphoproliferative disease
	Reaction to drugs and chemicals
	For example hydantoins and related chemicals, beryllium
	Hyperthyroidism

Fig. 11.29 Lymphadenopathy: causes.

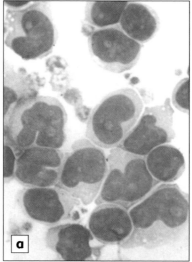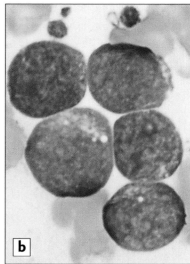

Fig. 11.30a and b Fine needle lymph node aspirates in non-Hodgkin lymphoma: (a) mantle cells ('centrocytes') and (b) large B cell lymphoma ('centroblasts'). (May-Grünwald–Giemsa stain.)

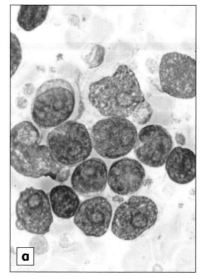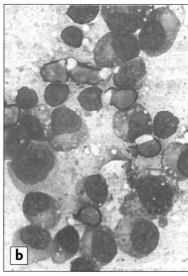

Fig. 11.31a and b Fine needle lymph node aspirates in non-Hodgkin lymphoma: (a) large B cell lymphoma; (b) large B cell lymphoma showing plasmacytic differentiation. (May-Grünwald–Giemsa stain.)

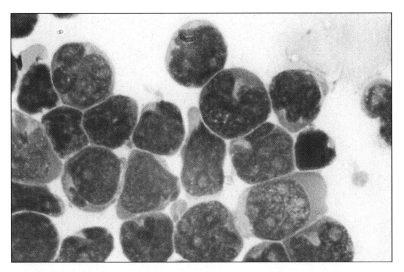

Fig. 11.32 Fine needle lymph node aspirate: lymphoblastic lymphoma. (May-Grünwald–Giemsa stain.)

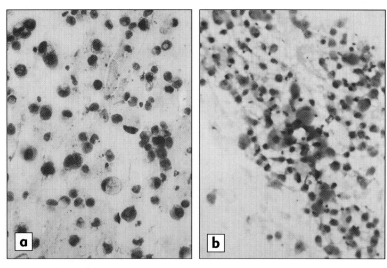

Fig. 11.33a and b Metastatic adenocarcinoma of the stomach in a fine needle aspirate of a supraclavicular lymph node: (a) tumour cells with cytoplasmic mucin, which (b) stains positively by the periodic acid–Schiff technique.

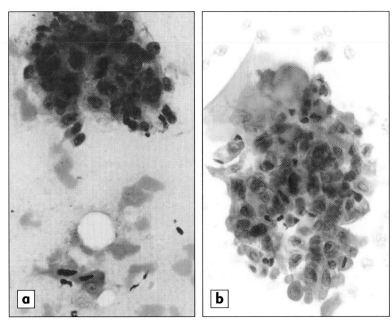

Fig. 11.34a and b Metastatic squamous cell carcinoma of the oesophagus: fine needle aspirate of lateral cervical lymph node. (a) Poorly differentiated squamous tumour cells. The two isolated cells show typical hyperchromatic nuclei and cytoplasmic keratinization. (b) Keratinization is better seen with Papanicolaou staining.

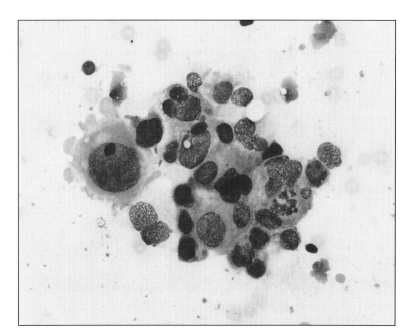

Fig. 11.35 Metastatic renal adenocarcinoma: Fine needle aspirate of an inguinal lymph node showing very large pleomorphic tumour cells. A diagnosis of poorly differentiated renal carcinoma was confirmed at nephrectomy.

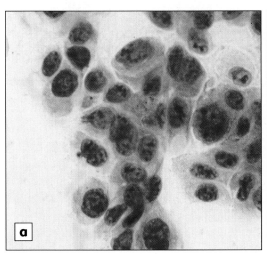
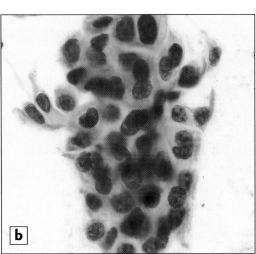

Fig. 11.36a and b Metastatic transitional cell carcinoma: (a, b) fine needle aspirate of inguinal lymph node showing poorly differentiated transitional cells. The patient's history included a previous tumour of the bladder. [(a) H & E; (b) Papanicolaou stain.]

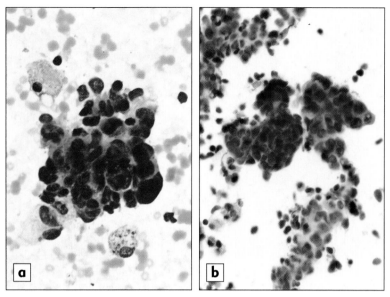

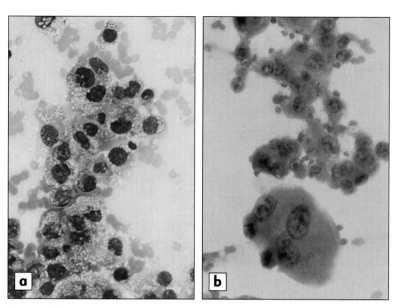

Fig. 11.37a and b Metastatic serous cystadenocarcinoma of the ovary: (a, b) fine needle aspirates of an inguinal lymph node showing papilliform clusters of pleomorphic tumour cells.

Fig. 11.38a and b Metastatic carcinoma of the lung: (a, b) fine needle aspirate of cervical lymph node. The pleomorphic tumour cells show abundant vacuolated cytoplasm typical of adenocarcinoma. [(a) May-Grünwald–Giemsa stain; (b) Papanicolaou stain.]

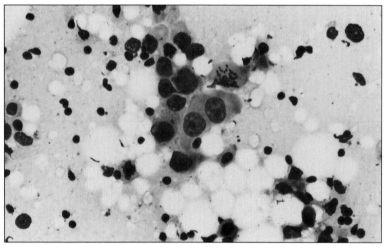

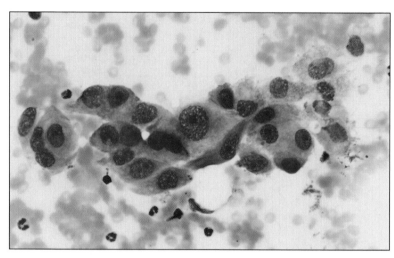

Fig. 11.39 Metastatic carcinoma of the breast: fine needle aspirate of axillary lymph node showing metastatic large nucleolated tumour cells, a mitotic figure and lymphocytes.

Fig. 11.40 Metastatic adenocarcinoma of the stomach: fine needle aspirate of a supraclavicular lymph node showing a cluster of large adhesive pleomorphic tumour cells with prominent nucleoli.

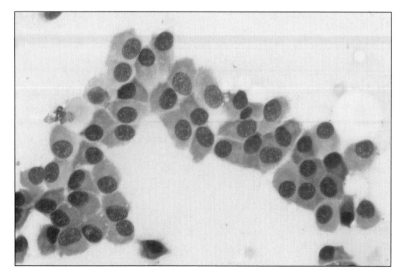

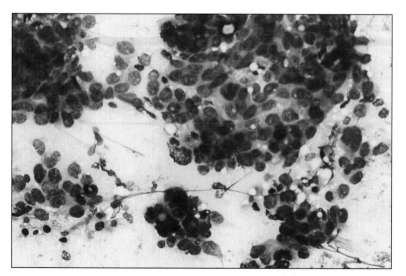

Fig. 11.41 Adenocarcinoma of the pancreas: fine needle aspirate of a para-aortic mass showing a loosely adhesive group of well-differentiated glandular cells with uniform nuclei and basophilic cytoplasm.

Fig. 11.42 Metastatic carcinoma of the lung: fine needle aspirate of cervical lymph node showing sheets of poorly differentiated large tumour cells with no obvious keratinization.

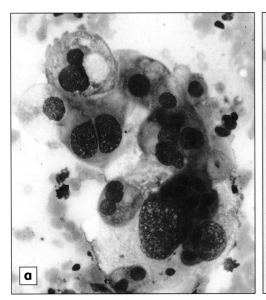

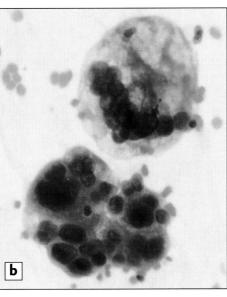

Fig. 11.43a and b Metastatic adenocarcinoma of the colon: (a, b) fine needle aspirate of inguinal lymph node showing clusters of poorly differentiated large tumour cells with mucin-containing cytoplasmic vacuoles.

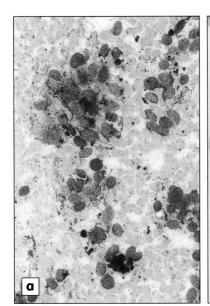

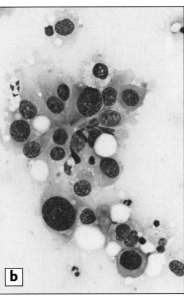

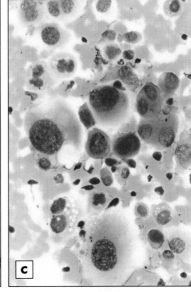

Fig. 11.44a–c Metastatic malignant melanoma in fine needle aspirates of cervical lymph node. (a) Group of tumour cells with prominent intracellular and free melanin pigment; (b, c) two examples showing greater cellular pleomorphism and anaplasia with no obvious melanin pigmentation.

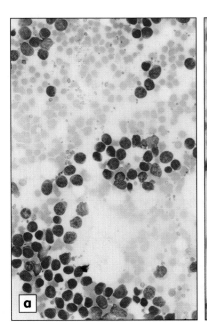

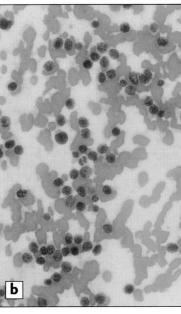

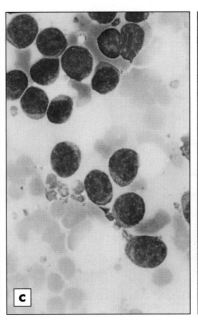

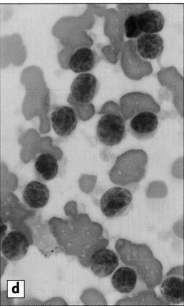

Fig. 11.45a–d Metastatic carcinoma of the lung in a fine needle aspirate of cervical lymph node: (a–d) trails of tumour cells with a high nuclear:cytoplasmic ratio and some resemblance to lymphoid cells are seen. This appearance is typical of a small cell carcinoma of the lung. [(a, c) May-Grünwald–Giemsa stain; (b, d) Papanicolaou stain.]

Merkel cell carcinoma (*Figs 11.46 and Fig. 11.47*) may occasionally cause diagnostic difficulty. Lymph node involvement frequently indicates disease in organs for which the node is a lymph drainage site. Metastatic disease often serves as the earliest indication of the malignant disorder, particularly in cervical and supraclavicular regions (e.g. carcinomas of the stomach, pharynx, lung and thyroid). Metastatic papillary carcinoma of the thyroid (*Fig. 11.48*) may present as lateral cervical node enlargement without palpable disease of the thyroid gland.

Finally, tumours of the salivary glands (*Fig. 11.49*) may be confused with lymphadenopathy. Parotid tumours may resemble enlargement of lymph nodes around the angle of the jaw and in the pre-auricular region, while those of the submandibular gland may be confused with anterior cervical lymphadenopathy. Occasionally, deep epidermoid cysts (*Fig. 11.50*), Merkel cell tumour and leiomyosarcoma (*Fig. 11.51*) may present as node-like enlargements in areas in which peripheral lymphadenopathy is expected.

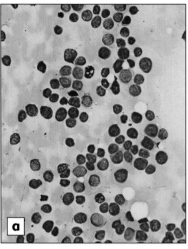
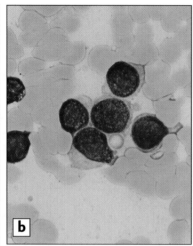

Fig. 11.46a and b Merkel cell carcinoma in a fine needle aspirate of posterior cervical mass: (a) medium-sized cells are seen with features reminiscent of lymphoid cells (high nuclear:cytoplasmic ratio, a fine chromatin pattern and pale blue cytoplasm); (b) at higher magnification, a cohesive nest of tumour cells is seen.

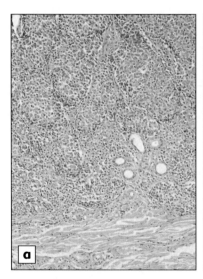
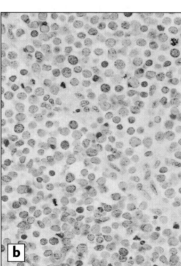
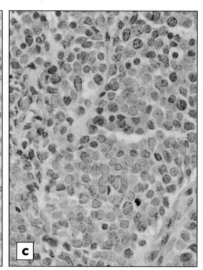

Fig. 11.47a–c Histological section of the Merkel cell carcinoma shown in *Fig. 11.46*: (a) infiltration of the lower dermis by uniform tumour cells; (b) the tumour cells show cytoplasmic positivity for low molecular weight keratin (antibody CAM 5.2); (c) the tumour cells show cytoplasmic positivity for neurone-specific enolase. [Paraffin sections, immunoperoxidase stain (b, c).]

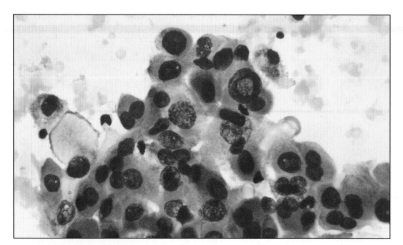

Fig. 11.48 Metastatic papillary carcinoma of the thyroid in a fine needle aspirate of cervical node: a papillary group of tumour cells showing pleomorphism, moderate amounts of pale cytoplasm and a prominent intranuclear inclusion vacuole.

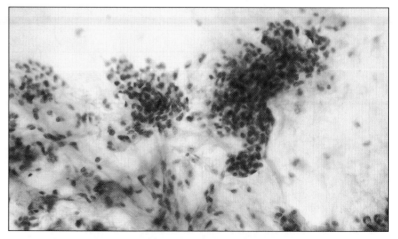

Fig. 11.49 Pleomorphic salivary adenoma in a fine needle aspirate of an interior cervical mass: groups of epithelial tumour cells and characteristic thick 'chondroid' stroma. (Papanicolaou stain.)

Immunophenotyping

Immunostaining of tissue sections is particularly useful when a tissue sample is small, crushed and/or shows evidence of poor fixation. *Fig. 11.52* lists the markers that can be used both to confirm a suspected diagnosis of non-Hodgkin lymphoma (e.g. to distinguish it from a carcinoma) and to establish the subtype. These markers can all be detected in paraffin-embedded tissue, and representative examples of staining are shown in *Figs 11.53–11.56*. If frozen tissue is available, a wider range of markers can be evaluated and labelling may be stronger.

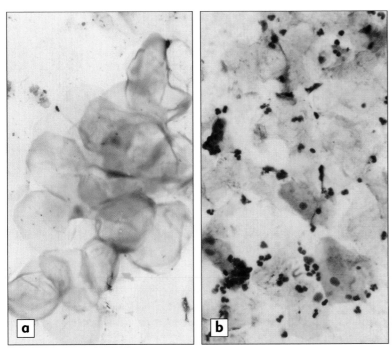

Fig. 11.50a and b Single epidermoid cyst in a fine needle aspirate of a lateral cervical mass: (a, b) mature squamous cells (mainly anucleate) and degenerate neutrophils. [(a) May-Grünwald–Giemsa stain; (b) Papanicolaou stain.]

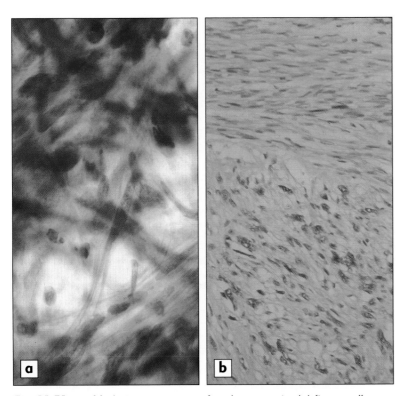

Fig. 11.51a and b Leiomyosarcoma of saphenous vein: (a) fine needle aspirate of an inguinal mass showing elongated cells with large fusiform and spindle-shaped nuclei. (b) Histological section shows smooth muscle tumour cells with similar features. [(a) Papanicolaou stain; (b) H & E stain.]

Markers for immunohistological labelling of paraffin-embedded lymphoma biopsies		
Markers for	**Markers**	**Comment**
B cells	CD20	Virtually B cell specific, but negative on precursor B cells
	CD45RA	Antigen also found on some T cells
	CDw75	Antigen found on mature B cells, but also found on epithelial cells
	CD79a	B cell specific
	Ig	B cell specific, but may be obscured by background Ig
T cells	CD2	T cell specific
	CD3/TCR	T cell specific, but lost by some neoplastic cells
	CD4	Specific for helper cells
	CD8	Specific for cytotoxic and/or suppressor cells
	CD45RO	Also present on myeloid cells, macrophages and some B cells
	Cytotoxic granules	Cytotoxic T cells
Myeloid cells	CD15	Also found on Reed–Sternberg cells, epithelium, etc.
	CD66	Also present on some epithelial cells
	CD68 (PG-M1)	Pan-macrophage
	CD68 (KP1)	Specific for macrophages and neutrophil lineage
		Elastase specific for neutrophil lineage
	Lysozyme	Neutrophil and/or macrophage marker, also found in secretory cells
	Myeloperoxidase	Neutrophil lineage
Miscellaneous	TdT	Marker of lymphoblasts
	CD21	Follicular dendritic cell marker
	CD30	Marker of Reed–Sternberg cells and anaplastic large cell lymphoma
	CD31	Megakaryocyte and/or platelet and endothelial marker
	CD45 (LCA)	Essential for carcinoma and/or lymphoma distinction
	CD61 (GPIIIA)	Marker of platelets and megakaryocytes
	CD74/major histocompatibilty complex Class II	Marker of B cells, some macrophages, and interdigitating dendritic cell
	Cyclin D1	Marker of mantle cell lymphoma
	DBA.44	Marker of hairy cell leukaemia

Fig. 11.52 Markers: immunohistological labelling of paraffin-embedded lymphoma biopsies.

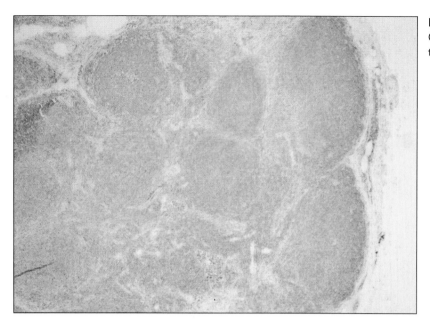

Fig. 11.53 Mantle cell lymphoma immunostained for the B cell marker CD20: antibody L26 reveals a nodular growth pattern as demonstrated in this lymph node biopsy. (Paraffin section, immunoperoxidase stain.)

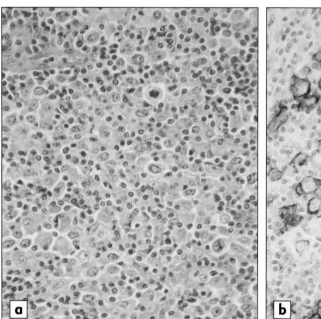

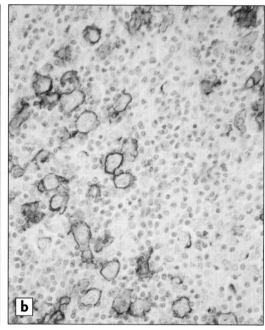

Fig. 11.54a and b Immunostaining of a follicular lymphoma: (a) lymph node biopsy showing extensive replacement of normal architecture by neoplastic centrocytes and centroblasts; (b) the tumour cells express the B cell marker CD20 (antibody L26). (Paraffin section, immunoperoxidase stain; courtesy of Dr JE McLaughlin.)

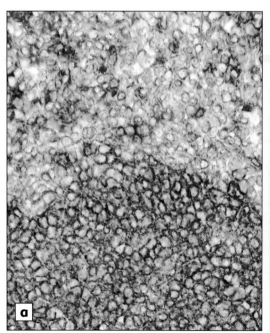

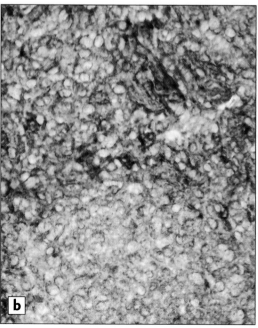

Fig. 11.55a and b Demonstration of monoclonality in a non-Hodgkin lymphoma by immunostaining: a lymph node biopsy shows (a) cytoplasmic positivity for κ light chains in the malignant lymphoid nodule; (b) no labelling for λ light chains is seen in the nodule (lower field). (Paraffin section, immunoperoxidase stain.)

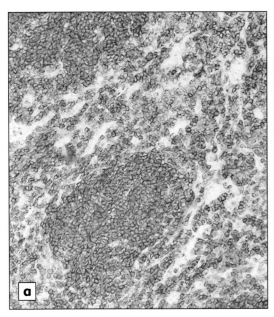
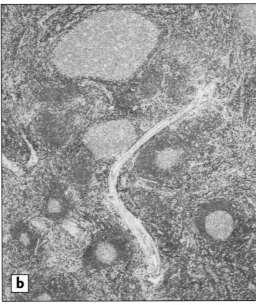

Fig. 11.56a and b Immunohistological detection of BCL-2 protein in reactive and neoplastic lymphoid cells: (a) a follicular lymphoma is positive, reflecting activation of the BCL-2 gene by the (14;18) translocation; (b) in reactive lymphoid tissue unstained germinal centres are surrounded by numerous positive mantle zone B and T cells. (Cryostat section, APAAP immunoalkaline phosphatase stain.)

Classification of lymphoma

History

The histological classification of non-Hodgkin lymphoma and Hodgkin lymphoma has posed a problem for pathologists for many years. It is now evident that there are more than 40 different categories of non-Hodgkin lymphoma, of differing cell origin, so the initial separation by Rappaport into tumours arising from lymphoid cells, from histiocytes, or from a mixture of the two was an oversimplification, albeit an understandable one. Furthermore, molecular markers are crucial, since they not only allow the major categorization into B and T/NK cell neoplasms, but also subclassification according to maturation stage and subpopulation. For these reasons the current understanding of non-Hodgkin lymphoma represents the culmination of many years of study.

By the late 1970s two classification schemes had come to be widely used, one proposed by Lennert and his colleagues (the Kiel classification) and the other from Lukes and Collins. Many pathologists and clinicians, however, still used the simple scheme that had been proposed by Rappaport more than a decade previously. A laudable attempt, which involved the review by a team of pathologists of a large number of cases, was made in the early 1980s to see if the obvious incompatibility between these schemes arose simply because of differing terminology; it was hoped that the clinical data available on the cases would clarify the confusion. However, the compromise classification that emerged (the Working Formulation), although it came to be widely used, particularly in the USA, proved unsatisfactory in practice and did not correspond to the experience of most seasoned haematopathologists.

The Revised European–American Lymphoma (REAL) and World Health Organization (WHO) schemes

In 1994 a group of approximately 20 pathologists ('The International Lymphoma Study Group') proposed a consensus categorization of lymphomas, the REAL scheme. It corresponds closely to the Kiel classification, but it eliminates two distinctions that pathologists had found impossible to make reliably in practice: namely, the subdivision of peripheral T cell lymphoma on the basis of cell size, and the controversial separation of large B cell lymphomas into 'centroblastic' and 'immunoblastic' subtypes. It covered both nodal and extranodal lymphomas and, for the first time, included both Hodgkin lymphoma and non-Hodgkin lymphoma in a single scheme.

The REAL classification of non-Hodgkin lymphoma is given in *Fig. 11.57*, and the proposed WHO classification is given in *Fig. 11.58*. The REAL scheme, like the Kiel classification, distinguishes two broad

---

The REAL classification of non-Hodgkin lymphoma

B cell neoplasms

Precursor B lymphoblastic leukaemia and/or lymphoma

B cell chronic lymphocytic leukaemia and/or prolymphocytic leukaemia and/or small lymphocytic lymphoma

Immunocytoma and/or lymphoplasmacytic lymphoma

Mantle cell lymphoma

Follicle centre lymphoma, follicular

Marginal zone B cell lymphoma

Hairy cell leukaemia

Plasmacytoma and/or plasma cell myeloma

Diffuse large B cell lymphoma

Burkitt's lymphoma

T and NK cell neoplasms

Precursor T lymphoblastic leukaemia and/or lymphoma

T cell chronic lymphocytic leukaemia and/or prolymphocytic leukaemia

Large granular lymphocytic leukaemia

Mycosis fungoides and/or Sézary syndrome

Peripheral T cell lymphomas, unspecified

Angioimmunoblastic T cell lymphoma

Angiocentric lymphoma

Intestinal T cell lymphoma

Adult T cell lymphoma and/or leukaemia

Anaplastic large cell lymphoma

Fig. 11.57 Non-Hodgkin lymphoma: the REAL classification. (Adapted with permission from Harris NL, Jaffe ES, Stein H, *et al. Blood.* 1994;84:1361–92.)

categories of non-Hodgkin lymphoma, based on phenotype – B cell and T cell and/or NK cell neoplasms. It is so similar to the Kiel classification that it is not necessary to give both here. However, it differs to a major degree from the Working Formulation, and so a comparison between the two schemes is shown in *Fig. 11.59*.

The REAL scheme has come to be widely used by pathologists and clinicians, and a clinical evaluation of its utility published in 1997 (The NHL Classification Project) concluded that the REAL classification can

World Health Organization classification of neoplastic diseases of the lymphoid tissues (provisional)

B cell neoplasms

Precursor B cell lymphoblastic leukaemia/lymphoma

Peripheral B cell neoplasms

B cell chronic lymphocytic leukaemia/small lymphocytic lymphoma
variant: with monoclonal gammopathy/plasmacytoid differentiation

B cell prolymphocytic leukaemia

lymphoplasmacytic lymphoma (immunocytoma)

mantle cell lymphoma
variant: blastic

follicular lymphoma
variants: Grade I, centroblasts comprise <50% of the follicle surface area
Grade II, centroblasts comprise >50% of the follicle surface area

cutaneous follicle centre lymphoma

marginal zone B cell lymphoma of mucosa-associated lymphoid tissue
(MALT-type)

nodal marginal zone lymphoma +/– monocytoid B cells

splenic marginal zone B cell lymphoma (+/– villous lymphocytes)

hairy cell leukaemia
variant: hairy cell variant

diffuse large B cell lymphoma
variants: centroblastic
immunoblastic
T cell or histiocyte-rich
anaplastic large B cell

diffuse large B cell lymphoma, subtypes:
mediastinal (thymic) large B cell lymphoma
intravascular large B cell lymphoma
primary effusion lymphoma in HIV patients

Burkitt's lymphoma
variants: endemic
sporadic
atypical (pleomorphic)
atypical, with plasmacytoid differentiation (AIDS-associated)

Immunosecretory disorders (clinical or pathological variants)

monoclonal gammopathy of undetermined significance (MGUS)

plasma cell myeloma (multiple myeloma)
variants: indolent myeloma
smouldering myeloma
osteosclerotic myeloma (POEMS syndrome)
plasma cell leukemia
non-secretory myeloma

plasmacytomas:
solitary plasmacytoma of bone
extramedullary plasmacytoma

Waldenström's macroglobulinaemia (immunocytoma, see above)

heavy chain disease (HCD):
gamma HCD
alpha HCD
Mu HCD

immunoglobulin deposition diseases:
systemic light chain disease
primary amyloidosis

T cell neoplasms

Precursor T cell lymphoblastic leukaemia/lymphoma

Peripheral T cell and NK cell neoplasms

T cell prolymphocytic leukaemia
variants: small cell
cerebriform cell

T cell large granular lymphocytic leukaemia

aggressive NK cell leukaemia

NK/T cell lymphoma, nasal and nasal-type (angiocentric)

Sézary syndrome

mycosis fungoides
variants: pagetoid reticulosis
MF-associated follicular mucinosis
granulomatous slack skin disease

angioimmunoblastic T cell lymphoma

peripheral T cell lymphoma (unspecified)
variants: lymphoepithelioid (Lennert's)
T zone

adult T cell leukaemia/lymphoma (HTLV-1+)
variants: acute
lymphomatous
chronic
smouldering
Hodgkin-like

anaplastic large cell lymphoma (ALCL; T and null cell types)
variants: lymphohistiocytic
small cell

primary cutaneous CD-30 positive T cell lymphoproliferative disorders
variants: lymphomatoid papulosis (type A and B)
primary cutaneous anaplastic large cell lymphoma (ALCL)
borderline lesions

subcutaneous panniculitis-like T cell lymphoma

enteropathy-type intestinal T cell lymphoma

hepatosplenic γ/δ T cell lymphoma

Hodgkin lymphoma (Hodgkin's disease)

Nodular lymphocyte predominance Hodgkin lymphoma

Classical Hodgkin lymphoma

Hodgkin lymphoma, nodular sclerosis (Grades I and II)

classical Hodgkin lymphoma, lymphocyte-rich

Hodgkin lymphoma, mixed cellularity

Hodgkin lymphoma, lymphocyte depletion

Fig. 11.58 Non-Hodgkin lymphoma: provisional WHO classification of neoplastic diseases of the lymphoid tissues. (Courtesy of the members of the Steering Committee for the WHO: Drs ES Jaffe, NL Harris, J Diebold, K Muller-Hermelink, J Vardiman, G Flandrin.) See also Harris NL et al. The Hematology Journal. 2000; 1:53–66.

Comparison between the REAL classification and the Working Formulation

Working formulation	REAL classification	
Low grade	**B cell neoplasms**	**T cell neoplasms**
A. Small lymphocytic consistent with chronic lymphocytic leukaemia	B cell chronic lymphocytic and/or prolymphocytic leukaemia and/or small cell lymphocytic lymphoma	T cell chronic lymphocytic and/or prolymphocytic leukaemia
	Marginal zone and/or MALT	Large granular lymphocytic lymphoma
	Mantle cell	Adult T cell leukaemia and/or lymphoma
Plasmacytoid	Lymphoplasmacytoid	
	Marginal zone and/or MALT	
B. Follicular, predominantly small cleaved cell	Follicle centre, follicular, Grade I*	
	Mantle zone	
	Marginal zone and/or MALT	
C. Follicular, mixed small cleaved and large cell	Follicle centre, follicular Grade II*	
	Marginal zone and/or MALT	
Intermediate grade		
D. Follicular, large cell	Follicle centre, follicular, Grade III*	
E. Diffuse, small cleaved cell	Mantle zone	T cell chronic lymphocytic and/or prolymphocytic leukaemia
	Follicle centre, diffuse small cell	Adult T cell leukaemia
	Marginal zone and/or MALT Large granular lymphocytic lymphoma	Angioimmunoblastic
		Angiocentric and/or nasal
F. Diffuse, mixed small and large	Large B cell (T cell rich)	Peripheral T cell, unspecified
	Follicle centre, diffuse small cell	Adult T cell leukaemia and/or lymphoma
	Lymphoplasmacytoid	Angioimmunoblastic
	Marginal zone and/or MALT	Angiocentric and/or nasal
	Mantle cell	Intestinal T cell
G. Diffuse, large cell	Diffuse large B cell	Peripheral T cell, unspecified
		Adult T cell leukaemia and/or lymphoma
		Angioimmunoblastic
		Angiocentric and/or nasal
		Intestinal T cell
High grade		
H. Large cell immunoblastic	Diffuse large B cell	Peripheral T cell, unspecified
		Adult T cell leukaemia and/or lymphoma
		Angioimmunoblastic
		Angiocentric and/or nasal
		Intestinal T cell
		Anaplastic large cell
I. Lymphoblastic	Precursor B lymphoblastic	Precursor T lymphoblastic
J. Small non-cleaved cell		
Burkitt's	Burkitt's	
Non-Burkitt's	High grade B cell, Burkitt-like	Peripheral T cell, unspecified
Diffuse large B cell		

*The grading is highly subjective and varies within a single biopsy. It is not now part of the REAL classification (see page 210). In the WHO classification, two grades are recognized (see Fig. 11.58).

Fig. 11.59 Non-Hodgkin lymphoma: comparison between the REAL scheme and the Working Formulation.

B cell lymphomas: immunohistological phenotyping		
Neoplasm	**Immunology**	
B lymphoblastic leukaemia and/or lymphoma	TdT	+
	CD10 (cALLA)	+/–
	Cytoplasmic μ	–/+
	CD19, 79a	+
B cell chronic lymphocytic and/or prolymphocytic leukaemia and/or small lymphocytic lymphoma	Surface IgM	+ (week)
	CD5	+
	CD10	–
	CD19, 20, 79a	+
	CD22	+/–
	CD23	+
Immunocytoma and/or lymphoplasmacytic lymphoma	Surface IgM	+
	Cytoplasmic Ig	+
	CD5, 10	–
	CD19, 20, 22, 79a	+
Mantle cell lymphoma	Surface immunoglobulin (λ>κ)	+
	CD5	+
	CD10	–/+
	CD19, 20, 22, 79a	+
	CD23	–
	Cyclin D1	+
Follicle centre cell lymphoma	Surface Ig	+
	CD5	–
	CD10	+/–
	CD19, 20, 22, 79a	+
	BCL-2	+
Marginal zone B cell lymphoma (MALT-type, 'monocytoid B cell', splenic marginal zone B cell lymphoma)	Surface Ig	+
	CD5, 10	–
	CD19, 20, 22, 79a	+
	CD23	–
Hairy cell leukaemia	Surface Ig	+
	CD5, 10, 23	–
	CD11c, 25	+
	CD19, 20, 22, 79a	+
	CD103 (MLA)	+
Plasmacytoma and/or plasma cell myeloma	Surface Ig	-
	Cytoplasmic Ig	+
	EMA	–/+
	CD19, 20, 22	–
	CD79a (mb-1)	+/–
Diffuse large B cell lymphoma	Surface Ig	+/–
	Cytoplasmic Ig	–/+
	CD5, 10	–/+
	CD19, 20, 22, 79a	+
Burkitt's lymphoma	Surface IgM	+
	CD5,23	–
	CD10	+
	CD19, 20, 22, 79a	+

Fig. 11.60 B cell lymphoma: immunohistological phenotyping.

be reproducibly applied by haematopathologists. However, it also showed that the International Prognostic Index (see *Fig. 11.107*) defines clinical subgroups in neoplasms, such as large cell lymphoma, that have strikingly different prognoses, emphasizing that lymphoma diagnosis represents a collaboration between the clinician and the pathologist.

The World Health Organization classification
A comprehensive classification of all neoplasms of haemopoietic and lymphoid tissue has been prepared under the auspices of WHO, but had not been published in final form at the time of writing (the latest version relating to the primary lymphoproliferative disorders is given in *Fig. 11.58*). It contains no new entities with respect to the REAL scheme, and the list of lymphoid neoplasms in the WHO scheme is essentially identical to that of the REAL scheme. However, the WHO scheme includes a few rare disorders that were provisional categories in the REAL scheme (e.g. hepatosplenic γδ and panniculitic lymphomas among the T cell tumours, and nodal marginal zone lymphomas among the B cell neoplasms). The WHO scheme also subdivides some entities in the REAL scheme (e.g. distinguishing prolymphocytic B cell leukaemia from small lymphocytic B cell neoplasms, and listing plasmacytoma separately from plasma cell myeloma, and Sézary syndrome from mycosis fungoides).

B CELL NON-HODGKIN LYMPHOMA

B cell non-Hodgkin lymphoma neoplasms differ from each other because they represent different stages of B cell maturation, ranging from the lymphoblast at one extreme to the plasma cell at the other. To a lesser extent their heterogeneity may reflect compartmentalization into different local populations (e.g. mucosal B cells, splenic B cells). Several of them are encountered by haematologists rather than histopathologists (notably acute lymphoblastic and chronic lymphocytic leukaemia, hairy cell leukaemia and myeloma, which are discussed in Chapters 8, 10 and 12). The phenotype of B cell neoplasms is summarized in *Fig. 11.60* and the presumed cell of origin is shown in *Fig. 11.61*.

Precursor B cell acute lymphoblastic lymphoma/leukaemia
Lymphoblastic neoplasms of B cell type usually present as a leukaemia. They typically express markers, such as terminal transferase and CD10, found on early B cells. The CD79a antigen is of value, since it is often the only B cell marker expressed by these cells that is detectable in paraffin-embedded tissue. Although bone marrow and blood involvement is very common, a few cases are localized as solid tumours, usually in lymph nodes. The disease, though aggressive, can be cured, particularly when it occurs in children.

Small lymphocytic lymphoma and chronic lymphocytic leukaemia
Neoplasms composed of small lymphocytes may also present as either lymphomas or leukaemias. The leukaemias comprise both chronic lymphocytic leukaemia and the leukaemia of larger cells, which haematologists define as 'prolymphocytic' leukaemia.

Histologically, small lymphocytic neoplasms show a monotonous infiltration of small cells (*Figs 11.62–11.64*), but clusters of larger cells ('pseudofollicles or proliferation centres') are a common feature. Occasionally, the neoplastic cells may differentiate to the plasma cell stage, but this should not prompt a diagnosis of immunocytoma (see below). Small lymphocytic neoplasms usually express CD5 and CD23, in addition to 'pan-B cell' markers. They tend to follow an indolent course.

Lymphoplasmacytic lymphoma (immunocytoma)
The neoplastic cell in lymphoplasmacytic lymphoma (also known as immunocytoma) is a B lymphocyte, which shows a tendency to differentiate towards the plasma cell stage (*Fig. 11.65*). In the cells with plasmacytic features, IgM is detectable within the cytoplasm or as

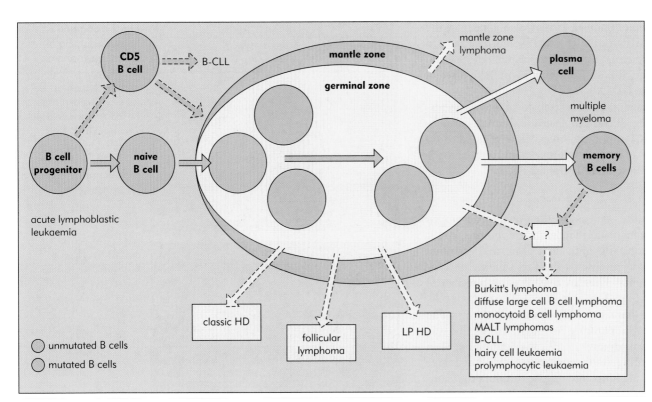

Fig. 11.61 B cell lymphoma: cellular origin in humans. (Adapted with permission from Klein U, Goossens T, Fischer M, *et al.* Somatic hypermutation in normal and transformed human B cells. *Immunol Rev.* 1998;162:261–80.)

Diagram labels: CD5 B cell → B-CLL; B cell progenitor; naive B cell; acute lymphoblastic leukaemia; mantle zone; germinal zone; mantle zone lymphoma; plasma cell; multiple myeloma; memory B cells; ?; classic HD; follicular lymphoma; LP HD; Burkitt's lymphoma; diffuse large cell B cell lymphoma; monocytoid B cell lymphoma; MALT lymphomas; B-CLL; hairy cell leukaemia; prolymphocytic leukaemia; unmutated B cells; mutated B cells

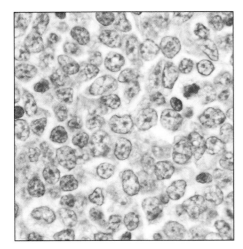

Fig. 11.62 Lymphoblastic lymphoma: the lymphoblasts have round or oval nuclei with delicate, evenly dispersed chromatin patterns and one to three nucleoli, and only a scanty rim of cytoplasm. The darker cells are small lymphocytes.

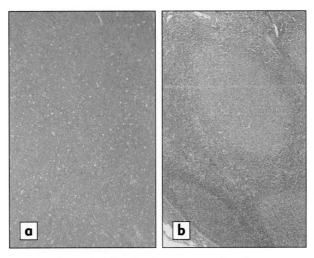

Fig. 11.63a and b Small cell lymphocytic lymphoma: (a) lymph node shows a diffuse pattern of involvement, with total replacement of the normal architecture by a uniform population of neoplastic lymphocytes; (b) lymph node showing a nodular or parafollicular pattern. [(a, b) May-Grünwald–Giemsa stain.]

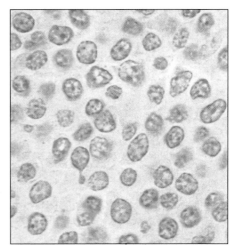

Fig. 11.64 Small cell lymphocytic lymphoma: a predominance of small lymphocytes with round nuclei that contain densely clumped heterochromatin.

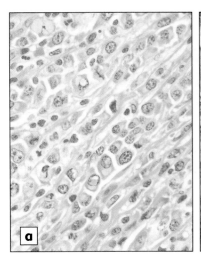
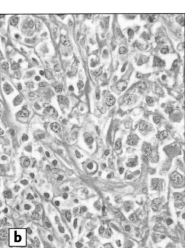
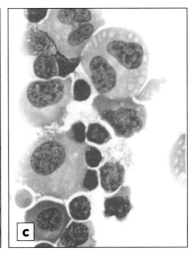

Fig. 11.65a–c Lymphoplasmacytic lymphoma (immunocytoma): (a) diffuse sheet of small lymphoid cells, some with plasmacytoid differentiation. (b) In lymphoplasmacytic lymphoma a periodic acid–Schiff (PAS) stain shows more marked plasma cell differentiation (centre) with an intranuclear inclusion (Dutcher body; these pink intranuclear inclusions are commonly encountered in lymphoplasmacytic lymphoma). Small scattered lymphocytes and lymphoplasmacytoid cells are also present. (c) Fine needle aspirate showing plasmacytic lymphoma. [(c) May-Grünwald–Giemsa stain.]

intranuclear inclusions (Dutcher bodies). It may also appear in the serum as a paraprotein, in which case the disease corresponds to Waldenström's macroglobulinaemia. Strong cytoplasmic IgM positivity can help to distinguish the disease from small lymphocytic neoplasms, as does the absence of CD5.

The disease is normally indolent, but may transform into an aggressive large cell lymphoma. Other B cell neoplasms (e.g. small lymphocytic lymphoma and MALT lymphoma) may show plasmacytoid differentiation, and a diagnosis of immunocytoma should only be made in cases that lack features of these other lymphomas.

Follicular lymphoma

Follicular lymphomas constitute, at least in the Western developed countries, one of the most frequent non-Hodgkin lymphomas, and it is clear that these are the neoplastic equivalent of normal germinal centres. This origin explains their title in the Kiel scheme of 'centroblastic–centrocytic' lymphoma. They are usually easy to recognize because of their follicular growth pattern (*Fig. 11.66*). The tumour cells are monoclonal and express either κ or λ light chains (*Fig. 11.67*). The tumour is graded I, II or III in the Working Formulation, but this was dropped in the REAL classification (*Fig. 11.59*). It is graded I or II in the WHO classification, according to the proportion of small and large cells. The cells occasionally transform into diffuse tumours that contain numerous large cells (centroblasts), and then fall into the group of 'large B cell lymphoma'. On occasion they may be found outside the lymphoid system. A rare cytological variant may contain numerous signet-ring cells (*Fig. 11.68*).

The (14;18) chromosomal translocation, present in two-thirds to three-quarters of cases, juxtaposes the BCL-2 gene to the Ig heavy chain gene, which is accompanied by expression of BCL-2 protein. This is in contrast to normal germinal centre B cells, which are BCL-2 negative (*see Fig. 11.56*). The disease is slowly progressive but essentially incurable.

Mantle cell lymphoma

Mantle cell lymphoma is the name now given to the tumour described by the Kiel group as 'centrocytic' lymphoma. It was argued that this tumour arose from germinal centres, and was related to follicular (centroblastic–centrocytic) lymphoma. However, it was noted even then that the tumour contains no centroblasts, and also shows other differences from follicular lymphoma, including an excess of male patients and frequent spread to blood and bone marrow.

Its pattern of antigenic expression is distinctive, as was first apparent more than 10 years ago. CD5 is commonly present (*Fig. 11.69*), but the disease differs from other CD5-positive B cell neoplasms (small lymphocytic lymphoma and/or leukaemia) in lacking CD23. Cyclin D1 expression is common and can be diagnostically valuable (*Fig. 11.69*).

The survival of cases of mantle cell lymphoma shows the steady fall characteristic of a relatively benign neoplasm (e.g. follicular lymphoma), reflecting a constant year-on-year mortality. However, the slope is steep, and there is little indication of a plateau, as seen in large cell lymphomas. More aggressive therapy is usually of little benefit and long-term survival is poor.

Mantle cell lymphoma is associated with a characteristic cytogenetic anomaly, the (11;14) reciprocal chromosomal translocation. This anomaly is present in the majority of cases and causes over-expression of the BCL-1 or PRAD 1 gene, which encodes cyclin D1 (*Fig. 11.69e*).

The disease usually presents with lymphadenopathy, but may be found at extranodal sites, notably the gastrointestinal tract (lymphomatous polyposis; *Fig. 11.70*). The neoplastic cells are usually of small-to-medium size and may have irregular or 'cleaved' nuclei (*Fig. 11.69; see also Fig. 11.30a*), or a more 'blastic' appearance (*Fig. 11.71*). The growth pattern is often nodular (*see Fig. 11.53*) and the neoplastic cells tend to 'home' to the mantle zones of lymphoid follicles.

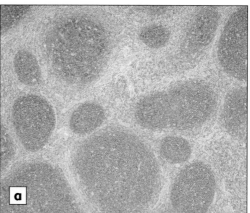
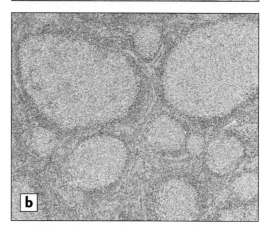

Fig. 11.66a and b Immunostaining of follicular lymphoma showing its typical nodular appearance: (a) CD20 is expressed by the tumour cells, whereas (b) CD3 is confined to reactive T cells. (Paraffin sections: APAAP immunoalkaline phosphatase stain.)

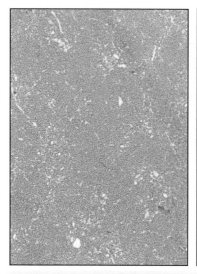
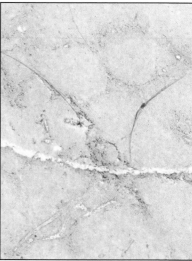

Fig. 11.67 Follicular lymphoma: tumour cells are monoclonal and express either κ or λ light chains. Here, APAAP immunoalkaline phosphatase stain for κ light chains shows a positive reaction, and a negative one for λ chains.

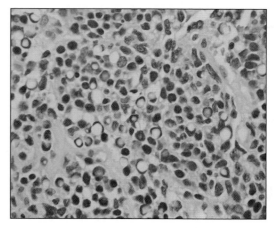

Fig. 11.68 Follicular lymphoma: rare signet-ring variant.

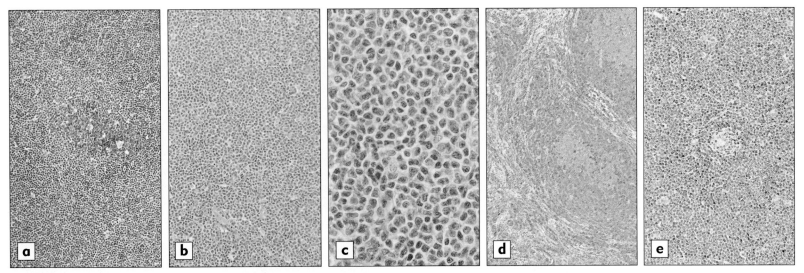

Fig. 11.69a–e Mantle cell lymphoma: (a) at low power the neoplasm is seen surrounding a naked reactive germinal centre, which gives a characteristic mantle zone distribution. (b) A medium power view shows diffuse growth pattern with some hyaline fibrosis around small vessels. (c) At high power irregular small lymphoid cells (small cleaved cells; centrocytes) typical of mantle cell lymphoma are seen. No large lymphoid cells are present (*see also Fig. 11.30*). (d) Immunoperoxidase stain for CD5 shows strong positivity. (e) Immunoperoxidase stain for cyclin D1 shows characteristic nuclear positivity.

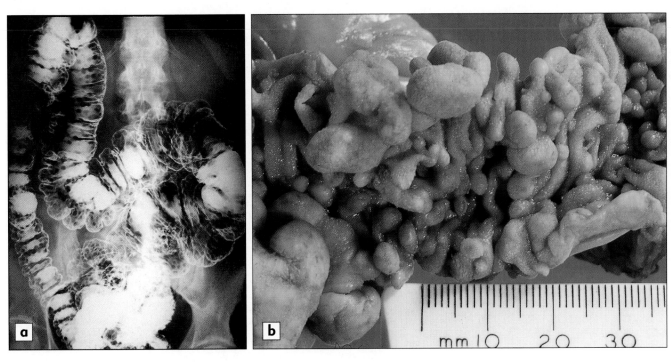

Fig. 11.70a and b Lymphomatous polyposis affecting the ileocaecal region: (a) barium study shows mucosal and mural involvement; (b) macroscopic appearances showing the presence of multiple mucosal polyps that range in size from a few millimetres to a few centimetres.

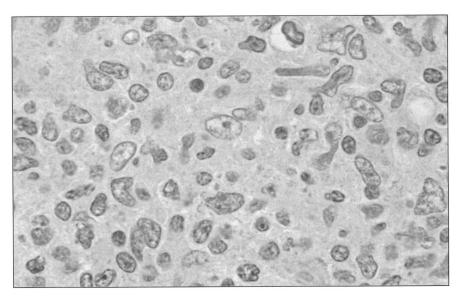

Fig. 11.71 Mantle cell lymphoma: large cells are seen with considerable nuclear pleomorphism and pale indistinct cytoplasm; the deformed nuclei have a light chromatin pattern and may contain nucleoli.

Marginal zone lymphomas

Marginal zone lymphomas are thought to represent the neoplastic equivalent of the marginal zone cells found in the spleen and lymph nodes, although, as in the case of mantle cell lymphoma, their origin is difficult to prove.

The only marginal zone neoplasm unequivocally recognized in the REAL scheme is 'MALT lymphoma'. This small cell lymphoma arises in the gastrointestinal tract (*Fig. 11.72*) or other extranodal sites (e.g. the skin, *Fig. 11.73*), glandular epithelial tissues (e.g. thyroid, bronchus and salivary glands; *Fig. 11.74*). These neoplasms derive from the B cells associated with epithelial tissues, and usually arise against a background of reactive lymphoid tissue, in which non-neoplastic germinal centres are prominent. Infection with *H. pylori* is thought to induce the lymphoid reaction in the stomach, and eradication of the infection may cause regression of the lymphoma.

When MALT lymphomas spread to mesenteric lymph nodes the appearance is often identical to that of the rare 'monocytoid B cell lymphoma' (*Fig. 11.75*). This latter disorder is a provisional entity in the REAL scheme and is said to arise from marginal zone B cells. The cell

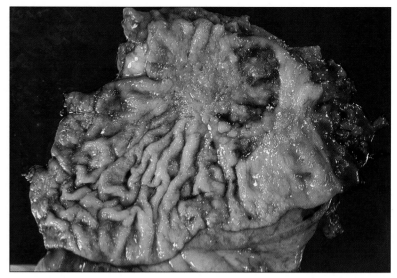

Fig. 11.72 Marginal zone lymphoma: partial gastrectomy specimen showing mucosal irregularity and lymphoma infiltration.

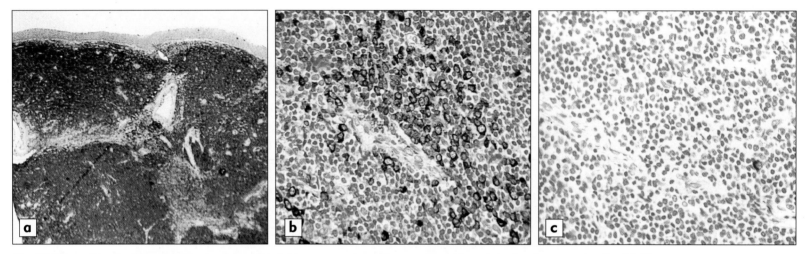

Fig. 11.73a–c Marginal zone lymphoma of the skin: (a) low-power view of immunoperoxidase stain showing extensive B cell infiltrate; (b, c) clonality of tumour cells (showing plasma cell differentiation) shown by (b) kappa positivity and (c) rare lambda positivity.

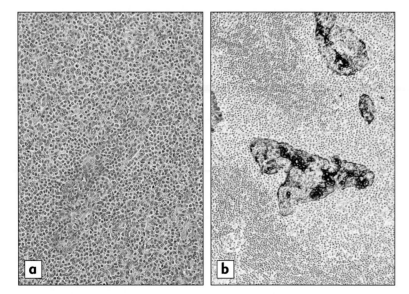

Fig. 11.74a and b Marginal zone lymphoma of salivary gland: (a) sheets of marginal zone B cells and formation of a lymphoepithelial lesion; (b) immunoperoxidase stain for low molecular weight cytokeratin (MNF116) shows positive staining of normal epithelial cells infiltrated by lymphoma.

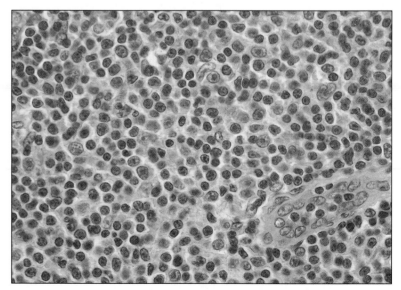

Fig. 11.75 Nodal marginal zone lymphoma (monocytoid B cell lymphoma): high power view of a lymph node shows an admixture of small-to-medium sized B cells with abundant clear cytoplasm and scanty, admixed, large transformed lymphoid cells. A venule with high endothelial cells is present, as typically encountered in this form of lymphoma.

morphology is sometimes, but by no means always, 'monocytoid'. This indolent neoplasm, in keeping with its putative normal counterpart, typically infiltrates lymph node sinuses.

Splenic marginal zone lymphoma was included in the REAL scheme as another provisional subtype of marginal zone lymphoma. However, although the evidence that this is a true clinicopathologic entity is now good, it is by no means certain that the neoplasm arises from marginal zone cells in the spleen. A major difference from marginal zone lymphoma of the MALT type is the high incidence of bone marrow disease at presentation. This disease corresponds to the rare form of chronic leukaemia known by haematologists as 'splenic lymphoma with villous lymphocytes' (see page 185).

Hairy cell leukaemia

Hairy cell leukaemia is characterized by cells with fine villous surface projections and bean-shaped nuclei, which are seen in the circulation, in the bone marrow and in the red pulp of the spleen (see page 183). The latter sites of involvement account for pancytopenia and marked splenomegaly. Lymph node infiltration is rare.

The cells express, in addition to typical B cell antigens, the receptor for interleukin 2 (CD25) and the CD103 integrin (a cell adhesion molecule). In paraffin sections a distinctive pattern of markers can be detected, and these may be of diagnostic value (e.g. when the marrow shows a low level of infiltration). In addition to pan-B markers such as CD20 and CD79a, the neoplastic cells often express CD68 (as cytoplasmic dots) and are labelled by antibody DBA.44. The disease tends to follow an indolent course.

Burkitt's lymphoma

Burkitt's lymphoma was first found in young African children and has an unusual predilection for massive jaw lesions (see Fig. 11.11), extranodal abdominal involvement and ovarian tumours (see Fig. 11.12). It is typically made up of medium-sized B cells with a high proliferation fraction interspersed with macrophages that contain cellular debris, which gives the characteristic 'starry sky' appearance (Fig. 11.76).

The immunophenotype is that of a peripheral B cell, although CD10 is also often present, which has prompted suggestions that it derives from germinal centre cells. In most 'endemic' African cases Epstein–Barr virus (EBV) viral DNA is found in the malignant cells. Histologically and phenotypically identical cases are also seen occasionally in the Western developed countries. These may arise in patients with acquired immunodeficiency virus, and EBV is detectable in almost half of these cases. Non-African 'sporadic' cases also arise in the absence of immune impairment, and EBV is detectable in less than a quarter of these cases.

Almost all cases, from whatever country, show a chromosomal translocation involving the c-MYC gene on chromosome 8 and the gene for the Ig heavy chain or, less commonly, one of the two Ig light chain genes (see Fig. 11.2). The disease may respond to aggressive therapy.

Diffuse large B cell lymphoma

The Kiel scheme postulated two categories of diffuse high grade B cell neoplasms: 'centroblastic lymphoma' and 'immunoblastic lymphoma'. However, no evidence for the validity of the distinction between 'centroblastic' and 'immunoblastic' lymphomas is convincing. It has been claimed that 'centroblastic' and 'immunoblastic' lymphomas show different survival curves, but this has not been confirmed in most studies. Furthermore, no specific chromosome or genetic changes can distinguish between these two diseases. Equally importantly, pathologists have difficulty in reproducibly distinguishing between the proposed subtypes.

'Diffuse large B cell lymphoma' was therefore introduced in the REAL scheme to combine the 'centroblastic' and 'immunoblastic' categories (Figs 11.77 and 11.78; see also Fig. 11.30b). It is one of the

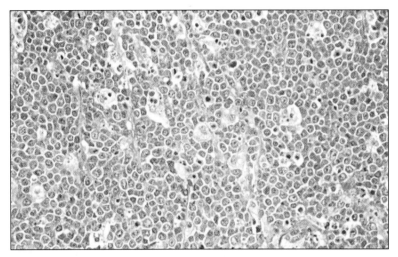

Fig. 11.76 Burkitt's lymphoma: section of lymph node showing sheets of lymphoblasts with prominent nuclear membranes and 'starry sky' tingible-body macrophages.

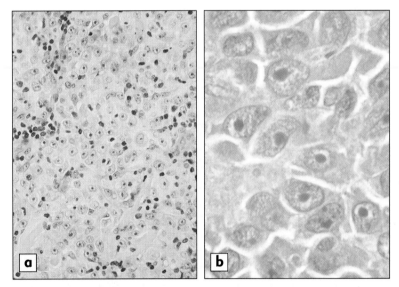

Fig. 11.77a and b Diffuse large B cell lymphoma: (a) large neoplastic cells with a single prominent central nucleolus and abundant, darkly staining cytoplasm; (b) at higher magnification, similar cells from another case showing immunoblastic cytology.

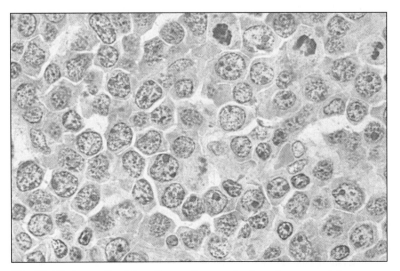

Fig. 11.78 Large B cell lymphoma: the neoplastic cells are much larger than normal lymphocytes and have a round nucleus with prominent nucleoli, many of which are adjacent to the nuclear membrane ('centroblasts'). A number of mitotic figures are seen.

most common categories of non-Hodgkin lymphoma. Pan-B cell markers are expressed, and in a minority of cases the (14;18) chromosomal translocation is present, which suggests an origin from follicular lymphoma. The disease usually requires aggressive treatment, but may respond well, at least for a period.

The REAL scheme recognizes primary mediastinal (thymic) lymphoma as a rare subtype of large B cell lymphoma. The neoplastic cells often have a characteristic pale cytoplasm and are thought to arise from intrathymic B cells.

Plasmacytoma and multiple myeloma

Plasma cells are the cells characteristic of multiple myeloma or plasmacytoma (see Chapter 12), the former term being used when the neoplasm is found in the bone marrow, causing skeletal destruction, and the latter for the rarer tumours that arise in soft tissue.

Generally, B cell surface antigens are absent, in keeping with their loss by normal mature plasma cells, but cytoplasmic Ig (of a single light chain type) is present, accompanied in about 50% of cases by CD79a, one of the two chains of the molecule associated with Ig in B cells. The chromosome abnormality associated with mantle cell lymphoma, the (11;14) translocation, is found in some cases.

Rare and provisional B cell entities

Lymphoma is a relatively rare disease – some entities are so uncommon that they are seen only occasionally even in specialist centres or are poorly

defined. These include intravascular large B cell lymphoma (*Fig. 11.79*), primary effusion B cell lymphoma, T cell rich B cell lymphoma (*Fig. 11.80*), anaplastic lymphoma kinase (ALK)-positive 'immunoblastic' B cell lymphoma, diffuse large cell lymphoma with anaplastic cytology (*Fig. 11.81*) and lymphomatoid granulomatosis (*Fig. 11.82*).

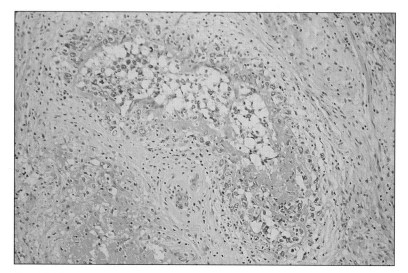

Fig. 11.79 Intravascular B cell lymphoma: section of cervix showing vascular distension by large lymphoid cells.

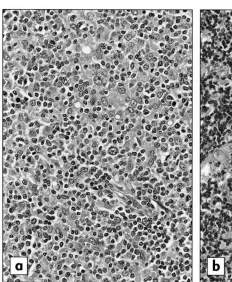 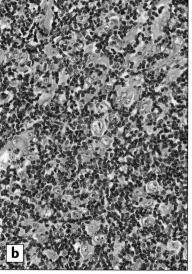 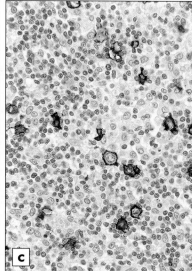

Fig. 11.80a–c T cell rich B cell lymphoma: (a) low-power view showing diffuse architecture with scattered large cells admixed with numerous small lymphocytes; (b) high-power view showing large blast cells with immunoblastic cytology; (c) immunostain for CD20 showing neoplastic large B cells.

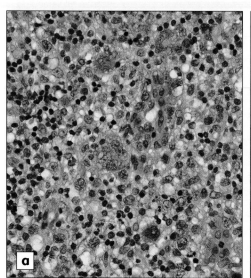 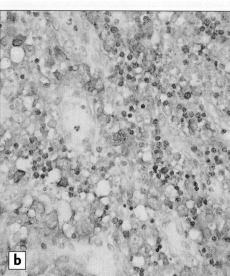

Fig. 11.81a and b Diffuse large B cell lymphoma with anaplastic cytology: (a) bizarre tumour cells infiltrating a lymph node; (b) showing CD30 surface antigen on tumour cells. (Immunoperoxidase stain.)

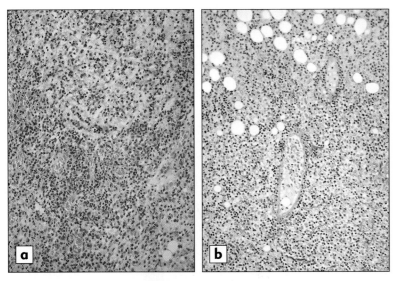

Fig. 11.82 Lymphomatoid granulomatosus: lung sections (a) showing prominent blood vessels with (b) thickened walls and areas of necrosis. (Elastic van Gieson stain; courtesy of Dr JE McLaughlin.)

T AND NK CELL NEOPLASMS

T and NK cell neoplasms differ, as do B cell tumours, in terms of the maturation stage from which they arise. However, there is also a greater degree of subdivision into different local populations (e.g. cutaneous T cells associated with the skin, gastrointestinal tract, etc.). As in the case of B cell neoplasms, those diseases diagnosed by haematologists rather than histopathologists (acute lymphoblastic, chronic lymphocytic and large granular lymphocytic leukaemia) are discussed in Chapters 8 and 10. The phenotype of T and NK cells is summarized in *Fig. 11.83*.

Precursor T cell acute lymphoblastic lymphoma and/or leukaemia
The morphology of lymphoblastic neoplasms of precursor T cell origin is usually indistinguishable from that of B cell lymphoblastic neoplasms. They typically present as acute leukaemias but occasionally give rise to tumours in the lymph node or thymus. T cell antigens are present although CD3, because of the immaturity of the cells, is usually only found in the cytoplasm. The disease is potentially curable with aggressive therapy.

Chronic T cell chronic lymphocytic leukaemia
T cell lymphomas of small lymphocytes resemble small lymphocytic B cell neoplasms in that they often involve the peripheral blood, and their morphology is similar. The nucleoli may be more prominent and the cytoplasm more abundant, so some cases would be classified haematologically as 'prolymphocytes' – this category includes cases that haematologists would categorize as T cell prolymphocytic leukaemia. However, debate as to whether there is a true distinction between prolymphocytic and chronic lymphocytic leukaemia of T cell origin is largely academic, given their rarity and the generally poor prognosis.

Unlike small lymphocytic B cell lymphoma, pseudofollicles that contain larger cells are not seen. These lymphomas express pan-T cell antigens and also CD7, and are commonly CD4 positive. The disease tends to follow a more aggressive course than do small lymphocytic B cell tumours.

Large granular lymphocytic leukaemia
Neoplasms that arise from 'large granular lymphocytes' can be subdivided, on the basis of phenotype, into those that arise from T cells and those that probably derive from NK cells. The former type is usually

Immunological phenotyping of T and NK cell lymphomas		
Neoplasm	**Immunophenotype**	
T lymphoblastic leukaemia and/or lymphoma	TdT	+
	CD1a	+/−
	CD3	+/−
	CD7	+
	CD4 ±	8 +
T cell chronic lymphocytic and/or prolymphocytic leukaemia	CD2, 3, 5, 7	+
	CD4	+
	CD8	−/+
Large granular lymphocytic leukaemia	CD2	+
	CD3, 8	+/−
	CD16	+
	CD56, 57	−/+
Mycosis fungoides and/or Sézary syndrome	CD2, 3, 4, 5	+
	CD7, 8, 25	−
Peripheral T cell lymphoma,	CD3	+/−
	Variable expression of other T cell markers	
Angioimmunoblastic T cell lymphoma	T cell phenotype; large follicular dendritic cell clusters around proliferating venules	
Angiocentric lymphoma	CD2, 56	+
	CD3	−/+
	CD5, 7	+/−
	CD4 or 8	+/−
Intestinal T cell lymphoma	CD3, 7	+
	CD8	+/−
	CD103 (MLA)	+
Adult T cell lymphoma and/or leukaemia	CD2, 3, 4, 5, 25	+
	CD7	−
Anaplastic large cell lymphoma	T or null phenotype	
	CD30	+
	EMA	+/−
	ALK	+/−

Fig. 11.83 T and NK cell lymphomas: immunological phenotyping.

indolent, and the prognosis is usually good, whereas patients with the NK cell type are usually younger with more acute symptoms and they have a poorer prognosis.

Mycosis fungoides and Sézary syndrome
Mycosis fungoides is a T cell lymphoma seen most commonly in the skin, but it is referred to as Sézary syndrome when the characteristic cells are also found in the circulation. The neoplastic cells accumulate in the epidermis, where they may form localized pockets, referred to as 'Pautrier's micro-abscesses' (*see Fig. 11.88*), and have a typical convoluted cerebriform nuclear morphology. The disease usually evolves through three stages:

- premycotic stage with lesions similar to eczema or psoriasis (*Fig. 11.84*);
- infiltrative or plaque stage (*Fig. 11.85*), sometimes with generalized exfoliative erythroderma (*Figs 11.86*) and invasion of the blood by typical convoluted neoplastic lymphoid cells (*see Figs 10.61–10.64*; the so-called Sézary syndrome); and
- nodular or tumour stage associated with deeper invasion by the tumour (*Fig. 11.87*) and infiltration of lymph nodes and other organs (*Fig. 11.88*).

The cells express pan-T cell antigens and are almost always of CD4 'helper' subtype (*Fig. 11.89*).

Peripheral T cell lymphoma, unspecified

Although a number of well defined categories of T cell neoplasia have come to be recognized over the years (e.g. mycosis fungoides or Sézary syndrome), many T cell tumours have none of the features of these subtypes. They were often referred to as 'pleomorphic' or 'polymorphic' T cell neoplasms, reflecting their wide variation in cell morphology. A revision of the Kiel scheme in 1987 defined two subtypes of pleomor-

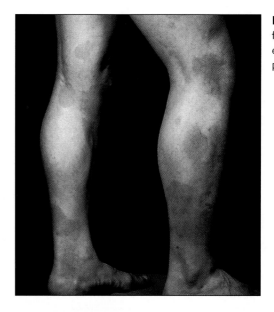

Fig. 11.84 Mycosis fungoides: typical eczematoid lesions at presentation.

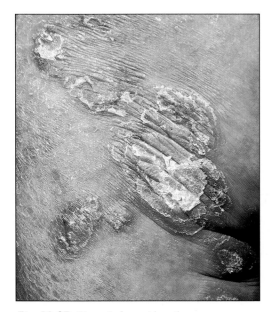

Fig. 11.85 Mycosis fungoides: these psoriasiform plaques appeared 6 months later (same patient as shown in *Fig. 11.84*).

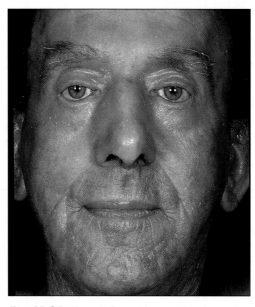

Fig. 11.86 Mycosis fungoides: erythroderma in advanced disease.

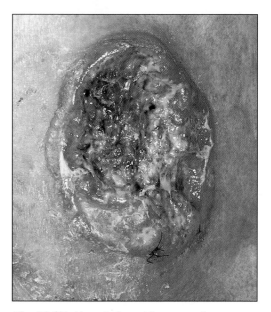

Fig. 11.87 Mycosis fungoides: extensive ulceration of the abdominal skin indicative of the invasive tumour stage.

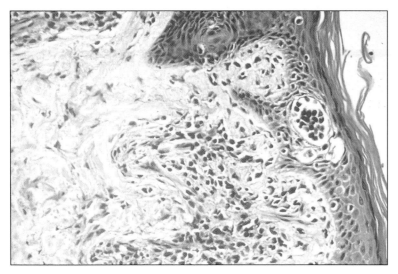

Fig. 11.88 Mycosis fungoides: typical histological pattern, showing a focal intraepidermal collection of abnormal lymphoid cells (Pautrier's abscess) and similar groups of tumour cells in the papillary dermis.

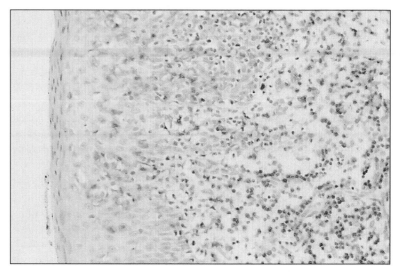

Fig. 11.89 Mycosis fungoides: malignant lymphoid cells in a skin biopsy show cytoplasmic positivity for the T cell marker CD45RO (antibody UCHL1; see *Fig. 11.52*). (Immunoperoxidase stain; courtesy of Dr JE McLaughlin.)

phic T cell neoplasms, one (of low grade) made up of small cells and the other (of high grade) containing medium and large lymphoma cells. A category of immunoblastic T cell neoplasia was also proposed. However, many pathologists found it difficult to apply this new aspect of the Kiel classification scheme to diagnostic samples. For this reason the REAL scheme created a single category of 'peripheral T cell lymphoma'. The word 'unspecified' was added to indicate that this category may comprise several entities.

These neoplasms typically contain a mixture of small and large neoplastic cells, often with irregular nuclei (Figs 11.90–11.93). There may be a marked infiltration of non-neoplastic cells, including macrophages and eosinophils. In some cases, clusters of epithelioid histiocytes, characteristic of so-called 'Lennert's' or lymphoepithelioid T cell lymphoma, are seen (Fig. 11.93). A variety of patterns of T cell antigen expression is found, CD4 being more frequent than CD8. Peripheral T cell lymphomas are for some reason seen with greater frequency in the Far East, than in Europe and the US where they account for <20% of non-Hodgkin lymphomas. The prognosis is very variable.

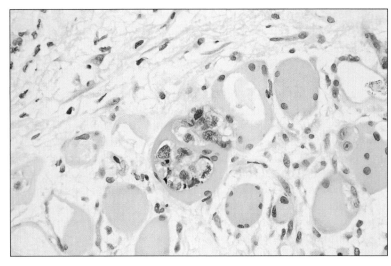

Fig. 11.90 Peripheral T cell lymphoma: neoplastic cells are invading striated muscle.

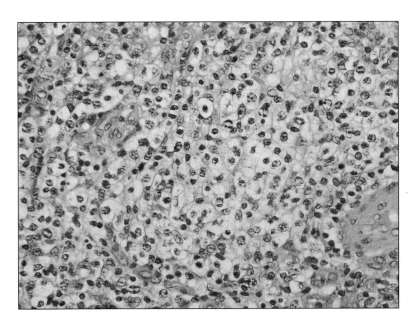

Fig. 11.91 Peripheral T cell lymphoma: high-power view of a peripheral T cell lymphoma of clear type showing a focus of neoplastic T cells with water-clear cytoplasm, which are commonly encountered in malignant lymphomas of peripheral T cell lineage.

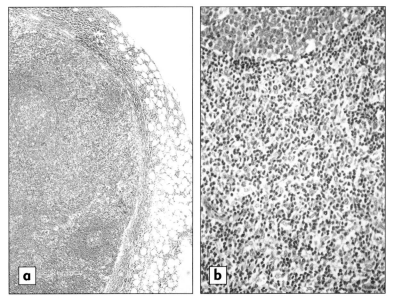

Fig. 11.92a and b Peripheral T cell lymphoma: (a) expansion of paracortical region with wide separation of germinal follicles; (b) high power shows many T lymphocytes with clear cytoplasm, eosinophils and prominent venules. This pattern is referred to as 'T-zone lymphoma' in the Kiel scheme but there is no evidence that it is an entity that can be differentiated from other peripheral T cell lymphomas. (Courtesy of Dr JE McLaughlin.)

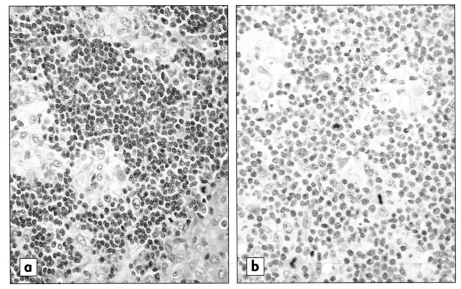

Fig. 11.93a and b Peripheral T cell lymphoma showing nodular accumulations of macrophages: (a, b) this appearance is given the title 'lymphoepithelioid lymphoma' in the Kiel scheme (and is also sometimes known as 'Lennert's lymphoma'), although no evidence indicates that this entity can be differentiated from other T cell lymphomas. Clumps of epithelioid cells are interspersed with a mixed population of small and large lymphocytes with occasional mitoses and large atypical cells that resemble Reed–Sternberg cells. The small cells show irregular angular nuclei. The tumour T cells are thought to produce lymphokines that cause epithelioid cell formation from histiocytes. [(a, b) Courtesy of Dr JE McLaughlin.]

T/NK nasal-type (angiocentric) lymphoma

A feature of angiocentric lymphoma, which is also referred to as 'nasal' or 'nasal-type' lymphoma (*Fig. 11.94*), is a tendency to invade the walls of blood vessels, accompanied in many cases by blockage of vessels by lymphoma cells, often associated with ischaemic necrosis of normal and neoplastic tissue (*Fig. 11.95*). The cell morphology is very variable, and admixed inflammatory cells may cause difficulty in diagnosing early cases. EBV is almost always present in the neoplastic cells (*Fig. 11.96*). The neoplastic cells are probably of NK cell rather than T cell origin: surface CD3 is absent in many cases (although cytoplasmic CD3 epsilon chain is present) and CD56 is often expressed (*Fig. 11.97*).

The disease is rare in the US and Europe, but is much more common in Asia and often involves the nose, palate and skin, but other soft tissues may also be involved. The distinction from Asian neoplasms of large granular lymphocytes is not always clear. The clinical course ranges from indolent to aggressive.

Intestinal- and/or enteropathy-associated T cell lymphoma

Small intestinal lymphomas have long been recognized as a complication of gluten-induced enteropathy (coeliac disease). They were first thought to be a heterogeneous group of tumours, but later studies suggested a histiocytic origin. In the early 1980s it became clear that they were T cell lymphomas of widely varying morphology.

This neoplasm is often associated with small bowel ulceration. The typical histological features of coeliac disease, though often present, may be absent because of the phenomenon of 'latency' recently recognized in coeliac patients. In keeping with this, some patients have a history of documented coeliac disease (*Figs 11.98–11.100*) while others present with the lymphoma. The neoplastic cells express pan-T cell markers (*Fig. 11.99*) and, in most cases, the CD103 integrin molecule found on normal intestinal T lymphocytes. The clinical outlook is poor since the neoplasm is frequently multifocal.

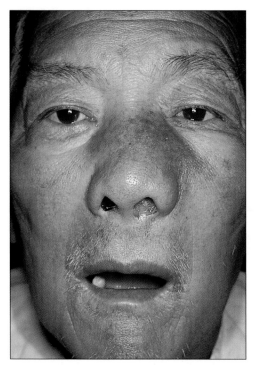

Fig. 11.94 T/NK nasal type (angiocentric) lymphoma: mid line nasal swelling. (Courtesy of Dr Liang.)

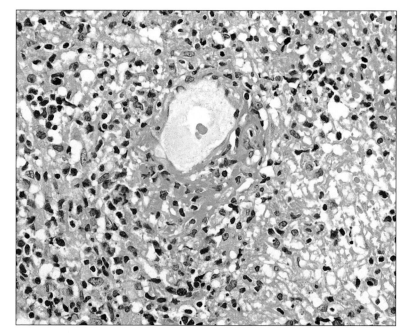

Fig. 11.95 T/NK nasal type (angiocentric) lymphoma: typical lesion with angiocentricity and marked necrosis. (Courtesy of Dr Liang.)

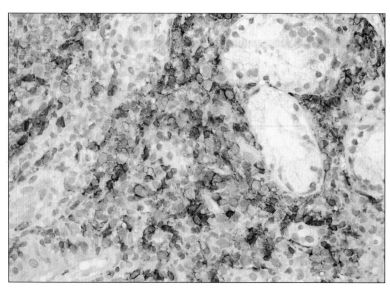

Fig. 11.96 T/NK nasal type (angiocentric) lymphoma: positive immunoperoxidase stain for EBER. (Courtesy of Dr Liang.)

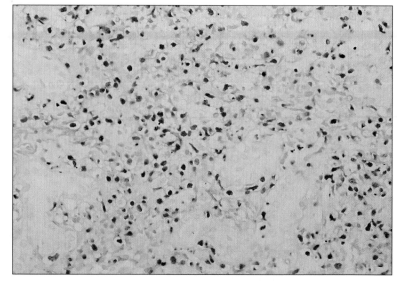

Fig. 11.97 T/NK nasal type (angiocentric) lymphoma: positive immunoperoxidase stain for CD56. (Courtesy of Dr Liang.)

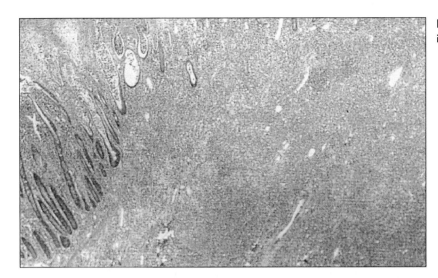

Fig. 11.98 Enteropathy-associated T cell lymphoma: ulceration of small intestinal mucosa and infiltration into the smooth muscle below.

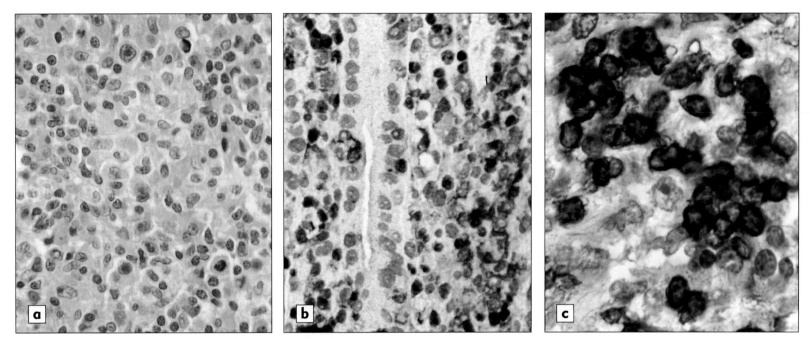

Fig. 11.99a–c Enteropathy-associated T cell lymphoma: (a) high-power view showing pleomorphic and polymorphic infiltration of lymphoid cells; (b, c) APAAP immunoalkaline phosphatase stain shows that some but not all of the neoplastic cells express CD3.

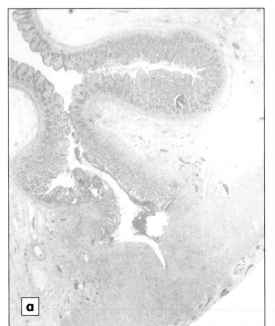

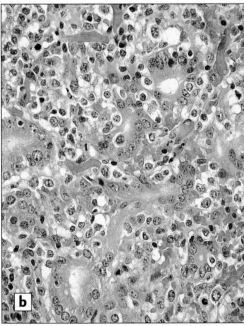

Fig. 11.100a and b Enteropathy-associated T cell lymphoma: (a) deep fissure formation and a flat small intestinal mucosa; (b) infiltration of small intestinal crypts by neoplastic cells.

Other peripheral T cell lymphomas

Other peripheral T cell lymphomas include subcutaneous panniculitis-like T cell lymphoma (*Fig. 11.101*) and hepatosplenic γ/δ T cell lymphoma (*Fig. 11.102*).

Angioimmunoblastic lymphadenopathy

Angioimmunoblastic T cell lymphoma was initially thought of as an abnormal immune reaction, but is now considered as a category of peripheral T cell lymphoma in which the neoplastic cells are mixed with and obscured by a complex histological picture that includes proliferating vessels, epithelioid histiocytes, plasma cells, eosinophils and hyperplastic clusters of follicular dendritic cells (*Figs 11.103 and 11.104*). The neoplastic cells are of variable morphology and include atypical 'clear' cells with indented nuclei and abundant pale cytoplasm. The cells carry T cell markers and are usually CD4 positive.

Patients often have systemic symptoms such as weight loss, fever, skin rash (*Fig. 11.105*) and a polyclonal hypergammaglobulinaemia. The disease is moderately aggressive and a high-grade lymphoma (usually of T but occasionally of B cell type) may emerge.

Adult T cell leukaemia/lymphoma

In the 1970s, an unusual T cell neoplasm was reported in southwest Japan which was subsequently shown to be confined to patients infected with the HTLV-1 retrovirus (see page 191). Identical cases were then found in other areas of HTLV-1 infection, notably the Caribbean.

The lymph node is diffusely replaced by neoplastic T cells, which vary widely in cell size and regularity, and neoplastic cells may also be seen in the peripheral blood (see Chapter 10). Patients often have aggressive disease, associated with lytic bone lesions, and hypercalcaemia, but the course is very variable, and indolent or smouldering cases are seen.

Anaplastic large cell lymphoma

In the 1980s, a monoclonal antibody ('Ki-1') raised against a Hodgkin cell line was found to react with the tumour cells in a group of non-Hodgkin large cell lymphomas. These neoplasms tended to share unusual morphological features (cohesive 'pseudo-carcinomatous' growth pattern, sinusoidal invasion, large bizarre cells), and the term 'anaplastic large cell lymphoma' was coined (*Fig. 11.106*). The (2;5)(q23;q35) chromosomal translocation was subsequently found to be associated

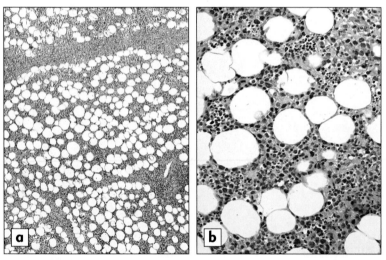

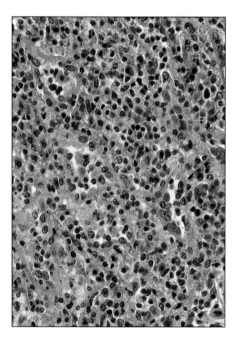

Fig. 11.102 Hepatosplenic γ/δ T cell lymphoma: infiltration of splenic pulp cords by medium-sized lymphoma cells. The cells showed clonal T cell receptor γ and δ rearrangements.

Fig. 11.101a and b Subcutaneous panniculitis-like T cell lymphoma: (a) low-power view showing lymphomatous infiltration between fat cells; (b) lymphomatous infiltration between fat cells with areas of apoptosis by lymphoma cells.

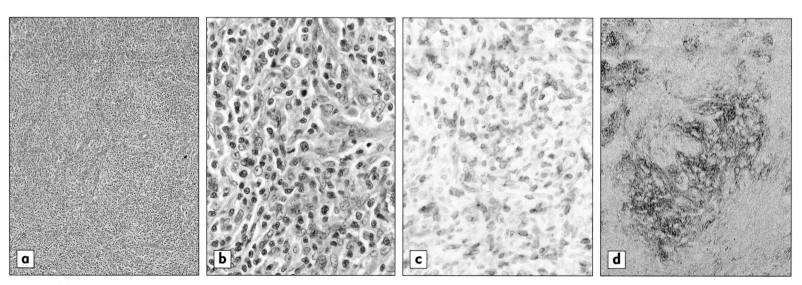

Fig. 11.103a–d T cell lymphoma: angioimmunoblastic lymphadenopathy type. (a) Low-power view showing prominent arborizing vascular pattern. (b) High-power view showing clear cell cytology of the neoplastic T cells. (c) Immunoperoxidase stain for CD3 showing positive staining of neoplastic T cells. (d) Immunoperoxidase stain for CD21 showing perivascular proliferation of follicular dendritic cells.

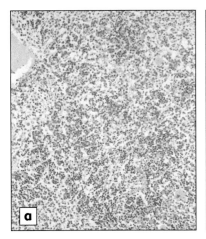

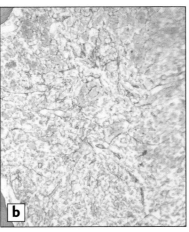

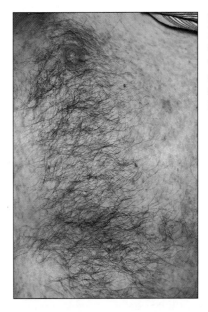

Fig. 11.105 Angioimmunoblastic lymphadenopathy: skin appearances of a 65-year-old man who presented with fever, an erythematous rash and lymphadenopathy, and who subsequently died of an overt lymphoma.

Fig. 11.104a and b Angioimmunoblastic lymphadenopathy: bone marrow trephine biopsy shows (a) extensive replacement of haemopoietic cells by abnormal lymphoid tissue, and (b) silver impregnation staining outlines the characteristic arborizing vascular pattern of the condition.

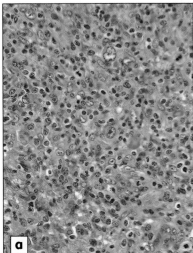

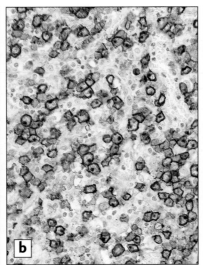

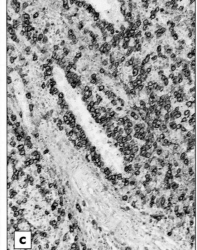

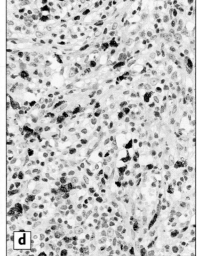

Fig. 11.106a–d Anaplastic large cell lymphoma, T or null cell type: (a) high-power view showing typical cytological features with large cells with prominent nucleoli, abundant cytoplasm and prominent Golgi zones; (b) immunoperoxidase stain for CD30 showing membrane and Golgi staining; (c) immunoperoxidase stain for CD30 showing perivascular accumulation of tumour cells; (d) immunoperoxidase stain for ALK-1 showing nuclear positivity in tumour cells.

with these lymphomas. This translocation creates the NPM-ALK fusion gene, encoding a hybrid tyrosine kinase. Variant translocations include t(1;2), t(2;3) and t(2;22, all of which are ALK positive.

It now appears that a distinct T or null cell lymphoma can be defined on the basis of NPM-ALK expression (*see Fig. 11.3*). Many cases express cytotoxic T cell markers, and B cell markers are not found. Patients tend to be children or young adults and chemotherapy is often curative. The term 'anaplastic large cell lymphoma' should be used, on the basis of current knowledge, for ALK-positive T or null cell lymphomas and for rare non-B cell ALK-negative cases with similar morphology (which express CD30 and EMA; *Fig. 11.106*).

The REAL classification does not include B cell neoplasms within the anaplastic large cell category and such tumours are probably diffuse large cell lymphomas (usually with a poorer prognosis than for ALK-positive tumours).

TREATMENT OF NON-HODGKIN LYMPHOMA

The Kiel scheme attempted to assist the clinician by dividing non-Hodgkin lymphoma into 'high-grade' and 'low-grade' categories. This tended to correlate with histology – most 'low-grade' neoplasms, associated with a good prognosis, were small cell tumours, whereas 'high-grade' neoplasms,

with a poorer outlook, were made up of large cells. The Working Formulation continued this idea of prognostic grading, but added a third 'intermediate' category.

With more recent experience it has become evident that each category of non-Hodgkin lymphoma tends to follow its own pattern of behaviour. There are exceptions to the 'small cell equals good, large cell equals bad' rule; for example mantle cell lymphoma carries a poor prognosis, despite being made up of small cells, whereas the tumour type containing the most aggressive and largest cells (anaplastic large cell lymphoma) is often curable (and may even rarely undergo spontaneous regression). It appears that those expressing genes characteristic of germinal centres have a far better prognosis than those expressing genes characteristic of activated peripheral blood lymphocytes. The REAL scheme does not categorize tumours into high- and low-grade neoplasms. However, the number of possible treatment options for non-Hodgkin lymphoma does not match the number of histological categories. Furthermore, many subtypes are rare (i.e. large B cell lymphoma and follicular lymphoma together account for about two thirds of all cases in Western developed countries), so clinical trials for some entities are difficult. For these reasons oncologists still tend to maintain a distinction between high-grade neoplasms, for which multidrug therapy is needed, and low-grade tumours that require less aggressive therapy.

Low-grade tumours

Optimal therapy for patients with non-Hodgkin lymphoma of 'favourable' histology is unclear and is palliative rather than curative. Some patients, particularly those with small lymphocytic lymphoma and/or leukaemia, may require no initial treatment. For those with localized Stage I or II disease local radiotherapy may produce disease-free survival at 5 years of up to 50%. Single alkylating agents, such as chlorambucil, are used if there are symptoms of advancing disease, and combination chemotherapy may be needed in later stages. Trials of α-interferon are in progress. Fludarabine (given alone or in combination with cyclophosphamide or with mitozantrone and dexamethasone) and 2-chlorodeoxyadenosine are newer drugs of value and deoxycoformycin has also proved of value in T cell lymphomas and some low-grade B cell lymphomas. The value of courses of intensive therapy followed by autologous stem cell transplantation after high-dose therapy is being explored.

High-grade neoplasms

Paradoxically, a greater potential for cure has been shown in large cell lymphomas than for the more indolent but usually incurable tumours such as follicular lymphoma. The best results are obtained with multiple cycles of intensive chemotherapy, using combinations of, for example, doxorubicin, cyclophosphamide, vincristine and corticosteroids (CHOP) initially. Other useful drugs include etoposide, bleomycin, mitozantrone, platinum, methotrexate and cytosine arabinoside. Autologous bone marrow (or peripheral blood stem cell) transplantation

International Prognostic Index	
Factor	**Adverse prognosis**
Age	≥60 years
Ann Arbor Stage	III or IV
Serum lactate dehydrogenase	Above normal
Number of extranodal sites	≥2
Performance status	ECOG 2 or equivalent

Fig. 11.107 International Prognostic Index. (Adapted with permission from The International Non-Hodgkin Lymphoma Prognostic Factors Project. A predictive model for aggressive non-Hodgkin lymphoma. *N Engl J Med.* 1993;329;987–94.)

after high-dose chemotherapy is used particularly in patients in second remission and for whom relapse is likely without further intensification of therapy. Haemopoietic growth factors (e.g. G-CSF or GM-CSF) may be used to accelerate myeloid recovery. Occasional patients with truly localized high-grade tumours are cured by high-dose radiotherapy with, for example, three cycles of CHOP.

Burkitt's lymphoma and lymphoblastic lymphoma

These patients tend to be treated with cyclical intensive chemotherapy programmes similar to those used to treat acute lymphoblastic lymphoma. Burkitt's lymphoma and B acute lymphoblastic leukaemia are now treated with different regimens using high-dose cytosine arabinoside and methotrexate as well as cyclophosphamide, etoposide, vincristine, vinblastine, anthracyclines and corticosteroids.

Histological grading and prognostic markers

Several attempts have been made to identify cell characteristics that enable subdivision of lymphomas into different prognostic categories. For example, it is well recognized that the relative proportions of large and small neoplastic cells (centroblasts and centrocytes, respectively) in follicular lymphomas differs from case to case. This has prompted attempts to correlate these histological features with clinical outcome and to 'grade' cases on the basis of percentage of large cells. However, it is now accepted that this assessment is highly subjective, and also there may be variability within a single biopsy. In consequence both the feasibility and the clinical relevance of histological grading in follicular lymphoma remains unclear, and so it is not incorporated into the REAL scheme. Two grades are recognized in the WHO scheme (*see Fig. 11.58*).

Also, evidence from several studies indicates that patients with diffuse large-cell non-Hodgkin lymphomas of T cell type fare worse than those with lymphomas of B cell origin, and this appears to be independent of other factors (e.g. the International Prognostic Index, *Fig. 11.107*).

Unclassified and reactive lymphoproliferative disorders

A number of rare or atypical lymphoid lesions, often of uncertain origin, fall outside the scope of this chapter. However, mention may be made of Castleman's disease (angiofollicular hyperplasia), since it is far from uncommon. This lymphoproliferative disorder typically affects mediastinal or axillary lymph nodes. In the hyaline vascular variant there are increased reactive follicles with prominent hyalinized central arterioles and whorls of mantle lymphocytes (*Fig. 11.108*). Patients with this

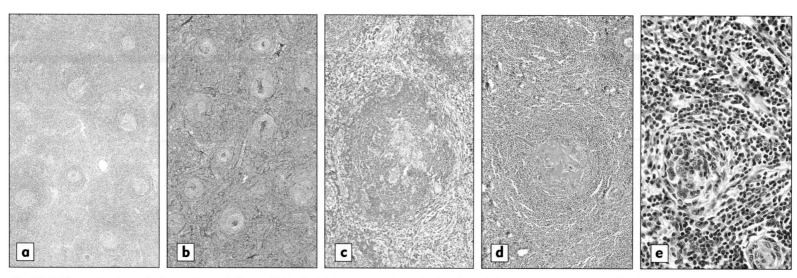

Fig. 11.108a–e Castleman's disease (angiofollicular hyperplasia): low-power views of a lymph node biopsy show increased follicular centres with prominent central arterioles and whorls of mantle lymphocytes in sections stained using (a) H&E and (b) silver impregnation for reticulin. (c) At higher power, prominent vascular proliferation in the centre of a follicle, (d) extensive hyalinization of central vessels and (e) whorling of mantle lymphocytes are seen. [(e) courtesy of Dr JE McLaughlin.]

variant are typically asymptomatic with localized disease that does not recur after surgical excision. In the rarer plasma cell type in which a marked increase in interfollicular plasma cells occurs (*Fig. 11.109*), the disease is usually multicentric and progressive with associated fever, weight loss, anaemia, neutropenia and thrombocytopenia. There may be bone marrow plasmacytosis and polyclonal gammaglobulinaemia, with frequent evolution to either malignant lymphoma or Kaposi's sarcoma.

True histiocytic lymphomas and other histiocytic proliferations

In the original Rappaport classification, 'histiocytic lymphoma' was a major class and included lymphomas made up of large cells with moderate or abundant cytoplasm and oval or round nuclei. However, subsequent studies showed that the vast majority of these tumours are diffuse large lymphoid cell neoplasms, most commonly of B cell origin, but including such T cell entities as peripheral T cell lymphomas (which contain many large cells), enteropathy-associated lymphoma and anaplastic large cell lymphoma. A rare example of dendritic cell sarcoma is shown in *Fig. 11.110*. Histiocytic medullary reticulosis was a term used to describe a disseminated malignant lymphoma with haemolytic anaemia resulting from phagocytosis of red cells by the tumour cells (*Fig. 11.111*). It is now known to be a poorly differentiated B cell lymphoma.

Monocytic leukaemia

The most frequently encountered tumours that arise from the monocyte–phagocyte system are tissue deposits of monocytic leukaemia (M5 variant of acute myeloid leukaemia), and these may mimic T cell lymphomas in their pattern of involvement of lymph nodes. The liver and spleen may also be involved. A rare example of monocytic (histiocytic) sarcoma of the bone marrow is illustrated in *Fig. 11.112*. Monocytic leukaemias are discussed in more detail in Chapters 8 and 10 and the classification of histiocytic disorders is given in *Fig. 7.34*.

HODGKIN LYMPHOMA (HODGKIN'S DISEASE)

Hodgkin lymphoma is one of the most common categories of lymphoid neoplasia and is closely related to the other malignant lymphomas.

Presentation and evolution

In many patients the disease at presentation is localized to a single peripheral lymph node region and studies of its natural history indicate that its subsequent progression is initially by direct contiguity within the lymphatic system.

With advanced disease, dissemination involves non-lymphatic tissue. The disease affects all age groups, but is particularly common in young and middle-aged adults. Most patients present with a painless, asymmetrical, firm and discrete enlargement of the superficial

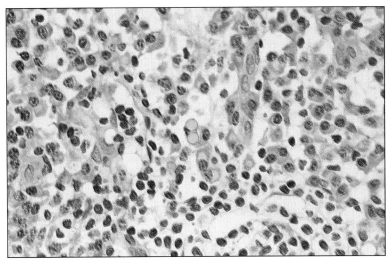

Fig. 11.109 Castleman's disease (angiofollicular hyperplasia), plasma cell variant: high-power view showing plasma cells, many of which contain Russell bodies; other fields showed typical follicular hyalinization.

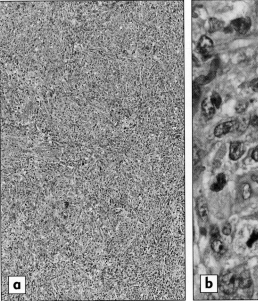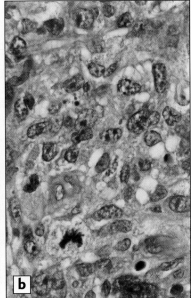

Fig. 11.110a and b Dendritic cell sarcoma: (a) lymph node biopsy showing complete replacement of normal architecture by pleomorphic oval and spindle-shaped cells with some areas showing a storiform ('cartwheel') appearance; (b) at higher magnification, the cells show irregular vesicular nuclei and pale cytoplasm within distinct borders. A prominent mitotic figure is seen here. Immunostaining was not carried out.

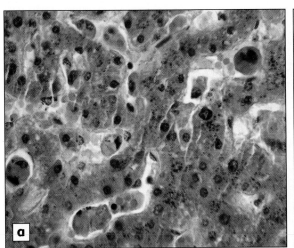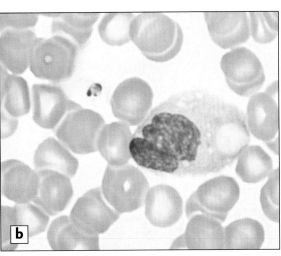

Fig. 11.111a and b 'Histiocytic medullary reticulosis': (a) liver biopsy showing Kupffer cell erythrophagocytosis; (b) peripheral blood film showing phagocytosed red cell in the cytoplasm of a monocyte. Tumours with this clinical and histological appearance are usually poorly differentiated B cell lymphomas.

lymph nodes (*Figs. 11.113 and 11.114*). Mediastinal disease, occasionally accompanied by an obstructed superior vena cava (*Fig. 11.115*), and involvement of retroperitoneal lymph nodes may be detected during staging procedures. Clinical splenomegaly occurs during the course of the disease in 50% of patients. Rarely, patients may present with lymphatic obstruction (*Fig. 11.116*).

The disease may involve the liver, skin (*Fig. 11.117*) and other organs, for example the gastrointestinal tract or brain and, in rare patients, the retina (*Fig. 11.118*). Depressed cell-mediated immunity is also present and is associated with an increased incidence of infections, particularly herpes zoster (*Fig. 11.119*), fungal diseases and tuberculosis.

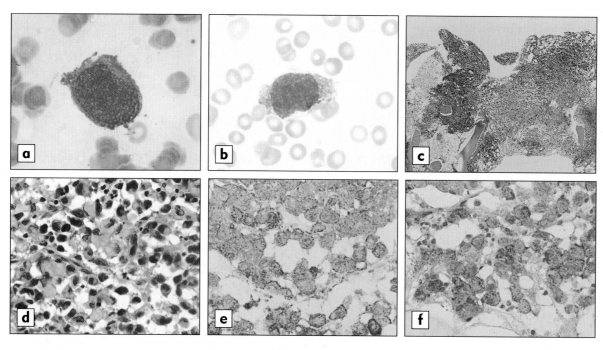

Fig. 11.112a–f Monocytic sarcoma: (a, b) two examples of the large atypical monocytoid cells in peripheral blood; (c) trephine biopsy showing extensive replacement of haemopoietic tissue and fat by tumour; (d) at higher magnification the atypical monocytoid cells are pleomorphic with hyperchromic nuclei and abundant cytoplasm, which in some cells show vacuolation. (e) Immunoperoxidase staining shows cytoplasmic positivity for CD68 and (f) lysozyme; the cells are also positive for CD45. [(a–f) Courtesy of Prof. PG Isaacson.]

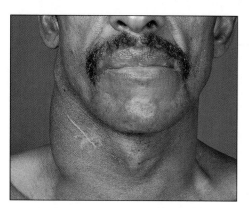

Fig. 11.113 Hodgkin lymphoma: right-sided cervical lymphadenopathy. The scar of previous biopsy incision is well healed.

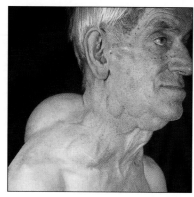

Fig. 11.114 Hodgkin lymphoma: massive cervical lymphadenopathy in a 73-year-old man who presented with extensive disease.

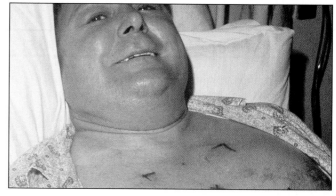

Fig. 11.115 Hodgkin lymphoma: cyanosis and oedema of the face, neck and upper trunk result from superior vena cava obstruction caused by mediastinal node involvement. The skin markings over the anterior chest indicate the field of radiotherapy.

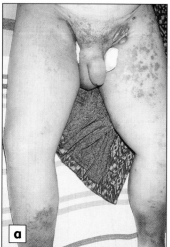

Fig. 11.116a and b Hodgkin lymphoma: (a) gross oedema of the legs, genitals and lower abdominal wall with umbilical herniation caused by lymphatic obstruction that resulted from extensive involvement of the inguinal and pelvic lymph nodes. A staphylococcal infection in the skin folds of the groins is present. (b) A close-up view of 'pitting' oedema of the abdominal wall is shown.

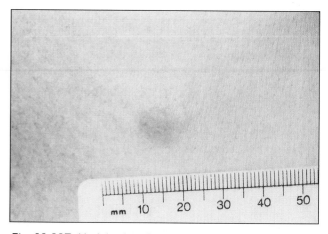

Fig. 11.117 Hodgkin lymphoma: a skin deposit approximately 1 cm in diameter is shown.

Occasionally the first indication of Hodgkin lymphoma follows fine needle aspiration of enlarged nodes (*Figs 11.120* & *11.121*). The diagnosis is usually made from histological examination of excised lymph nodes. The affected nodes are enlarged and show pale translucent cut surfaces (*Fig. 11.122*). Initially the nodes remain discrete, but later in the disease, they become matted together and there may be invasion of surrounding tissues. Hodgkin tissue in other organs has a similar pale, flesh-like appearance (*Fig. 11.123*).

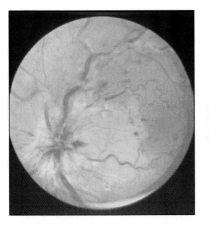

Fig. 11.118 Hodgkin lymphoma: extensive infiltration of the optic disc and surrounding retina.

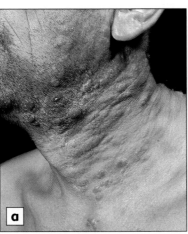

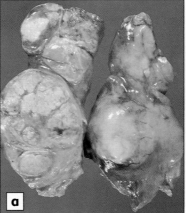

Fig. 11.119a and b Hodgkin lymphoma: (a) vesicular cutaneous eruption of the neck caused by herpes zoster; (b) atypical herpetic eruption of the palmar surface of the hand.

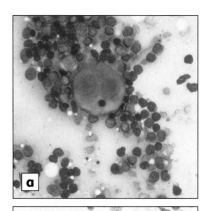

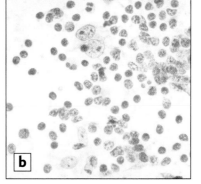

Fig. 11.120a and b Hodgkin lymphoma: fine needle aspirates of involved lymph nodes showing Reed–Sternberg cells stained by (a) May-Grünwald–Giemsa and (b) Papanicolaou techniques.

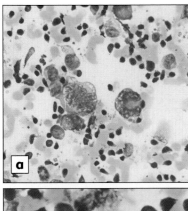
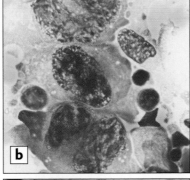
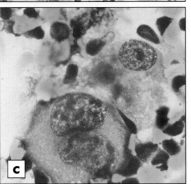
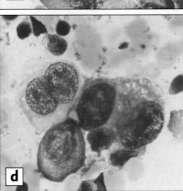

Fig. 11.121a–d Hodgkin lymphoma: (a) fine needle aspirate of lymph node showing Reed–Sternberg cells, a mitotic figure, histiocytes and lymphoid cells; (b–d) at higher magnification, further Reed–Sternberg cells from the same fine needle aspirate.

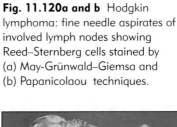
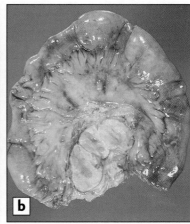

Fig. 11.122a and b Hodgkin lymphoma: (a) matted block of resected involved cervical nodes showing a cross-section of the pale, translucent, fleshy tumour tissue with areas of fibrosis and necrosis; (b) para-aortic lymph nodes removed at necropsy showing in cross-section the typical moist 'fish-flesh' appearance of this tumour.

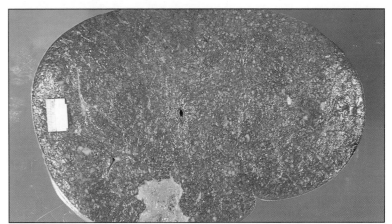

Fig. 11.123 Hodgkin lymphoma: cross-section of a spleen removed at laparotomy shows a single large Hodgkin deposit adjacent to the capsule. Numerous scattered focal greyish-yellow areas up to 4 mm in diameter are also present.

Histology

Hodgkin lymphoma is characterized by the presence of Reed–Sternberg cells, which are multinucleated cells, typically with prominent nucleoli and abundant violaceous cytoplasm (at least as seen in routine H & E stains; *Figs. 11.124–11.126*). The diagnosis of Hodgkin lymphoma is made when Reed–Sternberg cells are found against a background of lymphocytes, histiocytes, neutrophils and eosinophils (*Figs 11.125 and 11.126*), which distinguishes the disease from other conditions in which Reed–Sternberg cells may be found (viral infections, drug reactions, non-Hodgkin lymphomas).

Cell of origin

The malignant cells of Hodgkin lymphoma have a unique phenotype, being positive for CD15, CD30 and CD40, but negative for CD45 and all T cell markers. In about 60% of Hodgkin lymphoma cases, B cell markers (e.g. CD20) are expressed in a minority of the Reed–Sternberg cells, and in the lymphocytic predominant forms, B cell markers are expressed on all the tumour cells. Fascin antigen is expressed in the majority of cases; this antigen is a 55 kDa actin-bundling protein normally expressed in spleen and brain, but absent from normal B or T cells. Polymerase chain reaction tests for EBV have been reported positive in 30 to 70% of cases. Usually clonal rearrangement of Ig genes can be detected; occasionally, T cell receptor genes are clonally rearranged.

Classical Hodgkin lymphoma cells have a unique phenotype (*Fig. 11.127*), usually being positive for both CD15 and CD30 (*Fig. 11.128*).

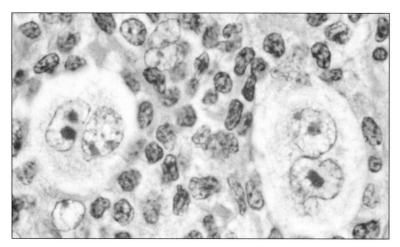

Fig. 11.124 Hodgkin lymphoma: high-power view of lymph node biopsy showing two typical multinucleate Reed–Sternberg cells surrounded by lymphocytes.

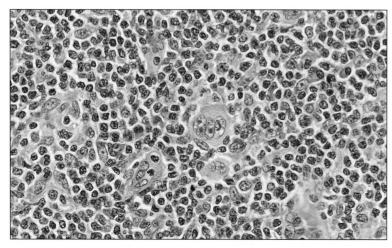

Fig. 11.125 Hodgkin lymphoma: lymph node biopsy showing multinucleate Reed–Sternberg cells surrounded by lymphocytes, histiocytes, neutrophils and eosinophils.

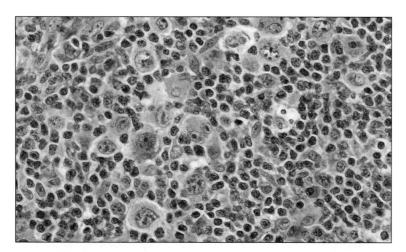

Fig. 11.126 Hodgkin lymphoma: lymph node biopsy showing multiple Reed–Sternberg cells surrounded by lymphocytes and other mononuclear cells in mixed cellularity disease.

Comparison of classic Reed–Sternberg cells with typical lymphocytic (L) and histiocytic (H) cells of lymphocyte predominance		
Marker classic	**Reed–Sternberg cells**	**L and H cells**
CD15	Usually positive	Usually negative*
CD20	Occasionally positive	Usually positive
Other B cell antigens (CD 19 and CD 22)	Rarely positive	Frequently positive
CD30 (Ki-1)	Positive	Sometimes positive [staining of this antigen in L and H cells is often seen only in frozen sections (i.e. not in paraffin material) and even then may be weak or negative]
CD45 (leucocyte common antigen)	Usually negative	Often positive
CD74 and CDw75 (LN2 and LN1, respectively)	Usually negative	Often positive
Epithelial membrane antigen	Usually negative	Often positive
Ig	Polytypic (i.e. for both κ and λ light chains, or negative, resulting from passive absorption of tissue fluid Ig)	Negative or monotypic
J chain	Negative	Positive
Epstein–Barr virus genome	Frequently positive	Infrequently positive

*There is evidence that this negative reaction is caused by sialylation of the CD15 hapten in L and H cells.

Fig. 11.127 Hodgkin lymphoma: comparison of classic Reed–Sternberg cells with typical lymphocytic (L) and histiocytic (H) cells of lymphocyte predominance.

It is now clear that in many cases a percentage of the abnormal cells also express B cell antigens, most commonly CD20 but occasionally others also, such as CD79a. This correlates with a growing body of evidence [from molecular biological studies of immunoglobulin (Ig) gene sequences in Reed–Sternberg cells] that they arise, at least in some cases, from germinal centre B cells.

Classification of Hodgkin lymphoma

The Rye classification (1966) defined four subtypes of Hodgkin lymphoma: lymphocyte predominance, nodular sclerosing, mixed cellularity and lymphocyte depleted (*Fig. 11.129*). It is now generally agreed that only the nodular sclerosing and mixed cellularity subtypes definitely fulfil the 'classic' criteria for Hodgkin lymphoma and are therefore recognized as such by and WHO classifications.

Nodular sclerosing Hodgkin lymphoma

Nodular sclerosing Hodgkin lymphoma is a nodular proliferation of Hodgkin lymphoma surrounded by birefringent collagen in a lymph node with a thickened sclerotic capsule (*Fig. 11.130*). A further diagnostic feature is the presence within the nodules of lacunar cells, which are Reed–Sternberg variants with friable cytoplasmic processes that open up into a 'lake-like' appearance when subjected to routine processing. (*Fig. 11.131*).

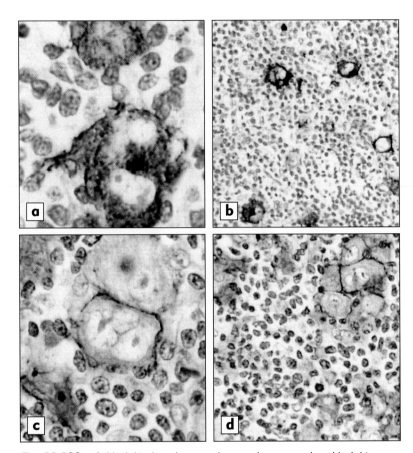

Fig. 11.128a–d Hodgkin lymphoma: abnormal mononuclear Hodgkin cells and binucleate Reed–Sternberg cells are positively labelled for (a, b) CD 15 and (c, d) CD30. [(a–d) Immunoperoxidase stain.]

Histological classification of Hodgkin lymphoma (Hodgkin's disease)

Type	Features
Nodular lymphocyte predominance Hodgkin lymphoma	Lymphocyte proliferation of irregular nodules that contain abnormal polymorphic B cells (L and H cells)
	Reed–Sternberg cells are absent
Classical Hodgkin lymphoma	
Nodular sclerosis	Tumour nodules surrounded by collagen bands extending from nodal capsule
Grades I and II (see text)	Characteristic 'lacunar cell' variant of Reed–Sternberg cell often seen
Mixed cellularity	Numerous Reed–Sternberg cells seen
	No sclerosis or fibrosis
	Intermediate numbers of lymphocytes
Lymphocyte rich	Scanty Reed–Sternberg cells; multiple small lymphocytes with few eosinophils and plasma cells; nodular and diffuse types
Lymphocyte depleted	'Reticular' pattern with predominant Reed–Sternberg cells and sparse lymphocytes or 'diffuse fibrosis' with disordered connective tissue, few lymphocytes and infrequent Reed–Sternberg cells
	This subtype is very rarely diagnosed currently

Fig. 11.129 Hodgkin lymphoma: WHO histological classification.

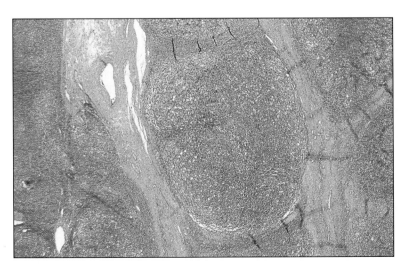

Fig. 11.130 Hodgkin lymphoma: lymph node biopsy showing abundant bands of collagenous connective tissue separating areas of abnormal Hodgkin tissue in the nodular sclerosis type.

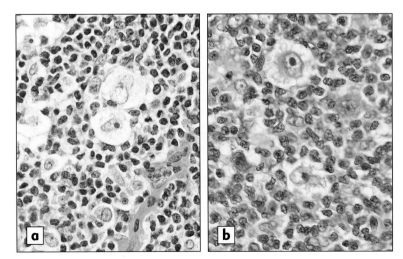

Fig. 11.131a and b Hodgkin lymphoma: (a, b) high-power views of 'lacunar' variants of Reed–Sternberg cells.

When Reed–Sternberg cells are particularly numerous, cohesive or pleomorphic (the criteria are subjective, but about 25% of the node or cells should be affected) the condition is believed to carry a worse prognosis and is graded by the British National Lymphoma Investigation group and WHO as Grade II. All other nodular sclerosing cases are Grade I. This grading is unclear, and many oncologists fail to find it of any prognostic value.

Mixed cellularity Hodgkin lymphoma

Mixed cellularity Hodgkin lymphoma represents all the other cases of classical Hodgkin lymphoma in which fibrosis, lacunar cells and sclerosis are lacking (*Fig. 11.132*). It may be that these variations reflect the lymph node regions within which Hodgkin lymphoma arises, that is B cell follicles in nodular sclerosing disease and the paracortex in mixed cellularity disease. Another hypothesis is that the architecture reflects cytokine production by Hodgkin cells.

Evidence for the presence of the EBV in Hodgkin cells occurs in over 50% of cases, especially in the mixed cellularity subtype. The virus may be detected by immunological and molecular tests (*Fig. 11.133*). It remains unclear whether the EBV is directly involved in the pathogenesis in some cases or is an innocent bystander.

Lymphocyte-rich classical Hodgkin lymphoma

The term lymphocyte-rich classical Hodgkin lymphoma (LRCHL) has been applied to morphological variants of Hodgkin lymphoma characterized by an abundance of small lymphocytes with relatively scanty classic Reed–Sternberg cells and very few eosinophils and plasma cells. LRCHL has been formally adopted as an entity in the WHO classification (*see Fig. 11.58*; and Stein H. Hodgkin's disease. *Am J Surg Pathol*. 1997;21:1361–92). This histologic subtype may be nodular (*Fig. 11.134a, b*) or diffuse (*Fig. 11.134c, d*). The nodular subtype corresponds closely to the entity of follicular Hodgkin lymphoma described by Isaacson and co-workers (Ashton-Key M, Thorpe PA, Allen JP *et al*. Follicular Hodgkin's disease. *Am J Surg Pathol*. 1995;19:1294–9), with infiltration of expanded mantle zones by Hodgkin and Reed–Sternberg cells. The diffuse subtype is characterized by a predominance of small T lymphocytes and shows no evidence of involvement of germinal centres.

Nodular lymphocyte predominance Hodgkin lymphoma

Lymphocyte predominance Hodgkin lymphoma of nodular type (nodular paragranuloma) is a distinct entity from classical Hodgkin lym-

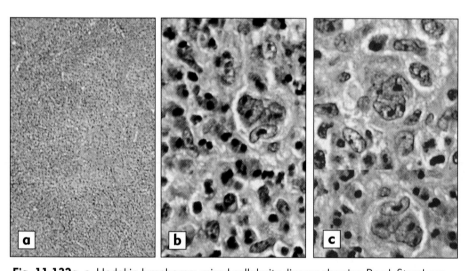

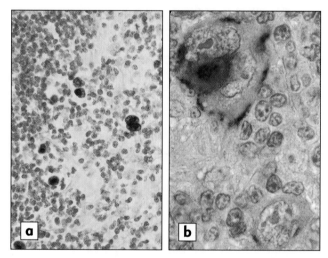

Fig. 11.132a–c Hodgkin lymphoma: mixed cellularity disease showing Reed–Sternberg cells surrounded by a mixed population of lymphocytes and eosinophils. (a) Low power; (b, c) higher powers.

Fig. 11.133a and b Mixed cellularity Hodgkin lymphoma: (a) *in situ* hybridization for EBV-encoded small nuclear RNAs (EBER1 and 2). Note the strong selective staining of the Hodgkin and Reed–Sternberg cells; (b) immunoalkaline phosphatase (APAAP) staining for the EBV-encoded latent membrane protein. Note the strong selective staining of the two Reed–Sternberg cells. (Courtesy of Prof. H Stein.)

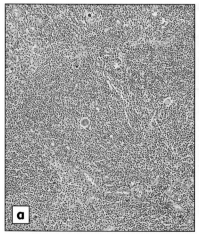
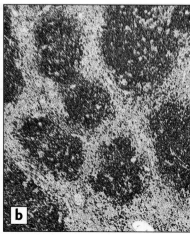
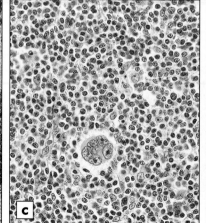
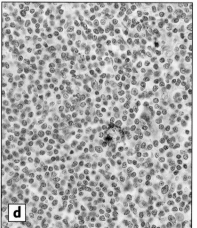

Fig. 11.134a–d Lymphocyte-rich classical Hodgkin lymphoma: (a) low-power view showing nodular growth pattern; (b) immunostain for CD20 shows the nodules are composed of small B cells; (c, d) diffuse growth pattern – a high-power view (c) shows a single Reed–Sternberg cell in a sea of small lymphoid cells and (d) immunostaining for CD30 highlights Hodgkin and Reed–Sternberg cells.

phoma. It has always been recognized as quite different from other types of Hodgkin lymphoma in view of its good prognosis with or without treatment and its unique histology (especially the lack of Reed–Sternberg cells). It usually presents in older patients as Stage I

disease. Immunohistological and molecular studies have shown convincingly that it is a proliferation of Ig-synthesizing germinal-centre B cells with a phenotype (IgM$^+$, IgD$^+$, CD5$^\pm$, CD20$^+$, CD79$^+$, J chain$^+$, CD15$^-$, CD30$^-$, p53$^-$, BCL-2$^-$, EBER$^-$) distinct from that of classical Hodgkin lymphoma. The abnormal polymorphic multinucleated cells were originally believed to be Reed–Sternberg cell variants, but they are B cells and lack both CD15 and CD30 (*Fig. 11.135*). There is usually a corona of T cells, CD3$^+$ and CD57$^+$.

Lymphocyte-depleted Hodgkin lymphoma

In lymphocyte-depleted Hodgkin lymphoma Reed–Sternberg cells are present as sheets or clusters within a fibrotic mass with no surrounding inflammatory cells (*Fig. 11.136*). It is rarely diagnosed in current clinical practice. Most lymphoma pathology groups that have reviewed their cases of lymphocyte-depleted Hodgkin lymphoma and applied immunostaining criteria have reclassified them as large B cell non-Hodgkin lymphoma or anaplastic large cell lymphoma. It usually occurs in patients over 50 years of age, with a high frequency of bone marrow disease, low complete remission rate and poor survival.

Staging techniques

The prognosis and selection of the optimum treatment depends on accurate staging of the disease (*Fig. 11.137*). After thorough clinical examination, a number of laboratory and radiological procedures are

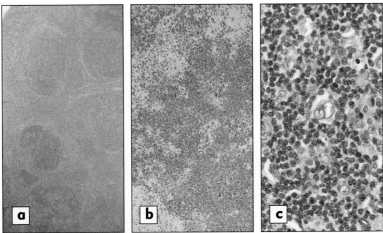
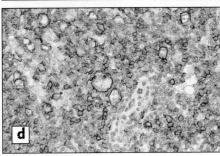
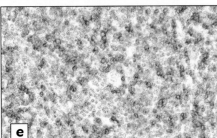
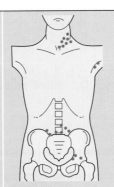
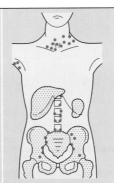

Fig. 11.135a–e Hodgkin lymphoma: nodular lymphocyte predominant. (a) Low-power view showing macronodular pattern. (b) Immunoperoxidase stain for CD20 showing B cell rich nodules; the larger L and H cells stand out in a corona of unstained T cells. (c) L and H cells show large lobulated nuclei. (d) L and H cells showing strong CD20 membrane in immunostaining. (e) Immunoperoxidase stain for CD3 showing corona of T cells surrounding L and H cells.

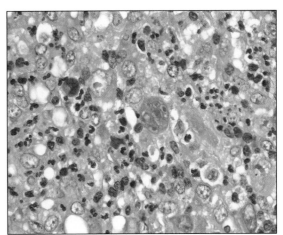

Fig. 11.136 Hodgkin lymphoma: lymphocyte depleted. Frequent Reed–Sternberg cells are present with a paucity of inflammatory cells. No immunostaining was carried out.

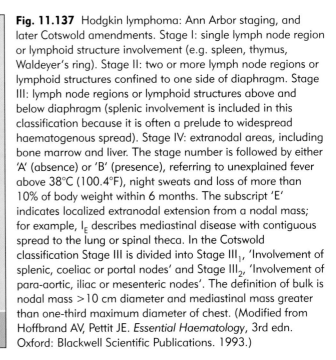

Fig. 11.137 Hodgkin lymphoma: Ann Arbor staging, and later Cotswold amendments. Stage I: single lymph node region or lymphoid structure involvement (e.g. spleen, thymus, Waldeyer's ring). Stage II: two or more lymph node regions or lymphoid structures confined to one side of diaphragm. Stage III: lymph node regions or lymphoid structures above and below diaphragm (splenic involvement is included in this classification because it is often a prelude to widespread haematogenous spread). Stage IV: extranodal areas, including bone marrow and liver. The stage number is followed by either 'A' (absence) or 'B' (presence), referring to unexplained fever above 38°C (100.4°F), night sweats and loss of more than 10% of body weight within 6 months. The subscript 'E' indicates localized extranodal extension from a nodal mass; for example, I$_E$ describes mediastinal disease with contiguous spread to the lung or spinal theca. In the Cotswold classification Stage III is divided into Stage III$_1$, 'Involvement of splenic, coeliac or portal nodes' and Stage III$_2$, 'Involvement of para-aortic, iliac or mesenteric nodes'. The definition of bulk is nodal mass >10 cm diameter and mediastinal mass greater than one-third maximum diameter of chest. (Modified from Hoffbrand AV, Pettit JE. *Essential Haematology*, 3rd edn. Oxford: Blackwell Scientific Publications. 1993.)

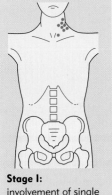
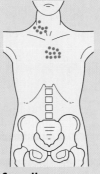

Stage I: involvement of single lymph node region or single extralymphatic site (I$_E$)

Stage II: involvement of two or more lymph node regions on same side of diaphragm; may include localized extralymphatic involvement on same side of diaphragm (II$_E$)

Stage III: involvement of lymph node regions on both sides of the diaphragm; may include spleen (III$_S$) or localized extranodal disease (III$_E$)

Stage IV: diffuse extralymphatic disease (e.g. in liver, bone marrow, lung, skin)

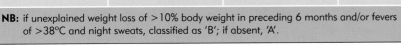

NB: if unexplained weight loss of >10% body weight in preceding 6 months and/or fevers of >38°C and night sweats, classified as 'B'; if absent, 'A'.

employed in the initial assessment (*Fig. 11.138*). Many patients have a normochromic normocytic anaemia with a leucocytosis and/or eosinophilia, and bone marrow aspirates and trephine biopsies may provide diagnostic material (*Figs 11.139–11.142*).

Mediastinal, hilar node or lung involvement may be detected by chest radiography (*Figs 11.143 and 11.144*), liver involvement by percutaneous biopsy, and para-aortic or pelvic lymph node involvement

by abdominal radiography (*Fig. 11.145*) and lymphangiography (*Figs 11.146 and 11.147*). Computed tomographic (CT) scanning and magnetic resonance imaging are now used extensively in the search for thoracic and abdominal lymph node and organ involvement (*Figs 11.148–11.150*). Gallium or positron-emission tomography scans can help to detect small areas of disease and to distinguish active areas of disease from scar tissue after therapy (*Fig. 11.151*).

Laboratory and radiological techniques for staging patients with Hodgkin lymphoma	
Laboratory	Full blood count
	Erythrocyte sedimentation rate
	Bone marrow aspirate and trephine biopsy
	Liver function
	LDH
	C-reactive protein
Radiology	Chest radiograph
	Computed tomography (thorax, abdomen, pelvis, neck)
	Ultrasound
Special tests	Magnetic resonance imaging
	Lymphangiography
	Bone scan
	Gallium scan
	Positron-emission tomography

Fig. 11.138 Hodgkin lymphoma: laboratory and radiological techniques for staging patients.

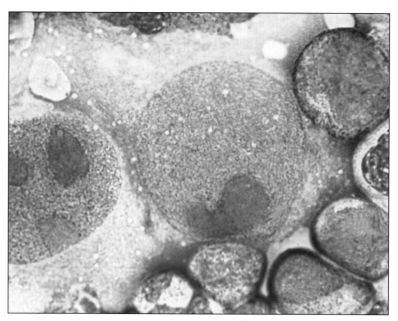

Fig. 11.139 Hodgkin lymphoma: high-power view of bone marrow aspirate, showing a Reed–Sternberg cell.

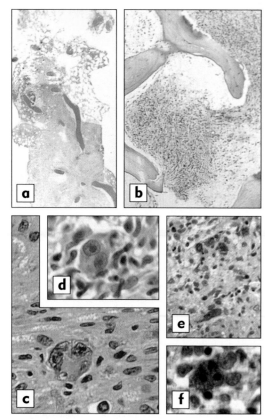

Fig. 11.140a–f Hodgkin lymphoma: trephine biopsy (a, b) showing Hodgkin tissue replacing normal haemopoietic elements; (c, d) higher power showing fibrosis and Reed-Sternberg cells labelled by (e, f) antibodies to CD30. (APAAP immunoalkaline phosphatase.)

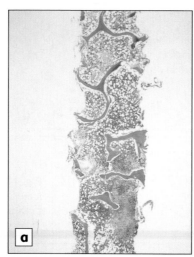

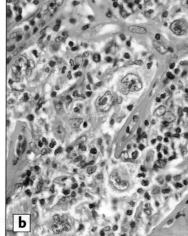

Fig. 11.141a and b Hodgkin lymphoma: bone marrow trephine biopsy. (a) Low-power view showing focal involvement. (b) High-power view showing mononuclear Hodgkin cells.

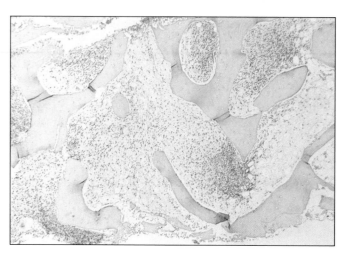

Fig. 11.142 Hodgkin lymphoma: trephine biopsy in the fibrotic variant of lymphocyte-depleted disease, showing almost complete replacement of haemopoietic tissue by Hodgkin deposits, along with abundant fibrous tissue in the intertrabecular space.

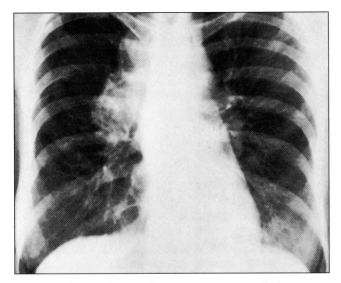

Fig. 11.143 Hodgkin lymphoma: chest radiograph showing prominent right paratracheal and hilar lymph node enlargement. The enlargement of the anterior mediastinal, subcarinal and left hilar nodes is less marked and the proximal regions of both major bronchi are significantly narrowed. Contrast material in the apical lymph node on the left is from previous lymphangiography.

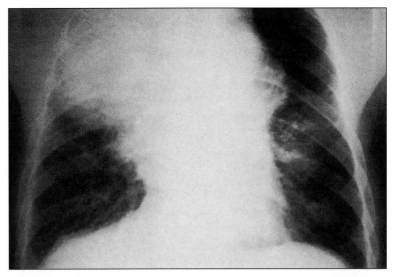

Fig. 11.144 Hodgkin lymphoma: chest radiograph showing widespread enlargement of hilar and mediastinal lymph nodes with associated collapse of the right upper lobe and infiltration or possibly pneumonic changes in the mid-zone of the left lung.

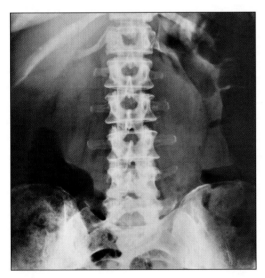

Fig. 11.145 Hodgkin lymphoma: plain abdominal radiograph showing bilateral massive para-aortic lymph node enlargement. (Courtesy of Dr D Nag.)

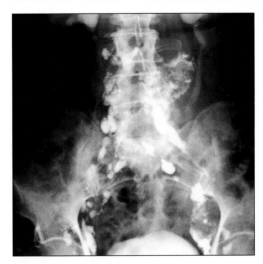

Fig. 11.146 Hodgkin lymphoma: lymphangiogram with intravenous pyelogram shows enlarged para-aortic lymph nodes (particularly on the left and lower left pelvis) with displacement of the ureter.

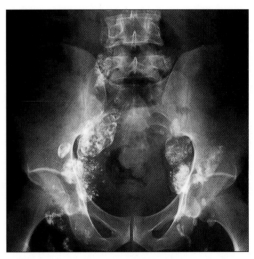

Fig. 11.147 Hodgkin lymphoma: lymphangiogram showing bilateral external iliac and lower para-aortic lymph node enlargement and filling defects.

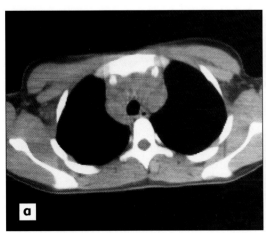
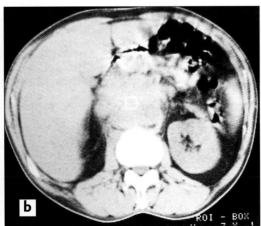
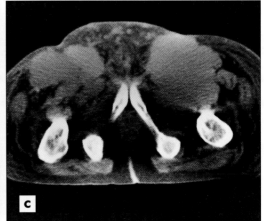

Fig. 11.148a–c Hodgkin lymphoma: CT scans of (a) chest showing paratracheal and anterior mediastinal lymph node enlargement; (b) abdomen showing massive para-aortic lymph node enlargement displacing the pancreas forwards; (c) pelvis showing massive bilateral inguinal and pelvic lymphadenopathy with marked oedema of the lower abdominal wall (see also Fig. 11.116).

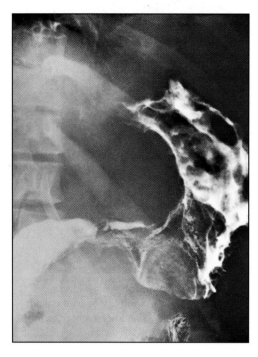

Fig. 11.149 Hodgkin lymphoma: barium meal demonstrating extensive mucosal and gastric wall involvement of the body and pyloris of the stomach. (Courtesy of Dr. D Nag.)

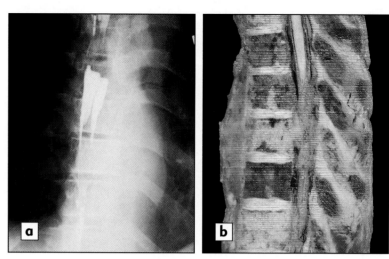

Fig. 11.150a and b Hodgkin lymphoma: (a) sisternogram showing partial block of contrast at the T4 level and a complete block at the lower part of T6; (b) sagittal section postmortem shows extradural extension of tumour from the body of T4 (uppermost) and more extensive cordal involvement at T7 and T9. There is patchy involvement of other vertebral bodies and spinous processes. Extensive paravertebral tumour is seen anteriorly below the T5 level.

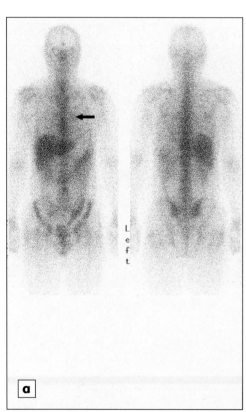

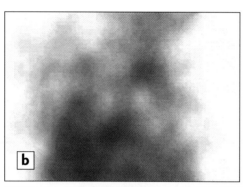

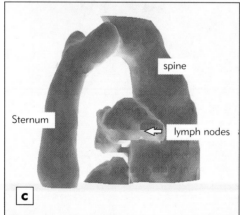

Fig. 11.151a–c Non-Hodgkin lymphoma: Stage IIb. Postchemotherapy with residual mediastinal mass see on CT scan. (a) Whole body scan 48 hours after injection of gallium-67 citrate, with subtle increased uptake in the mediastinum (arrow). (b) Tomographic image shows uptake in mediastinum. (c) Surface-rendered tomographic image confirms presence of active disease in hilar lymph nodes. (All courtesy of Dr AJW Hilson.)

Previously used staging procedures, such as laparotomy combined with abdominal node and liver biopsies, and splenectomy are very rarely carried out today.

Treatment

Wide-field radiotherapy and cyclical chemotherapy using different combinations of mustine hydrochloride, vincristine, vinblastine (V), etoposide, cyclophosphamide, dacarbazine (D), procarbazine, prednisolone, doxorubicin (adriamycin; A) and bleomycin (B) have resulted in dramatic increases in remission and cure. Patients with Stage IA are often treated with radiotherapy alone. Those patients with more advanced stages of disease or symptoms receive chemotherapy (e.g. ABVD or 'Stanford V') as primary treatment, but irradiation is used subsequently to treat sites of initial bulky tumour deposits. High-dose chemotherapy with autologous bone marrow or peripheral blood stem cell rescue is used if patients fail two chemotherapy regimens or are primarily resistant.

Myeloma and Related Conditions

MULTIPLE MYELOMA

In multiple myeloma there is a malignant neoplastic proliferation of plasma cells in the bone marrow, usually comprising over 15% of the marrow cell total in aspirates. In advanced disease the abnormal cell population may exceed half the total cell number (*Fig. 12.1*). The morphology of these cells is often abnormal, with more primitive features and a greater variation in size than found in classic plasma cells (*Figs 12.2–12.4*). Multinucleate cells may be frequent. As a result of abnormal immunoglobulin deposits, inclusion bodies may occur in the cyto-

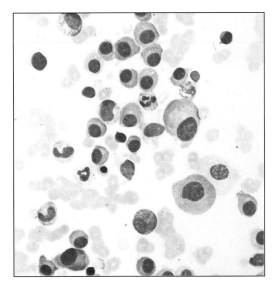

Fig. 12.1 Multiple myeloma: marrow cell trail. The majority of cells seen are atypical plasma cells.

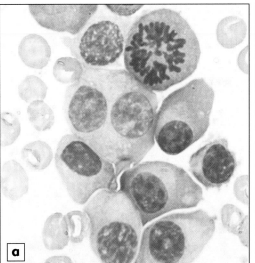
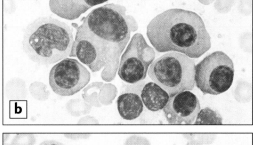
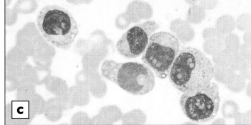

Fig. 12.2a–c Multiple myeloma: abnormal plasma cells in marrow in two cases. (a) Myeloma cells, one binucleate, with nucleoli, and one with a mitotic figure; (b) the nuclei in a binucleate cell vary greatly in size; (c) abnormal cytoplasmic and nuclear vacuolation.

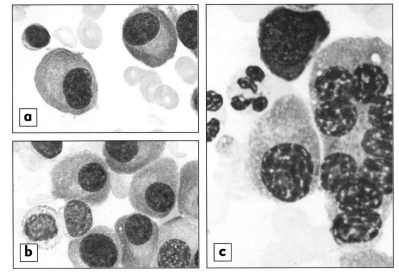

Fig. 12.3a–c Multiple myeloma: (a–c) abnormal plasma cells in bone marrow. Considerable variation occurs in nuclear size and cytoplasmic volume, and one of the myeloma cells is multinucleate (c).

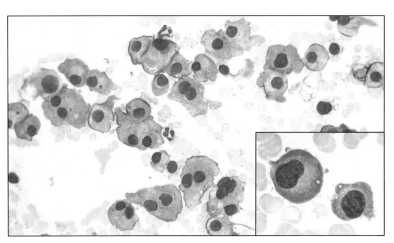

Fig. 12.4 Multiple myeloma: 'flaming' plasma cells in marrow with IgA M-protein in serum. There are numerous thesaurocytes, large plasma cells with small, sometimes pyknotic, nuclei and expanded fibrillary cytoplasm, which also shows 'flaming' of the cell rim (inset). Although 'flaming' occurs most frequently with IgA production, it may also be seen with M-proteins of other classes.

plasm (*Figs 12.5 and 12.6*). Trephine biopsy is not usually carried out, but shows a uniform infiltration by plasma cells and plasmablasts (*Figs 12.7 and 12.8*).

The majority of patients produce a monoclonal protein (M-protein or paraprotein), which may be demonstrated in the serum and/or urine. Typically, the serum protein is increased and electrophoresis shows an abnormal paraprotein in the globulin region (*Fig. 12.9*). Immunodiffusion techniques reveal which immunoglobulin fraction is increased, while the levels of the uninvolved classes of immunoglobulin are usually depressed. Immunoelectrophoretic techniques confirm the presence of an abnormal immunoglobulin and are able to establish the monoclonal nature of this protein (*Fig. 12. 10*).

In patients with complete monoclonal immunoglobulin in the serum, the synthesis of heavy and light chains in the neoplastic plasma cells is often imbalanced, with an excess production of light chains. The urine contains Bence–Jones protein in two-thirds of cases; this consists of free light chains, either κ or λ, of the same type as the serum M-protein. In about 17% of cases, Bence–Jones proteinuria is the sole

protein abnormality and complete abnormal immunoglobulin is not found in the serum. Occasionally, patients have two or more M-proteins while in <1% of patients no M-proteins are found in the serum or urine.

The advanced stage of this disease involves a normochromic normocytic anaemia, often with an associated neutropenia and thrombocytopenia, reflecting the development of bone marrow failure. The increased globulin in the serum is frequently associated with an increased erythrocyte sedimentation rate, and the blood may show marked red cell rouleaux formation and increased background staining (*Fig. 12.11*). In some cases a leucoerythroblastic blood picture is seen. Abnormal plasma cells appear in the blood film in about 15% of patients (*Fig. 12. 12*). Sensitive gene rearrangement studies, however, reveal typical cells of the malignant clone in the peripheral blood in a higher proportion of patients.

Skeletal radiology shows osteolytic lesions in 60% of patients and associated pain is characteristic. The lesions include the classic 'punched-out' lesions of the skull (*Figs 12.13 and 12.14*), lytic lesions and generalized bone rarefaction of the spine, ribs and pelvis, and

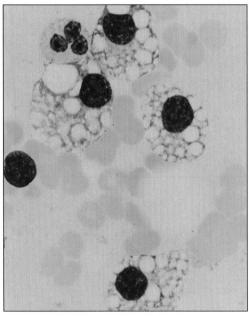

Fig. 12.5 Multiple myeloma: bone marrow aspirate showing abnormal plasma cells with many large cytoplasmic vacuoles ('Mott cells' or morular cells). Each vacuole is an accumulation of immunoglobulin. (Courtesy of Dr M Saary.)

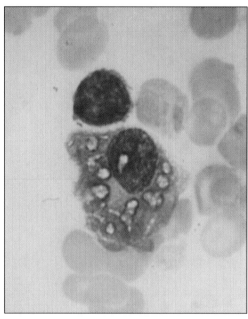

Fig. 12.6 Multiple myeloma: plasma cell showing crystalline pink inclusions of abnormal immunoglobulin. (Courtesy of Dr R Britt.)

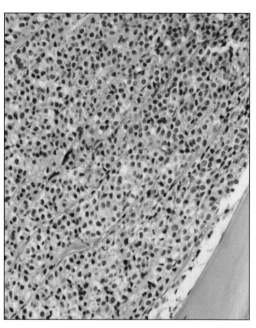

Fig. 12.7 Multiple myeloma: trephine biopsy shows almost complete replacement of haemopoietic tissue by sheets of abnormal plasma cells.

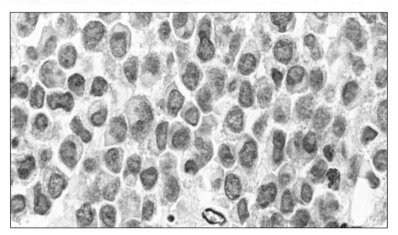

Fig. 12.8 Multiple myeloma/plasma cell leukaemia: trephine biopsy showing almost complete replacement of haemopoietic cells by plasma cells and plasmablasts. (Courtesy of Dr DM Swirsky.)

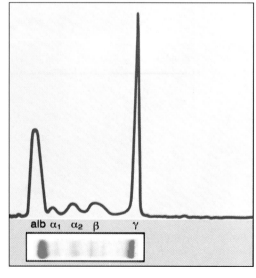

Fig. 12.9 Multiple myeloma: serum protein electrophoresis showing an M-protein in the γ-globulin region and reduced levels of background β- and α-globulins. This 'spike' and deficiency pattern is typical of patients with myeloma. (Total protein, 99 g/l; IgG M-protein component, 41 g/l.)

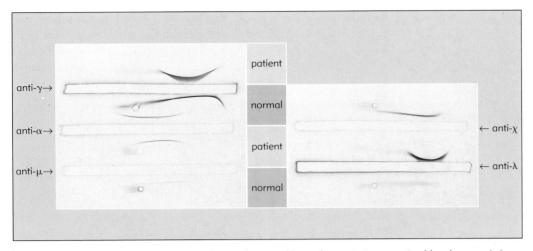

Fig. 12.10 Multiple myeloma: immunoelectrophoresis. Normal protein is recognized by characteristic arc patterns. In the reactions against anti-γ and anti-λ, the IgG-λ M-protein maintains its electrophoretic position, but appears as a 'bow' or thickened arc with a smaller than usual radius. Reduced levels of IgA and IgM are reflected in small or absent arcs in the reactions with anti-α and anti-μ.

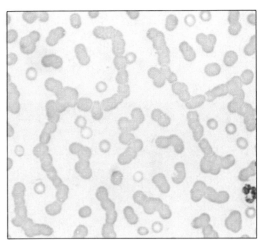

Fig. 12.11 Multiple myeloma: peripheral blood film shows marked rouleaux formation of red cells and increased background staining.

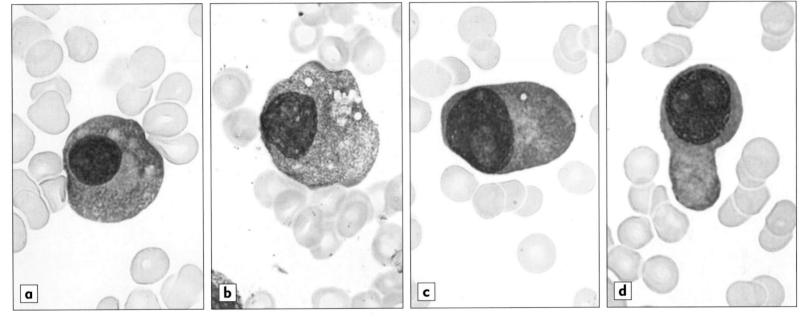

Fig. 12.12a–d Multiple myeloma: (a–d) isolated myeloma cells in peripheral blood films from two patients.

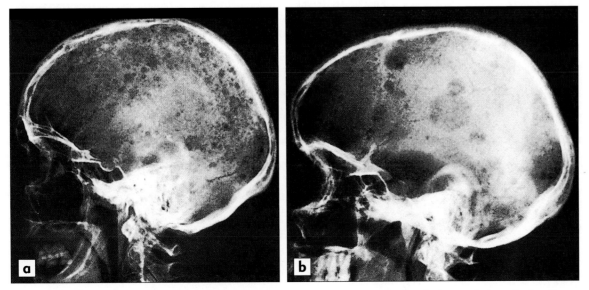

Fig. 12.13a and b Multiple myeloma: radiographs of skulls showing (a) typical multiple, small, 'punched out' osteolytic lesions; (b) a case in which the lesions vary much more in size.

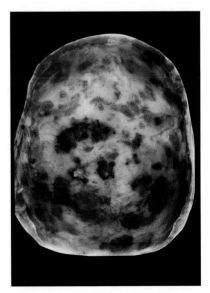

Fig. 12.14 Multiple myeloma: inside of the skull shows characteristic 'moth-eaten' osteolytic lesions.

pathological fractures (*Figs 12.15–12.18*). Extensive bone resorption (*Fig. 12.19*), thought to be caused by excessive production of osteoclast activating factor (OAF), probably a combination of tumour necrosis factor and interleukin-1, results in elevation of serum calcium in half the patients. In occasional patients, myeloma deposits may extend beyond the skeleton into surrounding soft tissues (*Figs 12.20 and 12.21*). Magnetic resonance imaging (MRI) may be valuable in assessing sites of tumour invasion (*Fig. 12.22*). Rarely, osteosclerosis

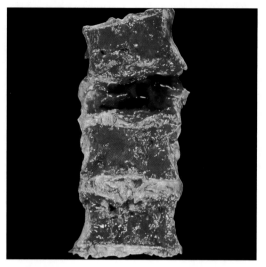

Fig. 12.15 Multiple myeloma: longitudinal section of lumbar spine shows a generalized replacement of normal medullary bone by vascular myeloma tissue. The body of L2 has collapsed and appears haemorrhagic.

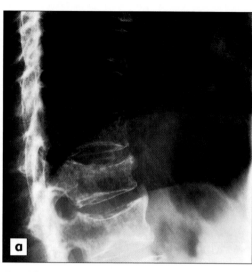
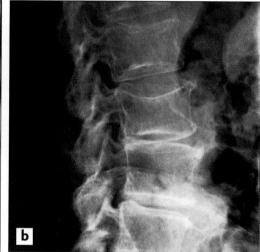

Fig. 12.16a and b Multiple myeloma: radiographs of (a) the lower thoracic and (b) lumbar spine show severe demineralization, with partial collapse of the vertebral bodies, most pronounced in T8–T12 and in L3.

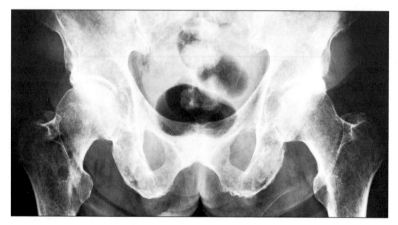

Fig. 12.17 Multiple myeloma: radiograph of pelvis with osteolytic lesions in the lower pelvic girdle and in the right femur.

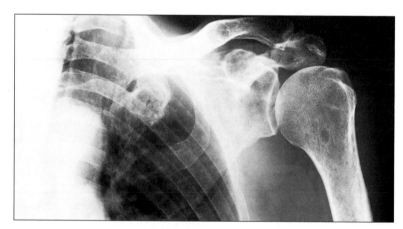

Fig. 12.18 Multiple myeloma: radiograph of left shoulder region shows a pathological fracture of the acromial process of the scapula and osteolytic lesions in the humerus, clavicle and ribs.

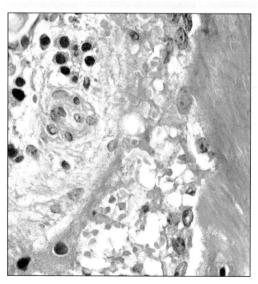

Fig. 12.19 Multiple myeloma: bone biopsy. Although plasma cells are seen in the upper left, osteoclasts (the multinucleate cells at the bone intertrabecular tissue interface) are the cells responsible for the bone absorption around the osteolytic lesion.

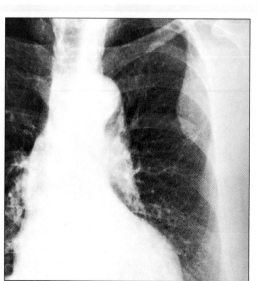

Fig. 12.20 Multiple myeloma: chest radiograph showing a prominent extrapleural soft tissue mass adjacent to the third left rib.

may occur. POEMS syndrome consists of polyneuropathy, osteosclerotic myeloma and systems involvement (e.g. endocrinopathy, skin pigmentation, clubbing and arthropathy, hepatosplenomegaly and lymphadenopathy; *Figs 12.23 and 12.24*).

Renal complications have an important influence on the course of multiple myeloma. Patients with persistent renal failure and blood urea in excess of 14mmol/l have a poor prognosis. Damage from heavy Bence–Jones proteinuria (*Fig. 12.25*), amyloid disease (*Fig. 12.26*),

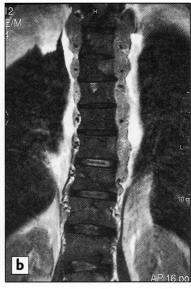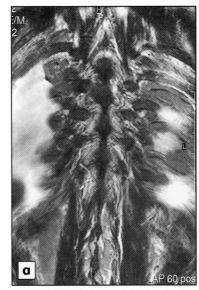

Fig. 12.22a and b Multiple myeloma: (a) T1 weighted parasagittal image from a 60-year-old man. All bones are abnormal (patchy, heterogeneous signal). There is an extensive extradural tumour in the spinal canal behind the spinal cord, compressing it from D3 to D8, with absence of cerebrospinal fluid. Incidental haemangioma at D4 stains as a bright signal. (b) T2 weighted coronal image of the thoracic spine in a 60-year-old man. The heterogeneous signal from the marrow is compatible with myeloma deposits with extraosseus soft tissue paraspinal masses of myeloma. [(a, b) Courtesy of Dr AD Platts.]

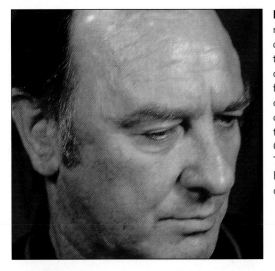

Fig. 12.21 Multiple myeloma: skull deposits have invaded the soft tissues and appear as lumps on the forehead. In this case, a proportion of marrow cells were positive for the surface antigen CD10 but negative for TdT. Such cells have been associated with aggressive disease.

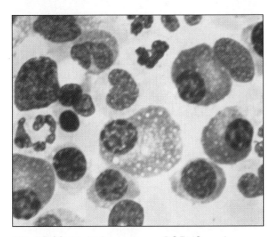

Fig. 12.23 Multiple myeloma: POEMS syndrome. The patient, a 39-year-old man, presented with lower limb weakness. Nerve conduction studies showed evidence of a peripheral neuropathy with demyelination. Endocrine screening was negative. Bone marrow shows excess plasma cells; serum IgG was raised (29.3 g/l) with Bence–Jones proteinuria. (Courtesy of Dr R Liang.)

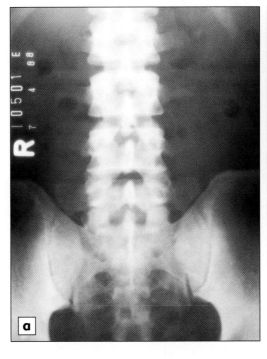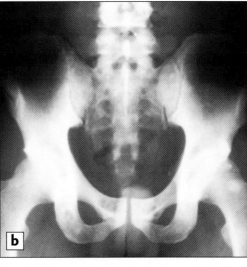

Fig. 12.24a and b Multiple myeloma: POEMS syndrome (same case as shown in *Fig. 12.23*). Radiographs of (a) lumbar spine, and (b) pelvis showing sclerosis and lytic areas with sclerotic rims. [(a, b) Courtesy of Dr R Liang.]

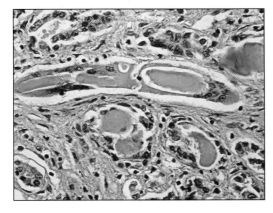

Fig. 12.25 Multiple myeloma: section of kidney showing acidophilic casts of myeloma protein blocking the renal tubules. There is surrounding giant cell reaction and interstitial fibrosis.

Fig. 12.26 Multiple myeloma: renal amyloid disease. Amyloid deposition in the glomeruli and associated arterioles is extensive. Congo red stain.

nephrocalcinosis (*Fig. 12.27*) and pyelonephritis (*Fig. 12.28*) may be important in the pathogenesis. A more generalized amyloid disease occurs in a small number of patients, and there may be macroglossia with tongue ulceration (*Figs 12.29–12.31*), 'carpal tunnel' syndrome (*Fig. 12.32*), skin deposits (*Figs 12.33 and 12.34*) and cardiac involvement resulting in cardiomegaly and congestive heart failure (*Fig. 12.35*).

Plasma cell leukaemia

Patients may present with large numbers of circulating plasma cells or this blood picture may arise during the course of the disease (*Figs 12.36–12.39; see also* page 185).

Treatment

Urgent initial therapy may be required to deal with hypercalcaemia, hyperviscosity or renal failure. There are a number of different approaches to chemotherapy of the underlying disease. In older patients an alkylating agent, such as melphalan or cyclophosphamide, is normally used, often in combination with a corticosteroid. In younger subjects, repeated courses of doxorubicin, vincristine and corticosteroids are often used to obtain a more prolonged clinical remission; high-dose melphalan, with autologous bone marrow rescue, appears to prolong remission. α-Interferon and biphosphonates both may be of value in prolonging remission, and biphosphonates may also reduce bone damage.

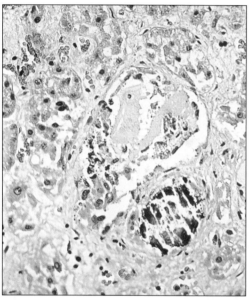

Fig. 12.27 Multiple myeloma: nephrocalcinosis. Irregular fractured haematoxylinophilic deposits of calcium are seen in the fibrotic renal tissue.

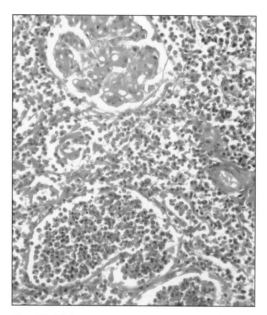

Fig. 12.28 Multiple myeloma: destruction of the renal parenchyma and acute inflammatory cellular infiltration of the interstitial tissues and tubular spaces in pyelonephritis.

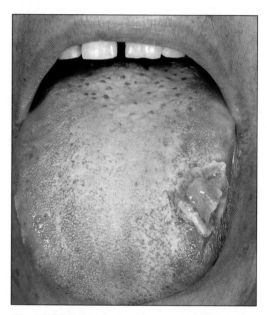

Fig. 12.29 Multiple myeloma: in amyloid disease, the tongue shows macroglossia and a deep ulcer on the upper and lateral anterior surfaces. The floor of the ulcer has the waxy appearance typical of amyloid deposition.

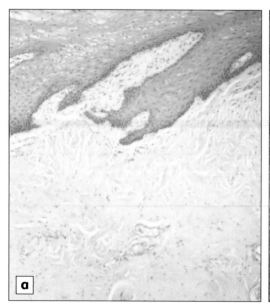

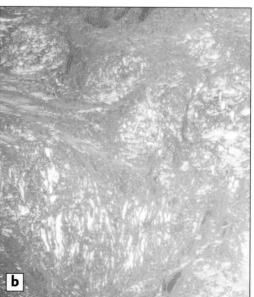

Fig. 12.30a and b Multiple myeloma: biopsy of the ulcer seen in *Fig. 12.29* shows (a) extensive deposition of pale-staining acidophilic material. (b) Stained with Congo red, this material shows the characteristic green birefringence of amyloid, when viewed with polarized light.

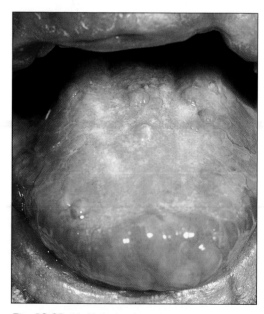

Fig. 12.31 Multiple myeloma: gross macroglossia. These nodular deposits of amyloid contrast with the diffuse enlargement in *Fig. 12.29*. Similar nodules are also evident in the lips.

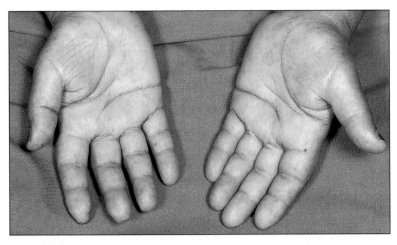

Fig. 12.32 Multiple myeloma: 'carpal tunnel syndrome' caused by deposition of amyloid in the flexor retinaculum and resulting in compression of the median nerve. The thenar muscles are wasting. The patient complained of paraesthesiae and weakness of both hands.

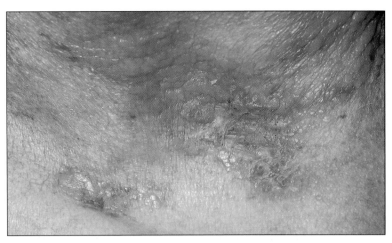

Fig. 12.33 Multiple myeloma: amyloid disease of the skin. There are plaque-like hyaline infiltrations of the skin folds in the supraclavicular area.

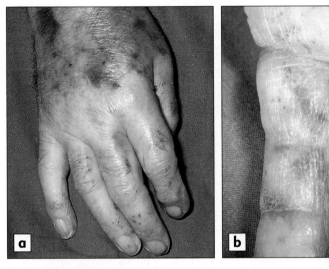

Fig. 12.34a and b Multiple myeloma: (a) amyloid disease on the back of the hand. Extensive diffuse and nodular deposits in the skin, subcutaneous tissues and tendon sheaths have resulted in irregular swelling over the metacarpal heads; the skin surface appears hard, tense and waxy; (b) extensive purpura, a characteristic feature, probably results from involvement of small cutaneous blood vessels.

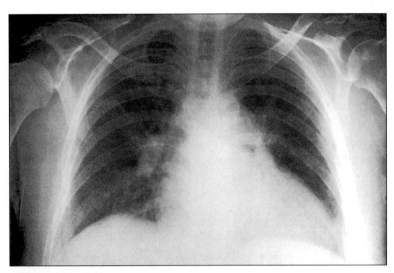

Fig. 12.35 Multiple myeloma: amyloid disease of the heart. This radiograph shows cardiomegaly and pulmonary congestion. Evidence of myeloma includes osteolytic lesions in the right humerus and ribs as well as pathological fractures of the left clavicle and the eighth right rib.

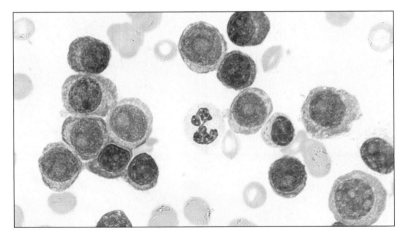

Fig. 12.36 Plasma cell leukaemia: peripheral blood film showing large numbers of plasma cells and/or plasmablasts. (WBC, 100 × 10⁹/l; courtesy of Dr DM Swirsky.)

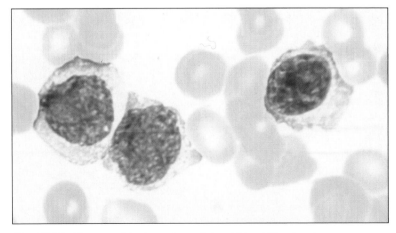

Fig. 12.37 Plasma cell leukaemia: peripheral blood film showing lymphocytoid plasma cells. The patient, a 44-year-old man, had been treated 1 year earlier for myeloma with six courses of intensive therapy [vincristine, doxorubicin (adriamycin) and methylprednisolone (VAMP)]. He relapsed with widespread lytic lesions and many circulating plasma cells. (Hb, 6.3 g/dl; WBC, 23.1 × 10⁹/l; plasma cells, 18.3 × 10⁹/l; platelets, 64 × 10⁹/l.)

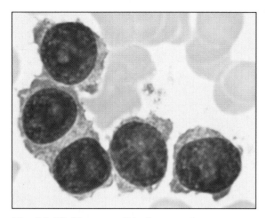

Fig. 12.38 Plasma cell leukaemia: bone marrow of same case as shown in *Fig. 12.37*.

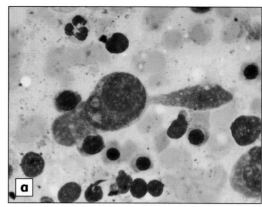

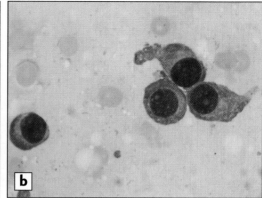

Fig. 12.39a and b Multiple myeloma with plasma cell leukaemia: (a, b) bone marrow showing cells with motility-associated features (pseudopods and long extensions). (Reproduced with permission from Berneman ZN, Chen ZZ, Peetermans ME. Morphological evidence for a motile behavior by plasma cells. *Leukemia.* 1990;4:53–9.)

Primary amyloidosis

Primary amyloidosis syndrome is dominated by clinical features caused by amyloid deposition in the tongue (*Fig. 12.40*), heart, tendon sheaths (*Fig. 12.41*) and skin. The disease can be assessed by serum amyloid P component scintigraphy (*Fig. 12.42*; *see also* page 308).

OTHER PLASMA CELL TUMOURS

Solitary and soft tissue plasmacytomas each comprise half of the 6% of plasma cell tumours which are not multiple myeloma.

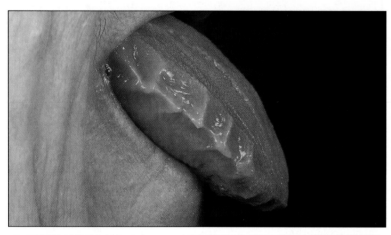

Fig. 12.40 Primary amyloidosis: tongue, enlarged, with a waxy smooth appearance.

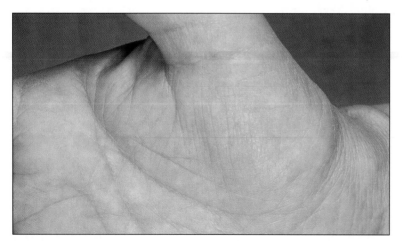

Fig. 12.41 Primary amyloidosis: flattening of thenar eminence caused by carpal tunnel syndrome. Same case as shown in *Fig. 12.40*.

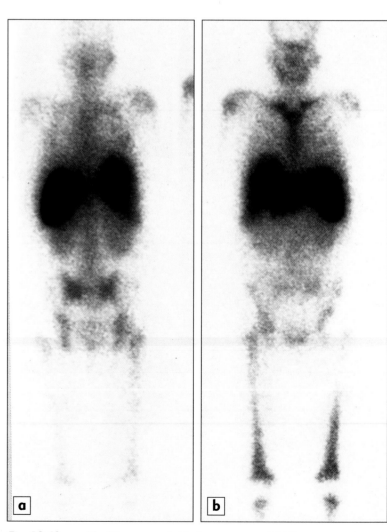

Fig. 12.42a and b Primary amyloidosis: serum amyloid P component scintigraphy. (a) Posterior and (b) anterior whole body scans obtained 24 hours after injection of ^{123}I-labelled serum amyloid P (SAP) component in a 62-year-old woman with systemic AL amyloidosis. The tracer has localized to amyloid deposits in the liver, spleen, kidneys and throughout the bone marrow. [(a, b) Courtesy of Dr PN Hawkins and Prof. MB Pepys.]

Solitary plasmacytoma of bone

In solitary plasmacytoma of bone (*Figs 12.43–12.48*), no plasma cell proliferation occurs in parts of the skeleton beyond the primary lesion; marrow aspirates distant from the primary tumour are usually normal. Associated M-proteins disappear following radiotherapy to the primary lesion.

Soft tissue plasmacytoma

Soft tissue plasmacytomas are found most frequently in the submucosa of the upper respiratory and gastrointestinal tracts, in the cervical lymph nodes and in the skin. They tend to remain localized and the majority are well controlled by excision or local irradiation.

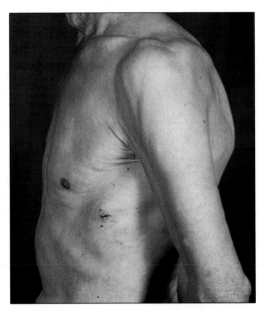

Fig. 12.43 Solitary plasmacytoma of bone: a firm ovoid mass, 9 cm in diameter, over the lower lateral aspect of the left chest wall. Protein studies, blood count and bone marrow were normal. No other skeletal lesions were detected by a radiological survey. (Courtesy of Dr S Knowles.)

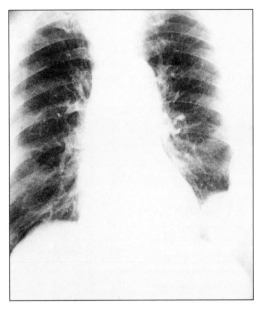

Fig. 12.44 Solitary plasmacytoma of bone: radiograph of the case in *Fig. 12.43* shows a well-defined mass approximately 5 cm in diameter, in the lower left chest, pleural in position and arising from the ninth rib.

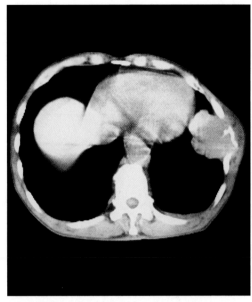

Fig. 12.45 Solitary plasmacytoma of bone: computed tomography scan of the case shown in *Fig. 12.43*, showing erosion of the rib, with soft tissue extension into both the pleural space and external soft tissues.

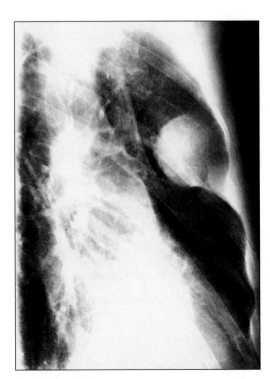

Fig. 12.46 Solitary plasmacytoma of bone: oblique radiograph of the left chest. There is expansion and destruction of the left fourth rib with an overlying soft tissue mass (the tumour).

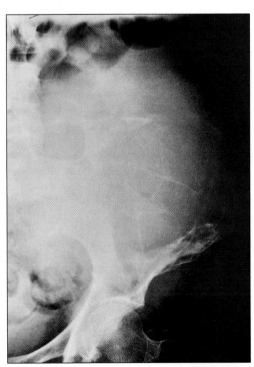

Fig. 12.47 Solitary plasmacytoma of bone: radiograph of left pelvic area shows massive destruction of the iliac bone and the tumour extending into the pelvis and abdomen. Linear residual streaks of bone produce the 'soap bubble' appearance seen in this type of tumour.

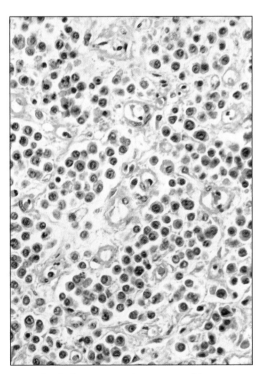

Fig. 12.48 Solitary plasmacytoma of bone: biopsy shows dense collections of plasma cells supported by a vascular stroma.

WALDENSTRÖM'S MACROGLOBULINAEMIA

Waldenström's macroglobulinaemia is a rare lymphoproliferative disorder that has similarities to both multiple myeloma and lymphocytic malignant lymphoma. There is a generalized proliferation of lymphocytes, many of which have plasmacytoid features (*Figs 12.49–12.52*).

Frequently, generalized lymphadenopathy is present and the liver and spleen are enlarged. The disease advances with extensive bone marrow involvement (*Figs 12.51 and 12.52*), and patients may present with evidence of bone marrow failure.

The proliferating cells produce an IgM M-protein that increases blood viscosity more than equivalent concentrations of IgG or IgA and may cause hyperviscosity. Clinically, the hyperviscosity syndrome is characterized by loss of vision, symptoms involving the central nervous system, haemorrhagic diathesis and heart failure; the most severely affected patients may present in coma. The retina may show a variety of changes, including engorged veins, haemorrhages, exudates and a blurred optic disc (*Fig. 12.53*).

The hyperviscosity syndrome may occur with multiple myeloma (*Fig. 12.54*) when there is polymerization of the abnormal immunoglobulin; a similar syndrome is occasionally caused by increased levels of blood components other than M-proteins (*Fig. 12.55*).

Patients with acute hyperviscosity syndrome benefit from plasmapheresis. Cyclophosphamide or chlorambucil, plus corticosteroids, have been used to reduce the tumour mass. Fludarabine and 2-chlorodeoxyadenosine are valuable newer agents

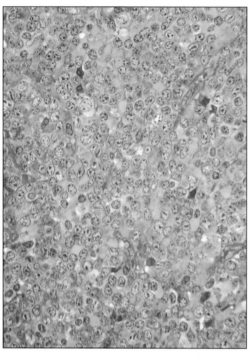

Fig. 12.49 Waldenström's macroglobulinaemia: biopsy of lymph node shows plasmacytoid lymphocytes. The nuclear chromatin has a 'clockface' pattern with coarse chromatin blocks alternating with open areas of clearing parachromatin. Very few cells can be identified as plasma cells. (Methacrylate-embedded section stained with phloxine.)

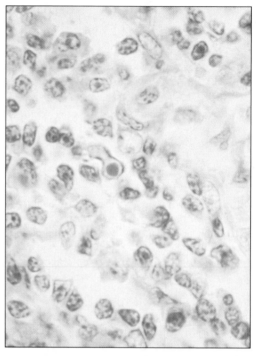

Fig. 12.50 Waldenström's macroglobulinaemia: biopsy of lymph node, periodic acid–Schiff (PAS) stain. In the centre is a large PAS-positive nuclear inclusion.

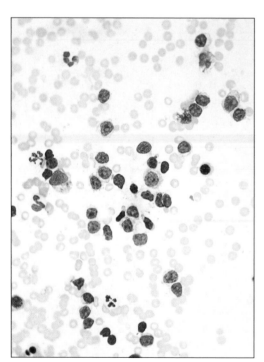

Fig. 12.51 Waldenström's macroglobulinaemia: bone marrow cell trail shows a predominance of lymphocytes and lymphoplasmacytoid cells.

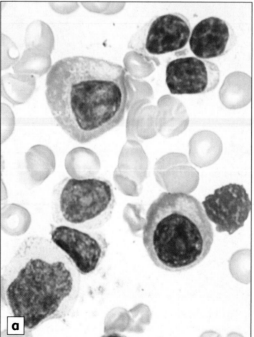
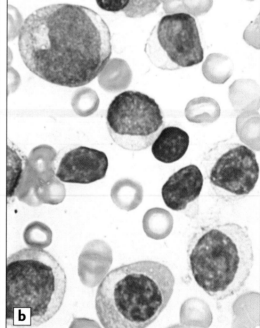

Fig. 12.52a and b Waldenström's macroglobulinaemia: (a, b) the cells have features varying between those of classic lymphocytes and plasma cells. The chromatin patterns in the larger nuclei are more open and primitive.

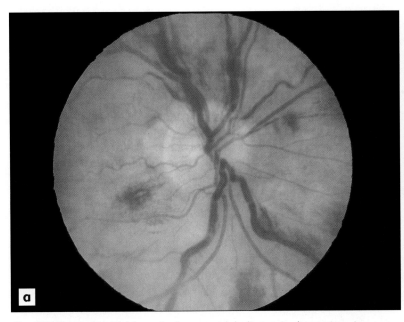

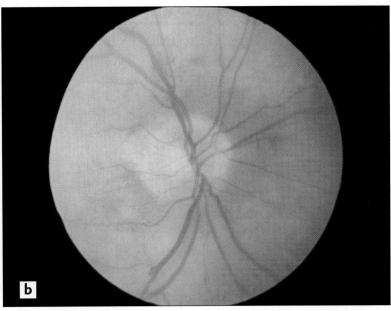

Fig. 12.53a and b Waldenström's macroglobulinaemia: hyperviscosity syndrome. The patient complained of blurred vision, headache and dizziness. (a) The retina before plasmapheresis shows gross distension of vessels, particularly the veins, which show bulging and constriction (the 'linked sausage effect'), and areas of haemorrhage; (b) following plasmapheresis, the vascular diameters are normal and the haemorrhagic areas have cleared.

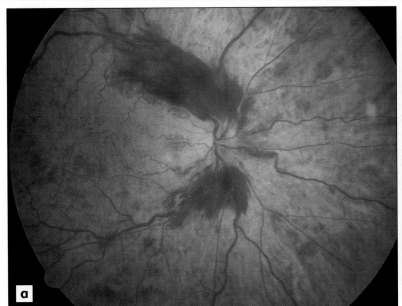

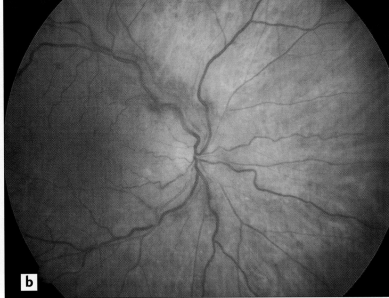

Fig. 12.54a and b Multiple myeloma: (a) distension of retinal veins and widespread haemorrhage in the hyperviscosity syndrome; (b) 2 months after plasmapheresis and chemotherapy the vessels are normal and almost all haemorrhage has cleared. The patient presented with some loss of vision and headache. [(a, b) Courtesy of Prof. JC Parr.]

Fig. 12.55 Causes of the hyperviscosity syndrome: M-proteins are the dominant cause, but others of importance are polycythaemia, leucostasis and hyperfibrinogenaemia.

Causes of hyperviscosity syndrome	
Causes	**Diseases**
M-proteins	Waldenström's macroglobulinaemia Multiple myeloma
Polycythaemia	Polycythaemia vera Severe secondary polycythaemia
Leucostasis	Chronic myeloid leukaemia Other leukaemias with very high white cell counts
Hyperfibrinogenaemia	Following factor VIII replacement therapy with large amounts of cryoprecipitate

OTHER CAUSES OF SERUM M-PROTEINS

The appearance of an M-protein spike during serum electrophoresis is usually associated with more than 5 g/l of that protein. Uncontrolled proliferation of an M-protein-producing clone, as in multiple myeloma or Waldenström's disease, is distinguished by a progressive increase in the serum M-protein concentration. Production of M-protein is controlled or stable in benign monoclonal gammopathy and chronic cold

Diseases associated with production of M-proteins
Malignant or uncontrolled production
Multiple myeloma
Waldenström's macroglobulinaemia
Malignant lymphoma
Primary amyloidosis
Heavy chain disease (λ, α and μ)
Benign or stable production
Benign monoclonal gammopathy
Chronic cold haemagglutinin disease
Transient M-proteins
Occasional association with carcinoma, connective tissue and skin disorders, human immunodeficiency virus infection, Gaucher's disease and many other conditions

Fig. 12.56 M-proteins: uncontrolled production of M-protein occurs with plasma cell dyscrasias, lymphoproliferative disorders and primary amyloid. The most common cause is benign monoclonal gammopathy with no apparent disease association. Benign controlled M-protein production has a number of causes, including human immunodeficiency virus and other infections, carcinoma and other tumours; 'benign' refers to the limited clone of M-protein-producing cells.

agglutinin disease (cold autoimmune haemolytic anaemia). Occasionally, production of M-protein is transient – for example, following recovery from infection or during a reaction to drug (*Fig. 12.56*).

Benign monoclonal gammopathy

Benign monoclonal gammopathy is the most common cause of a serum M-protein. Its benign nature is distinguished by the fact that the level of M-protein in the serum is stable over many years. It is not associated with Bence–Jones proteinuria, bone lesions or soft tissue plasma cell tumours (*Fig. 12.57*). The bone marrow may have 5–15% plasma cells, but patients are generally asymptomatic, with no evidence of bone marrow failure. When affected patients are followed for up to 10 years, 20–30% eventually develop myeloma or malignant lymphoma.

Although benign paraproteinaemia is usually symptomless, clinical features that may be associated include peripheral neuropathy, acquired von Willebrand's syndrome, papular mucinosis, cold haemagglutinin disease (*see* Chapter 4), amyloid (*see* Chapter 17) and cryoglobulinaemia. These syndromes may also occur, however, when the disease that causes the paraprotein is clearly malignant – for example, in lymphoma, myeloma or macroglobulinaemia.

Cryoglobulinaemia

Globulins that precipitate in the cold may occur in a primary disease (which may be monoclonal or oligoclonal; *Figs 12.58 and 12.59*) or in

Features of paraproteinaemia		
	Benign	**Malignant**
Bence–Jones proteinuria	Absent	May be present
Serum paraprotein concentration	Usually <25 g/l and stationary	Usually >25 g/l and rising
Immuneparesis	Absent	Present
Underlying lymphoproliferative disease or myeloma	Absent	Present

Fig. 12.57 Benign and malignant paraproteinaemia: distinguishing features.

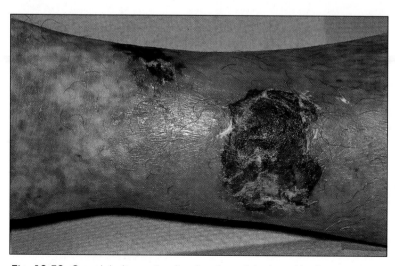

Fig. 12.58 Cryoglobulinaemia: discoloration of the leg with pigment deposition in a reticulated pattern because of vascular distension and haemorrhage. Areas of superficial necrosis and ulceration are seen. The patient showed a serum IgM paraprotein but no other evidence of myeloma or lymphoma.

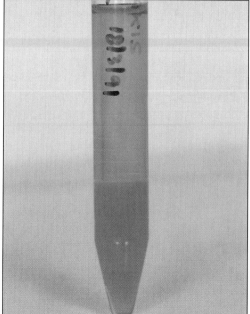

Fig. 12.59 Cryoglobulinaemia: same case as shown in Fig. 12.58. Serum from a patient with primary disorder, prepared from whole blood at 37°C, showing protein precipitation on cooling to room temperature. In this case the protein was monoclonal IgM.

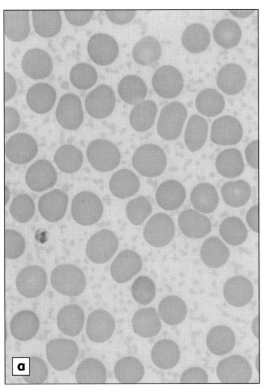

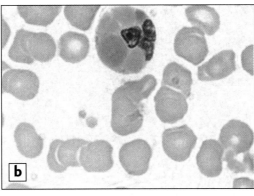

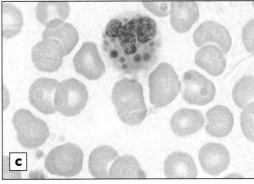

Fig. 12.60a–c Multiple myeloma: (a) cryoglobulin IgM protein – peripheral blood film showing pink staining aggregates of immunoglobulins between red cells; (b, c) neutrophils with multiple blue-staining inclusion bodies from ingested cryoglobulin. [(b, c) From Bain BJ. *Blood cells: A Practical Guide*. London: Gower; 1989.]

association with abnormal globulin production in myeloma (*Fig. 12.60*), macroglobulinaemia or non-Hodgkin lymphoma.

Heavy chain diseases

In the heavy chain diseases (HCDs), a rare group of disorders, the neoplastic cells secrete immunoglobulin heavy chains (γ, α or μ) without light chains attached to them. A single case of disease in which δ heavy chains were secreted has been described; the disease resembled myeloma. The secreted heavy chains in all types of HCD are usually incomplete.

Clinically, γ-HCD resembles a lymphoma. The protein usually consists of two γ heavy chains linked together. The variable region and part of the first domain of the constant region are sometimes deleted. The disease most often occurs in males, with a peak incidence in the seventh decade of life, with lymphadenopathy, fever and anaemia. The marrow shows a mixture of lymphocytes and plasma cells, often with eosinophilia, and the serum shows a monoclonal spike in the γ, α or β region.

The most common form of HCD, α-HCD, has a number of special features. It occurs largely in the Mediterranean area and Africa, often in patients with an Arabic genetic background, and in areas where intestinal parasites are frequent. It commences as a relatively benign plasma cell proliferation in the gastrointestinal tract (*Fig. 12.61*); subsequently, a poorly differentiated lymphoma of the small bowel develops and may spread, although usually within the abdominal cavity (*Fig.*

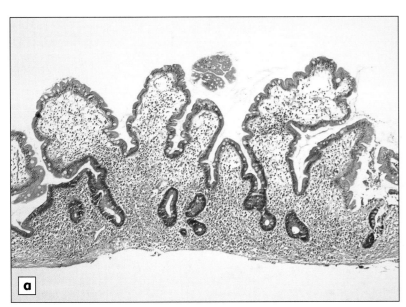

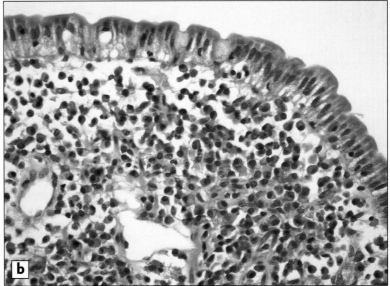

Fig. 12.61a and b α Heavy chain disease: this 25-year-old Algerian man presented in 1983 with a malabsorption syndrome, consisting of weight loss, chronic diarrhoea, steatorrhoea and hypocalcaemia, that responded to broad-spectrum antibiotics. (a) At this stage, small intestinal biopsy showed a diffuse infiltration of the lamina propria. (b) The cells were a mixture of lymphocytes, plasma cells and plasmacytoid cells. Immunocytochemical staining showed that a vast majority of these cells contained α heavy chains without κ or γ light chains. Serum and urine samples revealed a broad band in the α₂ globulin region, which precipitated with anti-IgA but showed no reactivity to anti-κ or anti-λ. [(a, b) Courtesy of Dr JE McLaughlin.]

12.62). The serum shows a monoclonal protein in the α_2 or β region in 50% of cases, and the protein may also be found in the urine. It consists of α heavy chains with an internal deletion.

A rare form of α-HCD occurs sporadically outside the areas in which intestinal infection is common and is characterized by a lymphoplasmacytoid infiltrate of the respiratory tract.

The rarest form is μ-HCD; the patients are usually African, particularly from parasite-infected zones (as for α-HCD). However, μ-HCD presents with a clinical picture that resembles chronic lymphocytic leukaemia or lymphoma, with enlargement of the liver and spleen and infiltration of the marrow with plasma cells. Light chains of one type may also be found in urine, but these remain separate from the μ heavy chain.

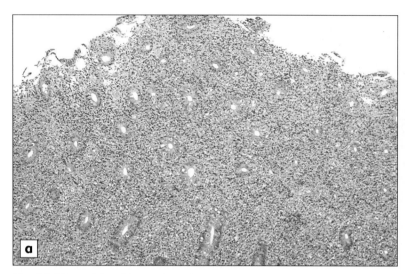

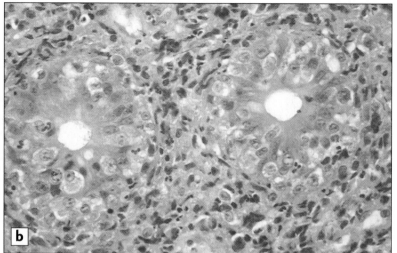

Fig. 12.62a and b α Heavy chain disease (same case as shown in *Fig. 12.61*): 2 years after presentation the patient developed small intestinal obstruction; intestinal resection revealed the small bowel to be heavily infiltrated by a large cell 'immunoblastic lymphoma' with an additional mixed infiltrate of neutrophils, plasma cells and macrophages. Despite intensive chemotherapy, the tumour relapsed, involving the large and small bowel, and intra-abdominal lymph nodes showed similar histological findings. The appearances of the rectal mucosa at (a) low and (b) high power show complete loss of normal architecture, with remaining crypt cells surrounded by the diffuse infiltrate consisting of immunoblasts and mixed inflammatory cells. The α heavy chain could still be detected in serum, but not in urine at this relapse. [(a, b) Courtesy of Dr JE McLaughlin.]

Non-Leukaemic Myeloproliferative Disorders

Polycythaemia vera, myelofibrosis and essential thrombocythaemia comprise the non-leukaemic myeloproliferative disorders. The endogenous proliferative process has features that suggest a process between benign hyperplasia and neoplasia. A clonal stem cell defect is thought to be responsible for the overlapping expansion of erythropoietic, granulopoietic and megakaryocytic components in the marrow (*Fig. 13.1*), although no aetiological features have been identified.

POLYCYTHAEMIA VERA

In classic cases of polycythaemia vera the marrow is hyperplastic. Examination of the blood reveals erythrocytosis and often a neutrophil leucocytosis and thrombocytosis; no primitive cells are seen in the peripheral blood film. The leucocyte alkaline phosphatase score is usually raised and there may be an increase in basophils. An invariable increase in total red cell volume is usually associated with mild-to-moderate degrees of splenomegaly and hepatomegaly, and extramedullary erythropoiesis is minimal. The main clinical problems are related directly to the increase in total blood volume and viscosity and to the hypermetabolism associated with myeloproliferation.

Polycythaemia vera is predominantly a disease of the middle-aged and elderly. The clinical features include plethora (*Figs 13.2 and 13.3*), headaches, lethargy, dyspnoea, fluid retention, bleeding symptoms, weight loss, night sweats, generalized pruritus made worse by hot baths,

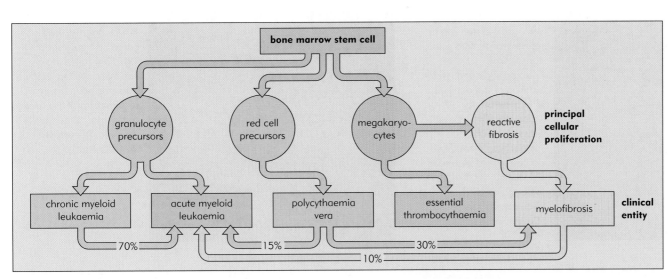

Fig. 13.1
Myeloproliferative disorders: their characteristic incidence of transformation.

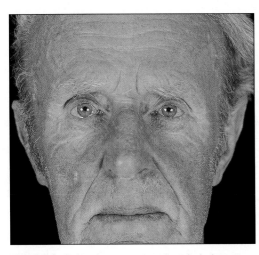

Fig. 13.2 Polycythaemia vera: facial plethora in a 65-year-old man. (Hb, 22 g/dl; WBC, 17 × 10⁹/l; platelets, 550 × 10⁹/l; total RCV, 65 ml/kg.)

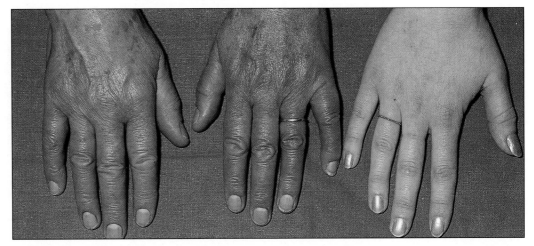

Fig. 13.3 Polycythaemia vera: the hands of a 50-year-old woman (on the left) appear congested and plethoric. (Hb, 20 g/dl; WBC, 15 × 10⁹/l; platelets, 490 × 10⁹/l.) The hand on the right is of a healthy 35-year-old woman. (Hb, 14.5 g/dl.)

acne rosacea (*Fig. 13.4*) and other non-specific forms of dermatitis. There is often suffusion of the conjunctivae (*Fig. 13.5*) and marked engorgement of the retinal vessels (*Figs 13.6 and 13.7*).

Mild-to-moderate splenomegaly is found in 70% of patients and the liver is palpable in 50% (*Fig. 13.8*). High blood uric acid levels are accompanied by gout (*Fig. 13.9*) in about 15% of cases. Major thromboses and haemorrhages dominate the course of untreated polycythaemia.

Portal or hepatic venous thrombosis is a serious complication, which occurs especially in women between the ages of 35 and 55 years.

Myelofibrosis develops in about 30% and death occurs in 10% of patients following the development of acute myeloid leukaemia (AML) late in the course of the disease.

Bone marrow aspirates typically show hyperplastic, normoblastic erythropoiesis and granulopoiesis with increased numbers of megakaryocytes

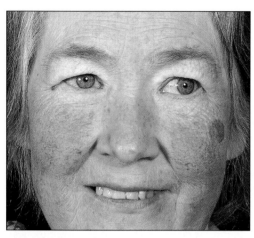

Fig. 13.4 Polycythaemia vera: acne rosacea in a middle-aged woman after treatment by venesection.

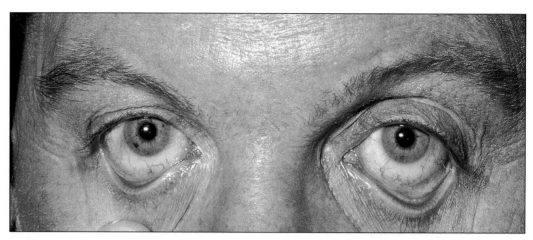

Fig. 13.5 Polycythaemia vera: facial plethora and conjunctival suffusion in a 40-year-old woman. (Hb, 19.5 g/dl.)

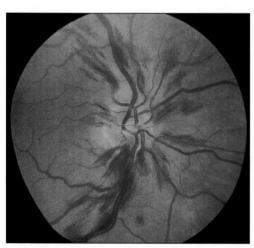

Fig. 13.6 Polycythaemia vera: gross distension of retinal vessels with conspicuous haemorrhage and mild swelling of the optic disc in hyperviscosity syndrome. The patient presented with headaches, lassitude, confusion and blurred vision. (Hb, 23.5 g/dl; WBC, 35 × 10⁹/l; platelets, 950 × 10⁹/l.) (Courtesy of Prof. JC Parr.)

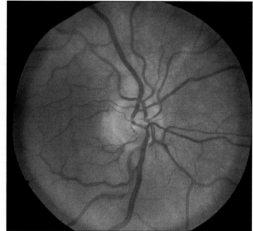

Fig. 13.7 Polycythaemia vera: same retina as shown in *Fig. 13.6* following venesection. The vessels and disc have returned to normal and the areas of haemorrhage have resolved. (Courtesy of Prof. JC Parr.)

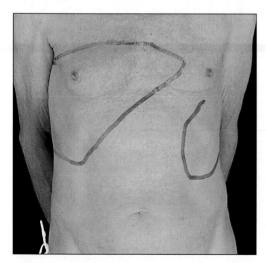

Fig. 13.8 Polycythaemia vera: enlarged liver and spleen of the patient shown in *Fig. 13.2*.

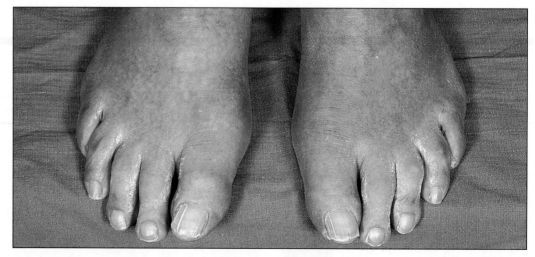

Fig. 13.9 Polycythaemia vera: acute gout with inflammation and swelling of the metatarsal and interphalangeal joints of the right great toe. The skin also shows a dusky plethora. (Hb, 21.5 g/dl; total RCV, 53 ml/kg; serum uric acid, 0.9 mmol/l.)

(*Figs 13.10 and 13.11*). Trephine biopsies confirm the hyperplastic haemopoiesis, and clusters of megakaryocytes are often prominent (*Figs 13.12 and 13.13*). In most patients haemopoietic tissue comprises 90% or more of the intertrabecular space. Silver impregnation techniques often show some increase in reticulin fibre density (*Fig. 13.14*).

Studies with radioactive iron usually demonstrate that erythropoiesis is confined to central skeletal sites without extramedullary activity (*Fig.*

13.15). Polycythaemia vera must be differentiated from other causes of polycythaemia (*Fig. 13.16*). The presence of splenomegaly, raised white cell and platelet counts and raised neutrophil alkaline phosphatase score are suggestive of polycythaemia vera. Additional helpful tests include the formation of spontaneous (in the absence of added erythropoietin) BFU-E and CFU-E colonies from the peripheral blood or bone marrow of patients with polycythaemia vera and the presence of

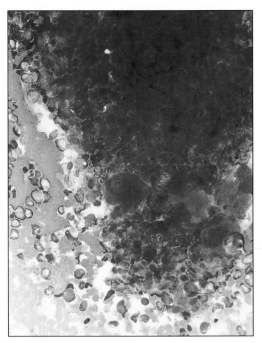

Fig. 13.10 Polycythaemia vera: bone marrow aspirate showing the edge of a hypercellular fragment. Marrow fat cells are absent.

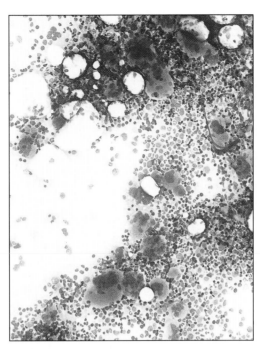

Fig. 13.11 Polycythaemia vera: bone marrow aspirate with hypercellular cell trails and bone marrow fragments, but incomplete replacement of marrow fat spaces. Megakaryocytes are especially prominent in the cell trails.

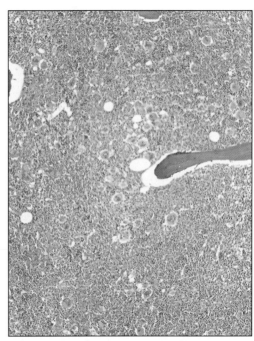

Fig. 13.12 Polycythaemia vera: trephine biopsy showing almost complete filling of the intertrabecular space with hyperplastic haemopoietlc tissue.

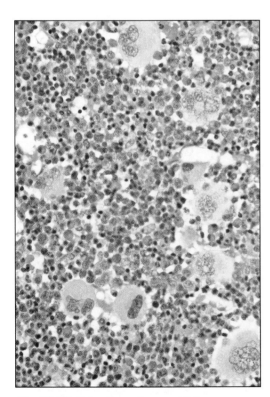

Fig. 13.13 Polycythaemia vera: higher power view of *Fig. 13.12* showing hyperplasia of erythropoiesis, granulopoiesis and megakaryocytes.

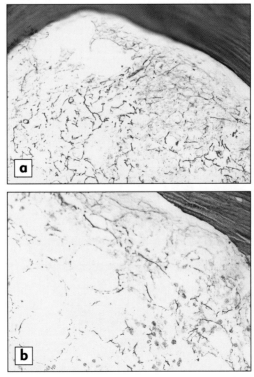

Fig. 13.14a and b Polycythaemia vera: silver impregnation staining shows (a) a moderate increase in the density of reticulin fibres compared with (b) normal bone marrow.

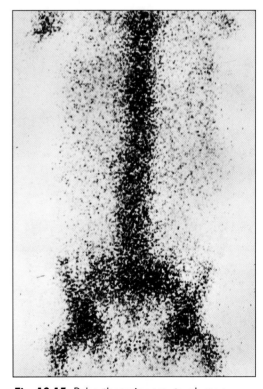

Fig. 13.15 Polycythaemia vera: trunk scan. Uptake of ^{52}Fe-labelled transferrin in the axial skeleton indicates that erythropoiesis is confined to the bone marrow.

Causes of polycythaemia		
Primary (increased red cell volume)	**Secondary (increased red cell volume)**	**Relative (normal red cell volume)**

Polycythaemia vera	As a result of compensatory erythropoietin increase in:
	
	  high altitudes
	  heavy smoking
	  cardiovascular disease
	  pulmonary disease and alveolar hypoventilation
	  increased affinity haemoglobins (familial polycythaemia)
	  methaemoglobinaemia (rarely)
	
	As a result of inappropriate erythropoietin increase in:
	
	  renal disease – hydronephrosis, vascular impairment,
	    cysts, carcinoma
	  massive uterine fibromyomata
	  hepatocellular carcinoma
	  cerebellar haemangioblastoma
		'Stress' or 'spurious' polycythaemia
		
		Dehydration:
		
		  water deprivation
		  vomiting
		  diuretic therapy
		
		Plasma loss:
		
		  burns
		  enteropathy

Fig. 13.16 Polycythaemia: causes.

raised levels of serum vitamin B$_{12}$ and/or of vitamin B$_{12}$ binding protein, transcobalamin I. Arterial oxygen saturation is normal. Relative polycythaemia is excluded by blood volume studies.

Treatment of polycythaemia vera is aimed at maintaining a normal blood count. Patients are usually managed by venesection or treated with cytotoxic drugs, usually hydroxyurea, or with radioactive phosphorus (^{32}P).

MYELOFIBROSIS

In myelofibrosis, a myeloproliferative disease that is also known as myelosclerosis, agnogenic myeloid metaplasia or non-leukaemic myelosis, the haemopoietic cell proliferation is more generalized, with splenic and hepatic involvement. This disorder is related closely to polycythaemia vera and a quarter of patients have a previous history of that disease. The associated increase in marrow fibre production is marked and the effectiveness of haemopoiesis decreases. Fibrosis is polyclonal, suggesting that it is a reaction to the underlying monoclonal marrow stem cell disorder.

Myelofibrosis usually occurs in the middle-aged and elderly. Most patients present initially with symptoms caused by anaemia, splenic enlargement (Fig. 13.17) or hypermetabolism such as night sweats, anorexia and weight loss. Some may complain of bone pain and gout (Fig. 13.18).

As a result of a hyperkinetic portal circulation, some cases of long standing develop portal hypertension and may present with bleeding oesophageal varices or ascites (Figs 13.19 and 13.20). Radiological surveys of the skeletal system frequently reveal no abnormality, although a minority of cases show generalized osteosclerosis (Fig. 13.21).

Most patients have a normochromic anaemia of moderate or marked severity. It may be macrocytic in those who are folate deficient or microcytic with associated iron deficiency. The peripheral blood usually shows florid leucoerythroblastic change and the number of nucleated red cells often exceeds the number of leucocytes. Marked polychromasia, anisocytosis and poikilocytosis with 'tear drop' red cells are typical changes (Fig. 13.22). In occasional patients with extensive osteosclerosis the blood film shows marked leucoerythroblastic change with circulating megakaryocyte fragments (Fig. 13.23). In contrast to polycythaemia vera, the serum lactic dehydrogenase level is raised.

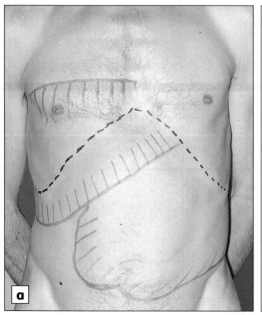
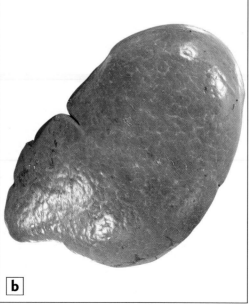
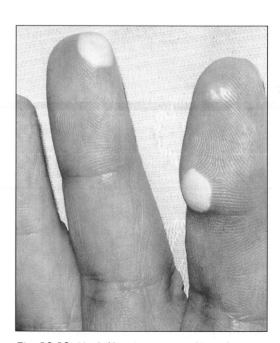

Fig. 13.17a and b Myelofibrosis: (a) splenohepatomegaly; (b) the patient's spleen shows a well-defined notch in the superior border. The prominent indent in the inferior border was palpable during clinical examination.

Fig. 13.18 Myelofibrosis: gouty tophi on the index and middle fingers of a 55-year-old man.

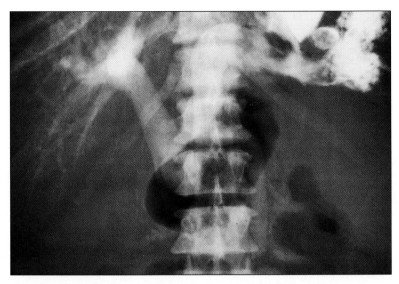

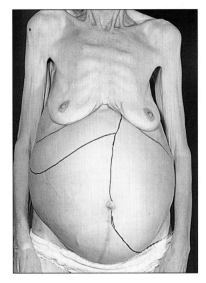

Fig. 13.20 Myelofibrosis: gross wasting and abdominal distension from massive splenomegaly, hepatomegaly and ascites.

Fig. 13.19 Myelofibrosis: trans-splenic portal venogram, showing gross dilatation of the splenic, inferior mesenteric and portal veins and increased bone density in the vertebral bodies. A great increase in splenic blood flow results in a hyperkinetic portal circulation which, together with the obstructive effects of extramedullary haemopoiesis, may be important in the pathogenesis of portal hypertension.

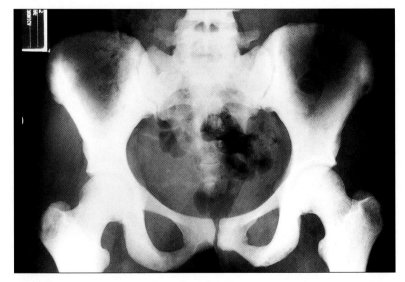

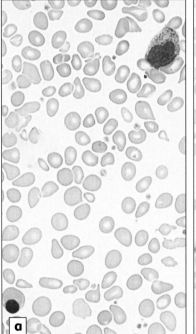

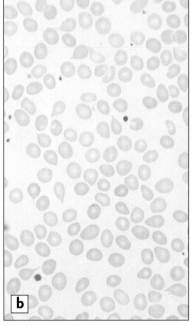

Fig. 13.21 Myelofibrosis: pelvic radiograph showing a generalized increase in bone density from osteosclerosis.

Fig. 13.22a and b Myelofibrosis: peripheral blood films showing (a) leucoerythroblastic changes with red cell polychromasia, anisocytosis and poikilocytosis, including 'tear drop' forms – the nucleated cells are an erythroblast and a late myelocyte; (b) red cell anisocytosis and poikilocytosis with 'tear drop' forms in early disease.

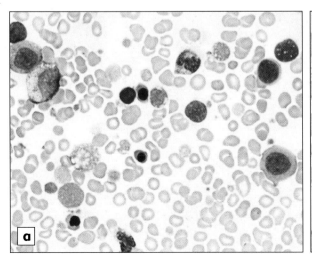

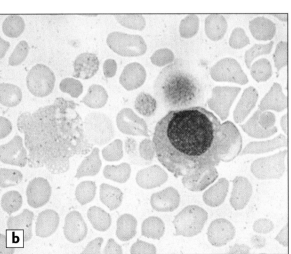

Fig. 13.23a and b Myelofibrosis/osteomyelofibrosis: peripheral blood films showing (a) myelocytes, erythroblasts and megakaryocyte fragments; (b) at higher magnification, megakaryocyte fragments.

Attempts at bone marrow aspiration are usually unsuccessful, but trephine biopsy of the iliac bone reveals a variable degree of haemopoietic cell activity and marrow fibrosis (*Figs 13.24–13.26*). Silver impregnation techniques show an increase in reticulin fibre density and thickness (*Figs 13.27 and 13.28*); only in advanced disease is there collagen deposition and, in 10% of cases, osteosclerosis (*Fig. 13.29*).

Radioisotope investigations may be used to determine the severity of the disease and may also help to elucidate the mechanism of the anaemia. Whole-body scanning techniques use cyclotron-produced ^{52}Fe to assess the distribution of the injected radioiron in the body (*Figs 13.30 and 13.31*). Extramedullary haemopoiesis may also be confirmed from a liver biopsy or after splenectomy (*Figs 13.32 and*

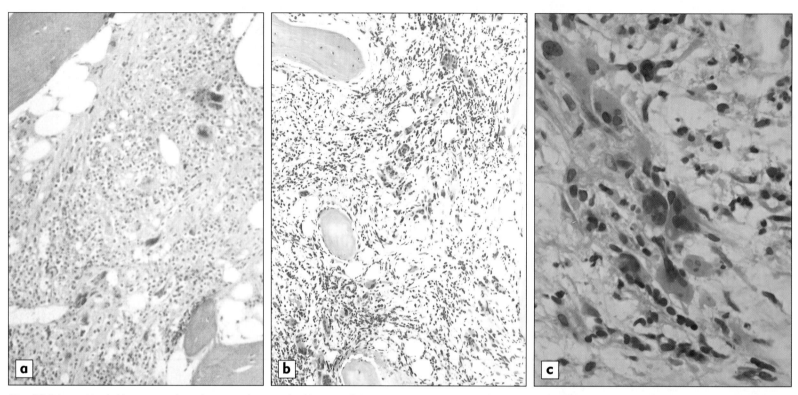

Fig. 13.24a–c Myelofibrosis: trephine biopsies showing (a, b) most of the intertrabecular space occupied by cellular loose connective tissue contains scattered haemopoietic cells including prominent megakaryocytes, fat cells comprising <15% of the intertrabecular space and extensive deposition of loose connective tissue around haemopoietic cells; (c) the prominence of megakaryocytes in the myelofibrotic tissue at higher magnification.

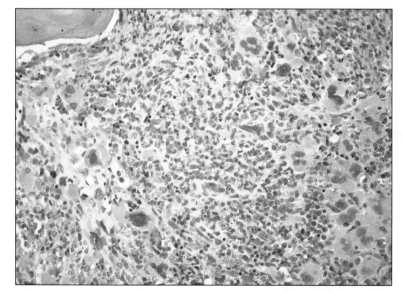

Fig. 13.25 Transitional myeloproliferative disease: trephine biopsy showing complete filling of intertrabecular space by hyperplastic haemopoietic tissue with large numbers of megakaryocytes and increased stromal connective tissue between haemopoietic cells. This patient has clinical features of both polycythaemia vera and myelofibrosis. The blood film showed leucoerythroblastic features and splenic enlargement extending 20 cm below the left costal margin. (Hb, 18.5 g/dl; WBC, 120 × 10⁹/l; platelets, 450 × 10⁹/l; total RCV, 49 ml/kg.)

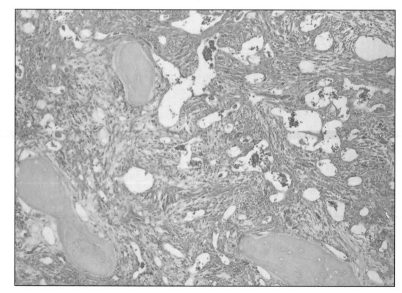

Fig. 13.26 Transitional myeloproliferative disease: trephine biopsy showing prominent dilated venous sinuses surrounded by hyperplastic and fibrotic haemopoietic tissue. The blood film showed leucoerythroblastic change. (Hb, 19.5 g/dl; WBC, 38 × 10⁹/l; platelets, 850 × 10⁹/l; total RCV, 44 ml/kg.)

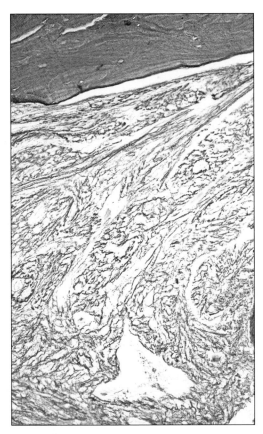

Fig. 13.27 Myelofibrosis: silver impregnation staining of the biopsy shown in *Fig. 13.24b* illustrates a gross increase in reticulin fibre density and thickness.

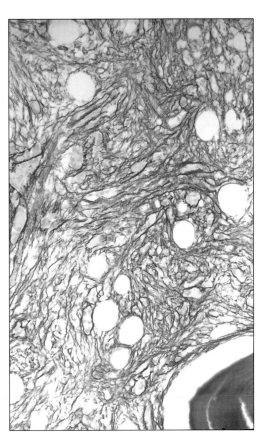

Fig. 13.28 Transitional myeloproliferative disease: silver impregnation staining of the biopsy shown in *Fig. 13.26* illustrates a marked increase in reticulin fibre density.

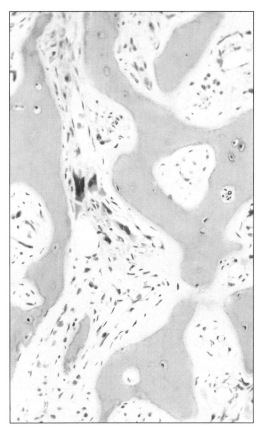

Fig. 13.29 Osteomyelofibrosis: trephine biopsy showing replacement of normal intertrabecular tissue by a fibrous connective tissue containing only isolated haemopoietic cells (the larger central cells are megakaryocytes). There is an increased amount of trabecular bone with an irregular lamellar pattern.

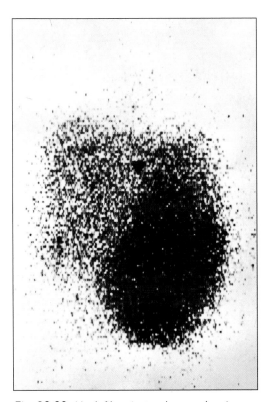

Fig. 13.30 Myelofibrosis: trunk scan showing dominant uptake of ^{52}Fe-labelled transferrin into the enlarged spleen and liver with no evidence of skeletal concentration, a pattern consistent with predominant extramedullary haemopoiesis.

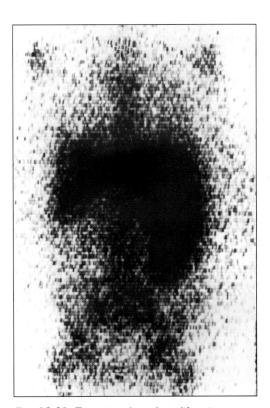

Fig. 13.31 Transitional myeloproliferative disease: trunk scan showing obvious uptake of ^{52}Fe-labelled transferrin in the liver and spleen, as well as in the central skeleton.

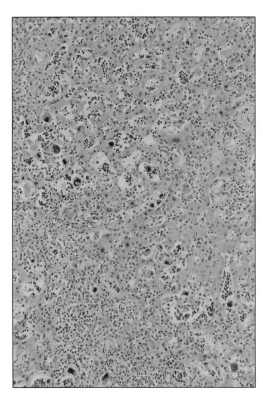

Fig. 13.32 Myelofibrosis: extramedullary haemopoiesis. Liver biopsy showing groups of erythroblasts, granulopoietic cells and multinucleate megakaryocytes in the sinuses.

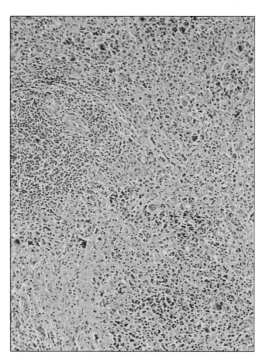

Fig. 13.33 Myelofibrosis: extramedullary haemopoiesis. Section of spleen following splenectomy showing similar groups of haemopoietic cells in the reticuloendothelial cords and sinuses.

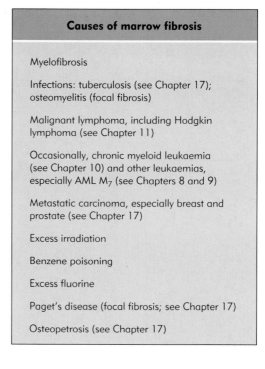

Causes of marrow fibrosis
Myelofibrosis
Infections: tuberculosis (see Chapter 17); osteomyelitis (focal fibrosis)
Malignant lymphoma, including Hodgkin lymphoma (see Chapter 11)
Occasionally, chronic myeloid leukaemia (see Chapter 10) and other leukaemias, especially AML M_7 (see Chapters 8 and 9)
Metastatic carcinoma, especially breast and prostate (see Chapter 17)
Excess irradiation
Benzene poisoning
Excess fluorine
Paget's disease (focal fibrosis; see Chapter 17)
Osteopetrosis (see Chapter 17)

Fig. 13.34 Reactive marrow fibrosis: causes.

13.33). Myelofibrosis must be differentiated from other causes of reactive marrow fibrosis (*Fig. 13.34*).

Treatment of myelofibrosis is unsatisfactory. Supportive red cell transfusions are required in severely anaemic patients. Alkylating agents, hydroxyurea and splenectomy may help in selected patients. Folic acid may be given to prevent deficiency.

ESSENTIAL THROMBOCYTHAEMIA

A diagnosis of essential thrombocythaemia is considered when a sustained rise in platelet count occurs, in some cases in excess of $1000 \times 10^9/l$, with no other underlying cause. There are usually abnormalities of platelet function and in severe cases the clinical course may be dom-inated by recurrent haemorrhage and thrombosis. In many patients, the raised platelet count is found on routine testing and there are no symptoms for many years, particularly in younger patients. In some patients this disorder is not easily distinguished from myelofibrosis and particularly polycythaemia vera, of which many investigators consider thrombocythaemia to be merely a variant. However, recent studies suggest that not all cases of essential thrombocythaemia are clonal. The dominant clinical problem is bleeding from the gastrointestinal tract and, less frequently, epistaxis, menorrhagia, haematuria or haemoptysis. Spontaneous bruising often appears (*Fig. 13.35*) and cere-brovascular accidents may occur in the elderly. Blockage of peripheral blood vessels may result in erythromelalgia (*Fig. 13.36*), ischaemia and gangrene (*Fig. 13.37*).

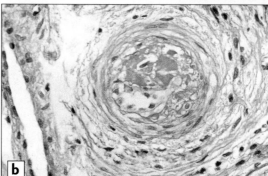

Fig. 13.35 Essential thrombocythaemia: haemorrhage into subcutaneous tissues following minor trauma. Gross defects of platelet aggregation with adenosine diphosphate, adrenaline and thrombin were found. (Platelets, $2300 \times 10^9/l$.)

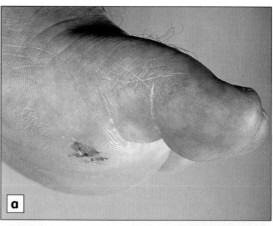

Fig. 13.36a and b Essential thrombocythaemia: erythromelalgia. (a) Severe burning pain and hot, red congestion of the forefoot and toes in a 39-year-old man. (Platelet count, $875 \times 10^9/l$.) (b) Section of a skin biopsy showing thrombotic occlusion of an arteriole with proliferative changes in the peripheral wall. [(a, b) Courtesy of Prof. JJ Michiels.]

The peripheral blood film shows a distinctive increase in platelet count and the platelets are often of abnormal morphology with many giant forms. Howell–Jolly bodies and other stigmata of splenic atrophy are found in a third of severe cases and careful search may reveal the presence of megakaryocyte fragments (*Figs 13.38–13.40*).

Aspiration of bone marrow may be difficult. There is usually a general hyperplasia of haemopoietic cells with a striking increase in the number of megakaryocytes (*Fig. 13.41*), which are often found in cohesive clusters (*Fig. 13.42*). The megakaryocytes tend to show many nuclear lobes and their average cell volume is above normal (*Figs 13.43 and 13.44*).

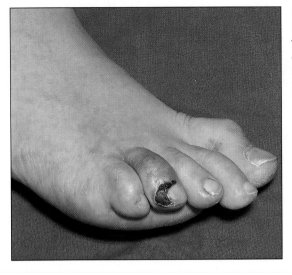

Fig. 13.37 Essential thrombocythaemia: gangrene of the left fourth toe. (Platelets, 1900 × 10⁹/l.)

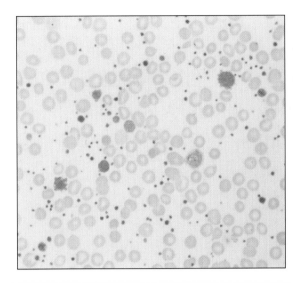

Fig. 13.38 Essential thrombocythaemia: peripheral blood film showing a gross increase in platelet numbers.

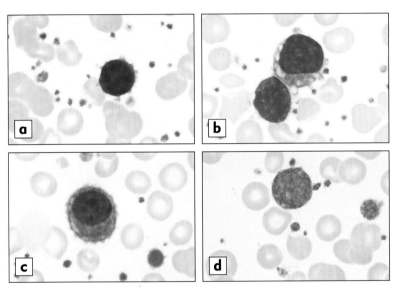

Fig. 13.39a–d Essential thrombocythaemia: (a–d) peripheral blood films showing circulating megakaryocyte fragments.

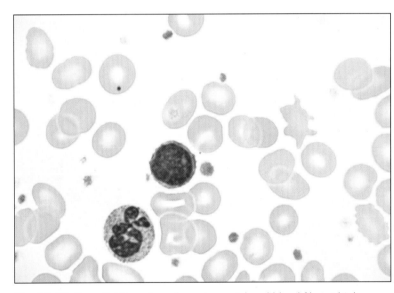

Fig. 13.40 Essential thrombocythaemia: peripheral blood film at high magnification showing features of splenic atrophy, including a Howell–Jolly body, red cell targetting, crenation and acanthocytosis.

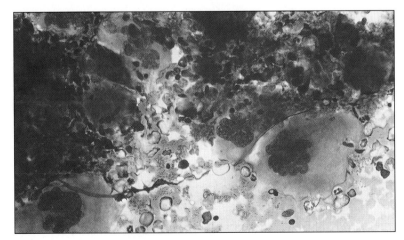

Fig. 13.41 Essential thrombocythaemia: bone marrow aspirate fragment showing a marked increase in the number of megakaryocytes.

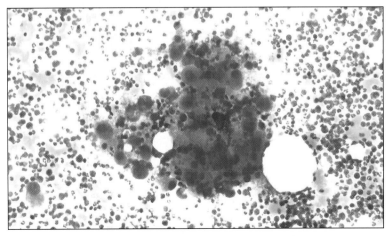

Fig. 13.42 Essential thrombocythaemia: bone marrow aspirate cell trail showing a prominent cluster of megakaryocytes.

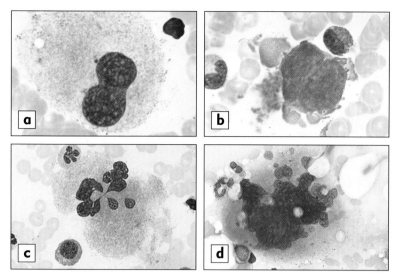

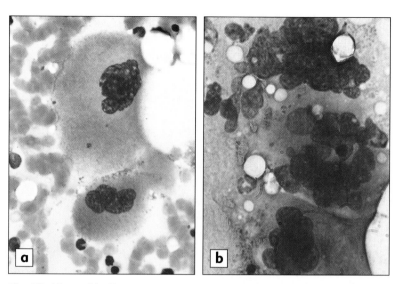

Fig. 13.43a–d Essential thrombocythaemia: bone marrow aspirate showing (a) binucleate megakaryocyte; (b) binucleate megakaryoblast with cytoplasmic differentiation; (c) relatively low and (d) high nuclear ploidy in hypersegmented megakaryocytes.

Fig. 13.44a and b Essential thrombocythaemia: bone marrow aspirates showing clumping of megakaryocytes with (a) definite cell borders and (b) lack of cytoplasmic separation.

In many patients the dominant feature is masses of adherent platelets that may be confused with marrow fragments (*Fig. 13.45*). Trephine biopsy preparations reflect the dramatic increase in the megakaryocyte population; large numbers of abnormal megakaryocytes are seen at all stages of development (*Fig. 13.46*). Silver impregnation techniques demonstrate an increase in reticulin patterns intermediate to those of polycythaemia vera and myelofibrosis.

Splenic atrophy (*Fig. 13.47*) often increases the severity of platelet elevation in the peripheral blood as obliteration of the splenic red pulp areas, in which platelet pooling normally occurs, results in the entire marrow platelet production being accommodated in the general circulation. Essential thrombocythaemia must be differentiated from other causes of a high platelet count (*Fig. 13.48*).

Hydroxyurea, busulfan (now largely obsolete), α_2-interferon and ^{32}P have been used to reduce platelet production. Trials of the drug anagrelide are in progress, since this has no leukaemogenic action compared with ^{32}P and hydroxyurea. Low-dose aspirin therapy may be used to reduce the risk of thrombosis in asymptomatic patients who show no evidence of excess bruising or haemorrhage.

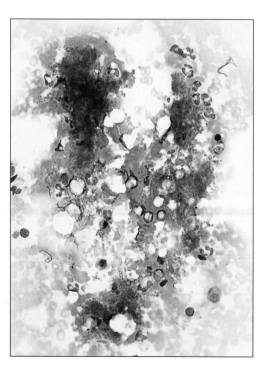

Fig. 13.45 Essential thrombocythaemia: bone marrow aspirate cell trail showing large masses of aggregated platelets.

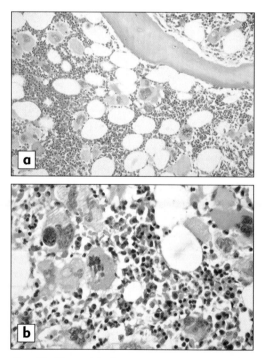

Fig. 13.46a and b Essential thrombocythaemia: trephine biopsy showing (a) that the overall cellularity of haemopoietic tissue is not greatly increased, but (b) large numbers of megakaryocytes, seen particularly well at higher magnification.

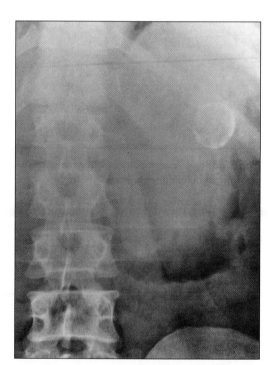

Fig. 13.47 Essential thrombocythaemia: abdominal radiograph showing a small spherical calcified mass (at upper right). The blood film showed features of splenic atrophy. At autopsy the fibrotic remnant of spleen weighed only 30 g and had extensive areas of dystrophic calcification.

Causes of a high platelet count	
Reactive	**Endogenous**
Haemorrhage	Essential thrombocythaemia
Trauma	Some cases of polycythaemia vera, myelofibrosis and chronic myeloid leukaemia
Postoperative	
Chronic iron deficiency	
Malignancy	
Chronic infections	
Connective tissue diseases	
Postsplenectomy with continuing anaemia and active marrow	

Fig. 13.48 High platelet count (thrombocytosis): causes.

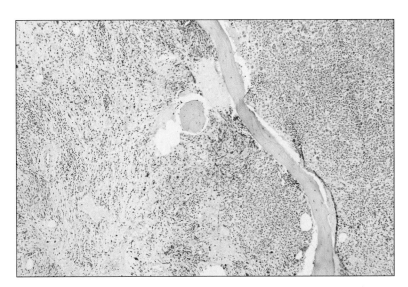

Fig. 13.49 Myelofibrosis transformed into acute leukaemia: trephine biopsy showing areas (left field) that are consistent with myelofibrosis, but the intertrabecular space (right field) contains sheets of closely packed mononuclear cells with no obvious stromal connective tissue.

LEUKAEMIC TRANSFORMATION OF POLYCYTHAEMIA VERA AND MYELOFIBROSIS

It is generally accepted that transformation is part of the natural history of the myeloproliferative syndrome. Transition to myelofibrosis from polycythaemia vera occurs in approximately 30% of cases and to acute leukaemia in about 15%. The latter is usually AML, but the occurrence of acute lymphoblastic leukaemia has been described. The incidence of leukaemia is similar in those treated with either ^{32}P or alkylating agents. Hydroxyurea is now used in preference to either as it is considered to be less likely to predispose to leukaemic transformation. Of patients with myelofibrosis, 10% develop a terminal leukaemia (*Figs 13.49–13.52*). Survival beyond leukaemic transformation in either condition is brief.

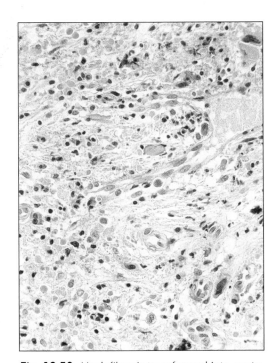

Fig. 13.50 Myelofibrosis transformed into acute leukaemia: higher power view of the left field in *Fig. 13.49* shows isolated haemopoietic cells surrounded by a loose fibrous connective tissue.

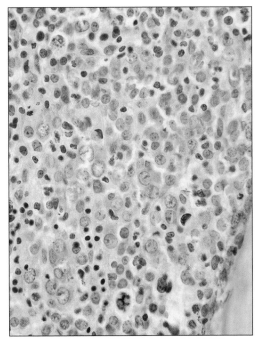

Fig. 13.51 Myelofibrosis transformed into acute myeloid leukaemia: higher power view of the right field in *Fig. 13.49* shows predominantly primitive myeloid blast cells and promyelocytes. Following a 9-year history of myelofibrosis, the patient had presented with a fever and bronchopneumonia. (Hb, 7.1 g/dl; WBC, 6 × 10^9/l; blasts, 4.5 × 10^9/l; neutrophils, 0.6 × 10^9/l; platelets, 40 × 10^9/l.)

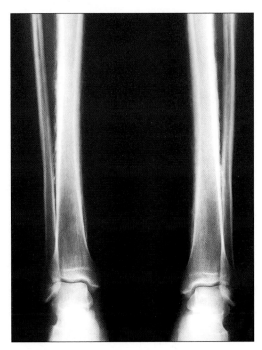

Fig. 13.52 Myelofibrosis transformed into acute myeloid leukaemia: radiograph of the lower legs of a middle-aged man showing extensive periosteal elevation caused by infiltration of myeloid blast cells from underlying medullary bone. Although the medullary cavities of these bones in adults usually contain only fat, haemopoietic tissue may extend to distal skeletal tissue in long-standing myeloproliferative disease.

ACUTE MYELOFIBROSIS

Patients with acute myelofibrosis present acutely with symptoms caused by anaemia, neutropenia or thrombocytopenia and show leucoerythroblastic changes in the peripheral blood. Attempts at marrow aspiration are unsuccessful, but trephine biopsies reveal evidence of myelofibrosis (*Figs 13.53 and 13.54*). Acute myelofibrosis is usually caused by the megakaryoblastic type of AML (FAB M$_7$; see page 143), but may also be caused by lymphoma, tuberculosis and other diseases. In typical cases the morphology and immunophenotype of the blast cells indicate that the condition is a megakaryoblastic variant of acute leukaemia (*Fig. 13.55*). The majority of patients do not have gross splenomegaly.

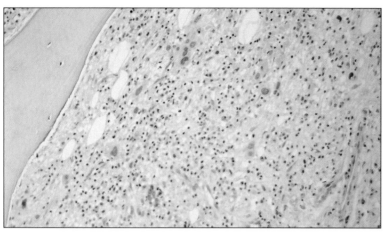

Fig. 13.53 Acute myelofibrosis: trephine biopsy showing abnormal haemopoietic tissue with predominant mononuclear cells, isolated megakaryocytes and an abundant fibrous stroma.

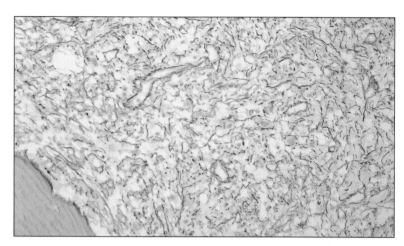

Fig. 13.54 Acute myelofibrosis: trephine biopsy with silver impregnation staining to illustrate a marked increase in reticulin fibre density.

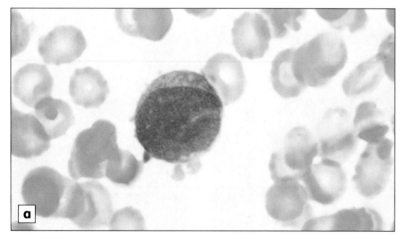

a

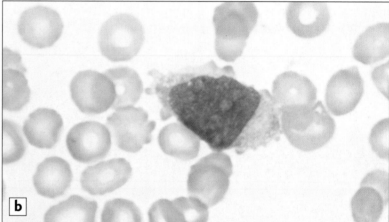

b

Fig. 13.55a and b Acute myelofibrosis, AML (FAB M$_7$): (a, b) peripheral blood films showing blast cells that are somewhat larger than classic myeloblasts and have irregular cytoplasmic borders. Electron microscopic studies and detection of platelet glycoproteins IIb/IIIa using monoclonal antibodies confirmed that these were megakaryoblasts. (Hb, 6.3 g/dl; WBC, 3 × 10^9/l; blasts, 1.2 × 10^9/l; neutrophils, 0.9 × 10^9/l; platelets, 65 × 10^9/l.)

14

Stem Cell Transplantation

STEM CELL TRANSPLANTATION

Stem cell transplantation may be carried out between siblings (allogeneic transplantation; *Fig. 14.1*) who are HLA identical and whose cells do not react in mixed lymphocyte culture or can be shown to be matching by a number of different techniques of DNA analysis. Syngeneic (identical twin), haploidentical, HLA-matched but unrelated donors and placental (cord) blood may also be used in appropriate cases (*Fig. 14.2*).

The recipient has severe aplastic anaemia, Fanconi anaemia, poor-prognosis leukaemia (e.g. poor or standard risk acute myeloid leukaemia in first remission, acute lymphoblastic leukaemia in second or subsequent remission or in first remission with poor prognostic features, or chronic myeloid leukaemia in chronic phase), a severe genetic abnormality (e.g. thalassaemia major) or an acquired marrow disorder (e.g. myeloma or myelodysplasia) (*Fig. 14.3*).

In autologous transplantation, the patient's own stem cells are used to rescue the patient from profound marrow ablation caused by high-dose chemotherapy, with or without total body irradiation, for malignant disease (*Fig. 14.4*).

Peripheral blood stem cells (PBSC) may be harvested using a cell separator (*Fig. 14.5*) and used instead of bone marrow both for allogeneic and autologous transplantation. Usually the patient is given cyclophosphamide and a 4–6 day course of granulocyte colony-stimulating factor (G-CSF) or granulocyte–macrophage CSF (GM-CSF) to mobilize PBSC. A collection of $>2.5 \times 10^6$/kg CD34$^+$ cells is regarded as adequate (*Fig. 14.5*). Stem cells appear similar to small or medium-sized lymphocytes (*Fig. 14.6*) and are contained in a CD34-enriched cell population (*Fig. 14.7*). Normal donors receive G-CSF but not cyclophosphamide. Recovery of platelets by PBSC is enhanced compared to the recovery of platelets after bone marrow transplantation.

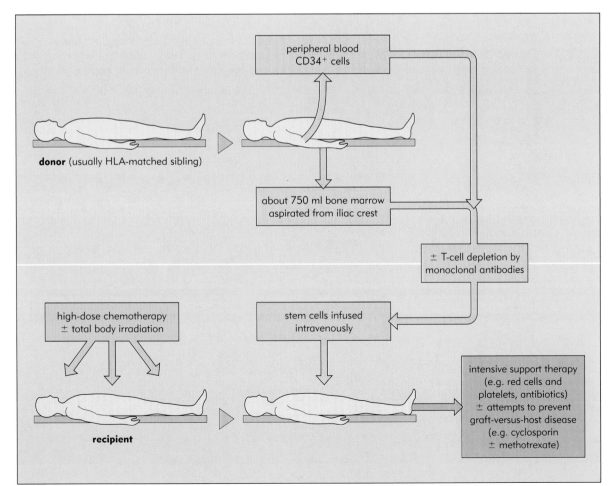

Fig. 14.1 Allogeneic stem cell transplantation: stem cells may be harvested from peripheral blood or bone marrow.

peripheral blood CD34$^+$ cells

donor (usually HLA-matched sibling)

about 750 ml bone marrow aspirated from iliac crest

± T-cell depletion by monoclonal antibodies

high-dose chemotherapy ± total body irradiation

stem cells infused intravenously

intensive support therapy (e.g. red cells and platelets, antibiotics) ± attempts to prevent graft-versus-host disease (e.g. cyclosporin ± methotrexate)

recipient

Stem cell transplantation – donors	
Type	**Donor**
Syngeneic	Identical twin
Allogeneic	HLA-matching brother or sister
	HLA-matching other family member (e.g. parent, cousin)
	HLA-matching unrelated volunteer donor (VUD or MUD)
Cord (placental) blood	
Autologous	

Fig. 14.2 Stem cell (bone marrow or peripheral blood) transplantation: donors

Fig. 14.3 Stem cell (bone marrow or peripheral blood) transplantation: indications.

Stem cell transplantation: indications

Allogeneic (or syngeneic)

Malignant

Acute myeloid leukaemia

Acute lymphoblastic leukaemia:
  poor prognosis: first remission
  second remission or subsequently

Chronic myeloid leukaemia

Chronic lymphocytic leukaemia

Other severe acquired disorders of the marrow
(e.g. Hodgkin's disease, non-Hodgkin's lymphoma,
myeloma, myelodysplasia)

Benign marrow disorders

Aplastic anaemia

Paroxysmal nocturnal haemoglobinuria

Thalassaemia major

Sickle cell anaemia

Kostmann's syndrome

Chronic granulomatous disease

Chediak–Higashi syndrome

Adhesion molecule deficiency

Glanzmann's disease

Bernard–Soulier disease

Osteoporosis

Congenital haemophagocytic syndrome

Immunodeficiency

Severe combined immunodeficiency

Wiscott–Aldrich syndrome

Metabolic storage diseases

Gaucher's disease (Type II)

Mucopolysaccharidosis

Autologous

Malignant lymphoma (Hodgkin's or non-Hodgkin's)
usually post first relapse

Other solid tumours (e.g. breast cancer)

Acute myeloid or lymphoblastic leukaemia
(in first or subsequent remission with or without
marrow purging)

Myeloma

Severe autoimmune disease (e.g. scleroderma)

For gene therapy (e.g. adenosine deaminase
deficiency)

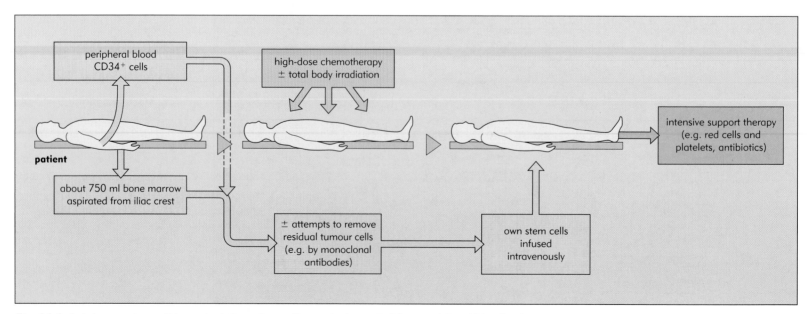

Fig. 14.4 Autologous stem cell transplantation: stem cells may be harvested from peripheral blood or bone marrow.

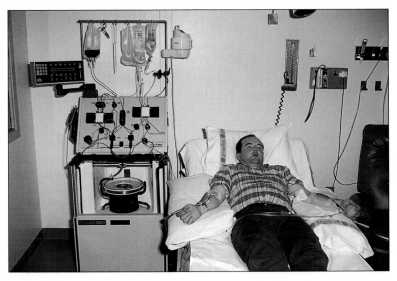

Fig. 14.5 Peripheral blood stem cell collection: blood is circulated from one arm to a cell separator and the buffy coat harvested, the red cells and plasma being returned to the donor.

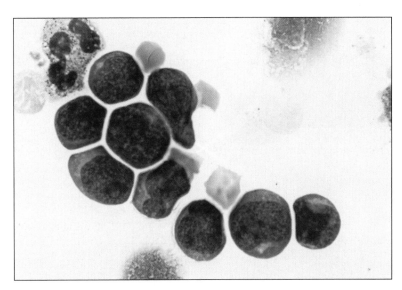

Fig. 14.6 Peripheral blood stem cell collection: enriched CD34$^+$ cells stained by May–Grunwald Giemsa. The cells have the appearance of small- and medium-sized lymphocytes. (Courtesy of Dr M Potter.)

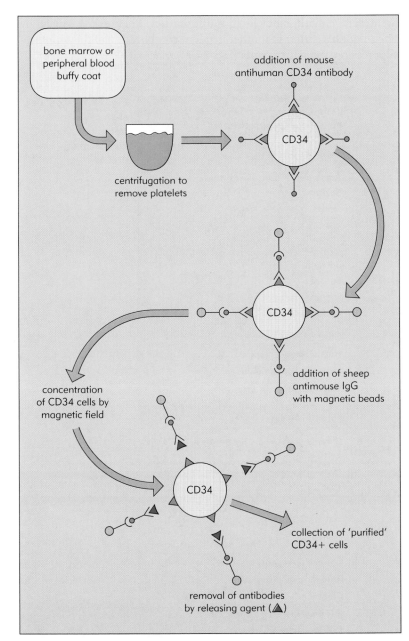

Fig. 14.7 Peripheral blood stem cell collection: steps in the Baxter system of purification of CD34$^+$ cells.

A typical haematological chart of a patient having allogeneic stem cell transplantation for aplastic anaemia is shown in *Fig. 14.8*.

Stem cell transplantation has also been carried out for certain benign congenital or acquired abnormalities of the marrow (e.g. thalassaemia major or paroxysmal nocturnal haemoglobinuria), the lymphoid system (as in severe combined immune deficiency) or the macrophage system (as in Hurler's disease) (*see Fig. 14.3*).

Failure of engraftment is unusual in well-matched transplants for leukaemia but is more common when the recipient has aplastic anaemia or when donor and recipient are not fully matched or when T-cell depletion has been carried out.

LOW INTENSITY CONDITIONING (LIC)-TRANSPLANTS

In 'LIC'-transplant procedures, the donor is treated with drugs and/or radiotherapy at a less intensive level than used for standard stem cell transplantation. The aim is to achieve immunosuppression sufficient for donor stem cells to be accepted into the marrow microenvironment, and to establish a durable graft without total marrow ablation by the conditioning treatment. Drugs used in different regimens include fludarabine, cyclophosphamide, anti-lymphocytic globulin, and busulphan. The aim is to establish chimerism between recipient and donor cells and for the donor immune competent cells to effect a cure by a graft versus leukaemia (myelodysplasia, myeloma or lymphoma) effect.

DONOR LEUCOCYTES

Donor leucocytes may be given after allogeneic stem cell transplantation if residual disease or recurrence of disease is evident. The best results are obtained if only minimal disease is present (e.g. chronic myeloid leukaemia detected by molecular methods or cytogenetics only, rather than from haematological relapse of the disease). Also, it is important that chimerism is still present (i.e. there is evidence of donor as well as recipient cells in the blood or bone marrow of the recipient).

COMPLICATIONS OF STEM CELL TRANSPLANTS

Allogeneic transplantation is not usually carried out for patients older than 45–50 years because of the increased incidence of complications

261

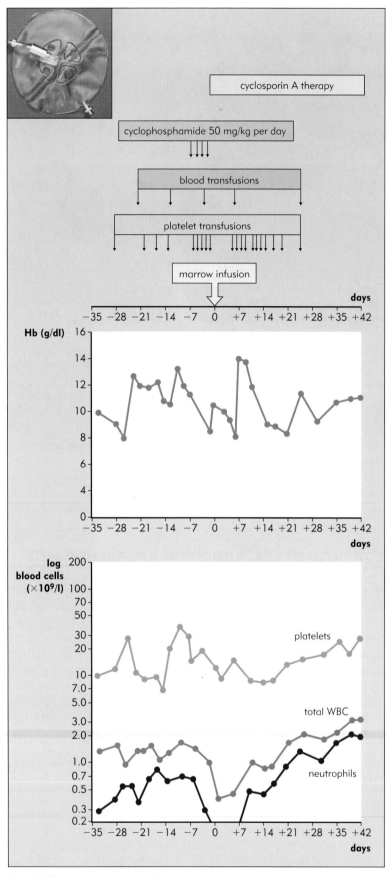

Fig. 14.8 Aplastic anaemia: haematological response to bone marrow transplantation. Marrow (500–1000 ml) is harvested from the pelvis of the donor. Red cells are removed and in some institutions T lymphocytes are also eliminated (e.g. by monoclonal antibodies) to prevent graft-versus-host disease (GVHD). Cyclosporin A is used to ameliorate GVHD and to enhance engraftment in aplastic anaemia. When the recipient has leukaemia, total body irradiation is usually used in addition to chemotherapy in the conditioning. The inset shows donor marrow depleted of red cells and T lymphocytes before infusion into the recipient. (Courtesy of Mr M Gilmore.)

(*Fig. 14.9*), but autologous transplantation is carried out for patients up to the age of 55–65 years. The recipient's marrow is first eliminated by intensive chemotherapy, which is usually combined in the case of leukaemia with total body irradiation. A least 2 weeks of pancytopenia follows before the infused donor pluripotent stem cells, having seeded the recipient's bone marrow, proliferate and differentiate sufficiently to produce new mature red cells, leucocytes and platelets.

Infections are a major hazard during the post-transplant period. Attempts at prevention include reverse-barrier or laminar-flow nursing, prophylactic non-absorbable antibiotics and antifungal agents, and early use of systemic antibiotics for febrile episodes. Prolonged antibiotic therapy however, increases the likelihood of fungal infections (*Figs 14.10 and 14.11*). Haemopoietic growth factors (e.g. G-CSF and GM-CSF) may be used to enhance granulocyte recovery (*see Fig. 1.13*).

Cytomegalovirus infection may result from reactivation of a previous latent infection or from transmission of the virus in blood products, and may result in severe pneumonitis and marrow suppression. Treatment is with ganciclovir alone or along with foscarnet (*Figs 14.12 and 14.13*).

Herpes simplex virus (e.g. HH-V6) infection is a frequent complication which tends to become generalized and may cause pneumonia, encephalitis, skin lesions (*Fig. 14.14*) or marrow suppression. Infection can be prevented by the use of prophylactic intravenous acyclovir. Treatment is with ganciclovir and foscarnet. Pneumonia caused by *Pneumocystis carinii* is another frequent complication of the immunosuppression and neutropenia (*Figs 14.15 and 14.16*).

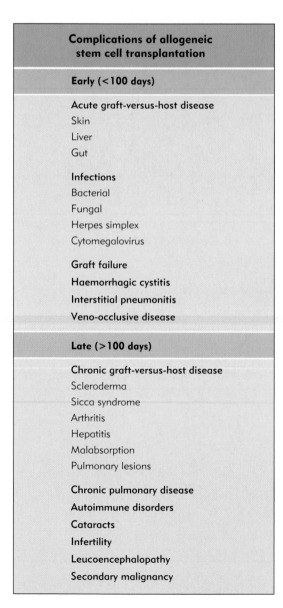

Fig. 14.9 Allogeneic stem cell transplantation: complications.

Complications of allogeneic stem cell transplantation
Early (<100 days)
Acute graft-versus-host disease
Skin
Liver
Gut
Infections
Bacterial
Fungal
Herpes simplex
Cytomegalovirus
Graft failure
Haemorrhagic cystitis
Interstitial pneumonitis
Veno-occlusive disease
Late (>100 days)
Chronic graft-versus-host disease
Scleroderma
Sicca syndrome
Arthritis
Hepatitis
Malabsorption
Pulmonary lesions
Chronic pulmonary disease
Autoimmune disorders
Cataracts
Infertility
Leucoencephalopathy
Secondary malignancy

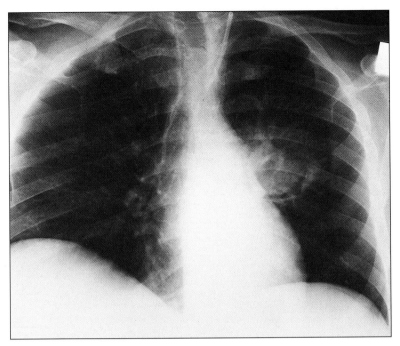

Fig. 14.10 Stem cell transplantation: chest radiograph showing an opacity in the upper left zone, with a cystic centre that contains a dense central zone, caused by aspergillosis.

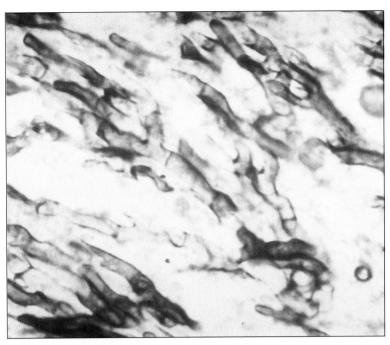

Fig. 14.11 Stem cell transplantation: cytology of sputum from the case shown in *Fig. 14.10* illustrates the typical branching septate hyphae of aspergilli. Methenamine silver stain.

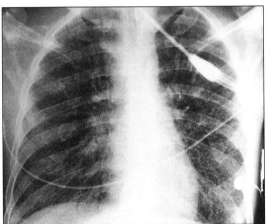

Fig. 14.12 Stem cell transplantation: chest radiograph showing widespread interstitial pneumonia. Sputum cultures and indirect immunofluorescence showed the presence of cytomegalovirus.

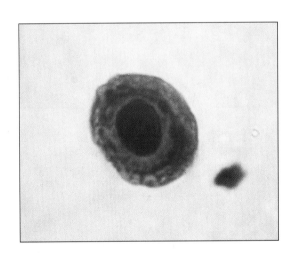

Fig. 14.13 Stem cell transplantation: sputum cytology shows a pulmonary cell with degenerative changes and a large intranuclear inclusion body typical of cytomegalovirus infection. Papanicolaou stain. (Courtesy of Prof. YS Erozan.)

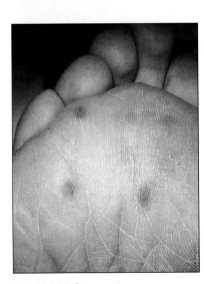

Fig. 14.14 Stem cell transplantation: herpes simplex virus infection with multiple widespread lesions on the skin of the sole of the foot. (Courtesy of Prof. HG Prentice.)

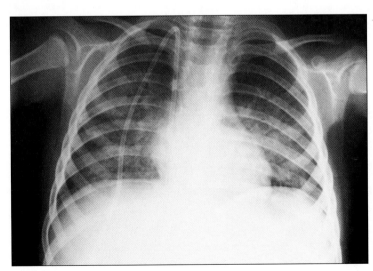

Fig. 14.15 Stem cell transplantation: chest radiograph showing typical 'bat wing' shadowing of both lung fields caused by *P. carinii* infection.

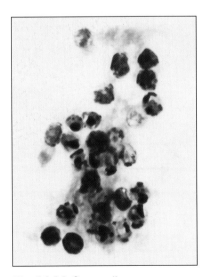

Fig. 14.16 Stem cell transplantation: high-power view of concentrated bronchial washings showing typical appearance of *P. carinii*. (Gram–Weigert stain; courtesy of Prof. YS Erozan.)

Total body irradiation itself may cause side effects that involve epithelial structures; damage to the nails and nail beds (*Fig. 14.17*) and temporary complete alopecia (*Fig. 14.18*) occur. Veno-occlusive disease (VOD) of the liver (*Fig. 14.19*) is an acute complication caused by chemotherapy and radiotherapy. Preceding chemotherapy and abnormal liver function may also predispose to VOD. Haemorrhagic cystitis may result from cyclophosphamide metabolites (mesna is given to try to prevent this) or from viral infection (e.g. adenovirus, cytomegalovirus or polyoma virus).

Graft-versus-host disease

Another major post-transplant complication is reaction of the immunocompetent cells in the graft against the tissues of the host, which causes GVHD that may be acute (occurring in the first 100 days post-transplant) or chronic. The risk factors for acute GVHD are given in *Fig. 14.20*. The triad of skin, mucous membrane and gut, and liver involvement is classified according to severity into Grades I, II, III and IV.

In acute cases of GVHD an erythematous itchy skin rash is widespread (*see Fig. 14.18*) and tends to be particularly severe on the hands and feet. In severe cases a bullous eruption and subsequent widespread exfoliation may occur (*Fig. 14.21*).

In chronic cases the lesions tend to be firm, red and plaque-like (*Fig. 14.22*) and ultimately may, in some patients, form a scleroderma-like picture with contractures and ulceration (*Fig. 14.23*) The hands and feet may continue to exfoliate (*Fig. 14.24*).

The mucous membranes may also be affected, with formation of lichen planus-like lesions in the mouth and pharynx (*Fig. 14.25*).

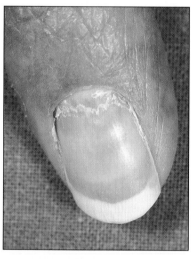

Fig. 14.17 Stem cell transplantation: this nail shows horizontal ridges and atrophy of the nail bed as a result of total body irradiation. (Courtesy of Prof. HG Prentice.)

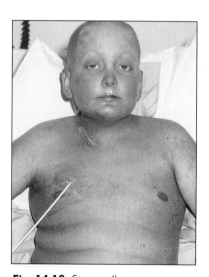

Fig. 14.18 Stem cell transplantation – acute GVHD: widespread erythematous skin rash. An indwelling central Hickman catheter is in place. (Courtesy of Prof. HG Prentice.)

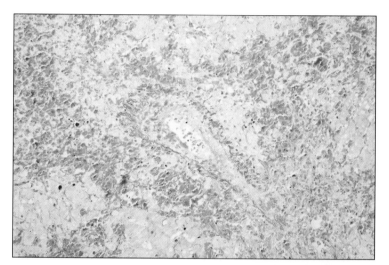

Fig. 14.19 Stem cell transplantation: VOD. Section showing a terminal hepatic venule with marked narrowing of its lumen. The deep-blue staining identifies the collagen of the original venule wall, while the inner paler blue area represents new collagen obstructing the lumen. Note the loss of hepatocytes in the perivenular area and the intense congestion of the sinusoids. (Chromotrope Aniline Blue × 40 stain; courtesy of Dr M Jarmulowicz.)

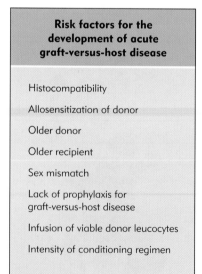

Risk factors for the development of acute graft-versus-host disease
Histocompatibility
Allosensitization of donor
Older donor
Older recipient
Sex mismatch
Lack of prophylaxis for graft-versus-host disease
Infusion of viable donor leucocytes
Intensity of conditioning regimen

Fig. 14.20 Stem cell transplantation: risk factors for the development of acute GVHD. (Adapted with permission from Atkinson K. *The BMT Data Book*. Cambridge: Cambridge University Press; 1998:464.)

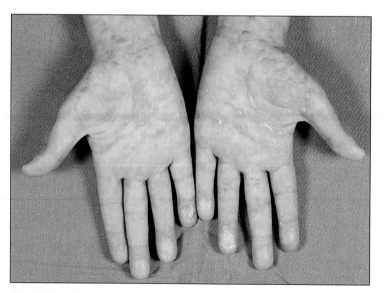

Fig. 14.21 Stem cell transplantation – acute GVHD: the palmar surfaces of these hands show an erythematous maculopapular eruption with bullous ulceration and denudation. (Courtesy of Prof. HG Prentice.)

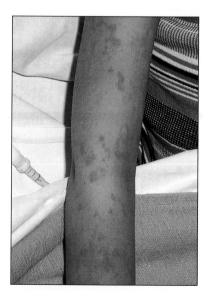

Fig. 14.22 Stem cell transplantation – chronic GVHD: these patchy raised erythematous skin lesions are characteristic. (Courtesy of Prof. HG Prentice.)

The histological appearances of GVHD are normally seen in life after skin or rectal biopsy. In acute GVHD the skin shows inflammatory changes with death of epidermal cells and a lymphoid infiltrate (*Fig. 14.26*) leading, in severe cases, to denudation.

The rectal mucosa also shows death of epithelial (crypt) cells and inflammatory changes (*Fig. 14.27*). When severe, there is loss of small and large intestinal mucosa (*Fig. 14.28*).

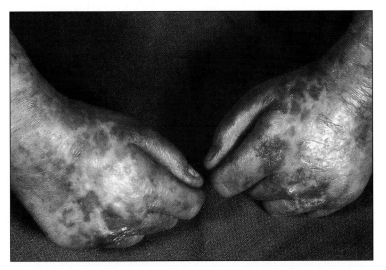

Fig. 14.23 Stem cell transplantation – chronic GVHD: scleroderma-like contractions of the hands with thickening of the skin and marked pigmentation. (Courtesy of Prof. HG Prentice.)

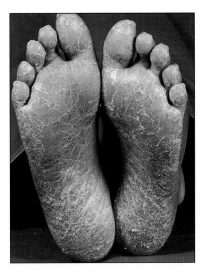

Fig. 14.24 Stem cell transplantation – chronic GVHD: erythema and exfoliation of the epidermis of the soles of the feet. (Courtesy of Prof. HG Prentice.)

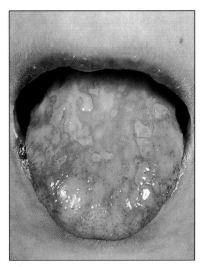

Fig. 14.25 Stem cell transplantation – chronic GVHD: lesions of the tongue and lips similar to those of lichen planus. (Courtesy of Prof. HG Prentice.)

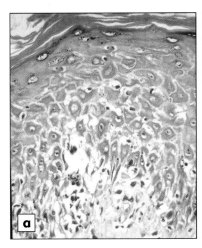

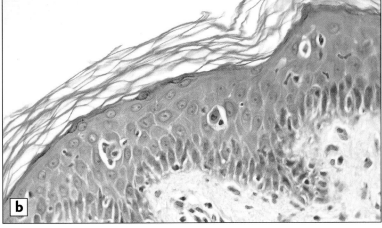

Fig. 14.26a and b Stem cell transplantation – acute GVHD: histological sections of skin in moderately severe (Grade II) acute GVHD, showing (a) vacuolation of the basal epidermal cells with inflammatory changes in the superficial dermis; (b) prominent vacuoles containing necrotic epidermal cells and lymphocytes, from an African patient.

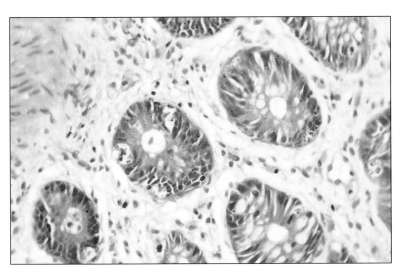

Fig. 14.27 Stem cell transplantation – acute GVHD: high-power view of rectal biopsy in Grade I acute GVHD showing individual crypt cell necrosis and oedema of the lamina propria.

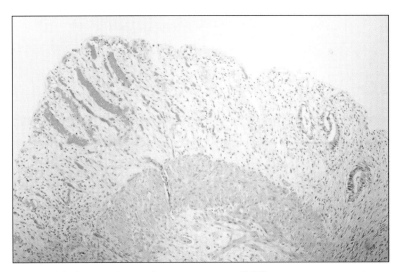

Fig. 14.28 Stem cell transplantation – acute GVHD: post-mortem section of colon in Grade IV acute GVHD showing almost complete denudation of the epithelium, with oedema and lymphocytic infiltration of the submucosa.

Liver function is abnormal in acute and chronic GVHD, except in mild cases. The histological appearances include damage to bile duct epithelial cells, inflammatory changes and cholestasis (*Fig. 14.29*). GVHD can be prevented in HLA-matched allogeneic transplantation if T lymphocytes are completely removed *in vitro* from donor bone marrow, but this may increase the risk of graft failure or of leukaemic relapse in some situations. Prevention of GVHD is usually carried out with cyclosporin with or without methotrexate; FK506 (tacrolimus) and mycophenalate mofetil are drugs under trials for prevention and treatment of GVHD.

A frequent post-transplantation complication is an interstitial pneumonia (*Fig. 14.30*), which is more common in GVHD but may also be related to lung irradiation and to infection, particularly with cytomegalovirus.

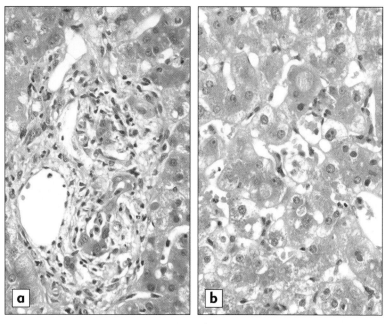

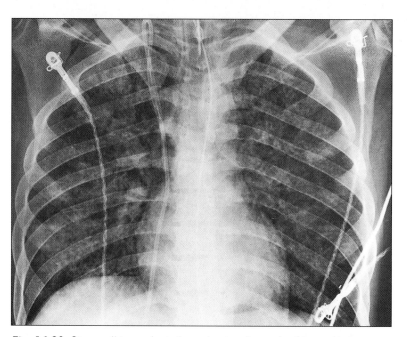

Fig. 14.29a and b Stem cell transplantation – acute GVHD: high-power views of liver biopsy showing (a) damaged, irregular and elongated bile duct epithelial cells with occasional pyknotic nuclei in the portal tract (there is a moderate infiltration of lymphocytes and neutrophils).
(b) Cholestatic changes include dilated bile canaliculi and pigmented hepatocytes. [(a, b) Courtesy of Prof. PJ Scheuer.]

Fig. 14.30 Stem cell transplantation: chest radiograph of interstitial pneumonitis showing widespread diffuse mottling. The patient had received total body irradiation and had Grade III GVHD. No infective cause of the pneumonitis was identified in this case.

15

Vascular and Platelet Bleeding Disorders

HAEMOSTASIS AND BLEEDING DISORDERS

The mechanism of normal haemostasis involves the interaction of blood vessels, platelets and coagulation factors (*Fig. 15.1*). The initial arrest of haemorrhage is the result of vasoconstriction and the elastic recoil of severed blood vessels, together with the formation of platelet plugs. This is followed by activation of blood coagulation factors, which convert the fluid blood into an insoluble fibrin clot, reinforcing the sealing effect. The coagulation cascade is detailed in Chapter 16.

The main function of the intact vessel wall is to prevent haemostasis and platelet aggregation (*Fig. 15.2*). A number of substances produced by the endothelium cause vasodilatation (e.g. nitric oxide), inhibit platelet aggregation [e.g. prostacyclin (epoprostenol)] or blood coagulation (e.g. antithrombin and protein C activator), or activate fibrinolysis (e.g. tissue plasminogen activator). Von Willebrand's factor (VWF), necessary for platelet–cell wall interaction, is also produced. A break in the vessel wall exposes clotting factors and platelets to the subendothelial connective tissue.

The platelet has a trilamellar surface membrane which invaginates into the cytoplasm to form an open canalicular system, giving a large surface (platelet factor 3) to which clotting factors may adsorb (*Fig. 15.3*). A mucopolysaccharide coat outside the membrane is important in platelet adhesion to the vessel wall and in aggregation and adsorption of clotting factors, especially fibrinogen and factor VIII. Glycoproteins (GPs) on the platelet surface include GP Ib (defective in Bernard–Soulier syndrome), and GP IIb–IIIa (defective in thrombasthenia). Both sites are important in the attachment of platelets to VWF and, hence, to vascular endothelium (*Fig. 15.4*). The binding site for GP IIb–IIIa is also

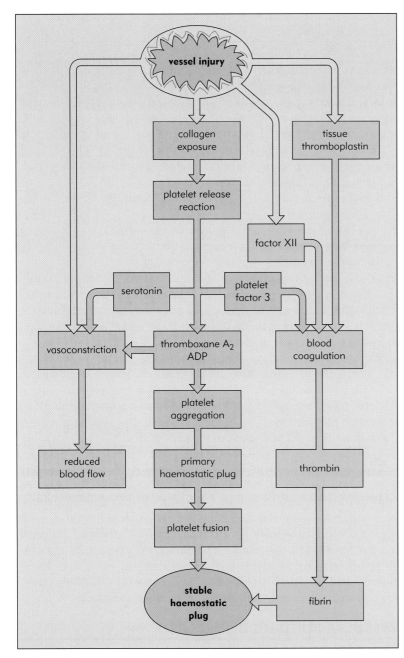

Fig. 15.1 Normal haemostasis: mechanisms.

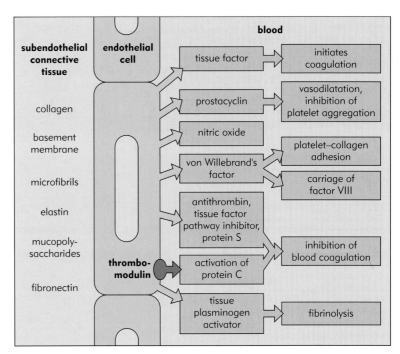

Fig. 15.2 Function of intact vessel wall: the endothelial cell forms a barrier between platelet and plasma clotting factors, and subendothelial connective tissues. Endothelial cells produce a variety of substances that cause vasodilatation, inhibit haemostasis or platelet aggregation, or activate fibrinolysis.

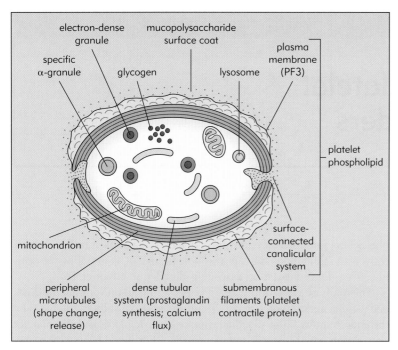

Fig. 15.3 Ultrastructure of a platelet: electron-dense granules contain adenine nucleotides, calcium and serotonin; specific α-granules contain growth factor, fibrinogen, factor V and von Willebrand's factor, fibronectin, β-thromboglobulin, heparin antagonist and thrombospondin; lysosomes contain acid hydrolases; the plasma membrane is the site of receptors for clotting factors and aggregating agents. (Courtesy of Dr RA Hutton.)

Fig. 15.5 Abnormal vascular bleeding: associated disorders.

Vascular bleeding disorders
Hereditary
Hereditary haemorrhagic telangiectasia
Ehlers–Danlos syndrome
Marfan's syndrome
Osteogenesis imperfecta
Fabry's syndrome
Infections
Bacterial
Viral
Rickettsial
Allergic
Henoch–Schönlein syndrome
Systemic lupus erythematosus
Drugs
Food
Atrophic
Senile purpura
Cushing's syndrome and corticosteroid therapy
Scurvy purpura
Dysproteinaemia
Amyloid
Miscellaneous
Simple easy bruising
Factitious
Autoerythrocyte sensitization
Fat embolism

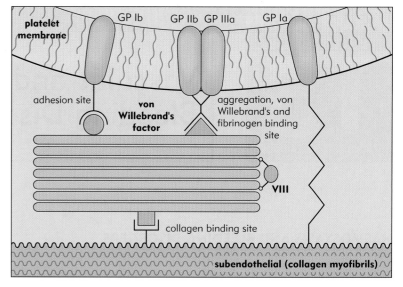

Fig. 15.4 Adhesion of platelets to vascular endothelium: this is mediated by von Willebrand's factor which also carries factor VIII coagulation factor (VIII:C). There are two binding sites on the platelet membrane for von Willebrand's factor: GP Ib and GP IIb–IIIa complex (see also Fig. 15.46). (Courtesy of Dr RA Hutton.)

the receptor for fibrinogen and, after conformational change, leads to platelet–platelet aggregation.

A submembranous microtubular system maintains the platelet shape; microfilaments distributed throughout the cytoplasm (including a complex mixture of muscle proteins) are involved in changes in platelet contraction and secretion, and clot retraction. The platelets also contain a number of organelles, including α-granules, which contain a variety of proteins (see Fig. 15.3):

- dense bodies (δ-granules), which contain calcium, adenine nucleotides and serotonin;
- lysosomes, which contain acid hydrolases;
- peroxisomes, which contain catalase;
- mitochondria; and
- a dense tubular system that contains substantial quantities of calcium and may be a site of synthesis of prostaglandins and thromboxane A_2.

The platelet attaches to subendothelial structures of damaged vessels, probably via attachment to VWF (see Fig. 15.4) which has binding sites for collagen microfibrils in the exposed subendothelium.

Bleeding disorders may be the result of abnormalities in blood vessels, qualitative or quantitative defects of blood platelets (dealt with in this chapter) or deficiencies of blood coagulation factors (dealt with in Chapter 16). They may present as excessive post-traumatic bleeding, epistaxis, menorrhagia, haematemesis, melaena, rectal bleeding, haematuria or as deep bleeding in muscles or joints.

Disorders of platelets and small blood vessels present as purpuras with pronounced cutaneous and mucosal bleeding. Prolonged bleeding from superficial cuts and abrasions is a feature of thrombocytopenia and disorders of platelet function. Gastrointestinal bleeding may occur. Menorrhagia is often the dominant clinical problem of women with severe thrombocytopenia or von Willebrand's disease. Repeated haemarthroses, deep dissecting haematomas and serious delayed excessive post-traumatic bleeding are more characteristic of severe deficiencies of blood coagulation factors. Initial haemostasis, in these cases, may be accomplished by vascular reaction and platelet plugs.

VASCULAR BLEEDING DISORDERS

Disorders associated with vascular bleeding are listed in *Fig. 15.5*.

Hereditary haemorrhagic telangiectasia

The small vascular malformations that are the essential lesion in hereditary haemorrhagic telangiectasia may be confused with petechiae. These bright red or purple spots are permanent and most noticeable on the face, nose, lips and tongue, and on plantar and palmar surfaces (*Figs 15.6–15.8*). Usually the lesions do not appear until adulthood, becoming more numerous with advancing age. Bleeding from the telangiectasia of the gastrointestinal mucosa produces a state of chronic severe iron deficiency.

Ehlers–Danlos syndrome

In Ehlers–Danlos syndrome the purpura arises from defective platelet aggregation because of an inherited abnormality of skin collagen. It is most marked in Type IV Ehlers–Danlos syndrome (*Fig. 15.9*), in which deficiency of Type III collagen occurs.

Senile purpura

Relative indolent purpuric ecchymoses are found frequently in the elderly, particularly on areas of skin exposed to sunlight – for example, on the backs of the hands and wrists (*Fig. 15.10*), the extensor surfaces of the forearms and the back of the neck. This condition may be caused by atrophy of dermal collagen and loss of subcutaneous fat, weakening the supporting tissue of the small blood vessels of the skin which then become more susceptible to shear strain.

Scurvy

Petechiae of perifollicular distribution (*Fig. 15.11*) are a feature of scurvy, probably because of a defect in the microvascular supporting tissue. Disordered platelet function may also be present.

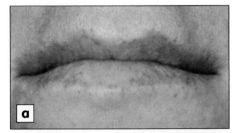
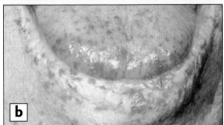

Fig. 15.6a and b Hereditary haemorrhagic telangiectasia: the characteristic small vascular lesions are obvious on (a) lips and (b) tongue.

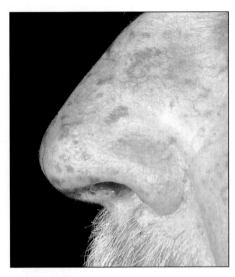

Fig. 15.7 Hereditary haemorrhagic telangiectasia: characteristic vascular malformations in the skin of the nose.

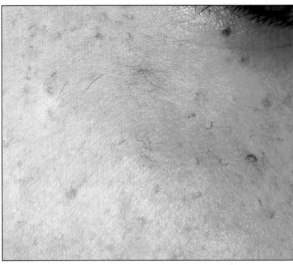

Fig. 15.8 Hereditary haemorrhagic telangiectasia: close-up view of the linear and punctate vascular lesions.

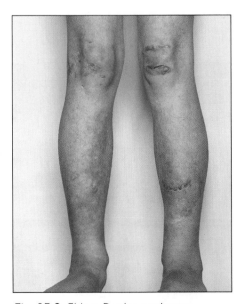

Fig. 15.9 Ehlers–Danlos syndrome: purpura into scars of the skin, especially around the knees, of a 16-year-old boy who also displayed hyperextensible joints, thin, easily torn skin and poor healing. The scars are raised into folds by the underlying bulging subcutaneous tissues. (Courtesy of Dr I Sarkany.)

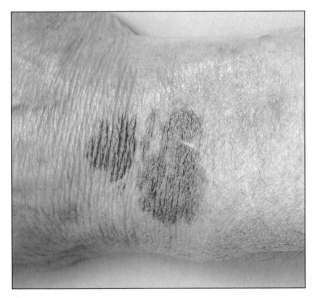

Fig. 15.10 Senile purpura: typical ecchymoses on the extensor surface of the wrist of an elderly man.

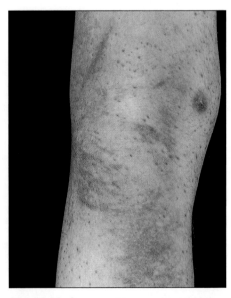

Fig. 15.11 Scurvy: widespread petechial perifollicular haemorrhages becoming confluent. Deeper haematomas were also present.

Purpura associated with abnormal proteins

Petechiae and ecchymoses may be seen in patients with multiple myeloma (*Fig. 15.12*), Waldenström's macroglobulinaemia, benign monoclonal gammopathy, cryoglobulinaemia or cryofibrinogenaemia. Many of the proteins involved in these conditions interfere with platelet function and fibrin formation.

Small vessel haemorrhages may also result from hyperviscosity of blood or from damage to the vessel upon precipitation of these proteins in the cooler parts of the skin. Similarly, patients with amyloidosis may show purpura caused by deposition of amyloid in the microcirculation (*Fig. 15.13*).

Allergic purpuras

The skin lesions in the allergic purpuras are more variable. Petechiae and ecchymoses associated with the Henoch–Schönlein syndrome may be accompanied by itching, tingling sensations, erythema and urticarial swelling. The lesions occur most commonly on the buttocks and legs (*Fig. 15.14*). In this syndrome there may be associated submucosal haemorrhage in the intestine (*Fig. 15.15*), haematuria and joint pain.

Some allergic drug reactions present as erythematous and purpuric skin eruptions (*Fig. 15.16*). The lesions may be generalized or may have a symmetrical proximal distribution. Extensive purpuric bleeding may also accompany severe vasculitis, as in systemic lupus erythematosus (SLE; *Figs 15.17 and 15.18*) and other connective tissue disorders.

Purpura associated with infection

Purpura associated with infection may be the result of toxic damage to the endothelium or of immune complex-type hypersensitivity. In some conditions, for example meningococcal septicaemia (*Fig. 15.19*), disseminated intravascular coagulation (DIC) is often associated. There may be extensive bleeding into the vesicular lesions of herpes zoster in patients with leukaemia (*Fig. 15.20*), and petechial haemorrhage of the palate in infectious mononucleosis (*Fig. 15.21*).

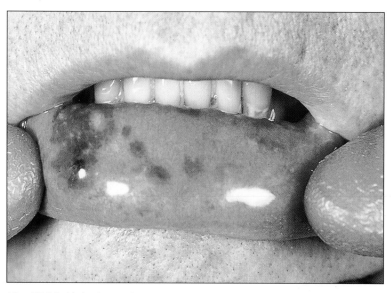

Fig. 15.12 Multiple myeloma: purpuric haemorrhages in the mucosal surface of the lower lip.

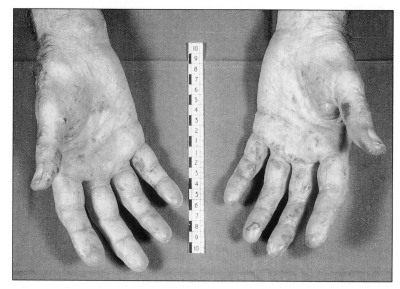

Fig. 15.13 Amyloidosis: purpura of the skin with characteristic smooth yellowish deposits secondary to multiple myeloma.

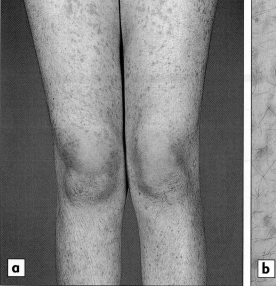
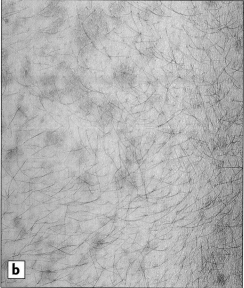
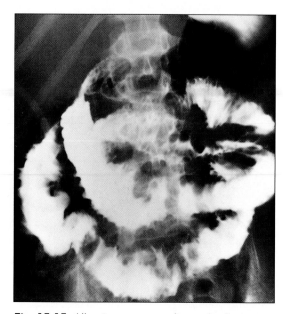

Fig. 15.14a and b Allergic purpura: (a) extensive purpura of the skin of the legs in Henoch–Schönlein syndrome; (b) the early lesions are more an urticarial erythema than true petechial haemorrhage.

Fig. 15.15 Allergic purpura: radiograph of Henoch–Schönlein syndrome with mucosal bleeding in the small intestine, indicated by the characteristic 'thumb printing' appearance of the barium pattern.

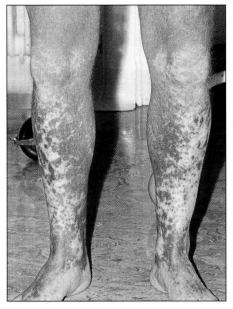

Fig. 15.16 Allergic purpura: symmetrical widespread erythematous and purpuric eruption as a hypersensitivity reaction to allopurinol.

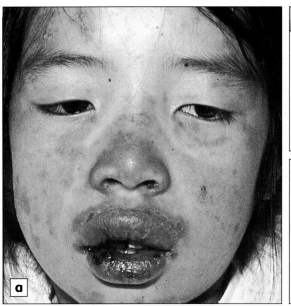

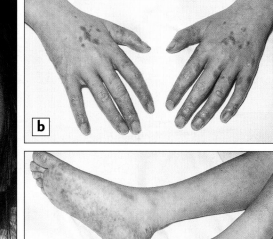

Fig. 15.17a–c Systemic lupus erythematosus: (a) typical fixed erythematous reaction over the 'butterfly area' of the face, and mucosal haemorrhage from the petechial lesions of the nasal and oral mucous membranes; skin of (b) the hands and (c) feet of the same patient shows erythematous and purpuric lesions. [(a, b) Courtesy of Dr MD Holdaway.]

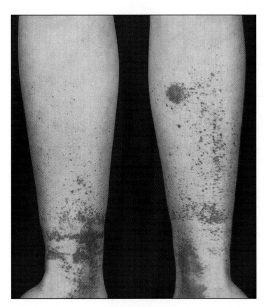

Fig. 15.18 Systemic lupus erythematosus: purpuric lesions over the shins of a 17-year-old girl (platelet count normal).

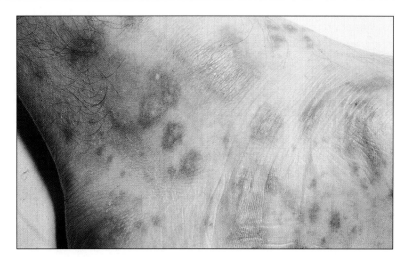

Fig. 15.19 Meningococcal septicaemia: typical purpuric skin lesions around the ankle in acute fulminating disease with disseminated intravascular coagulation.

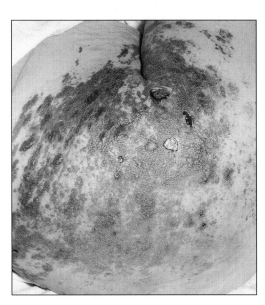

Fig. 15.20 Herpes zoster: haemorrhagic herpetic skin eruption over the lower back and upper thigh (lateral view) in a patient with acute leukaemia.

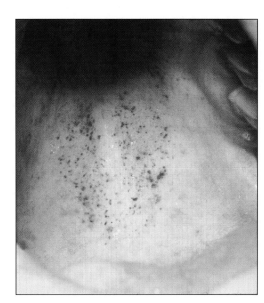

Fig. 15.21 Infectious mononucleosis: extensive petechiae in the mucosa of the palate.

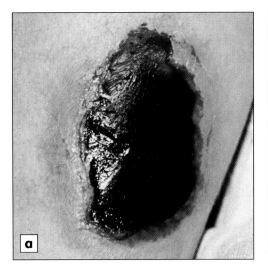
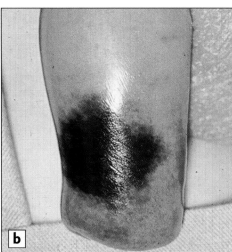

Fig. 15.22a and b Purpura fulminans: large necrotic ecchymoses of skin of (a) the leg and (b) penis of an infant, following varicella infection. [(a, b) Courtesy of Dr MD Holdaway.]

The rare condition known as purpura fulminans is characterized by the widespread development of painful, large, confluent and necrotic ecchymoses (*Fig. 15.22*). Almost any area of skin may be involved, but the face, extremities, buttocks and lower back are often the worst affected. Its occurrence is usually in children who are recovering from scarlet fever, varicella or other infections; in such cases it may result from the development of antibodies to protein C or protein S, or from excess consumption of them. Congenital deficiencies of protein C, protein S, or antithrombin in humans also underlie these conditions. Some patients have shown evidence of associated DIC with thrombocytopenia and coagulation factor deficiencies.

PLATELET BLEEDING DISORDERS

The most common cause of abnormal bleeding is a platelet disorder caused by either reduced numbers of platelets (thrombocytopenia; *Fig. 15.23*) or defective platelet function (*see Fig. 15.39*). It is characterized by spontaneous skin purpura (*Fig. 15.24*), mucosal haemorrhage and prolonged bleeding after trauma (*Fig. 15.25*).

Thrombocytopenia

Failure to produce platelets is the most common cause of thrombocytopenia. Drug toxicity or viral infections may result in selective megakaryocyte depression, while in aplastic anaemia, leukaemia, myelofibrosis, cytotoxic chemotherapy or marrow infiltrations decreased numbers of megakaryocytes may be part of a generalized bone marrow failure. Congenital deficiency of megakaryocytes can occur, in many cases with associated skeletal, renal or cardiac malformations – bilateral aplasia of the radii being the most common associated abnormality (*Fig. 15.26*).

Neonatal thrombocytopenia occurs in new-born infants as a result of intrauterine rubella or other infections, platelet antibodies, DIC, hereditary thrombocytopenias, giant haemangioma or congenital absence of megakaryocytes. Among the variety of hereditary thrombocytopenias, in the Wiskott–Aldrich syndrome there is associated immunodeficiency and eczema (*Fig. 15.27*); in some, such as the Bernard–Soulier syndrome, abnormalities of platelet morphology and function also occur, while other syndromes are better known for the associated abnormalities (e.g. May–Hegglin; Chédiak–Higashi; *see* Chapter 7).

Immune thrombocytopenic purpura

In immune thrombocytopenic purpura (ITP), a relatively common disorder, platelet sensitization with autoantibodies (usually IgG) leads to their premature removal from the circulation by cells of the

Causes of thrombocytopenia
Failure of platelet production
Generalized bone marrow failure   Leukaemia; myelodysplasia; aplastic anaemia; human immunodeficiency virus (HIV) infection; myelofibrosis; megaloblastic anaemia; uraemia; multiple myeloma; marrow infiltration (e.g. carcinoma, lymphoma)
Selective megakaryocyte depression   Drugs; alcohol; chemicals; viral infections
Hereditary thrombocytopenias   May–Hegglin, Wiskott–Aldrich, Bernard–Soulier syndromes; and others
Abnormal distribution of platelets
Splenomegaly
Increased destruction of platelets

Immune
  Alloantibodies – neonatal; post-transfusion
  Autoantibodies – primary; secondary (e.g. systemic lupus erythematosus, chronic lymphocytic leukaemia, post-infection, HIV infection, post-stem cell transplantation

Drug induced   Immune or because of platelet aggregation
Disseminated intravascular coagulation
Microangiopathic processes   Haemolytic–uraemic syndrome; thrombotic thrombocytopenic purpura; extracorporeal circulation; HELPP (haemolysis, elevated liver enzymes and low platelet count in association with pre-eclampsia) syndrome; post stem-cell transplantation Giant haemangioma (Kasabach–Merritt syndrome)
Dilutional loss
Massive transfusion of stored blood

Fig. 15.23 Thrombocytopenia: common causes.

reticuloendothelial system. Patients present with petechial haemorrhage, easy bruising or menorrhagia. The blood film shows reduced numbers of platelets, which are often large (*Fig. 15.28*), and the bone marrow has increased numbers of megakaryocytes (*Fig. 15.29*).

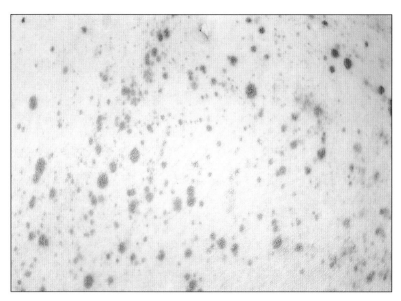

Fig. 15.24 Thrombocytopenia: abdominal skin purpura in myelodysplastic syndrome. The platelets are often functionally abnormal as well as reduced in number.

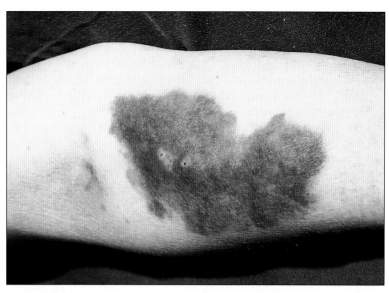

Fig. 15.25 Thrombocytopenia: large ecchymosis following performance of the Ivy bleeding-time test. The puncture marks of the stylet cutter are clearly seen.

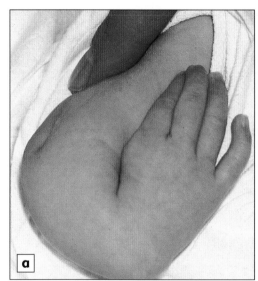

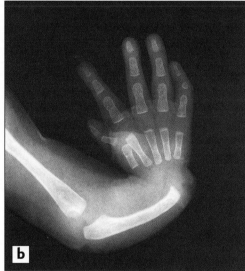

Fig. 15.26a and b Thrombocytopenia with absent radii syndrome: (a) the characteristic flexion deformity; (b) radiography shows complete absence of the radius.

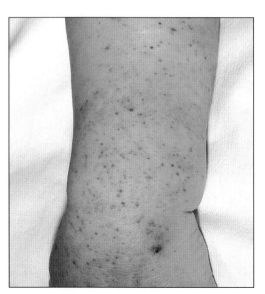

Fig. 15.27 Wiskott–Aldrich syndrome: eczema and skin purpura in an infant. (Courtesy of Dr U O'Callaghan.)

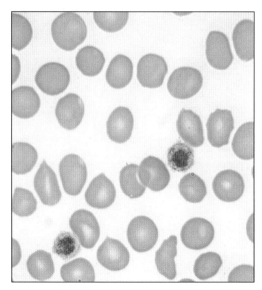

Fig. 15.28 Immune thrombocytopenia: blood film showing two large platelets.

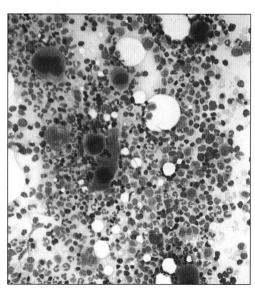

Fig. 15.29 Immune thrombocytopenia: bone marrow aspirate showing increased numbers of megakaryocytes.

The disease may occur alone (primary) or be accompanied by autoimmune haemolytic anaemia (Evans' syndrome). Also, ITP may occur in patients with other diseases, such as systemic lupus erythematosus (*Fig. 15.30*), human immunodeficiency virus infection and chronic lymphocytic leukaemia, and following stem cell transplantation.

Initial treatment is with high-dose corticosteroids; frequently splenectomy is performed in patients who do not respond to corticosteroids or who relapse when corticosteroids are withdrawn (*Fig. 15.31*). Sections of splenic tissue show prominent collections of macrophages with lipid-laden cytoplasm (*Fig. 15.32*). High-dose intravenous immunoglobulin has produced substantial rises in platelets in about 75% of cases of chronic ITP (*Fig. 15.33*). This therapy is most useful during the later stages of pregnancy to control acute bleeding episodes or in preparation of the patient for surgery, since the improvement is usually only marked for about 4 weeks. It is often valuable in children and infants. The mechanism of action may be either blockage of Fc receptors on macrophages or inhibition of the antiplatelet antibody biosynthesis.

Drug-induced immune thrombocytopenia

An allergic mechanism has been demonstrated to be the cause of many drug-induced thrombocytopenias. Rapid removal of platelets from the circulation may result in severe thrombocytopenia and many patients present with mucosal haemorrhage (*Fig. 15.34*) in addition to skin purpura.

Disseminated intravascular coagulation, thrombotic thrombocytopenic purpura and haemolytic–uraemic syndrome

In these conditions, thrombocytopenia is the result of increased consumption of platelets. For a detailed discussion of DIC see Chapter 16. In thrombotic thrombocytopenic purpura (TTP), platelet aggregation and accretion in small blood vessels is widespread (*Fig. 15.35*), but plasma levels of coagulation factors are normal. The clinical course may be fulminant and fatal, with confluent purpura and ischaemic damage to many organs, such as the brain, kidneys and skin (*Figs 15.36 and 15.37*). The majority of patients have an associated microangiopathic haemolytic anaemia (*see* Chapter 4). The acquired form may have no obvious precipitating cause, but some cases follow an infection, occur in pregnancy or follow allogeneic stem cell transplantation, particularly with cyclosporin use. Inhibitory antibodies against the metalloprotease that cleaves VWF occur in the plasma of patients with acute TTP (*Fig. 15.38*). A familial form of TTP results from congenital deficiency of the protease. An unusual preponderance of large multimers of von Willebrand's factor occurs in the plasma of patients with TTP and of those with haemolytic–uraemic syndrome (HUS). It is likely that the unusual large multimers of von Willebrand's factor cause platelet aggregation in the microcirculation of TTP. Treatment is with plasma exchanges, which remove autoantibodies and also multimers of von Willebrand's factor, and provide the necessary protease. Antiplatelet drugs, corticosteroids, vincristine and splenectomy have also been used with varying success.

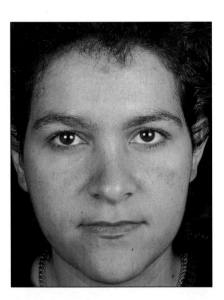

Fig. 15.30 Systemic lupus erythematosus: typical butterfly rash and frontal alopecia in a woman who also suffered from immune thrombocytopenia.

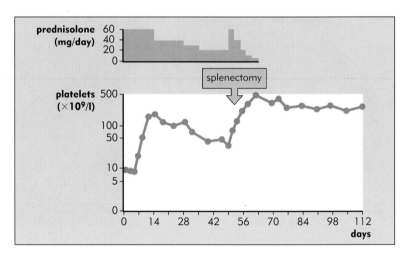

Fig. 15.31 Chronic immune thrombocytopenic purpura: response to prednisolone with subsequent relapse and response to splenectomy.

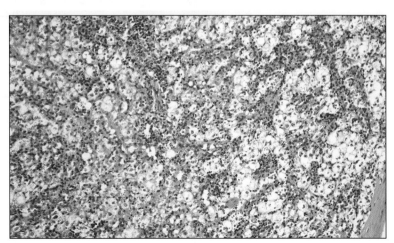

Fig. 15.32 Immune thrombocytopenic purpura: histological section of spleen showing prominent collections of lipid-filled macrophages caused by excessive breakdown of platelets in the splenic pulp.

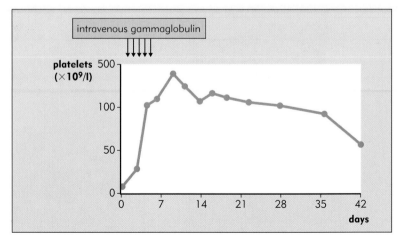

Fig. 15.33 Chronic immune thrombocytopenic purpura: typical response in platelet count to therapy with intravenous high-dose gammaglobulin (IVG) therapy (5-day course; 0.4 g/kg per day).

274

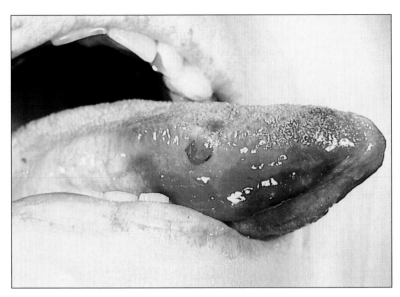

Fig. 15.34 Drug-induced thrombocytopenia: sublingual mucosal haemorrhage.

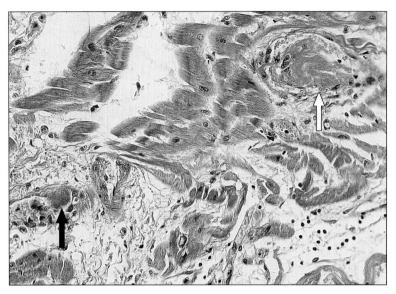

Fig. 15.35 Thrombotic thrombocytopenic purpura: fibrin thrombus (black arrow) in an arteriole of the heart and microthrombi (white arrow) of von Willebrand factor aggregate in another vessel. (Martius scarlet blue; courtesy of Prof. S Lucas.)

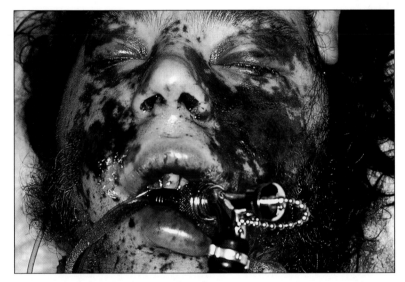

Fig. 15.36 Thrombotic thrombocytopenic purpura: widespread confluent and necrotic ecchymoses of the facial skin.

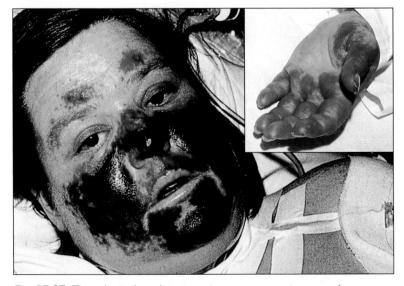

Fig. 15.37 Thrombotic thrombocytopenic purpura: massive area of haemorrhagic necrosis of the facial skin and extensive confluent ecchymoses on the hand (inset).

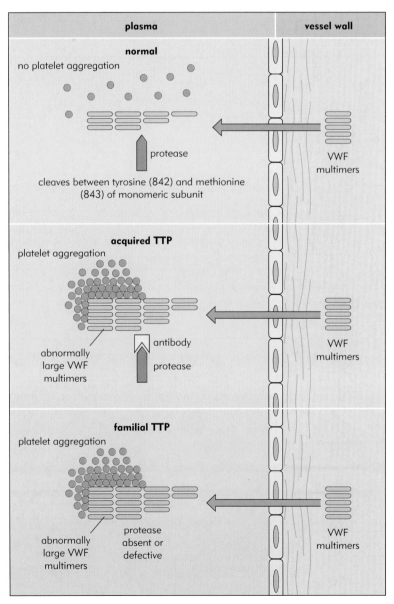

Fig. 15.38 Thrombotic thrombocytopenic purpura: postulated mechanism of how large von Willebrand's factor (VWF) multimers accumulate in plasma because of the lack of protease as a result of an immune mechanism or congenital deficiency.

Although HUS resembles TTP, it occurs mainly in infants and young children and is characterized by acute anaemia, thrombocytopenia and renal failure. Gastrointestinal symptoms include bloody diarrhoea and hypotension, and fits may occur. There is an association with infection by verotoxin-producing organisms, especially *Escherichia coli* O157:H57 strain and *Shigella dysenteriae* Types 1 and 24. The protease that cleaves VWF is present.

The HELPP syndrome occurs in late pregnancy and consists of haemolysis, elevated liver enzymes and low platelet count in association with pre-eclampsia; DIC may be present.

Disorders of platelet function

Many of the conditions associated with abnormal platelet function are listed in *Fig. 15.39*.

Hereditary disorders

The rare inherited disorders of platelet function may, at different phases of the reactions, produce defects in the formation of the haemostatic plug. In thrombasthenia (Glanzmann's disease), primary platelet aggregation fails, but platelet count, size and morphology are normal. There is deficiency of two closely associated membrane GPs, IIb and IIIa, on which receptors for fibrinogen and VWF are normally exposed during aggregation (*see Fig. 15.4*).

In Bernard–Soulier syndrome the platelets are large (*Fig. 15.40*) and are deficient in a surface GP (Ib) necessary for interaction between platelets and VWF (*see Fig. 15.4*); there is defective adhesion and diminished availability of platelet phospholipid. In the Hermansky–Pudlak syndrome, defective platelet aggregation is associated with oculocutaneous albinism and the accumulation of ceroid-like pigment in marrow macrophages (*Fig. 15.41*).

In storage pool disorders (SPD), defective platelet aggregation (*Fig. 15.42*) results from an intrinsic deficiency in the number of dense granules (δ-SPD). One type of SPD, the grey platelet syndrome (*Fig. 15.43*), is characterized by variable thrombocytopenia and large platelets that have a specific deficiency of α-granules (α-SPD).

In von Willebrand's disease, in addition to a platelet function defect the factor VIII clotting activity is low. The primary defect is reduced or abnormal synthesis of VWF, which results in defective platelet adhesion and defective *in vitro* aggregation activity with ristocetin (*Fig. 15.44*).

Acquired disorders

Intrinsic abnormalities of platelet function are found in many patients with essential thrombocythaemia (*see Fig. 13.35*) and other myeloproliferative diseases, uraemia, liver disease and hyperglobulinaemia. Aspirin and other non-steroidal anti-inflammatory drugs produce a

Disorders of platelet function
Inherited
Plasma membrane defects
Thrombasthenia; Bernard–Soulier syndrome; PF3 deficiency
Storage organelle deficiency
Dense body deficiency: idiopathic storage pool disease; Hermansky–Pudlak, Wiskott–Aldrich and Chédiak–Higashi syndromes
α-Granule deficiency: grey platelet syndrome
Cyclo-oxygenase and thromboxane synthase deficiencies
von Willebrand's disease
Acquired
Myeloproliferative disorders
Myelodysplastic syndromes
Acute myeloid leukaemia
Dysproteinaemias
Uraemia
Acquired storage pool deficiency
Disseminated intravascular coagulation; haemolytic–uraemic syndrome; thrombotic thrombocytopenic purpura; disseminated autoimmune disease
Acquired von Willebrand's disease
Drugs
For example aspirin; dipyridamole; sulfinpyrazone; prostacyclin; imipramine; non-steroidal anti-inflammatory

Fig. 15.39 Abnormal platelet function: causes.

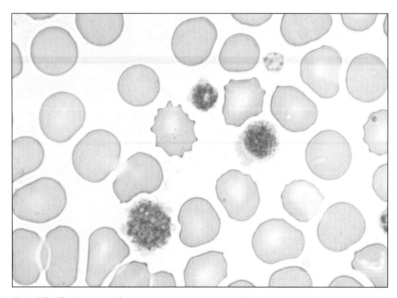

Fig. 15.40 Bernard–Soulier syndrome: blood film showing abnormally large platelets.

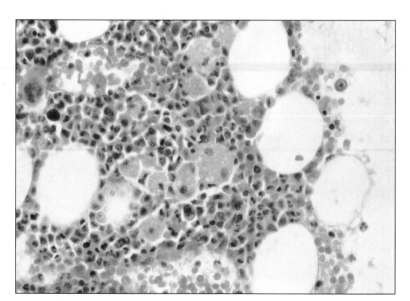

Fig. 15.41 Hermansky–Pudlak syndrome: bone marrow trephine biopsy showing prominent macrophages with ceroid-like pigment-laden cytoplasm. (Courtesy of Prof. EGD Tuddenham.)

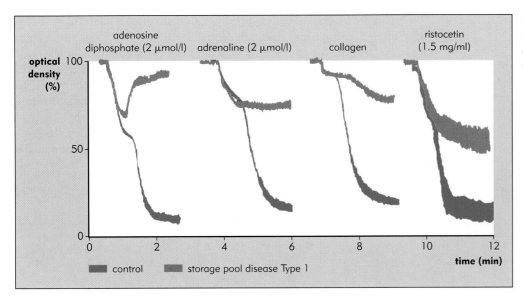

Fig. 15.42 Storage pool disease: platelet aggregation studies show defective primary and secondary aggregation with adenosine diphosphate, adrenaline and collagen. (Courtesy of Dr RA Hutton.)

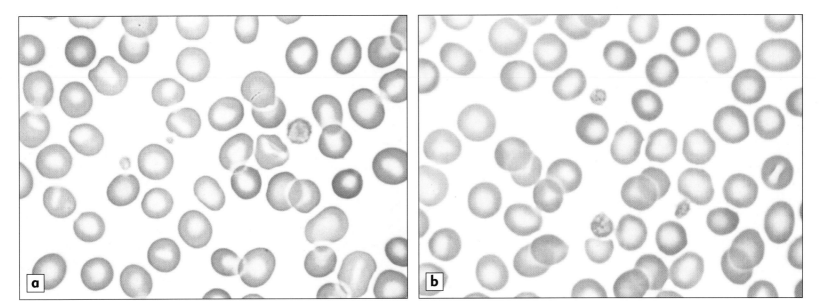

Fig. 15.43a and b Grey platelet syndrome: (a, b) typical large platelets that lack normal α-granules. [(a, b) Courtesy of Dr PC Shrivastava.]

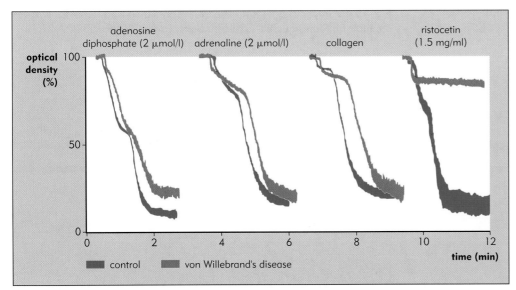

Fig. 15.44 Von Willebrand's disease: platelet aggregation studies show normal aggregation patterns with adenosine diphosphate, adrenaline and collagen, but no aggregation with ristocetin. (Courtesy of Dr RA Hutton.)

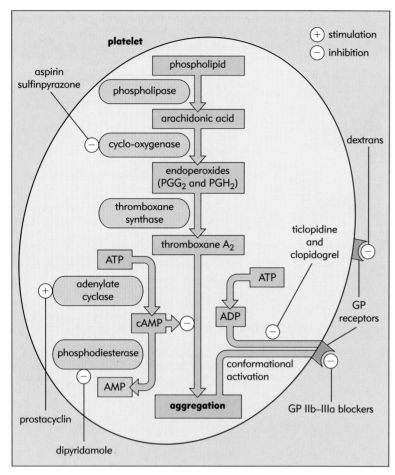

Fig. 15.45 Sites of action of antiplatelet drugs: aspirin acetylates the enzyme cyclo-oxygenase irreversibly. Sulfinpyrazone inhibits cyclo-oxygenase reversibly. Dipyridamole inhibits phosphodiesterase, increases cyclic adenosine monophosphate levels and inhibits aggregation. Inhibition of adenosine uptake by red cells allows adenosine accumulation in plasma which stimulates platelet adenylate cyclase. Prostacyclin stimulates adenylate cyclase. Ticlopidine and clopidogrel inhibit conformational activation of GP IIb–IIIa needed for platelet aggregation. Three GP IIb–IIIa blockers are licensed for human use – abciximab, eptifibatide and tirofiban. The lipid-soluble β-blockers inhibit phospholipase. Calcium channel antagonists block the influx of free calcium ions across the platelet membrane. Dextrans coat the surface, interfering with adhesion and aggregation. (ATP, adenosine triphosphate; ADP, adenosine diphosphate; cyclic adenosine monophosphate, c-AMP; PG, prostaglandin; modified from Hoffbrand AV, Pettit JE. *Essential haematology*, 3rd edn. Oxford: Blackwell Scientific Publications; 1993.)

platelet functional defect (*Fig. 15.45*), which often manifests as abnormal bleeding time; however, spontaneous haemorrhage during therapy, except for gastric mucosal bleeding caused by erosions, is not common. Antiplatelet drugs (usually aspirin) are used in the prevention of thrombosis, which reduces the risk of recurrence of myocardial infarct or of stroke in patients with transient ischaemic attacks.

Antiplatelet drugs that block the GP IIa–IIIb receptor (*Fig. 15.46*) – one of the integrin adhesion molecule receptors – are now used in the setting of percutaneous coronary intervention or acute coronary syndrome in patients on aspirin.

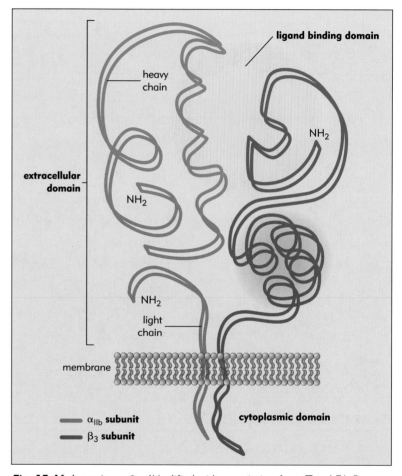

Fig. 15.46 Integrin $\alpha_{IIb}\beta_3$. (Modified with permission from Topol EJ, Byzova TV, Plow EF. Platelet GPIIb–GPIIIa blockers. *Lancet*. 1999;353:227–31.)

THE COAGULATION PATHWAY

The components of the blood coagulation cascade are proenzymes, procofactors and regulatory factors (*Fig. 16.1*). Following the initiation of blood coagulation, the coagulation factor enzymes are activated sequentially. The likely sequence *in vivo* is depicted in *Fig. 16.2*. The final steps involve the conversion of soluble plasma fibrinogen into fibrin by thrombin (*Fig. 16.2*). *In vitro*, the cascade has been divided into intrinsic and extrinsic pathways, which are useful for understanding the results of laboratory tests of coagulation. Physiological inhibitors of various components in the coagulation sequence include antithrombin, plasminogen activators, tissue factor pathway inhibition and proteins C and S.

HEREDITARY COAGULATION DISORDERS

Most inherited coagulation disorders involve deficiency of a single factor, with deficiencies of factor VIII (haemophilia A; von Willebrand's disease) and IX (haemophilia B) being the most common. All other hereditary disorders are rare.

Haemophilia

In haemophilia A, plasma factor VIII activity is absent or at a low level, because of either defective synthesis of the factor VIII molecule or synthesis of a structurally abnormal molecule (*Fig. 16.3*). The protein consists of three homologous regions, A1, A2 and A3, separated by a long

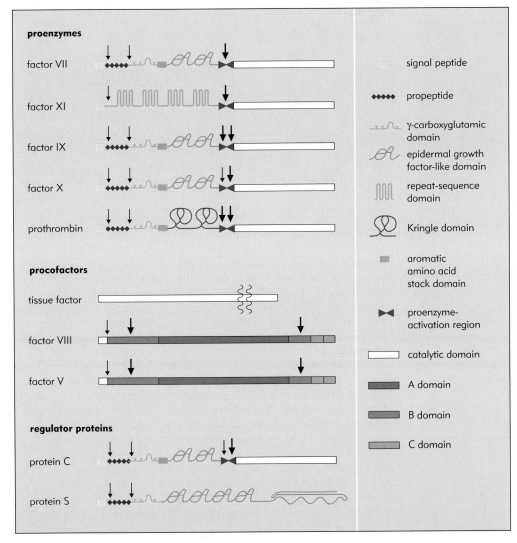

proenzymes

factor VII

factor XI

factor IX

factor X

prothrombin

procofactors

tissue factor

factor VIII

factor V

regulator proteins

protein C

protein S

signal peptide

propeptide

γ-carboxyglutamic domain

epidermal growth factor-like domain

repeat-sequence domain

Kringle domain

aromatic amino acid stack domain

proenzyme-activation region

catalytic domain

A domain

B domain

C domain

Fig. 16.1 Domains of the enzymes, receptors and cofactors involved in blood coagulation and regulation: the components are proenzymes, procofactors and regulatory proteins. The proenzymes, including protein C, contain a catalytic domain, an activation region and a signal peptide. The vitamin K-dependent proteins include a propeptide and a γ-carboxyglutamic acid domain. Other important domains include the epidermal growth factor-like domain, the Kringle domain and the repeat-sequence domain. Tissue factor is an integral membrane protein unrelated to other known proteins. Factors V and VIII have marked similarities in structure. Sites of intracellular peptide bonds cleaved during synthesis are indicated by thin arrows, and sites of peptide bonds cleaved during protein activation are indicated by thick arrows. The transmembrane domain of tissue factor is shown within the phospholipid bilayer. (Modified with permission from Furie B, Furie BC. Molecular and cell biology of blood coagulation. *N Engl J Med.* 1992;326:800–6.)

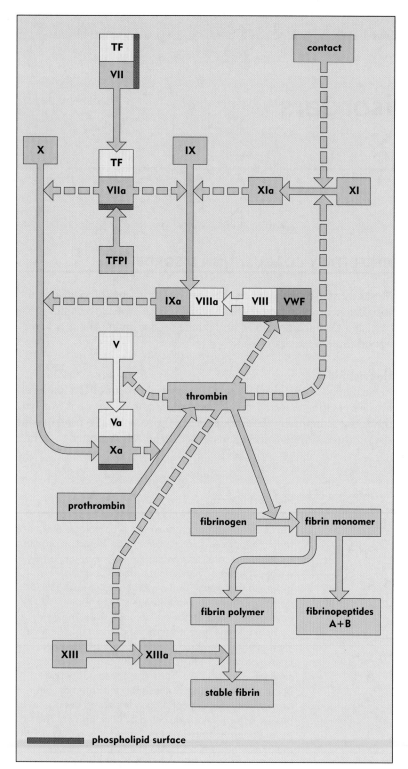

Fig. 16.2 Physiologic pathways of blood coagulation: blood coagulation is initiated by tissue factor (TF) expressed on the cell surface. When plasma comes in contact with tissue factor, factor VII (VII) binds to this receptor. The complex of TF and activated VII (VIIa) activates factors IX (IXa) and X (Xa). Tissue factor pathway inhibitor (TFPI) is an important inhibitor of TF–VIIa activity. The VIIIa–IXa complex greatly amplifies Xa production from X. The generation of thrombin from prothrombin by the action of the Xa–Va complex leads to fibrin formation. Thrombin also:

- activates factor XI, which increases IXa;
- cleaves factor VIII from its carrier molecule, von Willebrand's factor (VWF), so activating factor VIII and greatly augmenting Xa production by the VIIIa–IXa complex;
- activates factor V to Va; and
- activates factor XIII to XIIIa, which stabilizes the fibrin clot.

(Blue, enzymes in coagulation sequence; yellow, cofactors; orange, von Willebrand's factor; green, fibrinogen to fibrin pathway; dotted lines, activation or inhibition; solid lines, conversion of factor into a different form).

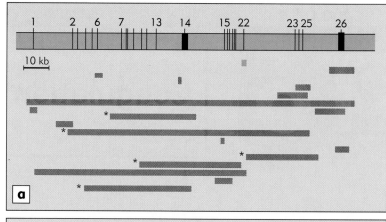

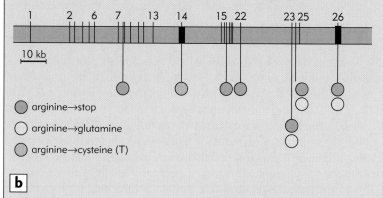

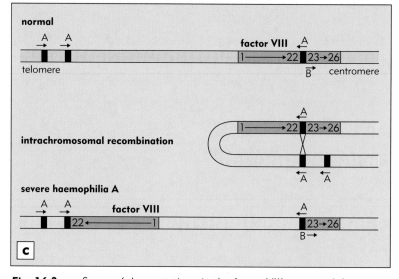

Fig. 16.3a–c Some of the mutations in the factor VIII gene and the region of chromosome X that contains it: (a) examples of deletion mutations. Bars beneath the representation of the factor VIII gene show the approximate size of DNA deletions that lead to haemophilia. The deletion in pink corresponds to a case of mild haemophilia; all other patients have severe disease. The asterisks correspond to gene deletion in haemophiliacs who have developed inhibitor antibodies. (b) Examples of point mutations. Nonsense (red) and missense (yellow and green) mutations have been discovered in parts of the factor VIII gene that normally encode the amino acid arginine. Many other examples of deletions, point mutations and deletions exist (see Anatorakis SE, Kazazian HH, Tuddenham EG. *Hum Mutat*. 1995;5:1–22). (c) The region of chromosome X q28 that contains the factor VIII gene. Inversion model of the recombination that accounts for approximately 45% of severe haemophilia A. (A, homologous promoter that is repeated; B, second promoter near A that is only in intron 22 and when active transcribes exons 23–26 – the opposing orientation of A sequences allows intrachromosomal homologous recombination.) [(a, b) Modified with permission from Hoffman R, Benz EJ, Shattil SJ (eds). *Hematology, Basic Principles and Practice*. New York: Churchill Livingstone; 1991:1286; (c) courtesy of Prof. KJ Pasi.]

B domain, rich in glycosylation sites and followed by two homologous C regions (*Fig. 16.4*). The A regions show homology with the copper-binding protein caeruloplasmin. Although the single-chain mature polypeptide has a molecular weight (MW) of about 267 kDa, it is cleaved by thrombin into two calcium-linked polypeptides of MW 90 kDa and 80 kDa, and it is in this activated form that it activates factor X. The gene maps to the distal band of the long arm of chromosome X (Xq28). Over 90 different large deletions and 77 unique small deletions (<100 bp) have been described, as well as 28 different sequence insertions (all associated with severe disease). Also, 309 different point mutations have been identified and these may be associated with severe or mild disease. In some of the cases with single-point mutations and with deletions, the patients develop a factor VIII inhibitor in plasma. Intrachromosomal rearrangement accounts for 45% of cases (*see Fig. 16.3c*). Von Willebrand's factor (VWF) activity is normal and VWF is present in normal amounts.

In haemophilia B (Christmas disease), either factor IX is absent or the factor IX molecule is structurally abnormal. The inheritance of both haemophilias is sex-linked (*Fig. 16.5*).

Major haemorrhage of the joints is the dominant problem in severe haemophilia A or B and most frequently affects the knees, elbows, ankles and wrists, although other synovial joints may be involved. Usually severe pain is present and the affected joint is tender, warm and may be grossly distended (*Figs 16.6 and 16.7*). Chronic joint haemorrhage results in degenerative joint changes and mechanical derangement of articular surfaces (*Figs 16.8 and 16.9*).

Demineralization, loss of articular cartilage, bone lipping and osteophyte formation produce deformity and crippling (*Figs 16.10 and 16.11*).

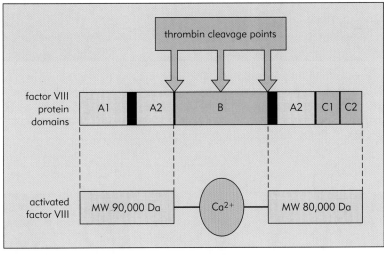

Fig. 16.4 Factor VIII clotting factor: structure.

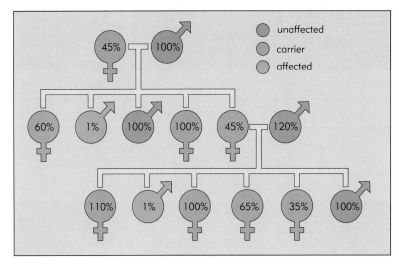

Fig. 16.5 Haemophilia: pattern of inheritance (family tree).

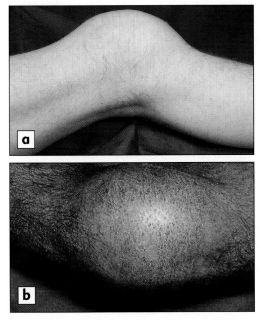

Fig. 16.6a and b Haemophilia A: (a, b) gross swelling from acute haemarthroses of the knee joints.

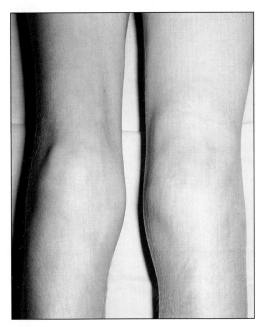

Fig. 16.7 Haemophilia A: acute haemarthrosis of the left knee joint, with swelling of the suprapatellar area. The quadriceps muscles are wasted, particularly that on the patient's right thigh.

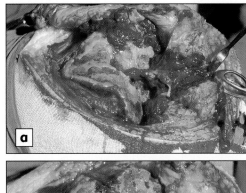

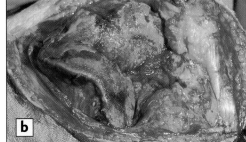

Fig. 16.8a and b Haemophilia A: (a) opened knee joint showing the femoral condyles and hypertrophied haemosiderin-stained synovium. Widespread erosion of the articular cartilage has exposed large areas of haemosiderin-stained bone; (b) removal of the synovium of the suprapatellar pouch and of the patella exposes the grossly damaged femoral articular surface.

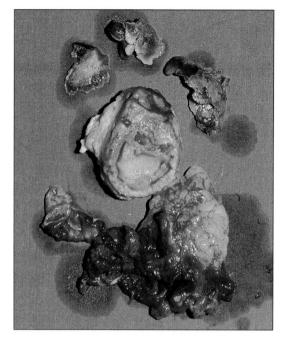

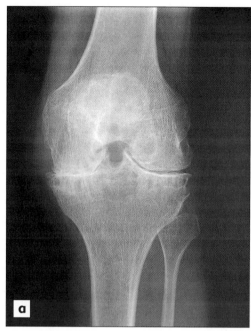

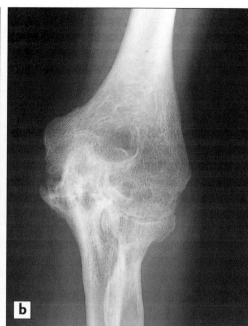

Fig. 16.9 Haemophilia A: resected material from the knee in *Fig. 16.8* included (from top to bottom) osteophytes from the arthritic femoral condyles, the patella, which shows haemosiderin-stained articular cartilage and secondary arthritic changes, and a portion of grossly haemosiderin-stained synovium of the suprapatellar pouch.

Fig. 16.10a and b Haemophilia A: (a) radiograph of the knee joint, showing marked narrowing of the joint space (particularly medially), a widened intercondylar notch, prominent osteoarthritic changes and subchondral cyst formation, with erosion of the upper lateral border of the tibial plateau; (b) radiograph of the elbow joint, showing marked joint space narrowing, enlargement of the radial head, secondary osteoarthritic features and subchondral cyst formation.

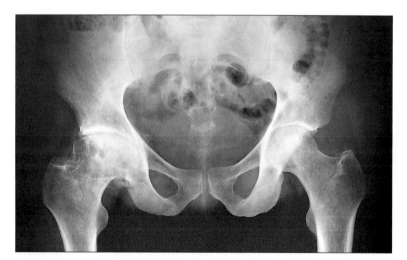

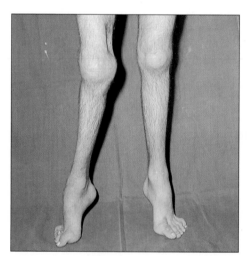

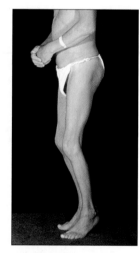

Fig. 16.11 Haemophilia A: radiograph of the pelvis, showing marked destruction and deformation of the right acetabulum and femoral head. Numerous subchondral cysts are present, and the right femoral neck is shortened and widened.

Fig. 16.12 Haemophilia A: gross crippling. The right knee is swollen, with posterior subluxation of the tibia on the femur. The ankles and feet show residual deformities of talipes equinus and some degree of cavus and associated toe clawing. Generalized muscle wasting is most marked on the right. The scar on the medial side of the right lower thigh is the site of a previously excised 'pseudotumour'.

Fig. 16.13 Haemophilia A: flexion deformities of the elbow, hip, knee and ankle joints following a 35-year history of multiple haemarthroses.

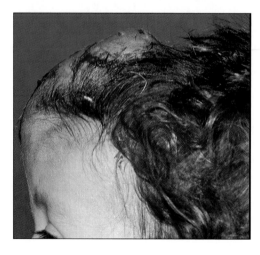

Fig. 16.14 Haemophilia A: extensive post-traumatic haematoma of the forehead in an infant.

The end result in poorly treated patients is permanent fixation of the affected joint or flexion deformities (*Figs 16.12 and 16.13*).

Traumatic and spontaneous soft tissue haemorrhage is another feature of haemophilia (*Figs 16.14–16.17*). Dissecting haematomas may involve large areas of muscle or deep fascial layers (*Fig. 16.18*). Haemorrhage into retroperitoneal fascial spaces or into the psoas muscle may produce considerable problems in differential diagnosis (*Figs 16.19–16.21*), since associated pain, tenderness and fever may suggest other causes of the acute abdomen.

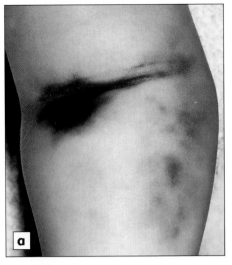

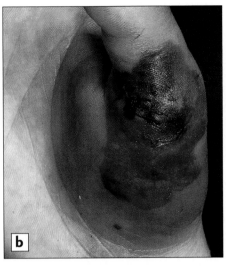

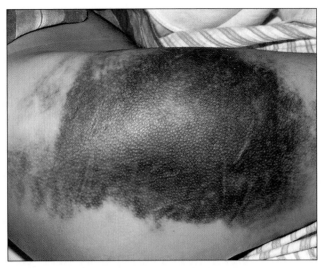

Fig. 16.15a and b Haemophilia B: (a) extensive subcutaneous haemorrhage about the elbow joint of an infant following venepuncture; (b) extensive bleeding into the thenar muscles and overlying subcutaneous tissue.

Fig. 16.16 Haemophilia A: massive haemorrhage in the area of the right buttock, following an intramuscular injection.

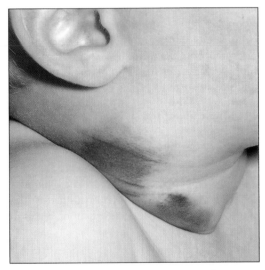

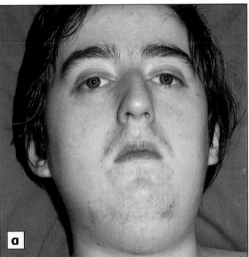

Fig. 16.17 Haemophilia B: extensive haemorrhage into the soft tissues of the neck following venepuncture of the external jugular vein.

Fig. 16.18a and b Haemophilia A: (a) marked submandibular swelling resulting from a large haemorrhage in the sublingual tissues; (b) the most superficial part of the sublingual haemorrhage is clearly visible beneath the mucosa of the floor of the mouth.

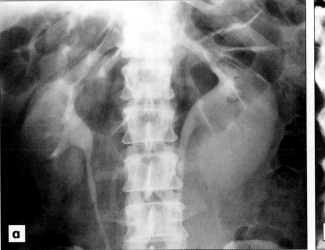

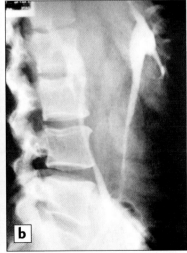

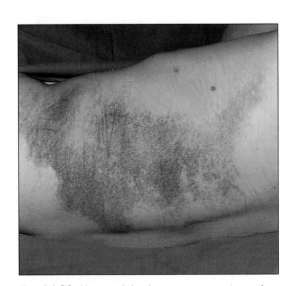

Fig. 16.19a and b Haemophilia A: intravenous pyelograms showing acute retroperitoneal haemorrhage. (a) A soft-tissue mass in the left flank has caused medial rotation of the left kidney and anteromedial displacement of the ureter. (b) The lateral view confirms the anterior displacement of both the kidney and ureter.

Fig. 16.20 Haemophilia A: acute retroperitoneal haemorrhage (same patient as shown in *Fig. 16.19*). The extensive subcutaneous bruising of the left flank appeared 24 hours after presentation.

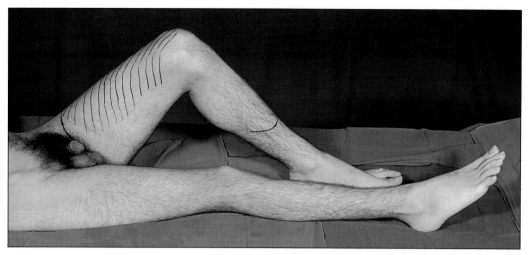

Fig. 16.21 Haemophilia A: acute retroperitoneal haemorrhage into the left psoas muscle. The lines indicate an area of anaesthesia over the distribution of the femoral nerve. There was also weakness of the quadriceps muscle and a flexion contracture at the left hip.

Haemophilic 'pseudotumours' are a serious complication of extensive fascial or subperiosteal haemorrhage. These blood-filled multiloculated cysts may cause extensive destruction of both soft tissue (*Fig. 16.22*) and bone (*Figs 16.23 and 16.24*) as they increase in size.

Ischaemic contractures may follow extensive haemorrhage into the muscles of the limbs (*Fig. 16.25*), for example Volkmann's contracture of the forearm (*Fig. 16.26*). Prolonged bleeding occurs after dental extractions and operative haemorrhage is life-threatening in both severely and mildly affected patients.

Spontaneous intracranial haemorrhage (*Fig. 16.27*), although an infrequent cause of bleeding in individuals, remains the most common cause of death in severe haemophilia.

The management of the haemophilias has been greatly improved by therapy with coagulation factor concentrates (factor VIII concentrates in haemophilia A and factor IX concentrates in haemophilia B) or factors made by recombinant DNA techniques. Prophylactic therapy and early treatment of bleeding episodes has reduced the occurrence of repeated and crippling haemarthroses and soft-tissue haemorrhage. With regular therapy even severely affected patients reach adult life without significant degenerative arthritis. In the majority of patients, replacement therapy with the appropriate coagulation factor concentrates has allowed even major surgical procedures to be undertaken without excessive risk.

Carrier detection and diagnosis

DNA analysis has improved carrier detection and prenatal diagnosis compared with the measurement of factor VIII antigenic and coagulation activity in plasma. Direct detection of the defect is possible in some cases but, more often, tracking of the abnormal gene is carried out by restriction fragment length polymorphism (RFLP) analysis using Southern blotting or polymerase chain reaction (PCR) technique (*Figs 16.28 and 16.29*).

Von Willebrand's disease

Von Willebrand's disease involves defective synthesis of VWF. This protein is an oligomer of units, each of MW 210,000. It carries factor VIII coagulation factor and is itself essential for the adhesion of platelets to damaged vessel walls (*see Fig. 15.4*).

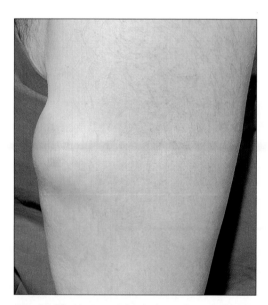

Fig. 16.22 Haemophilia A: 'pseudotumour' of the biceps, in fact a hard residual encapsulated swelling following incomplete resolution and repair of previous muscle haemorrhage.

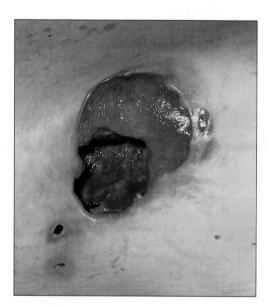

Fig. 16.23 Haemophilia A: large ulcer overlying the entrance to a multiloculated and cavernous pseudotumour of the right iliac bone and overlying soft tissues.

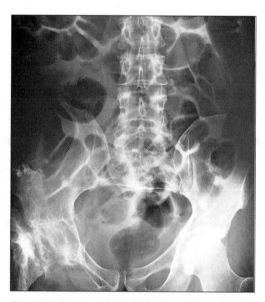

Fig. 16.24 Haemophilia A: pelvic radiograph (same patient as shown in *Fig. 16.23*). The pseudotumour destroyed a large area of the wing of the right iliac bone, including the anterior crest. The hip joint space on the right is obliterated and the femoral neck has a disunited fracture, with resultant pseudoarthrosis, gross deformity and shortening.

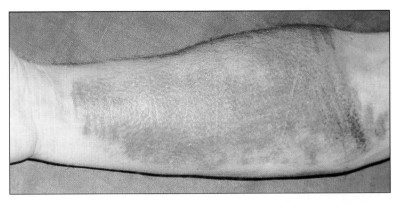

Fig. 16.25 Haemophilia A: subcutaneous bruising and extensive haemorrhage into the flexor muscles and associated soft tissues of the right forearm.

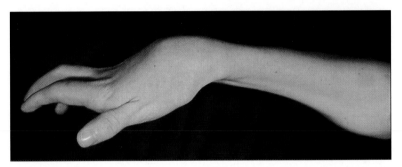

Fig. 16.26 Haemophilia A: Volkmann's contracture. The wasting and flexion deformities are a result of extensive repair and stricture formation in muscles damaged by repeated haematomas.

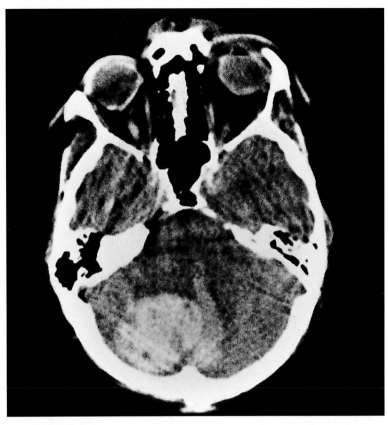

Fig. 16.27 Haemophilia A: computed tomography (CT) scan showing a large haematoma of the cerebellum.

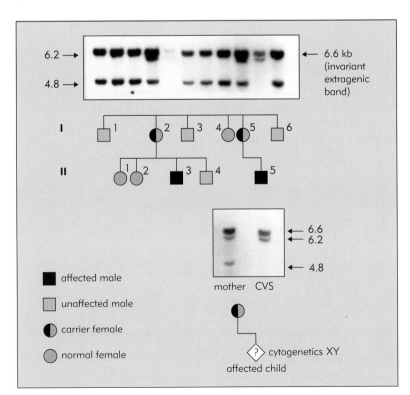

Fig. 16.28 Haemophilia A: antenatal diagnosis by chorion villous biopsy and RFLP DNA analysis. In this family, the haemophilia gene occurs in a 6.2 kb fragment after XbaI digestion; Southern blot analysis was carried out using a probe (p482.6) to the intron 22 of the factor VIII gene. The mother (I_2) has four children, including one affected (haemophilic) child (II_3), and wishes to know whether her present fetus is affected. Chorion villous sample analysis shows that the fetus has a 6.2 band alone, implying it is an affected male. Each track represents the DNA of the subject depicted below. (Courtesy of Prof. KJ Pasi.)

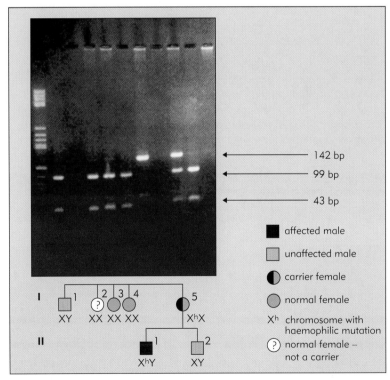

Fig. 16.29 Haemophilia A: carrier detection using PCR analysis (left-hand column gives molecular weight markers). Subject I_2 wishes to know whether she is a carrier because her sister (subject I_5) has a haemophilic son (II_1). The haemophilia gene is associated with a 142 base pair (bp) fragment in intron 18 of the factor VIII gene. Subject I_2 is homozygous for the 99 bp fragment, which indicates that she does not carry the haemophilia gene. (Courtesy of Prof. KJ Pasi.)

The inheritance pattern of von Willebrand's disease found in most patients is autosomal dominant. The disorder is characterized by operative and post-traumatic haemorrhage (*Fig. 16.30*), mucous membrane bleeding and excessive blood loss from both superficial cuts and abrasions. Spontaneous haemarthroses and arthritic changes are particularly rare, and occur only in homozygous patients (*Fig. 16.31*).

The molecular defects include point mutations or deletions (*Fig. 16.32*). The results of haemostasis tests in von Willebrand's disease and the haemophilias are given in *Figs 16.33 and 16.34*.

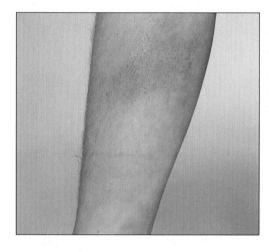

Fig. 16.30 Von Willebrand's disease: subcutaneous bruising overlying haemorrhage into the muscles and soft tissues of the left forearm.

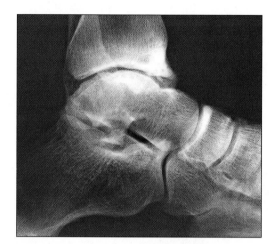

Fig. 16.31 Von Willebrand's disease: lateral radiograph of ankle joint showing loss of joint space, marginal sclerosis and a small subchondral cyst in the tibial epiphysis.

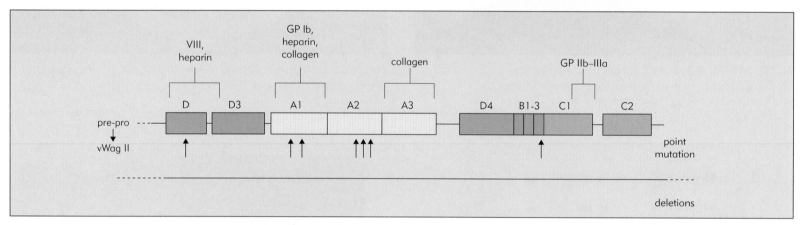

Fig. 16.32 Von Willebrand's disease: the mature VWF protein with the various domains. The portions that have been shown to interact with factor VIII, heparin, collagen and platelet glycoproteins GP Ib and GP IIb–IIIa are shown by square brackets. Point mutations identified in patients with von Willebrand's disease are shown by the arrowheads. The extent of deletions is indicated by the horizontal line. Pre-propeptide (pre-pro) and vWag II (antigen) are cleaved off the mature protein.

Haemostasis tests in hereditary coagulation disorders			
	Haemophilia A	Haemophilia B	von Willebrand's disease
Bleeding time	Normal	Normal	Prolonged
Prothrombin time	Normal	Normal	Normal
Activated partial thromboplastin time	Prolonged	Prolonged	Prolonged
Thrombin clotting time	Normal	Normal	Normal
Factor VIII	Low	Normal	Low or normal
Von Willebrand factor (VWF)	Normal	Normal	Low
VWF: ristocetin cofactor activity	Normal	Normal	Low
Factor IX	Normal	Low	Normal

Fig. 16.33 Haemostasis tests: typical results in the haemophilias and von Willebrand's disease.

Variants of von Willebrand's disease	
Type	Characteristics
1	Partial quantitative deficiency of VWF
2	Quantitative deficiency of VWF
2A	Decreased platelet-dependent function associated with absent high molecular weight multimers of VWF
2B	Variants with increased affinity for glycoprotein Ib
2M	As Type 2A but with high molecular weight multimers of VWF present
2N	Variants with decreased affinity for factor VIII
3	Virtually complete deficiency of VWF

Fig. 16.34 Von Willebrand's disease: variants.

Other hereditary coagulation disorders

Patients with inherited defects of coagulation factors other than VIII or IX often show easy bruising and spontaneous and excessive post-traumatic bleeding. Spontaneous haemarthroses and soft-tissue haematomas are, however, most unusual.

ACQUIRED COAGULATION DISORDERS

In clinical practice the acquired coagulation disorders (*Fig. 16.35*) are seen more often than the inherited disorders. Unlike the inherited diseases, there are usually multiple clotting factor deficiencies. Bleeding episodes that result from vitamin K deficiency, overdosage with oral anticoagulants or in association with liver disease and with disseminated intravascular coagulation (DIC) are seen most frequently.

Liver disease

Liver cell immaturity and lack of vitamin K synthesis in the gut are principal causes of haemorrhagic disease of the new-born. In adults, vitamin K deficiency may be the result of obstructive jaundice, or pancreatic or small bowel disease. Multiple haemostatic abnormalities contribute to increased surgical bleeding and may exacerbate haemorrhage from oesophageal varices. Biliary obstruction results in impaired absorption of vitamin K and decreased synthesis of factors II, VII, IX and X by the liver parenchymal cells. The hypersplenism associated with portal hypertension frequently results in thrombocytopenia. Patients in liver failure have deficiency of factor V and variable abnormalities of platelet function, and often produce functionally abnormal fibrinogen. As well as variceal bleeding and increased loss of blood during surgery, patients with severe liver disease may also suffer from spontaneous superficial haemorrhage (*Figs 16.36 and 16.37*).

Overdosage with anticoagulants

Overdosage with oral anticoagulants that are vitamin K antagonists results in severe deficiencies of coagulation factors II, VII, IX and X. Patients may present with extensive skin bruising (*Fig. 16.38*) or severe internal bleeding (*Fig. 16.39*).

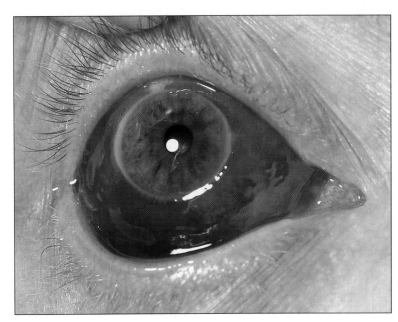

Acquired coagulation disorders
Liver disease
Deficiency of vitamin K-dependent factors
Haemorrhagic disease of the new-born
Biliary obstruction
Malabsorption of vitamin K, e.g. sprue, coeliac disease
Vitamin K-antagonist therapy, e.g. coumarins, indanediones
Disseminated intravascular coagulation
Inhibition of coagulation
Specific inhibitors, e.g. antibodies against factor VIII components
Non-specific inhibitors, e.g. antibodies found in systemic lupus erythematosus, rheumatoid arthritis
Miscellaneous
Diseases with M-protein production
L-Asparaginase
Therapy with heparin, defibrinating agents or thrombolytics
Massive transfusion syndrome

Fig. 16.35 The acquired coagulation disorders.

Fig. 16.36 Liver failure: extensive subconjunctival haemorrhage.

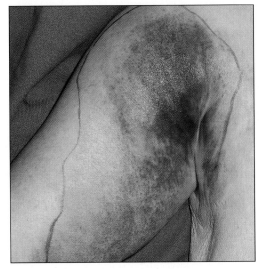

Fig. 16.37 Liver failure: subcutaneous haemorrhage of the upper arm following minor trauma. Laboratory tests revealed deficiencies of factors II, VII, IX and X as well as dysfibrinogenaemia.

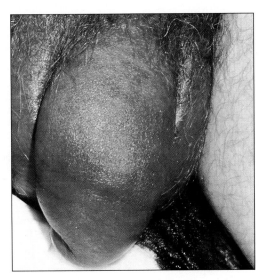

Fig. 16.38 Warfarin overdose: massive subcutaneous haemorrhage over the penis, scrotal and pubic areas following sexual intercourse.

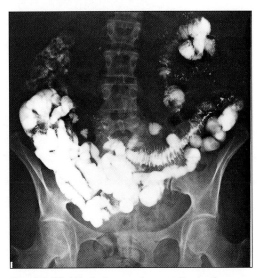

Fig. 16.39 Warfarin overdose: radiograph shows intramural bleeding in the small intestine with the characteristic 'stacked coin' pattern of barium distribution. (Courtesy of Dr D Nag.)

Similar skin lesions to those seen in homozygous protein C deficiency (*see Fig. 16.52*) may occur in patients commencing anticoagulant therapy with coumarin drugs. Selective severe protein C deficiency may occur temporarily before the levels of the vitamin K-dependent clotting factors fall (*Fig. 16.40*).

Disseminated intravascular coagulation

A consequence of many disorders, DIC causes widespread endothelial damage, platelet aggregation or release of procoagulant material into the circulation (*Fig. 16.41*). It is associated with widespread intravascular deposition of fibrin and consumption of coagulation factors and

platelets (*Fig. 16.42*). This may lead to both abnormal bleeding and widespread thrombosis, which is often fulminant (*Figs 16.43–16.46; see also* Chapter 15), although it can run a less severe, chronic course.

In the Kasabach–Merritt syndrome, a congenital haemangioma is associated with DIC (*Fig. 16.47*). The stimulus to intravascular coagulation is local, but the enhanced proteolytic activity of both coagulation and fibrinolytic systems probably becomes disseminated throughout the blood.

Acquired coagulation factor inhibitor

Occasionally patients present with a bleeding syndrome (*Fig. 16.48*) caused by circulating antibodies to coagulation factor VIII or to other

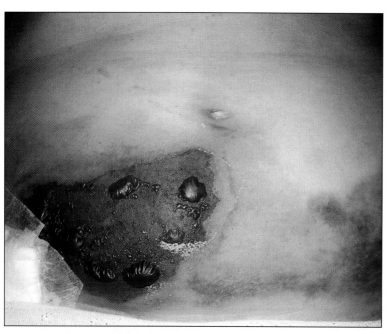

Fig. 16.40 Warfarin skin necrosis: these lesions over the abdomen developed in the first few days of warfarin therapy in a 40-year-old woman. Her protein C level was not measured but, in more recent examples of coumarin-induced skin necrosis, patients have been found to have reduced plasma levels of protein C. (Courtesy of Prof. SJ Machin.)

Conditions associated with disseminated intravascular coagulation	
Infections	**Hypersensitivity reactions**
Gram-negative and meningococcal septicaemia	Anaphylaxis
	Incompatible blood transfusion
Septic abortion and *Clostridium welchii* septicaemia	**Widespread tissue damage**
Severe falciparum malaria	Following surgery or trauma
Viral infection (purpura fulminans)	**Miscellaneous**
Malignancy	Liver failure
Widespread mucin-secreting adenocarcinoma	Snake and invertebrate venoms
	Severe burns
Acute promyelocytic leukaemia (AML M_3)	Hypothermia
	Heat stroke
Obstetric complications	Hypoxia
Amniotic fluid embolism	Vascular malformations (Kasabach–Merritt syndrome)
Premature separation of placenta	
Eclampsia; retained placenta	

Fig. 16.41 Disseminated intravascular coagulation: causes.

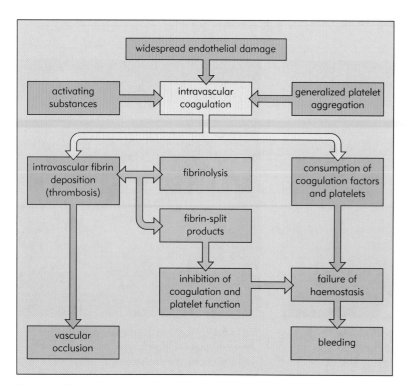

Fig. 16.42 Disseminated intravascular coagulation: pathogenesis.

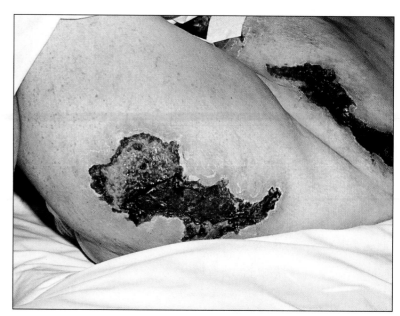

Fig. 16.43 Disseminated intravascular coagulation: later stages of skin necrosis (same patient as shown in *Fig. 16.45*). Loss of superficial necrotic tissue over the thigh and lateral abdominal wall has left large deep irregular ulcers with haemorrhagic areas of exposed tissue. (Courtesy of Dr BB Berkeley.)

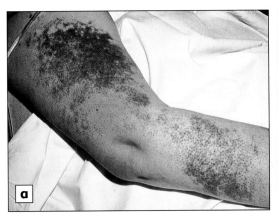

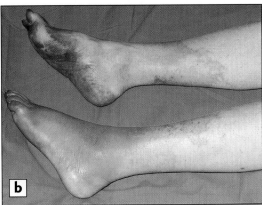

Fig. 16.44a and b Disseminated intravascular coagulation: (a) indurated and confluent purpura of the arm; (b) peripheral gangrene with swelling and discoloration of the skin of the feet in fulminant disease.

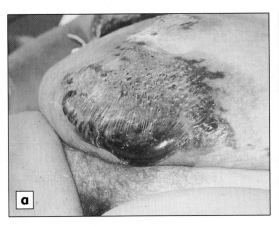

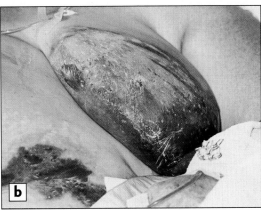

Fig. 16.45a and b Disseminated intravascular coagulation: extensive necrosis of the skin and subcutaneous tissues of (a) the lower abdominal wall and (b) breast in a grossly obese patient (same patient as shown in *Fig. 16.43*). [(a, b) Courtesy of Dr BB Berkeley.]

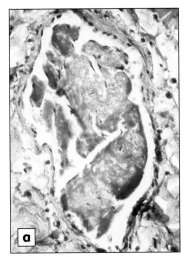

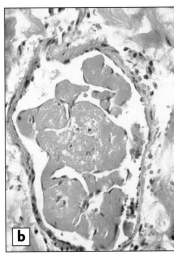

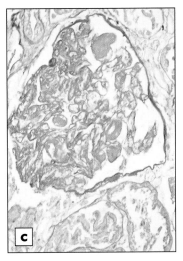

Fig. 16.46a–c Disseminated intravascular coagulation: (a, b) sections through a skin venule deep to an area of necrosis show occlusion by a thrombus composed mainly of fibrin; (c) necrosis of the glomerulus and the surrounding tubules with variable amounts of fibrinous material in the glomerular blood vessels. [(a) Martius scarlet-blue; (b) H & E; (c) periodic acid–Schiff stains.]

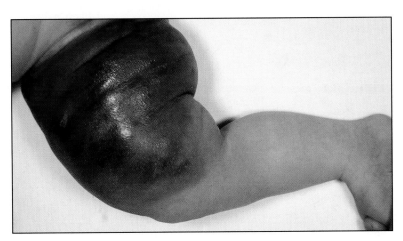

Fig. 16.47 Kasabach–Merritt syndrome: this giant congenital haemangioma of the thigh was associated with DIC.

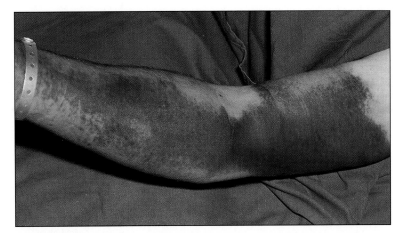

Fig. 16.48 Acquired coagulation factor inhibitor: extensive subcutaneous and deep soft-tissue haemorrhage in the arm because of circulating autoantibody to factor VIII.

clotting factors. These antibodies usually occur *post partum*, in systemic lupus erythematosus (SLE) associated with a malignancy and in old age.

Patients with SLE, other autoimmune disorders and, rarely, infections may also develop a less specific inhibitor, IgG or IgM, which is directed against phospholipid and is associated with a prolongation of the partial thromboplastin time not corrected by normal plasma. Patients with this 'lupus anticoagulant' may have no clinical symptoms, or may thrombose arteries or veins or suffer recurrent spontaneous abortions (see below). Results of haemostasis tests in the major acquired coagulation disorders are shown in *Fig. 16.49*.

THROMBOPHILIA

Multiple factors contribute to the pathogenesis of venous and arterial thrombosis, including genetic predisposition and many acquired risk factors (*Fig. 16.50*). Venous thrombosis occurs most frequently in the calf veins and/or iliac veins and may be complicated by pulmonary embolus.

Inherited thrombotic disorders

Protein C deficiency
Protein C is a vitamin K-dependent plasma protein synthesized by the liver. Its active form inhibits the active forms of coagulation factors V and VIII, and also increases lysis of clots by inactivating a protein that

normally destroys tissue plasminogen activator. Activation of protein C occurs via thrombin bound to a protein, thrombomodulin, on the surface of the endothelial cell (*Fig. 16.51*).

Heterozygous protein C deficiency predisposes affected individuals to recurrent venous thromboses, which tend to present at an early age, usually <30 years. Homozygous protein C deficiency results in neonatal purpura fulminans, characterized by superficial thromboses. The skin lesions are initially swollen and red or purple; they become blue–black and may necrose (*Fig. 16.52*). The blood shows features of DIC with low levels of factors V and VIII, antithrombin, fibrinogen and platelets.

Factor V Leiden
The factor V Leiden mutation (FV R506Q) is the most common cause of thrombophilia and is detected in about 30% of patients who present with venous thrombosis. The abnormal factor V is resistant to the action of activated protein C.

The mutation occurs at the site at which activated protein C normally cleaves factor Va (*Fig. 16.53*). Heterozygosity for this disorder is as high as 8% in some Caucasian populations. The global distribution is illustrated in *Fig. 16.54*. The risk of thrombosis is eight times greater than that of a control population; in the homozygous form of factor V Leiden the risk rises to at least 50 fold. The risks are compounded in women taking the contraceptive pill.

Haemostasis tests in acquired bleeding disorders				
	Platelet count	Prothrombin time	Activated partial thrombosplatin time	Thrombin time
Liver disease	Low	Prolonged	Prolonged	Normal (rarely prolonged)
Disseminated intravascular coagulation	Low	Prolonged	Prolonged	Grossly prolonged
Massive transfusion	Low	Prolonged	Prolonged	Prolonged
Heparin	Normal (rarely low)	Mildly prolonged	Prolonged	Prolonged
Circulating anticoagulant	Normal	Normal or prolonged	Prolonged	Normal

Fig. 16.49 Haemostasis tests: typical results in acquired bleeding disorders.

Causes of inherited thrombophilia
Established
Activated protein C resistance (factor V:R506Q, V Leiden)
Protein C deficiency
Protein S deficiency
Antithrombin deficiency
Hyperhomocysteinaemia
Elevated prothrombin levels (mutation G20210A)
Non-established as hereditary
Elevated factor VIII levels
Heparin cofactor II deficiency
Plasminogen deficiency
Elevated plasminogen inactivation inhibitor 1
Dysfibrinogenaemia

Fig. 16.50 Inherited thrombophilia: causes.

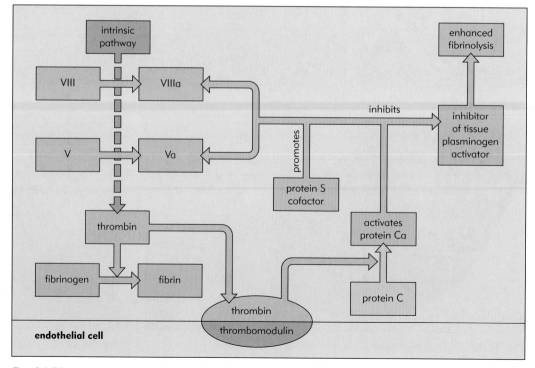

Fig. 16.51 Anticoagulant and fibrinolytic actions of protein C and protein S.

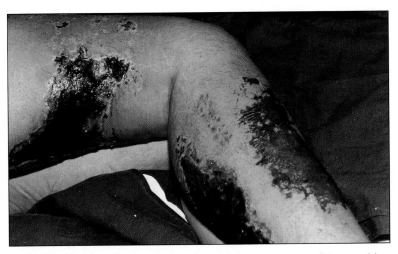

Fig. 16.52 Homozygous protein C deficiency: the patient, a 15-year-old girl, presented with skin necrosis and multiple venous thrombosis at 2 years of age.

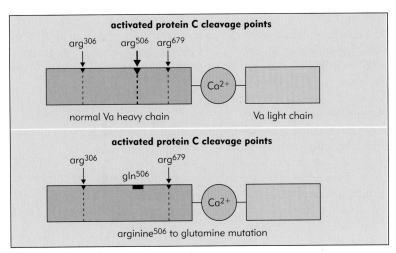

Fig. 16.53 Inactivation of factor Va: activated protein C inactivates membrane-bound factor Va through proteolytic cleavage at three points in the Va heavy chain. In the factor V Leiden mutation, arginine at position 506 is replaced by glutamine, which renders this position resistant to activated protein C cleavage. The mutant factor V molecule can still be inactivated, but more slowly, at the remaining cleavage sites.

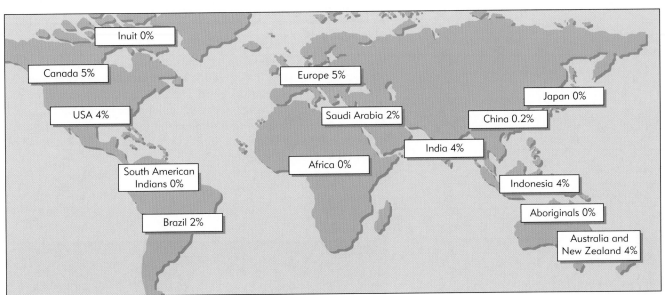

Fig. 16.54 Mutation FV:R506Q: distribution in the world population. (Modified with permission from Axelsson F, Rosén S. *Activated Protein C Resistance*. Product Monograph. Mölindal, Sweden: Chromogenix; 1997.)

Protein S deficiency

The anticoagulant activity of protein C requires a cofactor protein S, which is also vitamin K-dependent and exists in plasma as free and bound forms. Protein S deficiency, inherited probably as a dominant, presents as recurrent venous thromboses.

Antithrombin deficiency

Antithrombin is a potent inhibitor of the activated serum protease factors XIa, Xa, IXa, IIa and thrombin, forming high molecular weight inactive complexes with these proteins. Deficiency of antithrombin leads to recurrent venous thromboses which tend to be severe and present early in the homozygous form. The action of antithrombin is potentiated by heparin.

Hyperhomocysteinaemia

The plasma concentration of homocysteine is an important contributing factor in thrombosis and vascular disease, including peripheral vascular disease, myocardial infarct, stroke and venous thrombosis. Hyperhomocysteinaemia is, in part, genetically determined – several alterations in enzymes involved in homocysteine metabolism (*Fig. 16.55*) have been described (e.g. the mutation MTHFR C677T). The

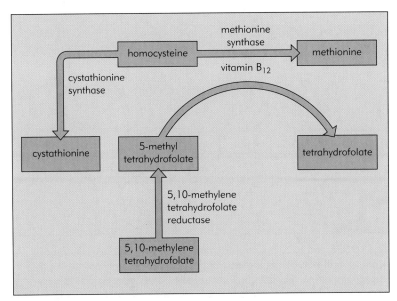

Fig. 16.55 Homocysteine metabolism: the roles of methionine synthase, cystathionine synthase and 5,10-methylene tetrahydrofolate reductase (*see also Fig. 3.10*).

mechanism of thrombosis is unclear, but endothelial cell damage may be important. Deficiencies of folate, vitamin B_{12} and vitamin B_6 also cause hyperhomocysteinaemia. The plasma level of homocysteine rises with age, is higher in men than in premenopausal women and is raised after liver or renal transplantation.

Hyperprothrombinaemia

The G20210A mutation of prothrombin causes high levels of prothrombin and is thrombogenic.

Other disorders

Although there are associations between thrombotic risk and high factor VIII levels, deficiency of heparin cofactor II and plasminogen, as well as with other fibrinolytic defects, the evidence for familial thrombophilia as a result of these conditions is inconclusive. Dysfibrinogenaemia is rarely a cause of thrombophilia.

Acquired thrombotic risk factors

Important acquired risk factors for thrombosis are given in *Fig. 16.56*.

Antiphospholipid antibodies

The antiphospholipid antibodies, 'lupus anticoagulant' and 'anticardiolipin antibody' are associated with predisposition to thrombosis, and are often both present in the same patient. The 'lupus anticoagulant' is associated with prolongation of activated partial thromboplastin time (APTT) that is not corrected by the addition of normal plasma. The antibodies react to phospholipids and β2-GP1. The reaction on the platelet surface is thought to be thrombogenic, even though *in vitro* tests such as the APTT appear to show anticoagulation.

The antibodies occur with SLE and other autoimmune disorders, but they may be 'primary' without associated disease. Patients may have no symptoms, but there is often a history of arterial (*Fig. 16.57*) and venous thrombosis, recurrent spontaneous abortion or persistent or relapsing thrombocytopenia.

DIAGNOSIS OF VENOUS THROMBOSIS

The techniques available include contrast CT (*Figs 16.58 and 16.59*), venography (*Figs 16.60 and 16.61*), and duplex and colour-coded Doppler ultrasonography (*Fig. 16.62*), which is also valuable in assessing deep veins (e.g. in the abdomen). Assay of D-dimer, a fragment specific for the degradation of fibrin, can also be used, and may be particularly valuable for the diagnosis of recurrent thromboses at the same site. For the diagnosis of pulmonary embolus, ventilation–perfusion (*see Fig. 5.77*) or spiral CT (*Fig. 16.63*) can be used.

Acquired risk factors for venous thrombosis
Advanced age
Heart disease, myocardial infarct
Immobility
Lupus anticoagulants
Malignancy
Obesity
Oral contraceptives (oestrogen)
Pregnancy and puerperium
Trauma and surgery
Varicose veins
Nephrotic syndrome
Hyperhomocysteinaemia
Hyperviscosity states
Myeloproliferative diseases
Paroxysmal nocturnal haemoglobinuria
Behçet's syndrome

Fig. 16.56 Venous thrombosis: acquired risk factors.

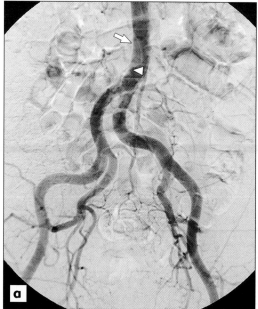
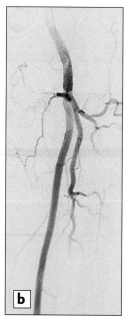

Fig. 16.57a and b Lupus anticoagulant syndrome: arteriogram of a 60-year-old man with non-Hodgkin lymphoma and a strongly positive lupus anticoagulant (APTT, 120 s; not corrected by a 50:50 mix with normal plasma). He developed pain and ischaemia in his left foot. (a) 'Saddle' embolus (arrow) at the aortic bifurcation and in the left common iliac artery (arrowhead); (b) the anterior tibial, peroneal and posterior tibial arteries are blocked by thrombi and do not fill with contrast below the mid calf level.

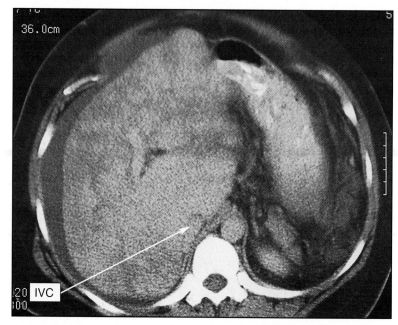

Fig. 16.58 Hepatic veno-occlusive disease (Budd–Chiari syndrome): dynamic contrast-enhanced CT showing the reticulated mosaic pattern of hepatic parenchymal enhancement with poor visualization of the hepatic veins. Typically, the caudate lobe enhances normally and appears hyperdense relative to the remaining liver parenchyma. Ascites is present and the inferior vena cava (IVC) is narrowed. (Courtesy of Drs IS Francis and J Tibballs.)

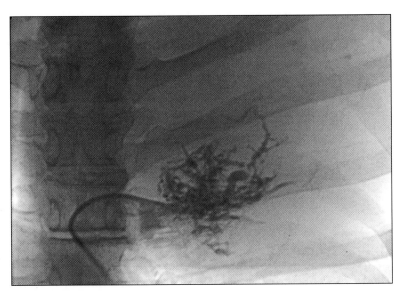

Fig. 16.59 Hepatic veno-occlusive disease (Budd–Chiari syndrome): using a transjugular approach, a catheter was introduced into the right hepatic vein. Direct injection of contrast shows a characteristic interlacing network of intrahepatic, portal and hepatic veins, with no flow exiting via the hepatic veins. This 'spider-web' appearance is unique to Budd–Chiari syndrome. (Courtesy of Drs IS Francis and J Tibballs.)

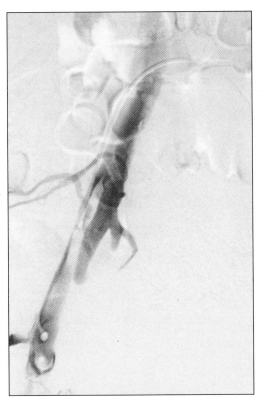

Fig. 16.60 Deep-vein thrombosis: a femoral venogram demonstrating extensive thrombus within the right external iliac vein extending into the right common iliac vein. (Courtesy of Drs IS Francis and AF Watkinson.)

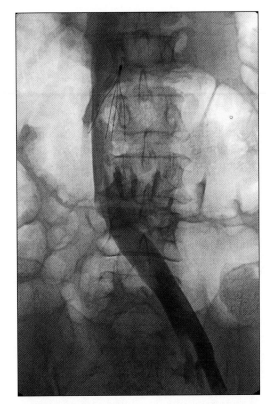

Fig. 16.61 Deep-vein thrombosis: A Gunther–Tulip filter positioned within the infrarenal IVC to prevent pulmonary embolism. Percutaneous access is via either the femoral or internal jugular vein. This particular device has a proximal hook, which permits its removal up to 2 weeks following placement. (Courtesy of Drs IS Francis and AF Watkinson.)

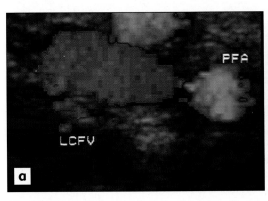
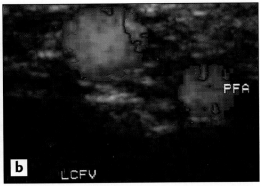
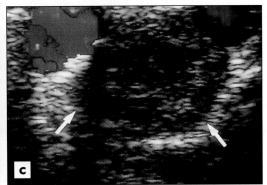

Fig. 16.62a–c Deep-vein thrombosis: Colour Doppler ultrasound. (a) Normal left common femoral vein (LCFV) without compression. (b) Normal left common femoral vein with compression. (c) Left common femoral vein with thrombosis (arrows); the vein is not compressible. [PFA, profunda femora artery; (a–c) courtesy of Dr IS Francis.]

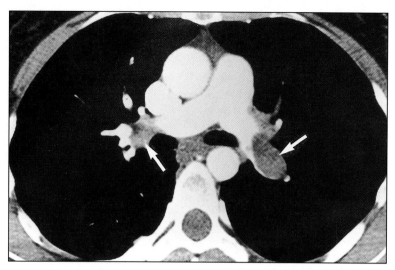

Fig. 16.63 Pulmonary embolus: contrast-enhanced spiral CT that shows filling defects within both main pulmonary arteries (arrows). These represent large pulmonary emboli. (Courtesy of Prof. DM Hansell.)

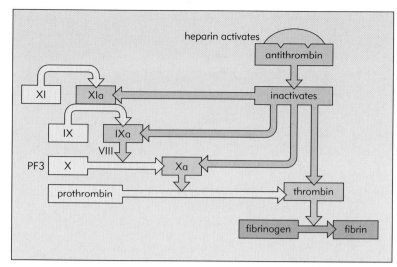

Fig. 16.64 The action of heparin: this activates antiprothrombin, which then forms complexes with activated serine protease coagulation factors (thrombin, Xa, IXa and XIa) and so inactivates them. (Modified with permission from Hoffbrand AV, Pettit JE. *Essential Haematology*, 3rd edn. Oxford: Blackwell Scientific Publications; 1993.)

ANTITHROMBOTIC THERAPY

Heparin

Heparin is an acid polysaccharide that potentiates (with antithrombin and heparin cofactor) inactivation of the serine protease coagulation factors (*Fig. 16.64*). Preparations are either unfractionated (standard heparin, MW 15–18 kDa) or fractionated (low molecular weight preparations, MW 4–8 kDa). Low molecular weight preparations are better able to inhibit factor Xa than thrombin (*Fig. 16.65*), interact less with platelets and may have a lesser tendency to cause bleeding (*Fig. 16.66*). Side effects of heparin include bleeding and thrombocytopenia, either Type I within 1–2 days because of agglutinates or Type II after 5 days or more because of platelet-activating autoantibodies directed against heparin-platelet factor 4 complexes. Type II is associated with thrombosis. Rarely, skin necrosis may occur because of local injection of heparin (*Fig. 16.67*) and osteoporosis is a late complication.

Oral anticoagulants

The oral anticoagulants are derivatives of coumarin and indanedione. Warfarin, a coumarin derivative, is used most widely. These drugs are vitamin K antagonists and therapy results in reduced activity of coagulation factors II, VII, IX and X.

The mechanism of action is shown in *Fig. 16.68*. The activity of warfarin can be enhanced or inhibited by a wide variety of drugs. The metabolism and therefore sensitivity to warfarin is also associated with polymorphisms in cytochrome P450 CYP2C9, the variant alleles being associated with a low-dose requirement.

Thrombin inhibitors

Thrombin inhibitors (*Fig. 16.69*) are effective against both free thrombin and thrombin bound to fibrin, but they do not inhibit thrombin generation. Hirudin and bivalirudin (hirulog) have been given clinical trials. Hirudin was originally extracted from the salivary glands of the medicinal leech *Hirudo medicinalis*. It is more effective than heparin in the prevention of venous thrombosis in high-risk patients and is licensed for use in heparin-induced thrombosis. The heparain analogue, darapanoid, may also be used for this. Inhibitors of thrombin that are of small molecular weight, including argatroban, efegatran and inogatran, are under evaluation in different settings.

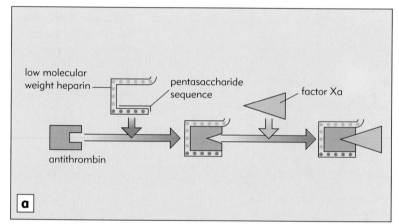

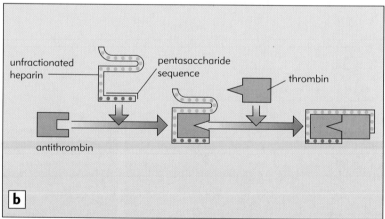

Fig. 16.65a and b Heparins (unfractionated and of low molecular weight): catalysis of antithrombin-mediated inactivation of thrombin or factor Xa. (a) the pentasaccharide sequence of both types of heparin causes a conformational change at the reactive centre of antithrombin when bound to it, which accelerates its reaction with factor Xa. (b) Catalysis of antithrombin-mediated inactivation of thrombin requires the formation of a ternary heparin–antithrombin–thrombin complex, which can be formed only by chains at least 18 saccharide units long. This explains why heparins of low molecular weight have less inhibitory activity against thrombin than unfractionated heparin. (Modified with permission from Weitz JI. Low molecular weight heparins. *N Engl J Med.* 1997;337:688–98.)

Comparison of the effects of unfractionated and low molecular weight heparins		
	Unfractionated	**Low molecular weight**
Mean molecular weight (kDa)	15	4.5
Inhibits	Xa and thrombin equally	Xa ± thrombin (2:1–4:1)
Platelet function	Inhibits	No inhibition
Protein binding	Yes	Reduced
Bioavailability	50%	100%
Elimination	Hepatic and renal	Renal
Half-life of anti-Xa, intravenous	1 h	2 h
Half-life of anti-Xa, subcutaneous	2 h	4 h
Frequency of heparin-induced thrombosis	High	Low
Osteoporosis	More frequent	Less frequent

Fig. 16.66 Heparins (unfractionated and of low molecular weight): comparison of effects.

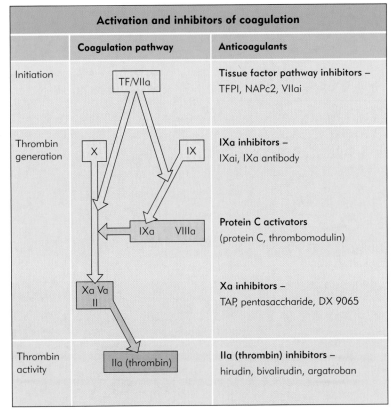

Fig. 16.67 Heparin: skin necrosis. After local subcutaneous injection of unfractionated heparin.

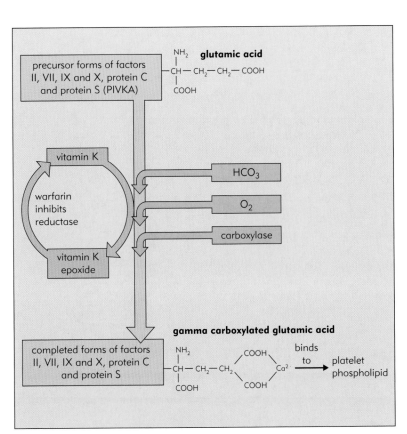

Fig. 16.68 The action of vitamin K in γ-carboxylation of glutamic acid in coagulation factors, which are then able to bind Ca^{2+} and attach to the platelet phospholipid. (Modified with permission from Hoffbrand AV, Pettit JE. *Essential Haematology*, 3rd edn. Oxford: Blackwell Scientific Publications; 1993.)

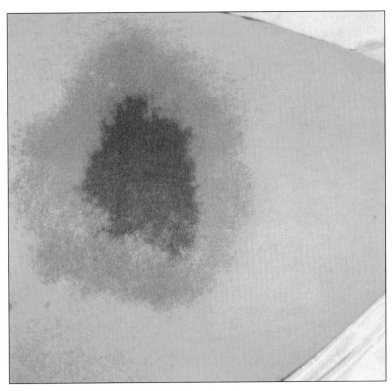

Fig. 16.69 Activation and inhibitors of coagulation: blood coagulation is initiated by the TF–VIIa complex, which induces thrombin generation by activating factors IX and X. New anticoagulants act by inhibiting the tissue pathway (initiation), blocking thrombin generation or inactivating thrombin. (TAP; tick anticoagulating peptide; IXai, active-site blocked factor IX; VIIai, active-site blocked factor VII; reproduced with permission from Hirsh J, Weitz JI. New antithrombotic agents. *Lancet*. 1999:353;1431–6.)

Fibrinolytic agents

Fibrinolytic agents act by enhancing conversion of the normal plasma constituent of plasminogen to plasmin, which degrades fibrin (*Fig. 16.70*). They are used to lyse fresh thrombi. They may be used systemically (e.g. for acute pulmonary embolus or iliofemoral thrombosis) or locally for acute peripheral arterial or venous (e.g. indwelling catheter) occlusion. The main side effect is haemorrhage.

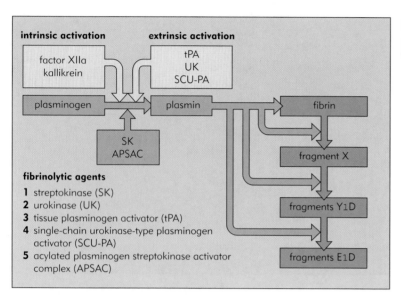

Fig. 16.70 The fibrinolytic system and fibrinolytic agents. (Modified with permission from Hoffbrand AV, Pettit JE. *Essential Haematology*, 3rd edn. Oxford: Blackwell Scientific Publications; 1993.)

17

Bone Marrow in Non-Haemopoietic Disease

Normal bone marrow appearances in paraffin sections of trephine biopsies are shown in *Figs 1.37* and *1.38*. In resin embedded sections a non-uniform distribution of haemopoietic precursors may be seen (*Fig. 17.1*).

The bone marrow may be involved in a number of disorders that are not primary diseases of the haemopoietic system. Aspirates or trephine biopsies may be used to assess bone-marrow involvement after primary diagnosis based on material from other sites, or may be responsible for the primary diagnosis itself. Magnetic resonance imaging (MRI) may be used to obtain an overall picture of marrow cellularity and to detect marrow infiltrations or deposits; the technique is reviewed at the end of this chapter.

METASTATIC BONE TUMOURS

The most common malignant tumours of bone are metastatic deposits from primary sites elsewhere in the body. Carcinomas of the breast, lung, kidney, thyroid and prostate are very likely to involve the marrow (*Figs 17.2–17.4*); stomach (*Figs 17.5a and 17.5b*), pancreas, colon (*Figs*

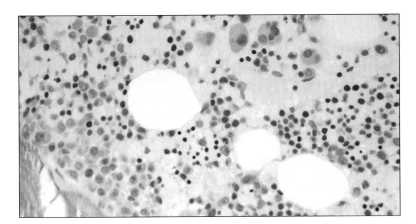

Fig. 17.1 Normal trephine biopsy, resin-embedded section: granulocyte precursors dominate close to the trabeculum (extreme left); erythroid precursors are mainly centrally placed (extreme right); and megakaryocytes are close to the central sinuses.

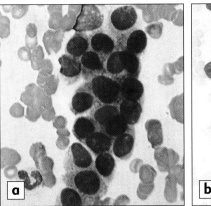
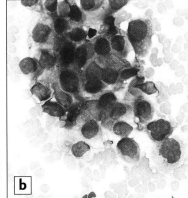

Fig. 17.2a and b Metastatic carcinoma: clusters of malignant epithelial cells in bone marrow. (a) An isolated group of small, fairly uniform, malignant epithelial cells (primary lung oat-cell carcinoma); (b) a clump of epithelial cells with features of a large undifferentiated cell carcinoma (primary carcinoma of breast).

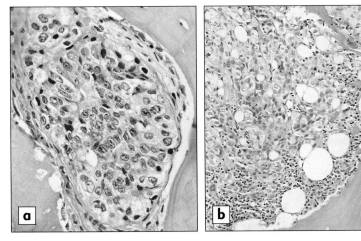

Fig. 17.3a and b Metastatic carcinoma: replacement of normal haemopoietic tissue in the intertrabecular areas by (a) nests of malignant epithelial cells (primary carcinoma of prostate) and (b) sheets of pleomorphic neoplastic epithelial cells (primary carcinoma of kidney).

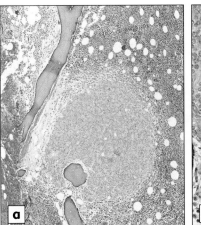
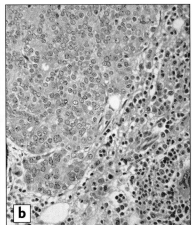

Fig. 17.4a and b Metastatic carcinoma: (a) a prominent paratrabecular deposit of neoplastic epithelial cells; the patient had chronic lymphocytic leukaemia and a primary carcinoma of the prostate. (b) Higher power shows a clear separation of malignant epithelial tissue from haemopoietic tissue that contains increased numbers of lymphocytes.

17.5c and 17.5d) and rectum tumours involve the marrow less frequently, but virtually any malignant tumour may metastasize to bone.

In advanced disease, leucoerythroblastic changes may be found in the blood film; there may also be evidence of bone marrow failure. The skeletal lesions are predominantly osteolytic, presenting as radiolucent areas on radiographic examination (Fig. 17.6). Extensive osteoclastic resorption of bone is often found in trephine biopsies (Fig. 17.7). Almost all tumours provoke some bone healing and sometimes new bone deposition; osteoblastic activity is most pronounced in metastatic spread from carcinoma of the prostate (Fig. 17.8) and breast (Fig. 17.9).

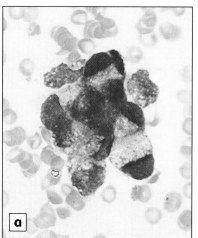
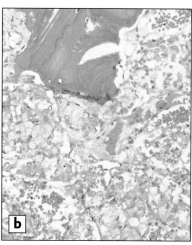
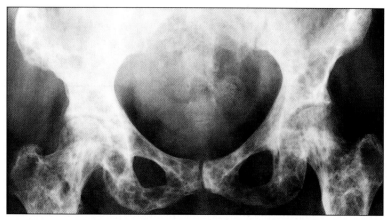
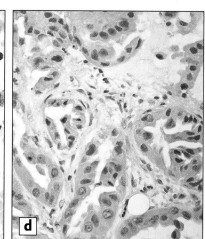

Fig. 17.5a–d Metastatic carcinoma: (a) a clump of distended and vacuolated neoplastic epithelial cells in a patient with microangiopathic haemolytic anaemia and laboratory evidence of disseminated intravascular coagulation; (b) sheets and acini of mucin-secreting adenocarcinoma in the same patient as described in (a), who had a primary tumour of the stomach; (c) a sheet of neoplastic columnar cells in bone marrow; (d) replacement of normal haemopoietic tissue by acini of neoplastic columnar cells in the same patient as described in (c), who had a primary carcinoma of the ascending colon.

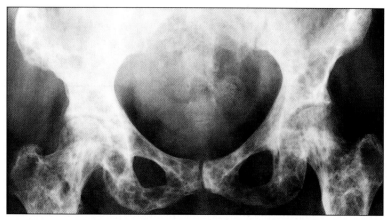

Fig. 17.6 Metastatic carcinoma: radiograph of the pelvis of a 58-year-old man with carcinoma of the lung. Metastatic deposits of tumour have produced widespread lytic lesions, most marked in the lower pelvis and upper parts of the femurs.

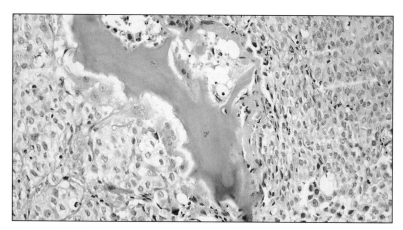

Fig. 17.7 Metastatic carcinoma: metastatic deposits from a carcinoma of the kidney. Sheets of neoplastic epithelial cell surrounding residual trabecular bone with osteoclasts adjacent to the scalloped edges.

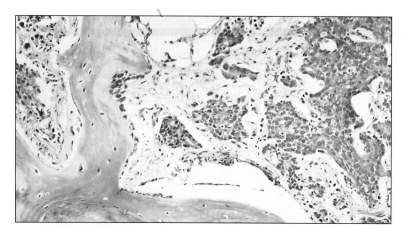

Fig. 17.8 Metastatic carcinoma: there is thickening of medullary trabecular bone and osteoblasts are prominent along the right-hand margin of the vertical trabecula. The intertrabecular space contains nests of malignant epithelial cells supported by an abundant fibrous stroma. The patient had carcinoma of the prostate.

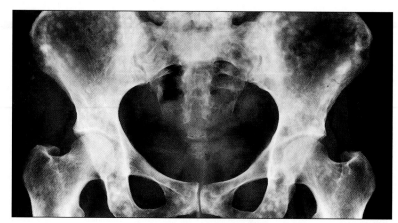

Fig. 17.9 Metastatic carcinoma: radiography of the pelvis of a 45-year-old woman with carcinoma of the breast. The widespread foci of increased bone density are the result of osteoblastic activity surrounding metastases.

Occasionally fragments of epidermis are carried into the marrow cavity during trephine biopsy (*Fig. 17.10*), but the well differentiated nature of such fragments allows easy distinction from metastatic carcinoma.

Involvement of bone marrow by tumours other than carcinomas also occurs. *Figs 17.11–17.13* demonstrate involvement by malignant melanoma, neuroblastoma and medulloblastoma. Bone marrow involvement arising from malignant lymphomas and histiocytic proliferative disorders is discussed in Chapters 7 and 11. Although the majority of primary bone tumours do not metastasize to parts of the skeleton distant from their origin, bone marrow examination may reveal evidence of dissemination in Ewing's tumour of bone (*Fig. 17.14*).

Metastatic tumours in the marrow may be detected using monoclonal antibodies and indirect immunofluorescence or alkaline phosphatase–anti-alkaline phosphatase (AP–AAP) techniques. Anti-milk fat globulin may detect breast carcinoma; anti-cytokeratin may detect epithelial carcinomas (*Fig. 17.15*); and anti-desmin (intermediate filaments) may detect mesenchymal tumours (*Fig. 17.16*).

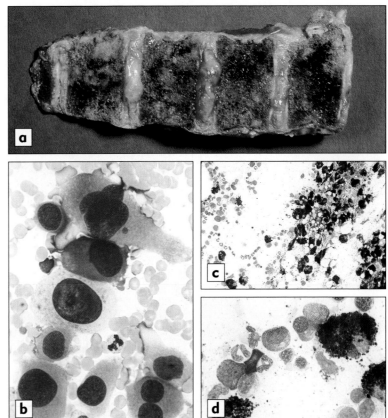

Fig. 17.11a–d Metastatic malignant melanoma: (a) post-mortem section of spine showing multiple black deposits; (b) large malignant melanoma cells of variable size with primitive chromatin patterns and nucleoli. (c, d) Lower and higher power views show no malignant cells, but numerous melanin-filled macrophages are evident. The patient had a malignant melanoma on the skin of the back. [(a) Courtesy of Dr R Britt.]

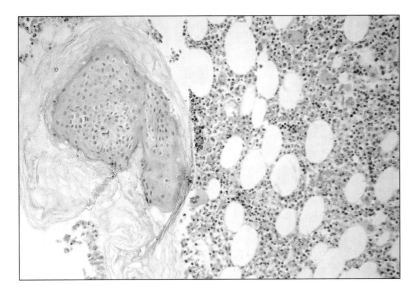

Fig. 17.10 Artefact on trephine biopsy: a small fragment of well-differentiated keratinized squamous epithelium has been carried into the bone marrow cavity. Normal haemopoietic tissue is on the right.

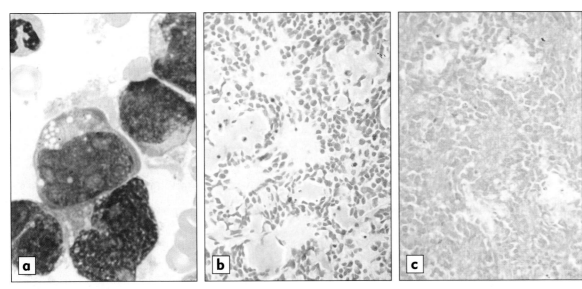

Fig. 17.12a–c Metastatic neuroblastoma: (a) bone marrow from a 3-year-old boy with neuroblastoma in the right thorax shows malignant 'neuroblasts', somewhat larger and more pleomorphic than haemopoietic blast cells and with fine chromatin patterns and prominent nucleoli; (b) rosettes of neuroblastoma cells, some pyriform or fibrillar, with neurofibrils within amorphous extracellular material; (c) staining for neuron-specific enolase, using an immunoperoxidase–avidin biotin complex technique, demonstrates the antigen within the cells and in the neurofibrillary extracellular material. [(b, c) Courtesy of Dr POG Wilson.]

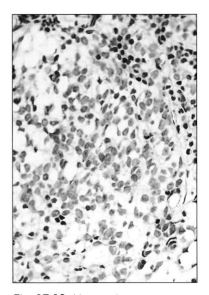

Fig. 17.13 Metastatic medulloblastoma: extensive replacement of haemopoietic tissue by small primitive cells with round nuclei, open chromatin and scanty cytoplasm.

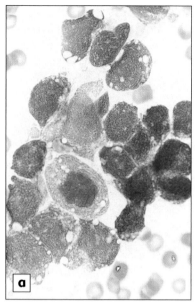
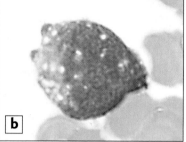
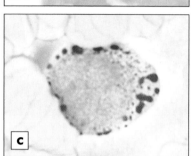
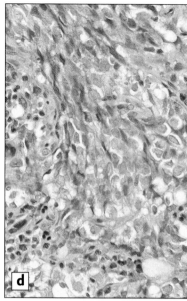

Fig. 17.14a–d Metastatic Ewing's sarcoma: (a) bone marrow aspirate showing vacuolated pleomorphic cells, including a cell in mitosis; (b) at higher magnification a tumour cell shows a fine chromatin pattern and vacuolated basophilic cytoplasm; (c) periodic acid–Schiff base (PAS) staining shows coarse blocks of positive material; (d) a trephine biopsy shows a sheet-like deposit of primitive cells with normal haemopoietic cells below.
[(a, b) May–Grünwald/Giemsa; (c) PAS; (d) H & E; (a, d) courtesy of Dr DM Swirsky.]

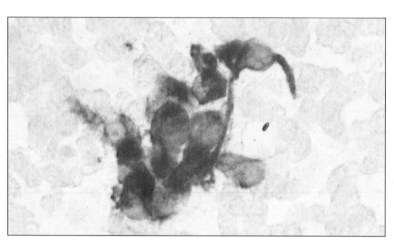

Fig. 17.15 Metastatic carcinoma: anti-cytokeratin antibody (AP–AAP technique). (Courtesy of Prof. DY Mason.)

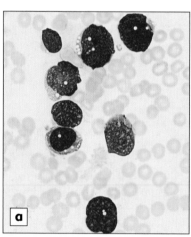
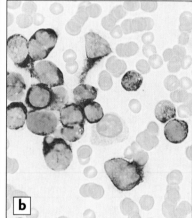

Fig. 17.16a and b Metastatic rhabdomyosarcoma: (a) May–Grünwald/Giemsa stain; (b) anti-desmin antibody (AP–AAP technique). [(a, b) Courtesy of Prof. DY Mason.]

MAST CELL DISEASE

Systemic mastocytosis is a rare disease of adults in which a persistent and progressive cutaneous eruption is a characteristic presentation (*Fig. 17.17*). Radiography usually reveals multiple, irregularly rounded, lytic lesions or new bone formation in the skeleton. In severe cases lymphadenopathy, hepatosplenomegaly and extensive infiltration of the bone marrow by mast cells may be present (*Fig. 17.18*). Evidence of disease may also be found in skin biopsies (*Fig. 17.19*) or at splenectomy (*Fig. 17.20*). Disease confined to the skin and bone marrow is frequently associated with prolonged survival, but patients who develop extensive reticuloendothelial involvement often die soon after diagnosis.

GRANULOMATOUS DISEASE

Sarcoidosis

This granulomatous disorder of unknown aetiology most frequently affects the middle-aged. It is characterized by widespread epithelioid cell granulomas, depression of delayed hypersensitivity and lymphoproliferation. Multisystemic involvement is characteristic – intrathoracic disease affects 90% of cases, ocular and skin involvement each occur in about 25% of cases, and erythema nodosum occurs in up to a third of cases.

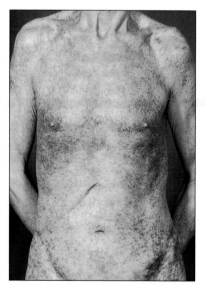

Fig. 17.17 Systemic mastocytosis: generalized pigmented and nodular cutaneous eruption seen after splenectomy (see *Fig. 17.20*) and psoralen and ultraviolet A (PUVA) therapy.

In different series, the reticuloendothelial system has been shown to be involved in up to 40% of patients. Evidence of disease may be found during bone marrow examination (*Fig. 17.21*) or at splenectomy (*Fig. 17.22*).

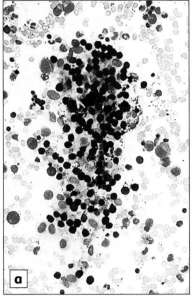

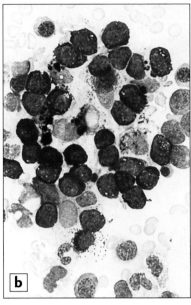

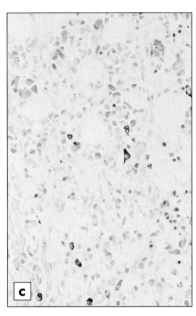

Fig. 17.18a–c Systemic mastocytosis: an extensive accumulation of mast cells at (a) low and (b) higher power; (c) the characteristic metachromatic staining reaction of the mast cells in the cytoplasm with toluidine blue stain.

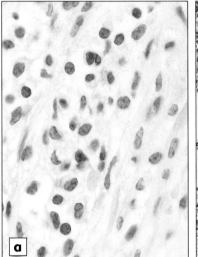

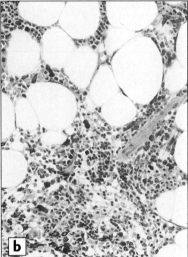

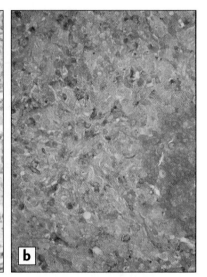

Fig. 17.19a and b Systemic mastocytosis: (a) bone marrow trephine biopsy showing mast cells, some of which have elongated nuclei that resemble fibroblasts; (b) low-power view showing perivascular distribution of mast cells – mast cells are also present around the edge of a lymphoid aggregate. [(a) Courtesy of Dr BJ Bain.]

Fig. 17.20a and b Systemic mastocytosis: sections of spleen showing mononuclear histiocyte-like cells on staining with (a) haematoxylin and eosin and (b) toluidine blue to demonstrate the cytoplasmic metachromasia. [(a, b) Courtesy of Dr JE McLaughlin.]

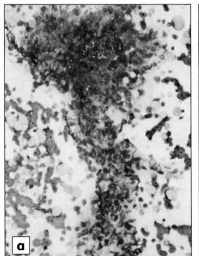

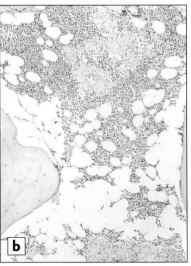

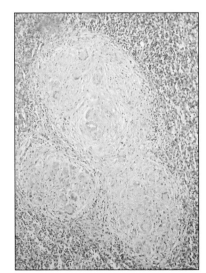

Fig. 17.22 Sarcoidosis: section of spleen showing granulomatous collections of epithelioid cells, including prominent multinuclear forms and peripheral lymphoid cells.

Fig. 17.21a and b Sarcoidosis: (a) a sheet of epithelioid histiocytic cells, scattered lymphocytes and myeloid cells; (b) two small granulomas comprising epithelioid cells and lymphocytes.

Tuberculosis

Blood-borne tubercle bacilli may lodge in the bone marrow; aspirates from patients with suspected miliary or other atypical haematogenous forms of tuberculosis may show characteristic epithelioid granulomas (*Fig. 17.23*). If left untreated the disease becomes extensive, particularly in the anterior aspects of the vertebral bodies and in the metaphyseal areas of the long bones. The tuberculous foci may progress, producing cystic areas of osteomyelitis that erode the endplates and involve the nearby joint spaces. Tuberculous spondylitis (Pott's disease) involves the anterior aspects of the vertebral bodies with subsequent wedging and eventual collapse (*Fig. 17.24*).

Other granulomas

Evidence of other granulomatous disease is occasionally found during bone marrow examination. Subsequent investigations may reveal the cause (e.g. brucellosis), although in many cases no cause is found (*Fig. 17.25*). Rarely foreign body granulomas are found during routine examination of trephine biopsies (*Fig. 17.26*).

KALA-AZAR (VISCERAL LEISHMANIASIS)

Kala-azar is distributed widely throughout tropical and warm regions of the world. The causal organism, *Leishmania donovani*, is transmitted by the bite of sandflies of the genus *Phlebotomus*. The non-flagellated amastigote forms of the organism are distributed widely through reticuloendothelial macrophages in the bone marrow, spleen and liver. Diagnosis is usually made by examining bone marrow (*Fig. 17.27*), splenic aspirates or biopsy specimens. Clinical features include prolonged fever, lassitude, weight loss, splenomegaly, hepatomegaly, anaemia, leucopenia and polyclonal increases in immunoglobulin.

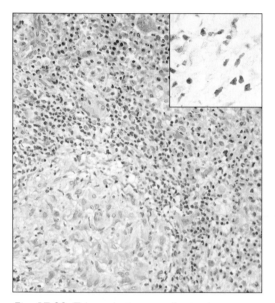

Fig. 17.23 Tuberculosis: a small granuloma surrounded by hyperplastic haemopoietic tissue; the inset shows small numbers of acid-fast bacilli. [(inset, Ziehl–Neelsen stain.]

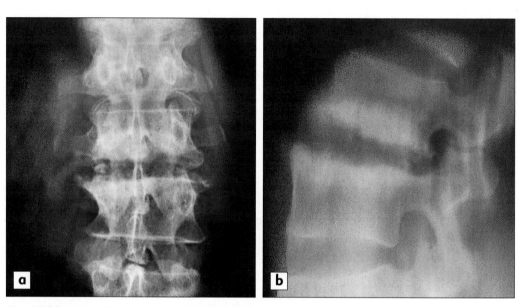

Fig. 17.24a and b Tuberculosis: radiographs of the lumbar spine seen in (a) anteroposterior view and (b) a lateral tomogram. Inflammatory changes are seen around the disc between the second and third lumbar vertebrae, with sclerosis of the adjacent vertebral endplates. [(a, b) Courtesy of Dr R Dick.]

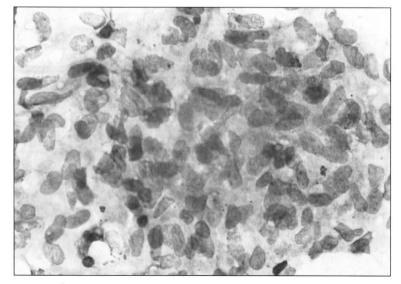

Fig. 17.25 Non-specific marrow granuloma: this small collection of epithelioid cells was found in a bone marrow cell trail that showed no other abnormality. No specific diagnosis was made.

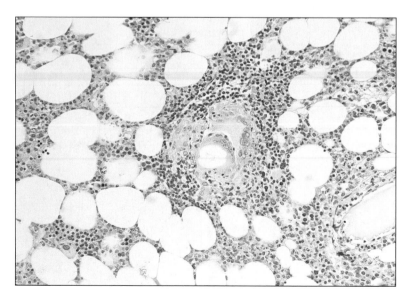

Fig. 17.26 Foreign body granuloma: an isolated granuloma with a central large vacuole that contains a refractile body of uncertain origin surrounded by giant cells.

OTHER INFECTIONS

Bone marrow examination has little part to play in the diagnosis and management of osteomyelitis, although (occasionally) initial evidence of a disseminated fungal infection may be uncovered (*Fig. 17.28*).

The bone marrow and spleen may be involved in cases of disseminated histoplasmosis. The *Histoplasma capsulatum* fungal organisms may be seen inside macrophages in stained aspirates or trephine biopsies (*Fig. 17.29*).

LYSOSOMAL STORAGE DISEASES

The lysosomal storage diseases of the reticuloendothelial system (*Fig. 17.30*) may result in pancytopenia, vacuolation or abnormal granulation of blood cells and the accumulation of degenerate foam cells in the bone marrow, liver and spleen. These lysosomal storage conditions result from defects in lysozymal hydrolytic enzymes (*Fig. 17.31*). The products of metabolism normally degraded by the specific enzyme that is defective disrupt the lysosomes and damage cell structure.

Gaucher's disease

Gaucher's disease is a relatively common familial disorder characterized by the accumulation of glucocerebrosides (especially glucosylceramide) in reticuloendothelial cells; it occurs because the enzyme glucocerebrosidase is deficient. Three types occur (*Fig. 17.32*):

- chronic adult;
- acute infantile neuropathic and;
- subacute neuropathic with onset in childhood or adolescence.

The gene is located on chromosome 1 band q21. There is a pseudogene 16 kb downstream from the glucocerebrosidase gene, which is

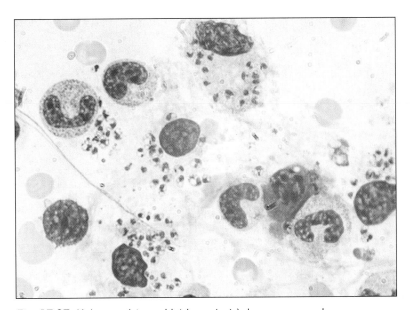

Fig. 17.27 Kala-azar (visceral leishmaniasis): bone marrow shows macrophages that contain Leishman–Donovan bodies. Also seen are neutrophil metamyelocytes and a plasma cell.

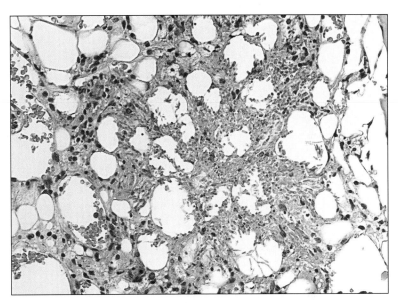

Fig. 17.28 Disseminated aspergillosis: biopsy taken after bone marrow transplantation shows hyphae of *Aspergillus* in an area of necrosis.

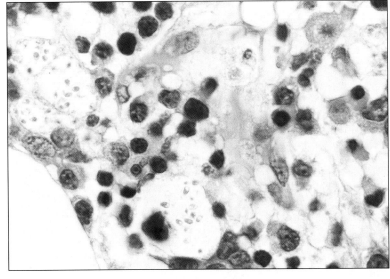

Fig. 17.29 Histoplasmosis: the encapsulated organisms are seen clearly inside the macrophages.

Lysosomal storage diseases	
Sphingolipidoses	**Diseases of complex carbohydrate metabolism**
Gaucher's disease	Sialidoses
Niemann–Pick disease	Mucolipidoses
Farber's disease	Fucosidosis
GM gangliosidoses	Mannosidosis
Mucopolysaccharidoses	Aspartylglucosaminuria
	Sialic acid storage disease
Hurler's, Scheie's and Hurler–Scheie disease	**Acid lipase deficiency**
Hunter's disease	
Sanfilippo's disease	Wolman's disease
Marquio syndrome	Cholesterol ester storage disease
Maroteaux–Lamy syndrome	
	Neuronal ceroid lipofuscinoses

Fig. 17.30 Lysosomal storage diseases.

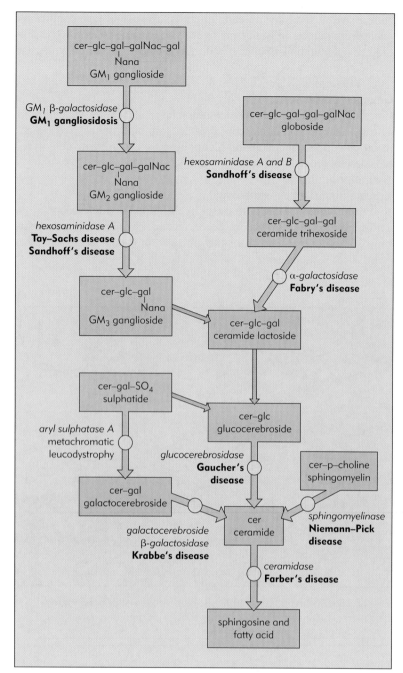

Fig. 17.31 Sphingolipid mechanism: pathways and diseases: the enzymes involved are given in italics, and below each is given the disease (in bold) that results from deficiency of that particular enzyme. [cer; ceramide; glc, glucose; gal, galactose; galNac, acetylgalactosamine; Nana, N-acetylneuraminic acid; adapted with permission from Kolodny EH, Tenembaum AL. In: Nathan DG, Oski FA (eds). *Hematology of Infancy and Childhood*, 4th edn. Philadelphia: Saunders; 1992:1452.]

Gaucher's disease – clinical types			
Clinical features	**Type 1**	**Type 2**	**Type 3**
Onset	Child/adult	Infancy	Juvenile
Hepatosplenomegaly	+	+	+
Hypersplenism	+	+	+
Bone crises/fractures	+	–	+
Neurodegenerative course	–	+++	+++
Death	Childhood/ adulthood	By 2 years	2nd to 4th decades
Ethnic predilection	Ashkenazi Jewish	Pan-ethnic	Pan-ethnic

Fig. 17.32 Gaucher's disease: the three clinical types. (Courtesy of Prof. G Gabrowski.)

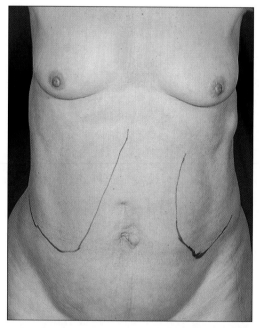

Fig. 17.33 Gaucher's disease: moderate enlargement of both the spleen and liver.

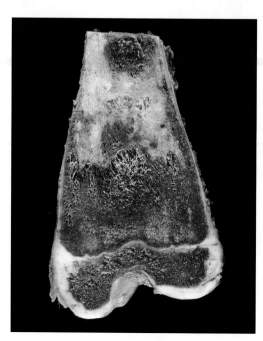

Fig. 17.34 Gaucher's disease: lower end of femur showing expansion of marrow cavity with thinning of cortical bone and multiple infarcted areas (white) giving typical Erlenmeyer flask deformity. There is subchondral bony collapse with osteonecrosis. (Courtesy of Prof. R Brady.)

95% homologous. The disease is caused by gene mutations or deletions or the formation of fusion genes between the functional gene and the pseudogene. The high prevalence in Ashkenazi Jews largely arises from a mutation at cDNA nucleotide 226 (amino acid 370). The chronic adult non-neuropathic form of the disease is accompanied by hepatosplenomegaly (*Fig. 17.33*) and bone lesions (*Fig. 17.34*), and sometimes by lymphadenopathy, skin pigmentation and pingueculae (*Fig. 17.35*). The most acute neuropathic forms present in infancy and survival beyond the first 3 years of life is rare. A juvenile form may present in childhood with features of the chronic adult form as well as progressive neurological dysfunction.

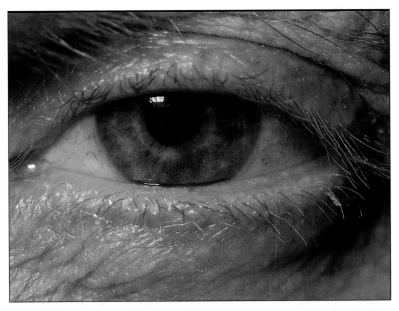

Fig. 17.35 Gaucher's disease: pingueculae, the brownish-yellow wedge-shaped thickenings of the bulbar conjunctiva.

A presumptive diagnosis of Gaucher's disease may be made when Gaucher's cells are detected in marrow aspirates (*Figs 17.36a and 17.36b*) and trephine biopsies (*Fig. 17.36c*). Diagnosis can be confirmed by demonstration of absence or severe deficiency of the enzyme glucosyl-ceramide β-glucosidase in fibroblast cultures. Gaucher's cells are also found in the liver and spleen (*Fig. 17.36d*). Most patients with this condition have elevated plasma acid phosphatase, serum angiotensin-converting enzyme (SACE), ferritin and transcobalamin II levels. Serum chitotriosidase is markedly raised and can be used to monitor efficacy of enzyme therapy. Over 50% of adult patients usually have asymptomatic radiographic changes, such as cortical expansion of the lower end of the femur, which produces a characteristic radiolucent area (*Fig. 17.37*).

It is now possible to replace the missing enzyme with aglucerase (Ceredase), an enzyme preparation prepared from human placenta in which the sugar moieties are designed to give maximum retention in the reticuloendothelial system. Alternatively, enzyme made using recombinant DNA techniques, such as imiglucerase (Cerezyme), may be given. Following therapy there is improvement in blood counts, reduction in liver and spleen size, and remodelling of the bones with reduction of osteoporosis (*Fig. 17.38*) which can be demonstrated by MRI scan (*Fig. 17.39*).

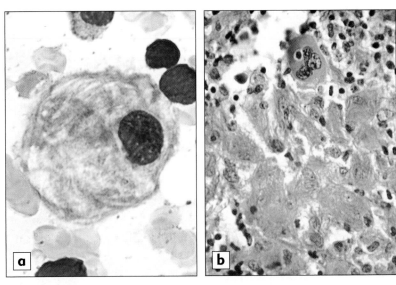
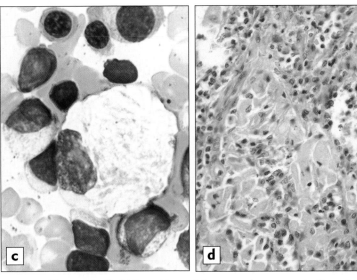

Fig. 17.36a–d Gaucher's disease: (a, b) characteristic histiocytic cells with a fibrillar or 'onion-skin' pattern of unstained inclusion material. In biopsy (c) these cells are bland histiocytes with a finely granular cytoplasmic PAS reaction. The markedly PAS-positive cell is a megakaryocyte. In the spleen (d) the histiocytic cells appear as pale clusters in the reticuloendothelial cords between the venous sinuses.

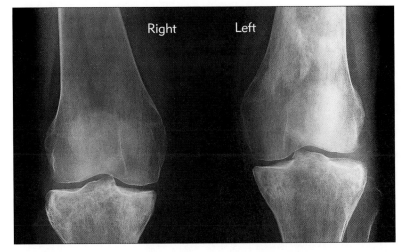

Fig. 17.37 Gaucher's disease: radiograph of the knee joints in a 45-year-old woman shows failure of correct modelling with expansion of the lower ends of the femurs. Bone thinning and loss of trabecular pattern are particularly apparent in the right femur. The sclerosis in the left femur and right tibia is caused by bone infarcts.

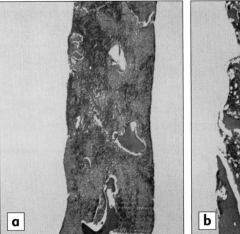
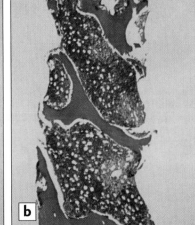

Fig. 17.38a and b Gaucher's disease: appearances of bone biopsy (a) before aglucerase therapy and (b) after 12 months of aglucerase therapy. [(a, b) Courtesy of Prof. R Brady.]

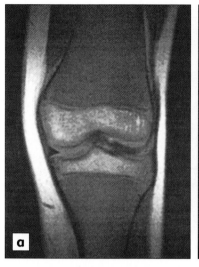 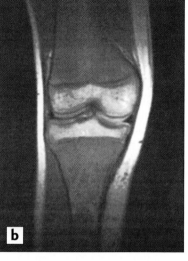

Fig. 17.39a and b Gaucher's disease: MRI scan of the left knee of an 11-year-old girl, (a) before treatment showing Erlenmeyer flask deformity with expansion of the marrow and thinning of the cortical bone – the bone marrow images have uniformly low intensity; (b) following 1 year of aglucerase therapy the bone marrow intensity is brighter, and remodelling of the bone is occurring (accompanying a growth spurt). [(a, b) Courtesy of Dr L Berger.]

Niemann–Pick disease

Niemann–Pick disease is a sphingomyelin lipidosis, is rarer than Gaucher's disease, and is characterized by extensive tissue storage of sphingomyelin, hepatic and splenic enlargement, and large lipid-filled macrophages in the bone marrow. In its best-defined forms there is an inherited deficiency of the enzyme sphingomyelinase, and sphingomyelin concentration in the tissues is up to 100 times higher than normal. As in Gaucher's disease, acute neuropathic and chronic non-neuropathic forms occur.

The disease is suspected in young children with hepatosplenomegaly when bone marrow aspirates show the presence of foam cells (*Fig. 17.40*). Confirmation is by showing low levels of sphingomyelinase in fibroblasts cultured from skin or bone marrow. In less severe adult forms of the disease, large numbers of sea-blue histiocytes may be found in bone marrow aspirates, in addition to the classic foam cells (*Fig. 17.41*).

Sea-blue histiocyte syndrome

Patients with the rare sea-blue histiocyte syndrome usually present with splenomegaly and thrombocytopenic purpura, in some cases with associated hepatic cirrhosis. The inheritance pattern is autosomal recessive. Bone marrow aspirates contain large numbers of 'sea-blue' histiocytes (*Fig. 17.42*). Phospholipids and sphingomyelin accumulate

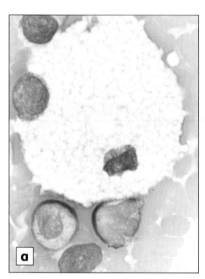 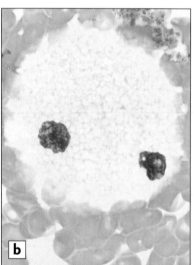 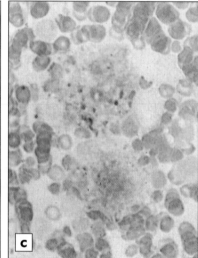 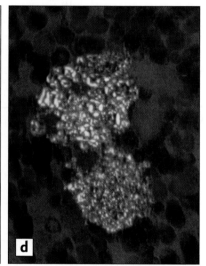

Fig. 17.40a–d Niemann–Pick disease (infantile): bone marrow showing (a, b) typical histiocytic cells with foamy deposits in the cytoplasm; (c) the histiocytic cells stain weakly with Sudan black stain for lipid; (d) in polarized light, strong red birefringence is present in the Sudan stain. [(c, d) Reproduced with permission from Hann IM, Lake BD, Pritchard J, Lilleyman J. *Colour Atlas of Paediatric Haematology*, 2nd edn. Oxford: Oxford University Press, 1990.]

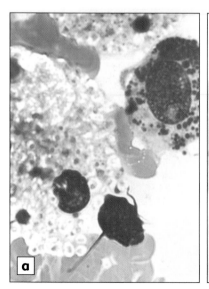 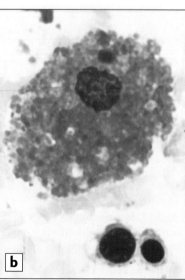 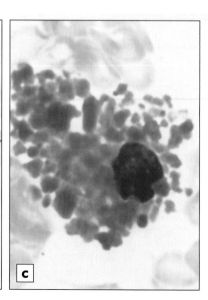

Fig. 17.41a–c Niemann–Pick disease (adult): bone marrow showing (a) typical foam cells, and (b, c) prominent histiocytes with sea-blue cytoplasm.

in tissue, and reduced levels of cellular sphingomyelinase activity have been reported. The syndrome is a variant of Niemann–Pick disease.

Other causes of sea-blue histiocytes in the bone marrow or spleen are listed in *Fig. 17.43*.

CYSTINOSIS

In this recessively inherited disease cystine crystals are deposited in the reticuloendothelial and corneal tissues. In its more severe form (cystinosis with Fanconi's syndrome or the de Toni–Fanconi–Lignac syndrome) progressive renal degeneration is fatal during early childhood. Children with this syndrome usually present with anorexia, thirst, polyuria, failure to thrive, rickets or photophobia. Laboratory tests reveal glycosuria, proteinuria, low serum bicarbonate, hypokalaemia or hypophosphataemia. The diagnosis is established by the demonstration of cystine crystals in macrophages in bone marrow aspirates (*Fig. 17.44*).

PRIMARY OXALURIA

In this fatal autosomal recessive metabolic disorder, there is widespread deposition of calcium oxalate crystals in the kidneys and elsewhere in the body, including the liver, spleen and bone marrow (*Figs 17.45 and 17.46*). A number of different enzyme deficiencies have been implicated as causal factors.

OSTEOPETROSIS (ALBERS–SCHÖNBERG OR MARBLE BONE DISEASE)

Osteopetrosis is a rare familial disorder that is characterized by an increase in density of all bones because of a functional defect in osteoclasts, with failure of bone resorption and remodelling. Severe forms of the disease present in infancy with anaemia and hepatosplenomegaly (*Fig. 17.47*). These children have little or no bone marrow; haemopoiesis

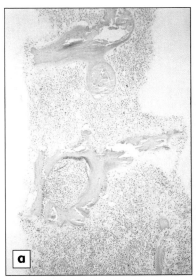

Fig. 17.42 Sea-blue histiocyte syndrome: bone marrow showing typical cells in the cell trails.

Causes of sea-blue histiocytes
Frequent, in marrow
Sea-blue histiocyte syndrome
Niemann–Pick disease
Occasional, in marrow
Hyperlipoproteinaemia
Hereditary acetyltransferase deficiency
Wolman's disease
Other lipid storage disorders
Chronic myeloid leukaemia
Polycythaemia vera
Chronic immune thrombocytopenia
Thalassaemia
Sickle cell disease
Sarcoidosis
Chronic granulomatous disease

Fig. 17.43 Sea-blue histiocytes in the bone marrow or spleen: causes.

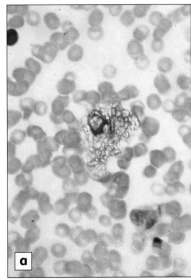
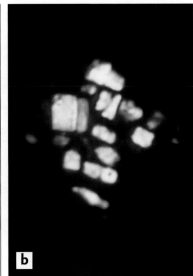

Fig. 17.44a and b Cystinosis: bone marrow containing (a) histiocytic cells, which (b) under polarized light show the characteristic birefringence of cystine crystals.

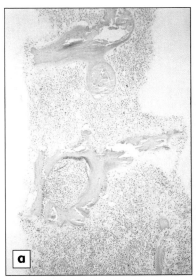
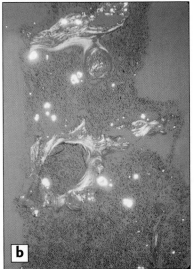

Fig. 17.45a and b Primary oxaluria: (a) normal and (b) polarizing microscopy shows birefringent calcium oxalate monohydrate crystals (and normal birefringent cortical bone). The patient, a 3-month-old boy, presented with renal failure. [(a, b) Courtesy of Dr S Milkins.]

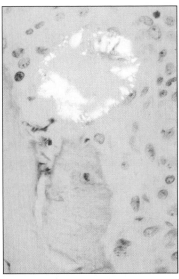

Fig. 17.46 Primary oxaluria: higher power (polarized) view of *Fig. 17.45* shows the oxalate crystals.

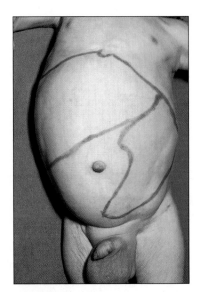

Fig. 17.47 Osteopetrosis: massive hepatosplenomegaly in a 14-month-old infant. Bilateral inguinal hernias are present because of raised intra-abdominal pressure.

is chiefly extramedullary and blood transfusions are required to sustain life. The typical radiographic appearances are shown in *Fig. 17.48*; characteristic microscopic abnormalities are found in trephine bone biopsies (*Figs 17.49 and 17.50*) and leucoerythroblastic changes are seen in the blood (*Fig. 17.51*). Failure to resorb bone results in optic atrophy, deafness and hydrocephalus. Milder cases may present later in childhood or in adult life with retarded growth, anaemia and splenomegaly (*Figs 17.52 and 17.53*).

AMYLOIDOSIS

Amyloidosis is a deposit of linear, non-branching protein fibrils laid down in a pleated β-conformation structure. Polysaccharides may form complexes with the protein. Amyloid deposits contain a non-fibrillar glycoprotein P component that is derived from a normal plasma precursor structurally related to C reactive protein. Primary amyloid is discussed in Chapter 12.

Amyloidosis occurs in a number of conditions (*Fig. 17.54*). In cases associated with immunocyte proliferation, immunoglobulin light chains appear to be the principal protein component (*see* Chapter 12); in the reactive type the major protein is not derived from immunoglobulins, but from protein A derived from serum amyloid, a protein that is an apolipoprotein. One important cause for this is familial Mediterranean fever, which is now thought to result from mutation in the gene MEFV that codes for pyrin. It has been postulated that pyrin inhibits nuclear transcription of inflammatory promoters. There are reduced activities of proteins, especially C5a, involved in the inactivation of chemotactic factors. Polymerization of the protein subunits involved in both types yields a characteristic fibrillary structure, visible by electron microscopy, with a distinct yellow–green dichromic birefringence under polarization microscopy after Congo red staining. In some patients, particularly those with reactive systemic amyloidosis, a trephine bone marrow biopsy may reveal the first evidence of amyloidosis (*Fig. 17.55*).

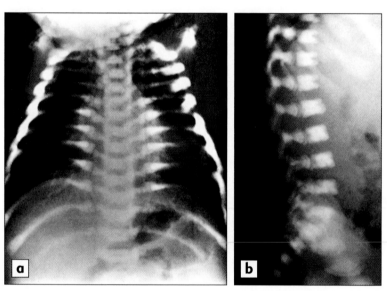

Fig. 17.48a and b Osteopetrosis: radiographs of (a) the chest and (b) lower spine of an infant with a gross generalized increase in bone density. The changes are most marked at the upper and lower margins of the vertebral bodies. The vertebrae also show the characteristic 'bone-in-bone' appearance.

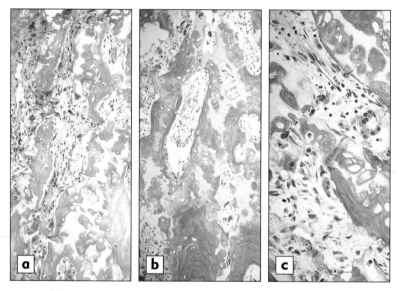

Fig. 17.49a–c Osteopetrosis: (a) compacted intramedullary osseous tissue and relatively little haemopoietic tissue; cores of cartilaginous matrix are bordered by areas of primitive bone; (b, c) persistence of cartilage, lack of bone modelling and primitive osseous tissue at the edges of and within the cartilage. [(b, c) Picro–Mallory stain.]

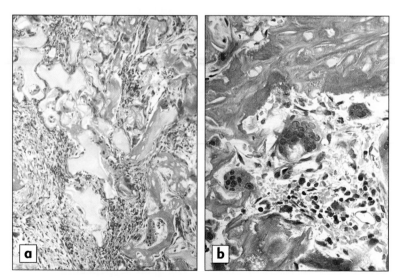

Fig. 17.50a and b Osteopetrosis: (a) biopsy (same case as shown in *Fig. 17.49*) shows large numbers of osteoclasts, (b) better seen at high power. There is little evidence of bone resorption, and no trabeculae or haemopoietic marrow spaces are seen. [(a, b) Picro–Mallory stain.]

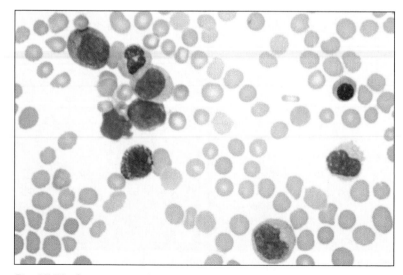

Fig. 17.51 Osteopetrosis: leucoerythroblastic changes. The red cells show anisocytosis and poikilocytosis; the nucleated cells include a myeloblast, a promyelocyte, a myelocyte and an erythroblast.

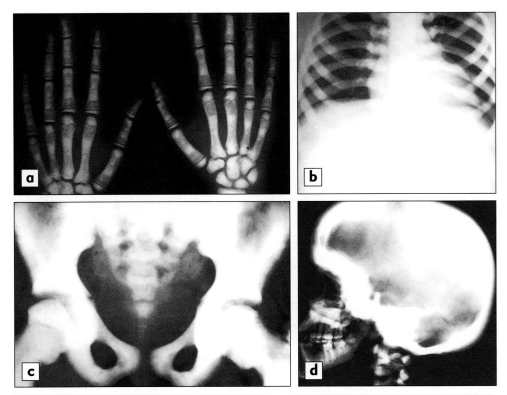

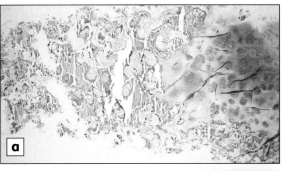

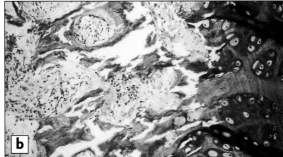

Fig. 17.52a–d Osteopetrosis: radiographs of (a) the hands, (b) chest, (c) pelvis and (d) skull of a 14-year-old girl who presented with retarded growth, leucoerythroblastic anaemia and massive splenomegaly. The bones are dense with coarse trabeculation and lack the usual corticomedullary demarcation. The mandible appears normal.

Fig. 17.53a and b Osteopetrosis: biopsy of the posterior iliac crest (same case as shown in *Fig.17.52*), seen at (a) low and (b) high power, shows persistence of cartilage in the cortex and medulla and architecturally disordered marrow with islands of haemopoietic tissue surrounded by sheets of primitive osteochondroid material. [(a, b) Courtesy of Dr JE McLaughlin.]

Classification of amyloidosis						
Acquired				**Hereditary**		
Type	**Disease associations**	**Chemical nature**	**Distribution**	**Dominant organ involved**		**Chemical nature**
Immunocyte-related:				Peripheral nerves		TTR, apoliprotein
systemic	Myeloma, Waldenström's macroglobulinaemia, monoclonal gammopathy, etc., primary amyloidosis	Immunoglobulin light chains and/or parts of their variable regions (AL)	Tongue, skin, heart, nerves, connective tissue, kidneys, liver, spleen	Cranial nerves		Gelsolin
				Brain:		
local (nodular amyloidosis)	Associated with local immunocyte dyscrasia	AL	Skin, respiratory tract etc.	cerebral amyloid angiopathy		β Amyloid protein, cystatin C
Reactive systemic	Chronic inflammatory diseases	Amyloid A protein, acute reactive (AA)	Liver, spleen, kidneys, bone marrow	familial Alzheimer's disease		β Amyloid protein
	Chronic/recurring infections					
	Malignant neoplasms			familial Creutzfeldt–Jacob disease		PrP
Other systemic amyloidoses	Dialysis-associated	β₂ Microglobulin	Osteoarticular tissues or systemic	Viscera		Lysosyme, Apo A1, fibrinogen
	Senile systemic	Transthyretin (TTR)	Systemic			
	Type II diabetes mellitus	Islet amyloid polypeptide	Systemic	Heart		TTR
Other focal amyloidoses:				Familial Mediterranean fever; distribution as reactive systemic, especially renal		AA
central nervous system	Alzheimer's disease, Down's syndrome, sporadic cerebral amyloid angiopathy	β Amyloid protein	Central nervous system			
	sporadic Creutzfeldt–Jacob disease, kuru	Prion protein (PrP)	Central nervous system			
endocrine	Associated with APUDomas	Peptide hormones or fragments of them	Endocrine tumours			
	Medullary cell carcinoma of thyroid					
cutaneous	Islet cell tumour	?Keratin	Skin			
senile		Atrial natriuretic peptide	Atria of heart			
		Beta protein	Brain			
		Not known	Joints			
		β₂ Microglobulin	Prostate			
		Not known	Ocular, orbital			

Fig. 17.54 Amyloidosis: classification of types, structure and organ involvement.

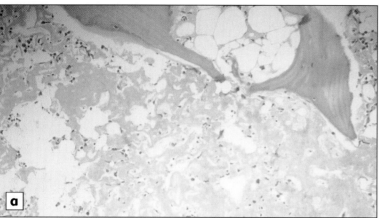
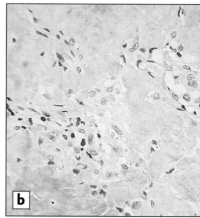
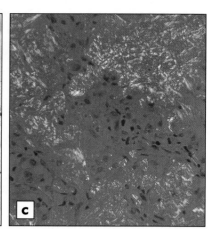

Fig. 17.55a–c Amyloidosis: biopsy from a patient with chronic bronchiectasis shows (a) extensive replacement of haemopoietic tissue by pale acidophilic material; (b, c) higher power views show the characteristic yellow–green birefringence of amyloid. [(b) Congo red stain; (c) with polarized light.]

RENAL OSTEODYSTROPHY AND OSTEOMALACIA

In uraemia there is resistance to the action of vitamin D and a compensatory parathyroid hyperplasia. Characteristic changes are found in the bony architecture on trephine biopsy examination (*Figs 17.56 and 17.57*). In mild disease the lesions are predominantly osteomalacic. Microscopically, the trabeculae are increased in thickness and in number, and the osteoid seams have defective mineralization, similar to the picture seen in dietary vitamin D deficiency. In severe disease evidence of osteitis fibrosa is also present.

PAGET'S DISEASE OF BONE (OSTEITIS DEFORMANS)

In Paget's disease of bone, which is of unknown aetiology, rapid bone formation and resorption occurs in the involved regions of the skeleton. The lesions are essentially local and asymmetrical in the early stages and frequently involve the weight-bearing bones, especially the sacrum and pelvis. Unsuspected disease may be found during trephine bone marrow biopsy examination (*Figs 17.58 and 17.59*). The plasma calcium and phosphorus levels are usually normal, while the alkaline phosphatase level is invariably high.

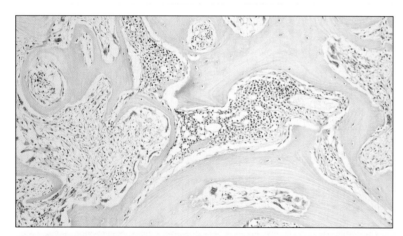

Fig. 17.56 Renal osteodystrophy and osteitis fibrosa cystica: extensive resorption of bone trabeculae with fibrous replacement. Osteoclasts lie adjacent to areas of active resorption.

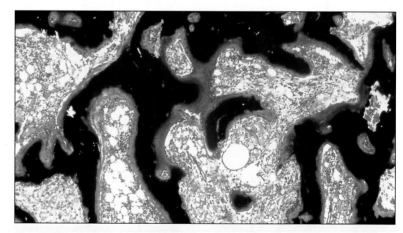

Fig. 17.57 Osteomalacia: thickened trabeculae with prominent layers of uncalcified osteoid on their outer borders. (Von Kossa stain; courtesy of Bullough PG, Vigorita VJ. *Atlas of Orthopedic Pathology*. New York: Gower Medical Publishing; 1984.)

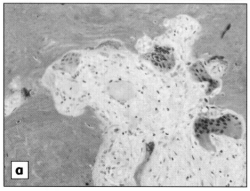
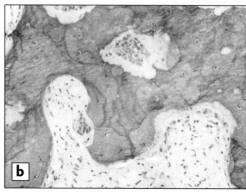

Fig. 17.58a and b Paget's disease of bone: (a) autopsy section shows increased osteoclastic and osteoblastic activity, with scalloping of the bone surface (green) adjacent to the osteoclasts. (b) In the biopsy of more advanced disease, the disturbed bone (undecalcified) architecture is obvious. Irregular cement lines separate the uneven bone sections, and osteoblasts and osteoclasts are prominent. [(a) Goldner's stain; (a, b) courtesy of Bullough PG, Vigorita VJ. *Atlas of Orthopedic Pathology*. New York: Gower Medical Publishing; 1984.]

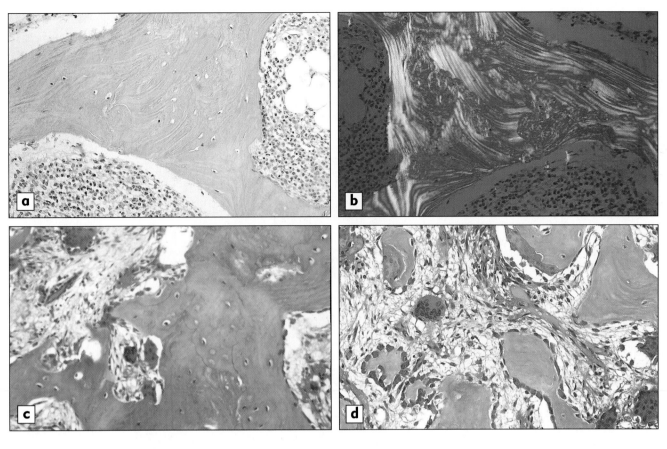

Fig. 17.59a–d **Fig. 17.59a–d** Paget's disease of bone: (a) thickened and irregular trabecular bone, (b) seen under polarized light; (c) intense bone resorption by osteoclasts; (d) bone apposition by osteoblasts during the active phase of the disease. The normal intratrabecular haemopoietic tissue has been extensively replaced by vascular loose connective tissues.

The bony trabeculae may have a striking mosaic appearance created by the pattern of cement lines. In areas of extensive repair the bone may be osteomalacic with wide osteoid seams. If extremely rapid absorption has occurred, areas of fibrosis and intensive osteoclastic activity may resemble the microscopical appearances of osteitis fibrosa.

ANOREXIA NERVOSA

These patients suffer from severe deficiency of carbohydrates, fats and calories, but little protein deficiency. The peripheral blood may reveal mild anaemia and thrombocytopenia with acanthocytes; the marrow is hypocellular, with fat cells replaced by acid mucopolysaccharides appearing as pink-staining extracellular material (*Fig. 17.60*). Similar appearances may occur in other causes of malnutrition, such as carcinomata (*Fig. 17.61*).

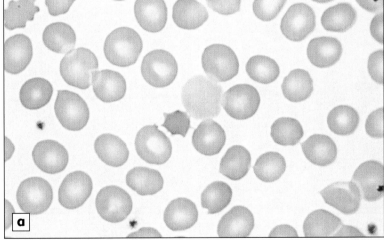

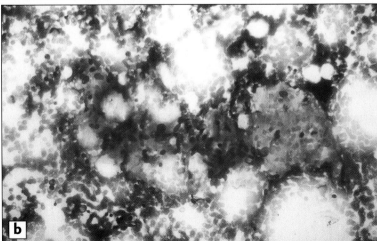

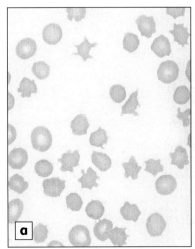

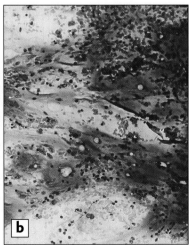

Fig. 17.60a and b Anorexia nervosa: (a) peripheral blood film showing occasional acanthocytes and a central, densely staining microcyte with spicules; (b) bone marrow showing extracellular homogeneous pink- and purple-staining material that replaces fat spaces and is composed of acid mucopolysaccharide.

Fig. 17.61a and b Cachexia caused by carcinomata: (a) peripheral blood film and (b) bone marrow showing similar appearances to those in *Fig. 17.60*. [(a, b) Courtesy of Dr D Simpson.]

SYSTEMIC LUPUS ERYTHEMATOSUS

In severe cases of acute systemic lupus erythematosus a marked pancytopenia often occurs. The bone marrow stromal tissue of patients may show evidence of degenerative changes (*Fig. 17.62*).

MAGNETIC RESONANCE IMAGING OF BONE MARROW

Magnetic resonance imaging of bone marrow is a non-invasive technique that can complement bone marrow biopsy in providing an overall picture. It can distinguish normal cellular marrow from aplastic (fatty) marrow or hypercellular marrow (*Fig. 17.63*), and can also be used to distinguish fibrotic from cellular marrow (*Figs 17.64–17.66*) and to diagnose deposits (e.g. lymphoma in the marrow; *Fig. 17.67*). Details of the technique are given in the articles by Rozman *et al.* (*Haematologica.* 1997;82:166–70; and *Br J Haematol.* 1999;104:574–80) and Moulopoulos and Dimopoulos (*Blood.* 1997;90:2127–47).

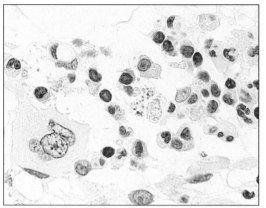

Fig. 17.62 Systemic lupus erythematosus: trephine biopsy showing stromal damage, small irregular fat cells and a centrally placed macrophage containing iron pigment and ingested nuclei. (Courtesy of Dr D Swirsky.)

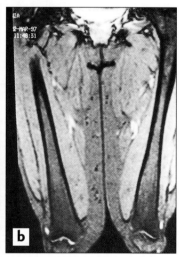

Fig. 17.63 Magnetic resonance imaging: dorsal vertebrae in T1 sequence. (a) In aplastic anaemia a marked increase of signal intensity can be observed in comparison with that of the spinal cord. (b) In chronic myeloid leukaemia the signal intensity is decreased in comparison with that of the spinal cord. [(a, b) Courtesy of Prof. C Rozman.]

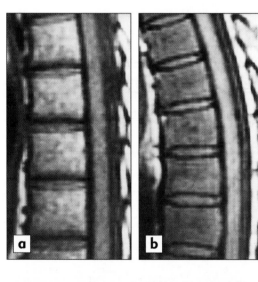

Fig. 17.64a and b Magnetic resonance imaging: T1 sequence. Dorsal vertebrae in (a) essential thrombocythaemia and (b) myelofibrosis. By comparison with the spinal cord, it can be seen that in (a) the vertebral signal is not decreased, whereas in (b) there is a marked decrease. [(a, b) Courtesy of Prof. C Rozman.]

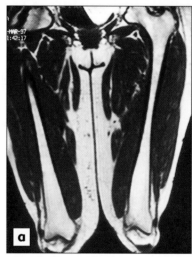

Fig. 17.65a and b Magnetic resonance imaging: essential thrombocythaemia – (a) T1 sequence and (b) T2 sequence. The femoral marrow is fatty (Grade 0). [(a, b) Courtesy of Prof. C Rozman.]

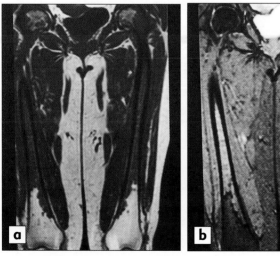

Fig. 17.66a and b Magnetic resonance imaging: myelofibrosis. Both femurs (except distal diaphyses) display a decreased signal in (a) the T1 sequence and (b) a corresponding increase in the T2 sequence. [(a, b) Courtesy of Prof. C Rozman.]

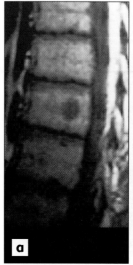
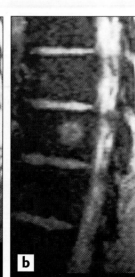

Fig. 17.67a and b Magnetic resonance imaging: Hodgkin lymphoma. The focal lesion in the tenth dorsal vertebra is (a) hypointense in the T1 sequence and (b) hyperintense in the T2 sequence. [(a, b) Courtesy of Prof. C Rozman.]

18

Parasitic Infections Diagnosed in Blood

MALARIA

The protozoal disease malaria has a distribution that is essentially world-wide in tropical and warm temperate regions. Mosquito-borne infection is caused by four species of the genus *Plasmodium* – *P. vivax* (benign tertian), *P. falciparum* (malignant tertian), *P. malariae* (quartan) and *P. ovale* (ovale tertian). Infections caused by *P. vivax* and *P. falciparum* are the most common and the latter is much more likely to be life threatening.

The malarial life cycle (*Fig. 18.1*) begins in the female mosquito after ingestion of human blood that contains the sexual forms (gametocytes) of the causal organisms. The resultant conjugate develops into infec-tive forms (sporozoites) within the mosquito, which are transmitted to humans when the insects feed.

The sporozoites pass to the liver parenchymal cells where they multiply and divide, producing merozoites in this pre-erythrocytic phase. When the liver cell ruptures, the parasites enter the red cells.

In the red cells, the parasites pass from early trophozoite or ring forms to actively amoeboid forms with malarial pigment (haemozoin), which then undergo chromatin division to form merozoites. The mature parasite is called a meront (schizont). The red cell ruptures, releasing into the plasma merozoites, which may enter other red cells and repeat the cycle, or form male and female sexual forms (gametocytes).

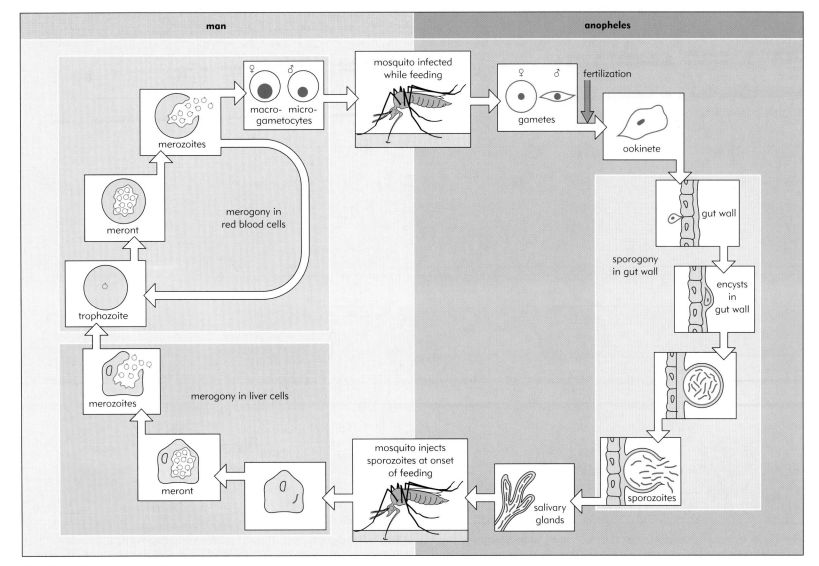

Fig. 18.1 Life cycle of a malarial parasite.

The four types of malaria organisms may be distinguished by their characteristic appearances within red cells (*Fig. 18.2*). In *P. vivax* infection (*Fig. 18.3*), the red cells are large (as they are young) and Schüffner's dots (degraded red cell microtubules) are present; the ring forms and meronts of the parasites are large, with up to 24 merozoites per meront.

In *P. falciparum* infections (*Fig. 18.4*), usually a heavy parasitaemia with small ring forms occurs, often with double chromatin dots; multiple ring forms may be found, some on the margins, within individual red cells, and the red cells may contain blue-staining Maurer's clefts. The gametocytes have a characteristic crescent shape and meronts are rarely seen.

As in *P. falciparum* infections, with *P. malariae* (*Fig. 18.5*) the red cells are not enlarged and do not contain pigment; the ring form tends to have an inverted chromatin dot. Occasionally, dust-like stippling (Ziemann's dots) are seen. The amoeboid trophozoites often show band forms and the merozoites may show a 'daisy-head' distribution.

Identification of malaria in peripheral blood				
	Plasmodium falciparum	*Plasmodium malariae*	*Plasmodium vivax*	*Plasmodium ovale*
Red blood cells (RBCs)				
Enlargement	None	None	Yes	Yes; oval shape; fimbriated edge
Inclusions (not always present)	Maurer's clefts	Ziemann's dots (rare)	Schüffner's dots (coarse red granules)	Red granules similar to Schüffner's dots
Ring form				
Size	Less than one third of RBC	Greater than one third of RBC	Greater than one third of RBC	Greater than one third of RBC
Multiple parasites in RBC	Common; often at margins	Rare	Rare	Rare
Shape	Delicate; often double chromatin dot	Tends to be compact; inverted chromatin dot	Rough; single chromatin dot	Rough; single chromatin dot common
Amoeboid forms	Absent	Common; often as band across RBC	Common	Common
Meront (schizont)				
Frequency	Very rarely seen	Common; dense, central, yellow/black haemozoin pigment	Common; with haemozoin pigment	Common
Configuration	Random	Daisy head	Random	Daisy head
Merozoite number	8–24	8–12	12–24	8–12
Gametocyte	Crescent forms; centrally placed chromatin	Small and round; eccentrically placed chromatin; occupies one half to two thirds of RBC	Large and round; eccentrically placed chromatin; fills RBC	Small and round; eccentrically placed chromatin; occupies one half to two thirds of RBC
Infections with two types of malarial parasite are common.				

Fig. 18.2 Identification of the different forms of malaria in the peripheral blood.

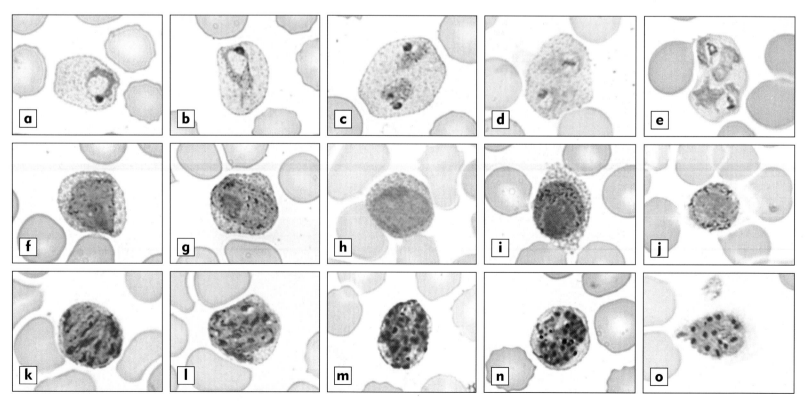

Fig. 18.3a–o Malaria: peripheral blood films showing various stages of *P. vivax*. (a) Early trophozoite or ring form; (b, c) young amoeboid trophozoites with Schüffner's dots; (d, e) developing trophozoites after asexual binary fission; (f–h) female gametocytes with localized eccentric chromatin; (i, j) male gametocytes with more diffuse chromatin; (k–o) early and later meronts with haemozoin pigment densities and many merozoites randomly distributed.

P. ovale (*Fig. 18.6*) infections are distinguished by the parasitized red cells being enlarged and oval shaped, but with fimbriated edges. The red cells show red granules similar to Schüffner's dots and the meronts have a daisy-head distribution.

Effects of malaria on various organs

Malaria may effect the structure and function of various organs. The most serious complication is cerebral malaria, which may prove fatal. Parasites in cerebral capillaries (*Figs 18.7 and 18.8*) may lead to

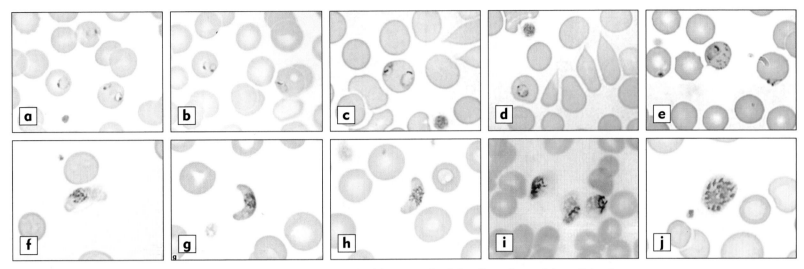

Fig. 18.4a–j Malaria: peripheral blood films showing various stages of *P. falciparum*. (a–d) Small ring forms; (e) small ring form showing Maurer's clefts, denatured red cell microtubules; (f–h) crescentic gametocytes with centrally placed chromatin; (i) rarely seen rounded 'pink flag' gametocytes; (j) rarely seen meront with randomly distributed merozoites. [(e) Courtesy of Dr S Knowles.]

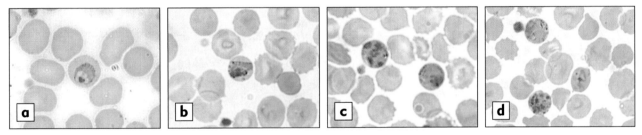

Fig. 18.5a–d Malaria: peripheral blood films showing various stages of *P. malariae*. (a) Ring form with inverted chromatin dot; (b) band-form amoeboid trophozoite; (c) developing trophozoite and female gametocyte; (d) from top left clockwise, male gametocyte, ring form and developing meront with daisy-head merozoite distribution. [(a, b) Courtesy of Dr S Knowles and Mr J Griffiths.]

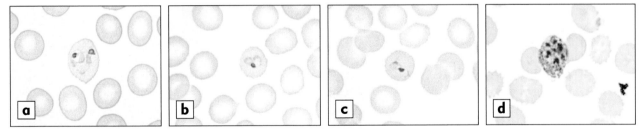

Fig. 18.6a–d Malaria: peripheral blood films showing various stages of *P. ovale*. (a–c) Ring forms in enlarged red cells with fimbriated margins and faint red granules; (d) meront with daisy-head merozoite distribution.

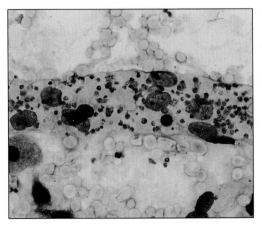

Fig. 18.7 Cerebral malaria: cerebral capillary. This high-power view shows abundant parasites within red cells. (Squash preparation of white matter stained with Giemsa; courtesy of Prof. S Lucas.)

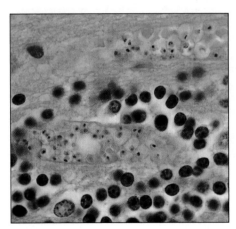

Fig. 18.8 Cerebral malaria: cerebral capillary. In this histological preparation, two capillaries are seen with parasitized red cells adherent to the endothelium (sequestration). (Courtesy of Prof. S Lucas.)

haemorrhage (*Figs 18.9 and 18.10*). The placenta may be infested with parasites, but they do not usually cross from the maternal to the fetal circulation (*Fig. 18.11*).

Anaemia is frequent, partly because parasitized red cells are prematurely destroyed and phagocytosed (*Fig. 18.12*). It may also arise from hypersplenism, since frequently there is splenic enlargement,

caused by the phagocytosis of infected red cells in splenic macrophages (*Fig. 18.13*).

Comparative methods for malaria diagnosis

In *Fig. 18.14* the sensitivities of the different methods for malaria diagnosis are compared. Thick films may improve sensitivity. Red cell lysis

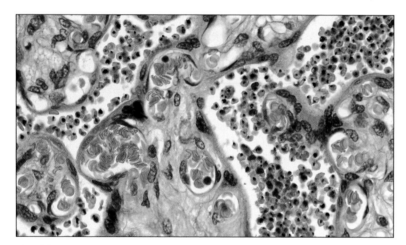

Fig. 18.9 Cerebral malaria: haemorrhage. Low-power view of brain white matter with three ring haemorrhages caused by obstructed vessels. (Courtesy of Prof. S Lucas.)

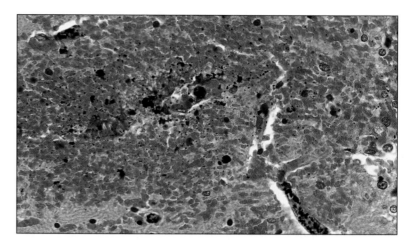

Fig. 18.10 Cerebral malaria: haemorrhage from vessel rupture by falciparum malaria. The intense pigmentation within the blood vessel indicates the heavy parasitaemia at this site. (Courtesy of Prof. S Lucas.)

Fig. 18.11 Placental malaria: placental villi and maternal sinus. Nearly all the red blood cells in the maternal sinus contain parasites and/or pigment. Note that the fetal vessels in the villi are not infected. (Courtesy of Prof. S Lucas.)

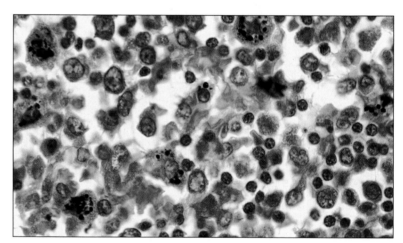

Fig. 18.12 Paediatric malaria: hypercellular bone marrow. Macrophages that contain brown-coloured haemozoin malaria pigment are plentiful. Parasites inside red blood cells are not seen in this field. (Courtesy of Prof. S Lucas.)

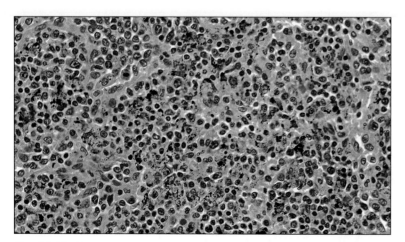

Fig. 18.13 Spleen: red pulp showing abundant macrophages that contain brown-coloured haemozoin malaria pigment. (Courtesy of Prof. S Lucas.)

Comparison of methods of malaria diagnosis	
	Limits of detection (parasites/ml)
Thin film	200
Thick film	10
Quantitative buffy coat	20*
Histidine-rich protein II antigen detection†	50
DNA hybridization	40
Polymerase chain reaction	<5

*The quantitative buffy coat method is as sensitive as thick film for *P. falciparum*, but less so for other species.
†Histidine-rich protein II antigen is in the red cell membrane and is secreted by red cells infected by *P. falciparum* (see *Fig. 18.9*).

Fig. 18.14 Malaria diagnosis: comparison of methods. (Courtesy of Dr W Erber.)

is carried out at pH 6.8 in phosphate buffers for 10 minutes. Thick films are made and stained with Giemsa at pH 7.2 for 30 minutes. *Fig. 18.15* shows positive films for *P. vivax* and *Fig. 18.16* a film with a heavy parasite load in *P. falciparum* infection. The antigen capture assay is also useful in the detection of *P. falciparum* infection.

TOXOPLASMOSIS

Toxoplasmosis, a common infection, is caused by the protozoan *Toxoplasma gondii*. Most human infections are acquired from cats. Affected patients may be symptomless or suffer a brief febrile illness with lymphadenopathy and fatigue. Severe infection, most commonly seen in the fetus (congenital toxoplasmosis) or in patients with

immunodeficiency, is associated with extensive damage to the brain, eyes, muscle, heart and lungs. Diagnosis is usually confirmed by positive serology, although a lymph node biopsy may be needed (*see* Chapter 7). Rarely, the trophozoite forms are present in blood monocytes (*Fig. 18.17*).

BABESIOSIS

Babesiosis is a tick-borne disease caused by protozoan parasites of the genus *Babesia*. Although the disease affects a number of animal species, it is only occasionally transmitted to humans. In most patients the illness is mild and characterized by fever, malaise, myalgia, mild hepatosplenomegaly and haemolytic anaemia. Occasionally, patients

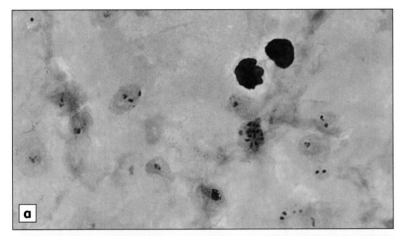

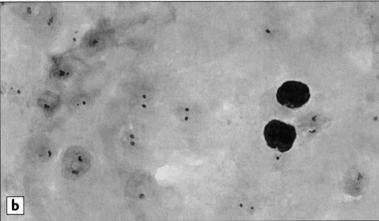

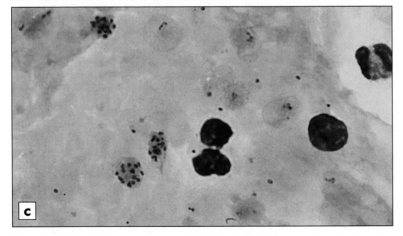

Fig. 18.15a–c Malaria diagnosis: thick films. (a) *P. vivax* trophozoites and schizonts; (b) *P. vivax* trophozoites; (c) *P. vivax* trophozoites and schizonts. [(a–c) Giemsa stain; courtesy of Dr W Erber.]

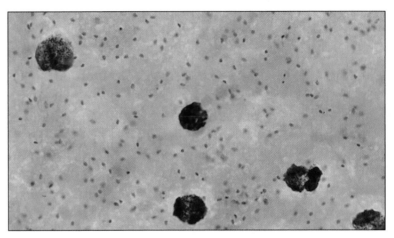

Fig. 18.16 Malaria diagnosis: thick film. *P. falciparum* (heavy infection). Chromatin dots of *P. falciparum* are easily seen in this thick film. (Giemsa stain; courtesy of Dr W Erber.)

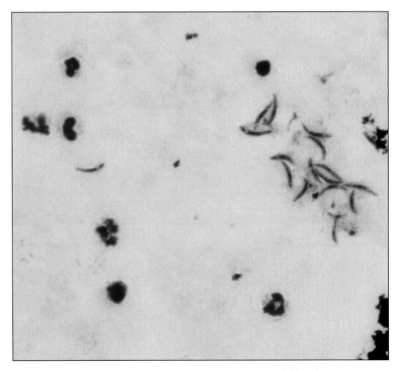

Fig. 18.17 Acute toxoplasmosis: thick peripheral blood film showing trophozoite forms of *Toxoplasma gondii* from a ruptured monocyte.

who have had previous splenectomy are known to have developed a more fulminating infection with massive intravascular haemolysis, which has sometimes proved fatal.

The majority of human infections are caused by *B. microti*, a species that usually infects rodents. Several cases in splenectomized patients result from *B. bovis*, a species associated with red water fever in cattle. Diagnosis is made by finding the trophozoites, which resemble small ring forms of *P. falciparum*, in the red cells (*Fig. 18.18*).

TRYPANOSOMIASIS

The East African and West African variants of trypanosomiasis are caused by *Trypanosoma brucei* and *T. brucei gambiense*, respectively. Both are transmitted by tsetse flies of the genus *Glossina*. The dominant clinical problems are related to involvement of the central nervous system. In the acute phase of the disease, organisms are found in the blood (*Fig. 18.19*).

American trypanosomiasis, or Chagas' disease, occurs widely in Mexico and in many countries in Central and South America. The causative organism, *T. cruzi*, is transmitted by a triatomid bug. During the acute febrile stage of the illness, flagellated parasites may be found in the blood (*Fig. 18.20*). In the chronic stage, which is associated with myocarditis, megacolon or megaoesophagus, nests of amastigote forms are found within the tissues.

BANCROFTIAN FILARIASIS

Bancroftian filariasis is a widespread disease that occurs throughout the tropical and subtropical regions of the world and is caused by *Wuchereria bancrofti*. A similar condition is caused by infection with the related *Brugia malayi*.

Both organisms are transmitted by infected mosquitoes. Larvae pass into the lymphatic vessels and lymph nodes, where they mature into adult worms (*Fig. 18.21*). The fertilized females release microfilariae via the lymphatic vessels into the bloodstream.

Many patients are asymptomatic, but others develop a febrile illness with headaches, muscle pains and lymphadenitis. Chronic inflammatory changes in the infected lymphoid system may lead to lymphatic obstruction and elephantiasis of the scrotum or lower extremities. Diagnosis is usually made by demonstrating microfilariae in the blood (*Figs 18.22 and 18.23*). Microfilaraemia is usually greatest at night.

LOIASIS

Infection with *L. loa* occurs in Central and West Africa. The adult worm causes subcutaneous swellings, but occasionally its passage through the subconjunctival tissues produces local pain and acute conjunctivitis. Microfilariae are found in the blood (*Fig. 18.24*) and infestation is via tabanid flies.

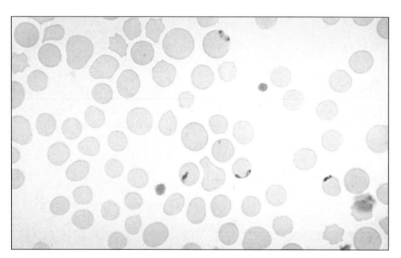

Fig. 18.18 Babesiosis: peripheral blood film showing red cell infestation with the typical small coccoid and dumbbell-shaped *Babesia* organisms. (Courtesy of Mr PJ Humphries.)

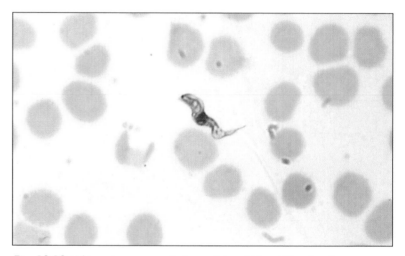

Fig. 18.19 African trypanosomiasis: peripheral blood film showing *T. brucei*.

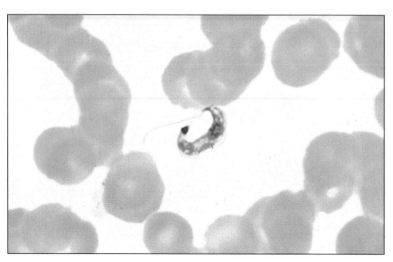

Fig. 18.20 Chagas' disease: peripheral blood film showing the flagellate form of *T. cruzi*. (Courtesy of Mr J Williams.)

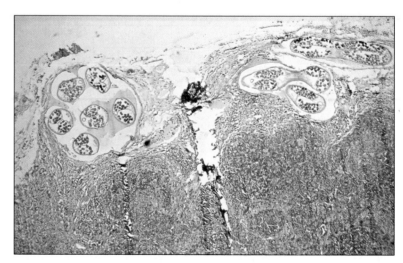

Fig. 18.21 Bancroftian filariasis: section of lymph node showing adult forms of *W. bancrofti* in the peripheral sinus area.

BARTONELLOSIS

Bartonella bacilliformis causes a severe febrile haemolytic anaemia. The disease occurs in inhabitants of the Andes mountains in Peru, Columbia and Ecuador. The characteristic rod-shaped coccobacilli are found in red cells (*Fig. 18.25*). The infection is also known as Oroya fever and Carrión's disease and is transmitted by *Phlebotomus* sandflies.

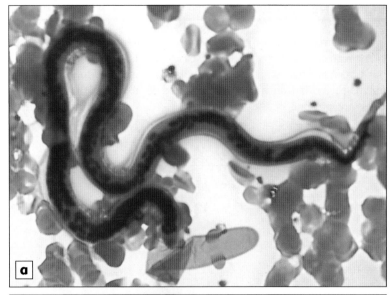

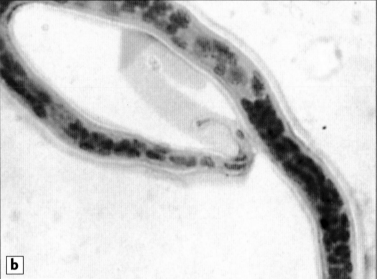

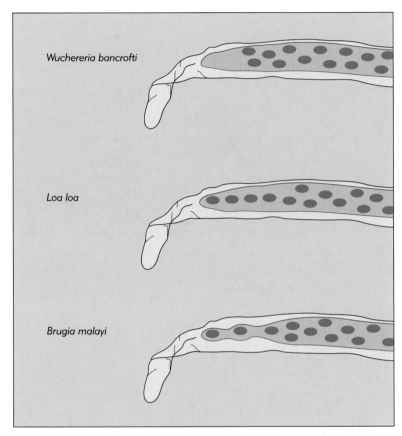

Fig. 18.22 Posterior ends of sheathed microfilariae found in blood. In *W. bancrofti* the nuclei do not extend to the tip of the tail; in *Loa loa* there is a continuous line of nuclei to the end of the tail; in *Br. malayi* the nuclei are not continuous, with two isolated nuclei at the tip of the tail.

Fig. 18.23a and b Filariasis: thick preparations of peripheral blood, showing the centre and tail portions of the microfilariae of (a) *W. bancrofti* and (b) *Br. malayi*. [(b) Courtesy of Dr AE Bianco.]

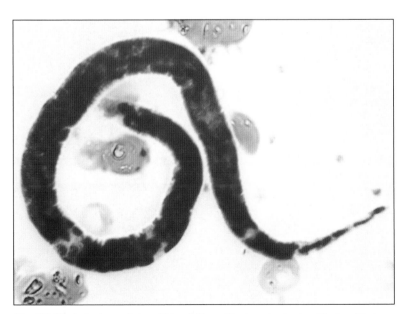

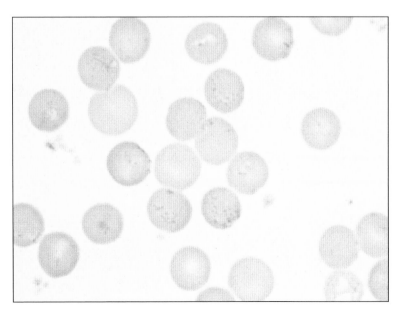

Fig. 18.24 Loiasis: peripheral blood film with sheathed microfilaria of *L. loa*.

Fig. 18.25 Bartonellosis: peripheral blood film showing rod-shaped coccobacilli of *Ba. bacilliformis* in the red cells in Oroya fever. (Courtesy of Mr H Furze.)

RELAPSING FEVER

Various spirochaetes of the genus *Borrelia* cause relapsing fever. Louse-borne relapsing fever is a human disease caused only by *Bo. recurrentis,* but tick-borne relapsing fever is a zoonosis caused by a number of different species. It is during the febrile period of the disease that the organisms are present in the blood (*Fig. 18.26*). With the production of antibodies, the *Borrelia* spirochaetes disappear and the patient becomes afebrile. Relapses occur, after 7–10 days, with the production of new antigenic variants of the organisms. In louse-borne relapsing fever a single relapse is usual, while in the tick-borne forms of the disease multiple relapses may occur.

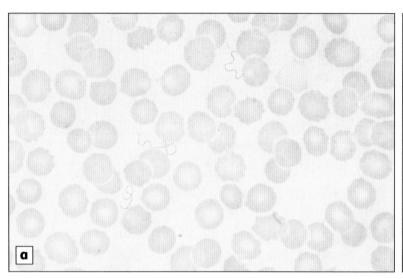
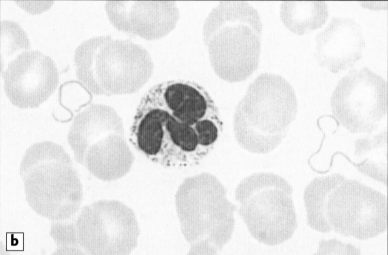

Fig. 18.26a and b Relapsing fever: (a, b) peripheral blood films showing the coiled spirochaetes *Borrelia recurrentis.*

Blood Transfusion

BLOOD TRANSFUSION

Blood transfusion involves transfusion of whole blood or a blood component from an individual (the donor) into the recipient. In the case of red cells, autologous (self) transfusion is also carried out. The major clinical need is for red cells, for which compatibility between donor red cell antigens and the antibodies in the recipient's plasma must be ensured.

Red cell antigens

Over 400 red cell antigens have been identified and the best characterized are listed in *Fig. 19.1*. They are inherited in a simple Mendelian fashion and are stable. Subjects who lack any antigen are likely to make antibodies to that antigen if they are exposed to it. The clinically important red cell blood group systems are detailed in *Fig. 19.2*.

Fig. 19.1 Red cell antigens: those best characterized are assigned to recognized blood group systems. Other antigens include Hh, Kx, Gerbich, Cromer, Knops, Indian, P, P^k, Sd^a, Bg (HLA on red cells). (Modified from Issett PD. *Applied Blood Group Serology*. Miami: Montgomery Scientific Publications; 1985:612–21.)

Blood group antigens									
ABO	**'Lewis'**	**I**	**P**	**Rh**		**MNS**		**Lutheran**	**Kell**
A	Le^a	I	P_1	D	CE	M	m^v	Lu^a	K
A_2	Le^b	i	P	C	D^w	N	m^A	Lu^b	$\bar{k}$
A_3	I^T	I^T	p^k	E	E^T	Hu	Sul	Lu^3	Kp^a
A_x			Luke	$\bar{c}$	Rh26	S	Sj	Lu^6	Kp^b
A_m		$\bar{p}$		e	cE	$\bar{s}$	m'	Lu^8	Kp^c
B				$\bar{f}$	hr^H	He	Kam	Lu^9	Ku
B_3				$C\bar{e}$	Rh29	Mi^a	En^aTS	Lu^{14}	Js^a
B_m				C^w	Go^a	U	En^aFS		Js^b
B_w				C^x	hr^b	M^c	En^aFR	probably	K^w
H				V	Rh32	V^w	Shier	Lu^4	KL
C				E^w	Rh33	Mg	N^A	Lu^5	Ul^a
				G	Rh34	Vr	U^Z	Lu^7	K11
				Rh^A	Rh35	M_1	AY	Lu^{11}	K12
				Rh^B	Be^a	Mur	FR	Lu^{16}	K13
				Rh^C	Rh37	M^e	JL	Lu^{17}	K14
				Rh^D	Rh38	Mt^a	'N'	Singleton	K16
				Hr_o	Rh39	St^a	U^x	Much	WK^a
				Hr	Rh40	Ri^a	S^D	Hughes	K18
				hr^S	Rh41	Cl^a	Can	Anton	K19
				VS	Rh42	Ny^a	Mit	Au^a	K20
				C^G		Tm	Dantu	Wj	K22
						Hut	Wr^b		
						Hil	En^aTK		
Lw	**Duffy**	**Kidd**	**Xg^a**	**Diego**	**Cartwright**	**Scianna**	**Dombrock**	**Colton**	**Chido/Rogers**
Lw^a	Fy^a	JK^a	Xg^a	Di^a	Yt^a	Sc1	Do^a	Co^a	Ch
Lw^b	Fy^b	JK^b		Di^b	Yt^b	Sc2	Do^b	Co^b	Rg
Lw^{ab}	Fy^x	JK^3				Sc3		Co^3	
	Fy^3								
	Fy^4								
	Fy^5								

Red cell antibodies causing haemolytic reactions and haemolytic disease of the new-born			
Blood group system	Frequency of antibodies	Haemolytic transfusion reactions	Haemolytic disease of the new-born
ABO	Very common	Yes (common)	Yes
Rh	Common	Yes (common)	Yes
Kell	Occasional	Yes (occasional)	May
Duffy	Occasional	Yes (occasional)	May
Kidd	Occasional	Yes (occasional)	May
Lutheran	Rare	Rare	No
Lewis	Common	Rare	No
P	Rare	Rare	No
MNSs	Rare	Rare	No
Ii	Rare	Unlikely	No

Fig. 19.2 Red cell antibodies: those that cause haemolytic reactions and haemolytic disease of the new-born.

Red cell antibodies

There are two types of red cell antibodies, 'natural' and 'immune'. Natural antibodies are a normal occurrence in plasma in the absence of transfusion or pregnancy. Immune antibodies develop in response to exposure to the antigen by transfusion or by exposure to red cells that cross the placenta during pregnancy. Natural antibodies, usually IgM, react best in the cold and include anti-A and anti-B. Immune antibodies, usually IgG, react best at 37°C and include Rhesus (Rh) antibody anti-D. Ig antibodies, but not IgM, cross the placenta.

ABO system

The structure of the A, B and H antigens is shown in *Fig. 19.3*. The relative incidence in the UK population is shown in *Fig. 19.4*. The A, B and H antigens occur in most body cells, including leucocytes and platelets, and in so-called secretors (80% of the population); they also occur in body fluids such as saliva, tears, semen and sweat.

Rh system

The Rh system is more complex than the ABO system. There are three closely linked loci with alternative antigens, Cc, D or no D (termed 'd', for which there is no antigen) and Ee (*Fig. 19.5*). They are immune

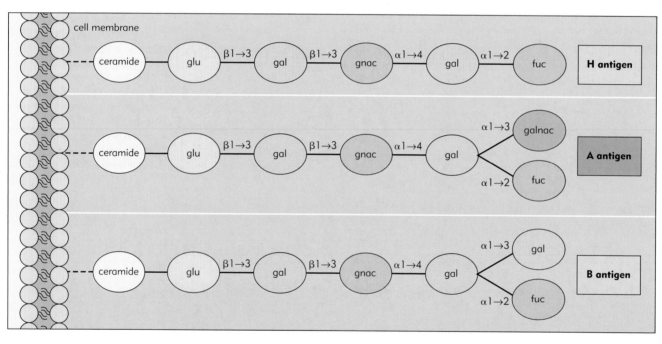

Fig. 19.3 Structure of the ABO blood group antigens: each consists of a chain of sugars, in α or β conformation, linked through different carbon atoms (numbered 1 to 4). The H antigen of the O blood group has a terminal fucose (fuc). The A antigen has an additional *N*-acetylgalactosamine (galnac), whereas the B antigen has an additional galactose (gal). (glu, glucose; gnac, *N*-acetylglucosamine.)

Incidence of different ABO blood groups in the UK population				
	Blood group			
	O	A	B	AB
Antigens on red (and other) cells	None	A	B	A+B
Antibody in serum	Anti-AB	Anti-B	Anti-A	None
Approximate percentage in UK population	47	42	8	3

Fig. 19.4 ABO blood groups: incidence in the UK population.

The Rh system			
CDE nomenclature	Short symbol	Caucasian frequency (%)	RhD status
cde/cde	rr	15	Negative
CDe/cde	R_1r	32	Positive
CDe/CDe	R_1R_1	17	Positive
cDE/cde	R_2r	13	Positive
CDe/cDE	R_1R_2	14	Positive
cDE/cDE	R_2R_2	4	Positive
Other genotypes		5	Positive (almost all)

Fig. 19.5 The Rh system: genotypes. (Modified from Hoffbrand AV, Pettit JE. *Essential Haematology*, 3rd edn. Oxford: Blackwell Scientific Publications; 1993.)

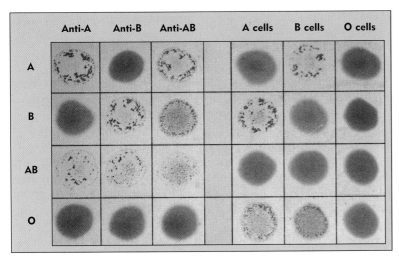

Fig. 19.6 ABO blood group testing: reactions observed. Agglutination denotes reactivity. The left hand three columns denote patient cells (A, B, AB or O) mixed with anti-A, anti-B or anti-AB. The right hand three columns denote plasma from the patients, mixed with A, B or O cells.

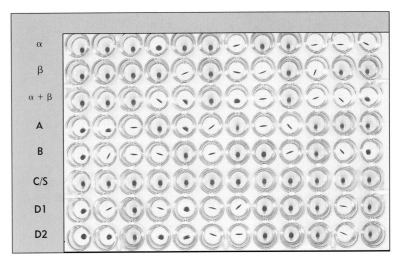

Fig. 19.7 ABO grouping: standard layout for 96-well microplate blood grouping (12 patients grouped on one plate). Symbols along the vertical side are: α, anti-A; β, anti-B; $\alpha+\beta$, anti-A+B; A, B, known A or B cells; C/S, patient cells and serum; D1, D2, two sources of anti-D. Sharp agglutination ('comma-like') shows a positive reaction, and no agglutination shows a negative reaction. (Courtesy of Mr G Hazlehurst.)

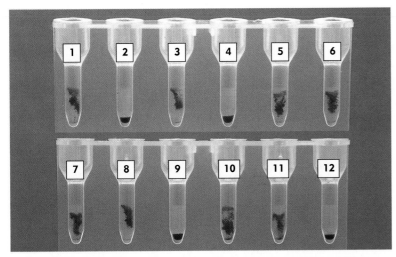

Fig. 19.8 Patient antibody screening using microcolumn (gel) system: ten tests with two controls (tube 11 is the positive control and tube 12 the negative control) are shown. Patient's serum is tested against screening cells with known red cell phenotype. Tubes 1, 3, 5, 6, 7, 8, and 10 show positive results. The patient's serum contained anti-Fy^a. (Courtesy of Mr G Hazlehurst.)

antibodies, and before the introduction of prophylaxis with Rh anti-D after delivery or miscarriage, anti-D was the dominant cause of haemolytic disease of the new-born.

Blood grouping and cross-matching

Blood grouping and cross-matching is carried out by a tile (*Fig. 19.6*), microplate (*Fig. 19.7*) or gel microtube (*Fig. 19.8*) technique. The patient's cells are mixed with known anti-sera and the patient's serum is mixed with cells of known A, B or O type (*Figs 19.6 and 19.7*). An indirect antiglobulin test (IAT) may be used to detect irregular red-cell antibodies in the patient's serum (*Fig. 19.9*). This technique can also be used to detect antibodies in the serum of the recipient that react against the donor red cells. For patients with antibodies, the selection

ABO grouping
IgM agglutination

patient's red cells

IgM anti-A reagent

visual agglutination = group A

monoclonal IgM antibodies are used for ABO and RhD grouping

a

detection of irregular antibodies
the indirect antiglobulin (Coombs') test (IAT)

human reagent red cells

+

IgG antibody in patient's serum

red cells become coated

washed four times +

anti-human globulin

visual agglutination = presence of antibody

IAT is used to identify irregular red cell antibodies in patient's serum; other techniques may be used (see Fig. 19.8)

b

Fig. 19.9a and b ABO grouping: (a) IgM agglutination. Monoclonal IgM antibodies are used for ABO and RhD grouping. (b) The indirect antiglobulin (Coombs') test (IAT). The IAT is used to identify irregular red cell antibodies in the patient's serum. [(a, b) Courtesy of Prof. M Contreras and North London Blood Transfusion Centre.]

Red cell units		
Specificity	**Clinical significance**	**Selection of units and compatibility testing**
Rh antibodies (reactive in IAT)	Yes	Antigen negative
Kell antibodies	Yes	Antigen negative
Duffy antibodies	Yes	Antigen negative
Kidd antibodies	Yes	Antigen negative
Anti-S, -s	Yes	Antigen negative
Anti-A_1, -P_1, -N	Rarely	IAT cross-match compatible at 37°C
Anti-M	Rarely	IAT cross-match compatible at 37°C
Anti-M IAT reactive at 37°C	Sometimes	Antigen negative
Anti-Le^a, anti-Le^{a+b}	Rarely	IAT cross-match compatible at 37°C
Anti-Le^b	No	Not clinically significant and can be ignored
High-titre low-avidity antibodies	Unlikely	Seek advice from blood centre
Antibodies against low high-frequency antigens	Depends on specificity	Seek advice from blood centre

Fig. 19.10 Red cell units: selection based on antigen specificity and clinical significance. (Courtesy of British Committee for Standardization in Haematology; 1996.)

of red cell units should be based on antigen specificity and clinical significance (*Fig. 19.10*).

Red cell components

The major types of red-cell components and their indications are listed in *Fig. 19.11*. SAG-M blood may be provided as buffy coat depleted red cells (*Fig. 19.12*) or as a multisatellite red cell pack (*Fig. 19.13*).

Clinical blood transfusion

A typical surgical blood ordering policy is detailed in *Fig. 19.14*, and the more complicated overall management of a patient with thalassaemia major who requires life-long transfusions for severe refractory anaemia is shown in *Fig. 19.15*. In some patients, especially those with sickle cell anaemia, exchange transfusion is needed, which can be carried out using a cell separator (*Fig. 19.16*) manually.

Red cell components				
Component	**Haematocrit**	**Volume**	**Main indication**	**Special comments**
Whole blood	0.35–0.45	510 ml	Acute massive blood loss	May require platelets ± labile clotting factor replacement if loss exceeds twice the blood volume
Red cells	0.55–0.75	Approximately 200 ml	Chronic blood loss or anaemia	None
Red cells in optimal additive solution (SAG-M)	0.55–0.70	Approximately 280 ml	Blood loss or anaemia	Do not use for neonatal exchange transfusion
Filtered blood			Non-haemolytic transfusion reactions and prevention of HLA immunization	Use in-line WBC depletion filters or pre-filtered red cells with 35-day shelf life
Frozen, thawed and washed red cells	Variable	Variable but usually < 200 ml	Patients with rare blood groups	Use within 24 hours of preparation

Fig. 19.11 Red cell components: comparison.

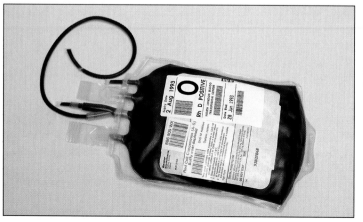

Fig. 19.12 Buffy coat depleted red cells: the average volume of this product, which contains CPDA-1 as the anticoagulant, is 280 ml. SAG-M additive solution (100 ml) is added to give a final haematocrit of 50–70%. The storage temperature of these red cells is 4 ± 2°C and the shelf life is 35 days. Reduction in the white cell content of red cell products reduces the incidence of reactions caused by human leucocyte antigen (HLA) alloimmunization. (Courtesy of Prof. M Contreras and the North London Blood Transfusion Centre.)

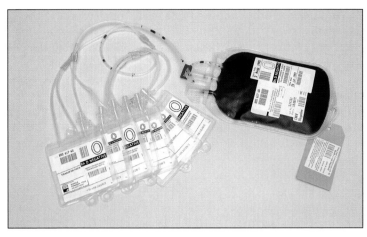

Fig. 19.13 Small volume neonatal transfusions: use of red cell concentrate, buffy coat depleted and supplemented with SAG-M additive solution. It is usually supplied as group O RhD-negative blood, which should be stored at 4°C for up to 35 days. It may be anti-cytomegalovirus antibody negative, HbS negative and have up to seven attached satellite bags. This enables a single unit of blood to be dedicated to an individual infant so that donor exposure is limited. (Courtesy of Prof. M Contreras and the North London Blood Transfusion Centre.)

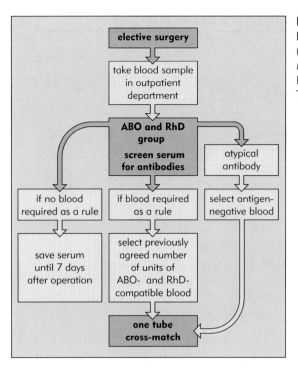

Fig. 19.14 Surgical blood ordering policy. (Courtesy of Prof. M Contreras and the North London Blood Transfusion Centre.)

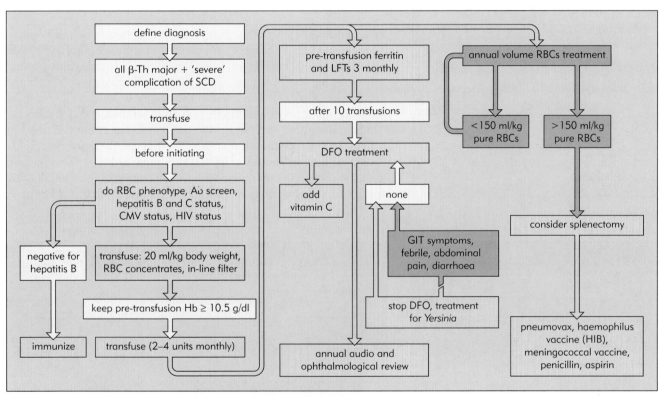

Fig. 19.15 Patients with haemoglobinopathies: transfusion management. (β-Th, β-thalassaemia; Ab, antibody; CMV, cytomegalovirus; DFO, desferrioxamine; GIT, gastrointestinal tract; Hb, haemoglobin; HIV, human immunodeficiency virus; LFT, liver function test; RBC, red blood cell; SCD, sickle-cell disease; courtesy of Dr B Modell.)

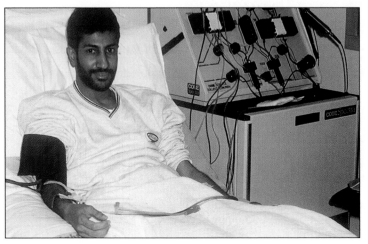

Fig. 19.16 Exchange transfusion: use of a cell separator to exchange red cells in a patient with sickle cell anaemia.

COMPLICATIONS OF BLOOD TRANSFUSIONS

Complications of blood transfusions include haemolytic reactions (immediate or delayed) as a result of red cell incompatibilities, and allergic or pyrogenic reactions to white cells, platelets or proteins (*Fig.* *19.17*). A number of other non-immune reactions may occur acutely (e.g. circulatory overload, air embolism, thrombophlebitis), as may complications of massive transfusions (e.g. clotting abnormalities, citrate toxicity, hyperkalaemia).

Infections

Immediate shock may occur after transfusion if the blood is infected, and a number of different infectious diseases may be transmitted. These may be bacterial, parasitic (*Fig. 19.18*), viral or possibly prions (*Fig. 19.19*).

Viruses

Viral infections are the most common, so blood donations are tested for these infectious agents (*Fig. 19.20*). Hepatitis B (*Fig. 19.21a*) was frequently transmitted. A typical course of an acute infection is illustrated in *Fig. 19.21b*. The sequelae may be cirrhosis and, in a minority of cases, hepatocellular carcinoma. A similar outcome may occur after hepatitis C infection (*see Fig. 5.34*). On the other hand, hepatitis G does not cause overt liver disease.

Transfusion-transmissible virus (TTV), which bears some structural relation to parvovirus, was first described in Japan in 1997. It is likely to be transmitted by blood products, but as yet (as for hepatitis G) there is no evidence that it causes disease.

Prion disease

Although no definite cases of Creutzfeldt–Jacob disease (CJD) have been caused by blood transfusion, it is clear that the disease can be transmitted by infectious agents (e.g. in pituitary-derived growth hormone and gonadotrophins). The cause of the disease is now considered to be an abnormal form of a naturally occurring protein, and the infection can be transmitted without nucleic acids and thus is not the result of a virus. In prion disease, it is considered that a natural protein (PrP) is converted into an abnormal form (PrP scrapie or PrP^{Sc}). This has the ability to convert the normal protein, which has a multiple helical structure, into the abnormal variant in which much of the backbone is

Complications of blood transfusions
Immunological

Sensitization to red cell antigens
    haemolytic transfusion reactions
        immediate (e.g. ABO)
        delayed (e.g. Rh)

Reactions as a result of white cell and platelet antibodies
    febrile
    post-transfusion purpura

Reactions as a result of plasma protein antibodies
    urticaria
    anaphylaxis (e.g. IgA deficient recipient)

Transfusion-related acute lung injury (TRALI; see Fig. 19.26)
Graft versus host disease (if host severely immunocompromised)
Non-immunological
Transmission of disease (see Figs 19.18 and 19.19)
Reactions as a result of bacterial pyrogens and bacteria
Circulation overload
Thrombophlebitis
Air embolism
Transfusion haemosiderosis
Complications of massive transfusion

Fig. 19.17 Blood transfusion: complications.

Bacteria and parasites transmissible by blood transfusion
Bacteria
Occasional bacterial contaminants (e.g. *Pseudomonas, Salmonella*)
Treponema pallidum (syphilis)
Brucellosis (donors giving a history are not accepted in the UK)
Parasites
Plasmodium spp. (malaria)

Trypanosoma cruzi (Chagas' disease)
    endemic in Latin America, this parasite is present in 75% of
    seropositive subjects; up to 22% of donors in Latin America
    may be seropositive

Toxoplasma gondii
    only a risk in granulocytes transfused to immunosuppressed
    seronegative recipients

Babesia microti (Nantucket fever)   potential risk in certain areas of North America

Fig. 19.18 Blood transfusion: transmissible bacteria and parasites. (Courtesy of Prof. M Contreras and the North London Blood Transfusion Centre.)

Viruses (and potentially prions) transmissible by blood transfusion
Plasma-borne viruses
Hepatitis B and delta agent; hepatitis B variants Hepatitis A (rarely) Hepatitis C Hepatitis G ?Other hepatitis viruses, e.g. transfusion-transmissible virus (TTV) Serum parvovirus B19 HIV-1 and HIV-2 (also cellular borne)
Cell-associated viruses
Cytomegalovirus Epstein–Barr virus (more than 95% of adults are immune) HTLV-I (causes human T-cell leukaemia and tropical spastic paraparesis) HTLV-II (clinical relevance not clear; may be more common than   HTLV-I in Western developed countries)
Prions
?Transmissible by blood transfusion

Fig. 19.19 Blood transfusion: transmissible viruses; prions are also potentially transmissible. (Courtesy of Prof. M Contreras and the North London Blood Transfusion Centre.)

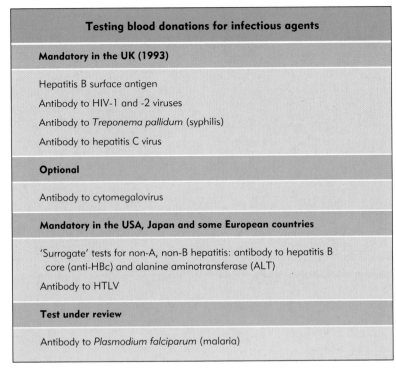

Testing blood donations for infectious agents
Mandatory in the UK (1993)
Hepatitis B surface antigen
Antibody to HIV-1 and -2 viruses
Antibody to *Treponema pallidum* (syphilis)
Antibody to hepatitis C virus
Optional
Antibody to cytomegalovirus
Mandatory in the USA, Japan and some European countries
'Surrogate' tests for non-A, non-B hepatitis: antibody to hepatitis B core (anti-HBc) and alanine aminotransferase (ALT)
Antibody to HTLV
Test under review
Antibody to *Plasmodium falciparum* (malaria)

Fig. 19.20 Blood donations: testing for infectious agents. (Courtesy of Prof. M Contreras and the North London Blood Transfusion Centre.)

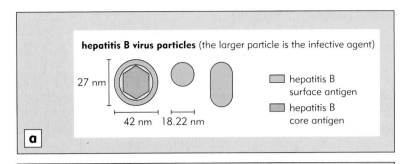
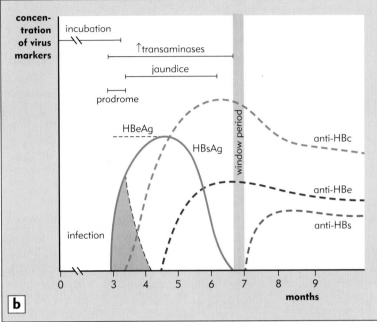

Fig. 19.21a and b Hepatitis B: (a) hepatitis B virus particles (the larger particle is the infective agent); (b) typical course of an acute infection with hepatitis B virus (HBV). [HbeAg, hepatitis Be antigen; HbsAg, hepatitis B surface antigen; HBc, hepatitis B core antigen; (a, b) courtesy of Prof. M Contreras and the North London Blood Transfusion Centre.]

straightened out. The abnormal PrP may arise by a random change in a normal protein, which probably accounts for sporadic CJD. In familial CJD, a point mutation occurs in the DNA coding for the protein. Thus there is the potential for transmission of the disease, if it is present in the blood of asymptomatic individuals, to recipients of the blood. New-variant CJD has been likened to bovine spongiform encephalitis (BSE; *Figs 19.22–19.25*). As yet, no human cases of CJD can be confidently attributed to transmission by infected blood products.

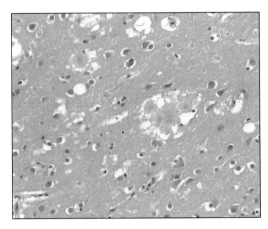

Fig. 19.22 New variant Creutzfeldt–Jacob disease (nvCJD): frontal cortex from a 22-year-old man with nvCJD showing the characteristic florid plaques (centre) which are composed of aggregates of the prion protein. (Courtesy of Dr JW Ironside.)

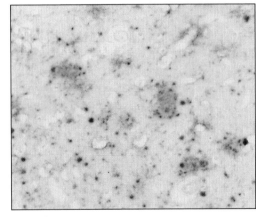

Fig. 19.23 New variant Creutzfeldt–Jacob disease: immunocytochemistry for PrP in the occipital cortex in nvCJD shows strong staining of individual plaques, with diffuse PrP deposits around neurons and blood vessels (KG9 monoclonal antibody). (Courtesy of Dr JW Ironside.)

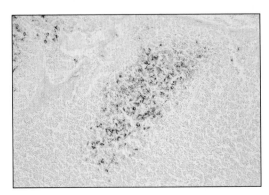

Fig. 19.24 New variant Creutzfeldt–Jacob disease: the tonsil in a 27-year-old woman with nvCJD shows positive staining for PrP within the germinal centre in follicular dendritic cells (KG9 monoclonal antibody). (Courtesy of Dr JW Ironside.)

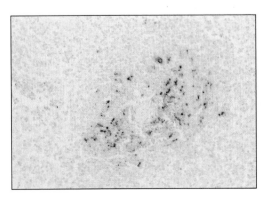

Fig. 19.25 New variant Creutzfeldt–Jacob disease: follicular dendritic cells in the spleen surrounding a small arteriole show strong positive staining for PrP in a 32-year-old woman with nvCJD (3F4 monoclonal antibody). (Courtesy of Dr JW Ironside.)

Iron overload

Iron overload may become a major clinical problem in multi-transfused and anaemic patients. In such cases, iron chelation therapy is required (*see Fig. 19.15*; *see also* Chapter 5).

Transfusion-related acute lung injury

Transfusion-related acute lung injury (TRALI) is an acute respiratory distress syndrome, resembling adult respiratory distress syndrome, that occurs within 4 hours (rarely, 1–2 days) of a blood transfusion. It is characterized by dyspnoea and hypoxia, with transient pulmonary infiltrates on chest radiographs (*Fig. 19.26*). Oxygen support is needed and mechanical ventilation is needed in more than 50% of patients. It is rare, occurring in about 1 in 5000 transfusions, and patients usually (>90%) recover. The aetiology is unclear; it may result from a combination of different mechanisms, including reaction of the recipient's neutrophils with HLA or neutrophil antibodies in donor plasma, which leads to increased permeability in the pulmonary circulation, or from cell membrane derived lipids in the donor plasma priming the recipient's neutrophils. The donors are often multiparous women and, once identified as the cause of a reaction, should be removed from the donor panel.

Graft-versus-host disease

Transfusion of viable lymphocytes to a heavily immunosuppressed host may result in 'grafting' of the lymphocytes, which may proliferate in the host and cause a disease similar to graft-versus-host disease (GVHD) in stem cell transplant recipients. Transfusion GVHD is rare, is likely to be associated with marrow aplasia and pancytopenia and is usually fatal. It is diagnosed by finding lymphocytes in the blood of the recipient that are of the HLA type of the donor, and it is prevented by irradiation of all blood products before transfusion into immunosuppressed patients.

OTHER BLOOD COMPONENTS

The preparation of blood components from whole blood is illustrated in *Fig. 19.27*.

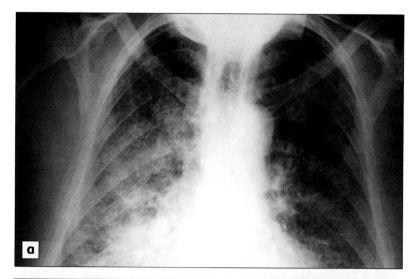
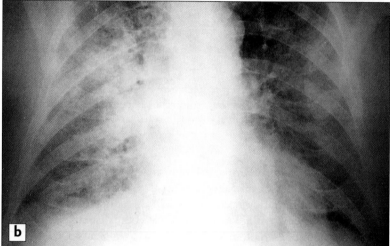

Fig. 19.26a and b Transfusion-related acute lung injury: chest radiographs (a) 3 hours and (b) 48 hours after onset of dyspnoea in a 55-year-old man receiving chemotherapy for acute myeloid leukaemia. The patient had received 1 unit of platelets 12 hours before the onset of symptoms, then 4 units of blood and a further unit of platelets 30 minutes before the onset. The patient was treated with high-dose corticosteroids and made a full recovery, with chest radiographs clear 7 days after onset of symptoms. [(a, b) Courtesy of Dr A Virchis.]

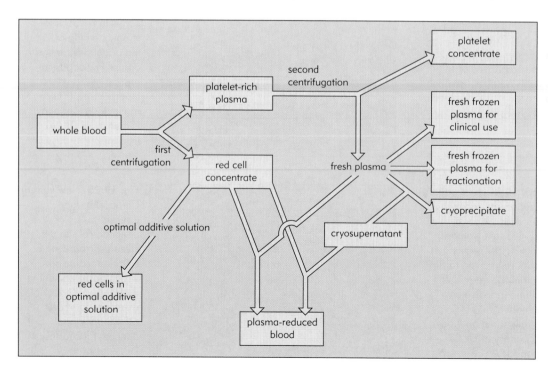

Fig. 19.27 Blood components from whole blood: preparation. [Adapted with permission from Contreras M, Hewitt PE. Clinical blood transfusion. In: Hoffbrand AV, Lewis SM, Tuddenham EGD (eds). *Postgraduate Haematology*, 4th edn. Oxford: Butterworth–Heinemann; 1999:215–34.]

Platelet concentrates

Platelet concentrates may be prepared from a donor pool (*Fig. 19.28*) or from a single donor (*Fig. 19.29*). They are required for patients with severe thrombocytopenia as a result of bone marrow failure (e.g. caused by acute leukaemia, myelodysplasia, aplastic anaemia, chemotherapy or radiotherapy). They are used:

- prophylactically (because the platelet count is extremely low, $<5 \times 10^9/l$, or likely to fall that low, or is $5–20 \times 10^9/l$ and associated with infection);
- before minor surgery (e.g. liver biopsy, insertion of indwelling catheter), or in patients with less severe degrees of thrombocytopenia and established haemorrhage) to raise the platelet count to $>50 \times 10^9/l$.

Patients with platelet functional defects require platelet support at higher platelet counts. Platelets express only HLA Class I antigens, whereas leucocytes express both HLA Class I and Class II antigens. Both are required to stimulate the reticuloendothelial system to make HLA antibodies. These antibodies may cause refractoriness to mixed-platelet packs. If this occurs, HLA-compatible simple donor packs may be needed.

Leucocytes

Leucocytes are not often used because of the difficulties in obtaining sufficient quantities, their short life span *in vivo*, the lack of data on a beneficial effect and the danger of transmission of disease (e.g. CMV). Buffy coat preparations or cells harvested by leucapheresis from patients with chronic myeloid leukaemia may have a restricted place in therapy, particularly in severely neutropenic patients with local infections.

Plasma components
Fresh frozen plasma

Fresh frozen plasma (FFP; *Fig. 19.30*) is used to replace clotting factors, for example in patients after massive transfusion or cardiopulmonary

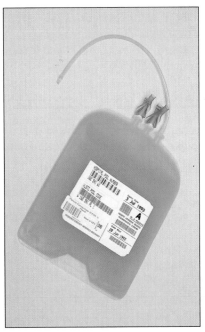

Fig. 19.28 Platelet pool: this may be derived from 4–6 donors depending on the place of manufacture. When produced by the buffy coat method a pool of platelets contains more than 250×10^9 platelets per unit. Such pools should be stored at 22°C and they have a shelf life of up to 5 days. (Courtesy of Prof. M Contreras and the North London Blood Transfusion Centre.)

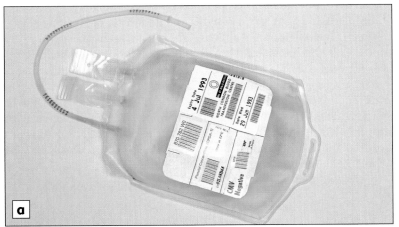

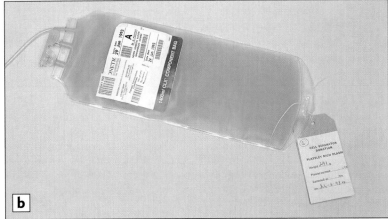

Fig. 19.29a and b Platelet concentrates: (a) from a single donor. These platelet concentrates are derived from a single blood donation and are approximately 50 ml in volume. The concentrate is derived from CPDA-1 plasma and contain platelets $>55 \times 10^9$ and leucocytes $<0.05 \times 10^9$ per unit. Platelets should be maintained at 22°C, and they have a shelf life of 5 days. (b) Platelet pack (pheresis): platelets may be collected by apheresis and an adult dose can be derived from a single donor. The volume of such a platelet concentrate is between 230 and 280 ml and contains ACDA anticoagulant. It contains more than 200×10^9 platelets and leucocytes from 0.01 to 0.05×10^9 per unit. These platelets should also be stored at 22°C, and they have a shelf life of 5 days. In addition, they may be HLA-matched or cross-matched to be compatible with recipient serum in cases of refractory patients. [(a, b) Courtesy of Prof. M Contreras and the North London Blood Transfusion Centre.]

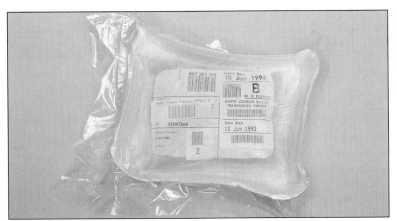

Fig. 19.30 Fresh frozen plasma: this can be provided in various volumes including adult (600 ml, 300 ml and 150 ml) and paediatric (70 ml and 20 ml) doses. It can be supplied in large volumes from volunteer plasmapheresis donors or recovered from routine blood donations. Illustrated here is a 150 ml FFP pack anticoagulated with CPDA-1. It should be stored at –30°C, and will then keep for up to 1 year. It should not be used as a plasma expander. Its use should be monitored with tests of coagulation when administered to correct a documented coagulation abnormality. (Courtesy of Prof. M Contreras and the North London Blood Transfusion Centre.)

by-pass, in liver disease, to reverse a warfarin effect or for plasma exchange in thrombotic thrombocytopenic purpura (*see* page 274). The dose is 15–20 ml/kg body weight, monitored by coagulation factor assays.

Cryoprecipitate (*Fig. 19.31*) is obtained by thawing FFP at 4°C, and is widely used as a replacement for factor VIII in haemophilia A.

Human albumin solution (4.5%) is used mainly to treat shock. Human albumin solution (20%) is used for patients with severe hypoalbuminaemia (e.g. with liver disease or nephrotic syndrome).

Clotting factor concentrates (e.g. factor VIII or factor IX) and Ig concentrates can also be made from human plasma (*Fig. 19.32*).

HUMAN LEUCOCYTE ANTIGEN SYSTEM

The short arm of chromosome 6 contains a cluster of genes known as the major histocompatibility complex (MHC) or the HLA region (*Fig. 19.33*).

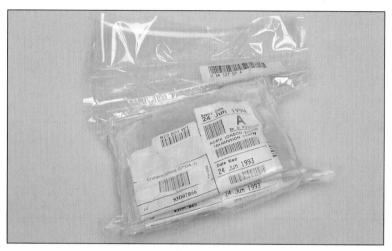

Fig. 19.31 Batched cryoprecipitate: individual cryoprecipitates from different donors may be batched together in groups of six to represent an adult dose. Each unit contains approximately 20 ml and is derived from CPDA-1 plasma. It contains fibrinogen >140 mg per unit and factor VIII >70 iu per unit. It should be stored at –30°C and has a shelf life of 1 year. In general, group A donors have higher levels of factor VIII than group O donors. (Courtesy of Prof. M Contreras and the North London Blood Transfusion Centre.)

Among the genes in this region are those that code for the proteins of the HLA antigens that are present on the cell membranes of many nucleated cells. As well as playing a major role in transplant rejection, these antigens are involved in many aspects of immunological recognition and reaction.

The MHC proteins are classified into three types. Class I proteins comprise two polypeptides, the larger of which is encoded by the MHC. The small component, a β_2-microglobulin, is encoded outside the MHC. Class II proteins comprise an α and a β chain, both of which are encoded by the MHC (*Fig. 19.34*). Class III proteins are the complement components encoded by the MHC region.

In humans, the main regions of the MHC gene complex are A, B, C and D. The Class I proteins encoded by the A, B and C regions act as surface recognition antigens, which can be identified by cytotoxic $CD8^+$ T lymphocytes. The D region genes encode Class II proteins, which are involved in cooperation and interaction between T helper $CD4^+$ lymphocytes and antigen-presenting cells. HLA-A, -B and -C antigens are present on all nucleated cells and platelets, and those encoded by the D region are present on B lymphocytes, monocytes, macrophages and some activated T cells.

Human leucocyte antigen nomenclature

The naming of antigens or types involves a letter to denote the locus and a number (given in chronological order of discovery) to denote a particularly specificity at that locus, determined originally by serology or cellular techniques (e.g. HLA-A1, -B8, -CW3, -DR1). Some HLA types were subsequently divided into two or more subtypes [e.g. DR13 and DR14 are splits of DR6, denoted DR13(6) and DR14(6)].

Molecular typing has now produced definition of alleles by DNA sequencing. Alleles are numbered using the letter that defines the locus and four digits (e.g. HLA-B27 is coded for by a number of alleles denoted B*2701, B*2702, etc.). The asterisk after the gene name indicates a particular allele. For Class II, the gene name includes a reference to the specific heavy or light chain locus (e.g. HLA-DQA1* or HLA-DQA2* for the two DQα chain loci. The DRB1 gene codes for the HLA-DR(1–18) antigens recognized serologically. DRB3 codes for the DR52 antigens, DRB4 for the DR53 antigens and DRB5 for the DR51 antigens (*Fig. 19.35*).

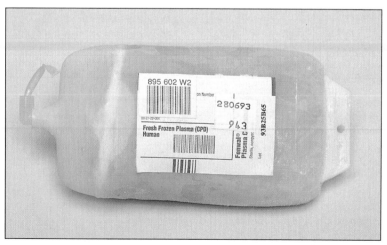

Fig. 19.32 Plasma for fractionation: plasma is also fractionated to make coagulation concentrates (FVIII and IX, etc.), albumin and Igs. It is supplied in a special pack that can be opened by BPL automatic machines. (Courtesy of Prof. M Contreras and the North London Blood Transfusion Centre.)

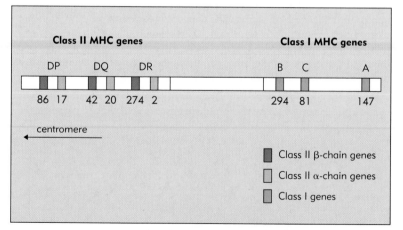

Fig. 19.33 Major histocompatibility complex polymorphism: the main genes that encode MHC Class I and MHC Class II molecules and their exceptional polymorphism (with approximate number of alleles). In practice, the genes that encode most of the three main types of the Class IIα and β chains are located at more than one locus and there are additional class I MHC loci. (Prepared by Steven GE Marsh.)

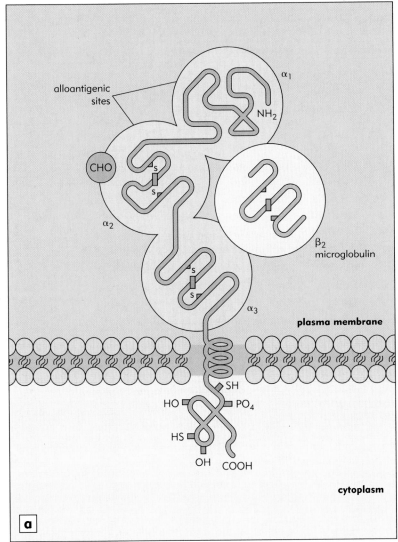
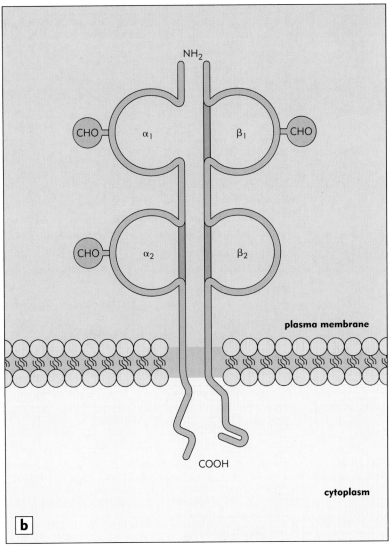

Fig. 19.34a and b Structure in the plasma membrane: (a) Class I and (b) Class II HLA antigens. The Class I MHC-encoded chain has three globular domains α_1, α_2 and α_3. A non-MHC-encoded peptide, β_2-microglobulin, is closely associated with the α_3 domain. Alloantigens occur on the α_1 and α_2 domains. The HLA-DR antigen consists of an α and a β peptide, non-covalently bound together. Each peptide has two globular domains, which are structurally related to Ig domains.

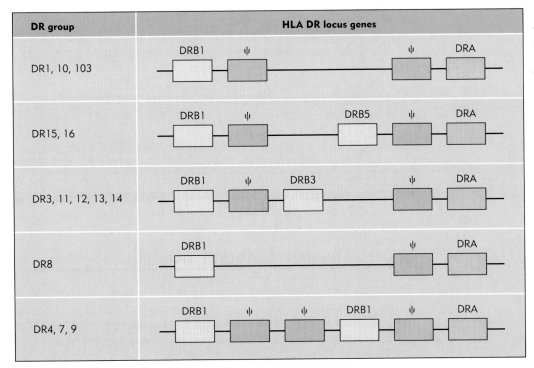

DR group	HLA DR locus genes					
DR1, 10, 103	DRB1	ψ		ψ	DRA	
DR15, 16	DRB1	ψ	DRB5	ψ	DRA	
DR3, 11, 12, 13, 14	DRB1	ψ	DRB3	ψ	DRA	
DR8	DRB1			ψ	DRA	
DR4, 7, 9	DRB1	ψ	ψ	DRB1	ψ	DRA

Fig. 19.35 Variable expression of genes according to HLA haplotype. (Yellow boxes, DRB genes; orange boxes, non-polymorphic DRA genes; purple boxes, pseudo-genes, ψ; adapted with permission from Mickelson E, Petersdorf EW. *Hematopoietic Cell Transplantation*, 2nd edn. Oxford: Blackwell Science; 1999.)

Genes of the human major histocompatibility complex

Name	Molecular characteristics	Name	Molecular characteristics
HLA-A	Class I α-chain	HLA-DQB1	DQA β chain as expressed
HLA-B	Class I α-chain	HLA-DQA2	DQ α-chain-related sequence, not known to be expressed
HLA-C	Class I α-chain	HLA-DQB2	DQ β-chain-related sequence, not known to be expressed
HLA-E	Associated with class I 6.2 kb Hind III fragment	HLA-DQB3	DQ β-chain-related sequence, not known to be expressed
HLA-F	Associated with class I 5.4 kb Hind III fragment	HLA-DOA	DO α chain
HLA-G	Associated with class I 6.0 kb Hind III fragment	HLA-DOB	DO β chain
HLA-H	Class I pseudogene associated with 5.4 kb Hind III fragment	HLA-DMA	DM α chain
HLA-J	Class I pseudogene associated with 5.9 kb Hind III fragment	HLA-DMB	DM β chain
HLA-K	Class I pseudogene associated with 7.0 kb Hind III fragment	HLA-DPA1	DP α chain as expressed
HLA-L	Class I pseudogene associated with 9.2 kb Hind III fragment	HLA-DPB1	DP β chain as expressed
HLA-DRA	DR α chain	HLA-DPA2	DP α-chain-related pseudogene
HLA-DRB1	DR βI chain determining specificities DR1, DR2, DR3, DR4, DR5, etc.	HLA-DPB2	DP β-chain-related pseudogene
HLA-DRB2	pseudogene with DR β-like sequences	TAP1	ABC (ATP binding cassette) transporter
HLA-DRB3	DR β3 chain determining DR52 and Dw24, Dw25, Dw26 specificities	TAP2	ABC (ATP binding cassette) transporter
HLA-DRB4	DR β4 chain determining DR53	LMP2	Proteasome-related sequence
HLA-DRB5	DR β5 chain determining DR51	LMP7	Proteasome-related sequence
HLA-DRB6	DRB pseudogene found on DR1, DR2 and DR10 haplotypes	MICA	Class I chain-related gene
HLA-DRB7	DRB pseudogene found on DR4, DR7 and DR9 haplotypes	MICB	Class I chain-related gene
HLA-DRB8	DRB pseudogene found on DR4, DR7 and DR9 haplotypes	MICC	Class I chain-related pseudogene
HLA-DRB9	DRB pseudogene, isolated fragment	MICD	Class I chain-related pseudogene
HLA-DQA1	DQA α chain as expressed	MICE	Class I chain-related pseudogene

Fig. 19.36 Human major histocompatibility complex: genes. (Adapted with permission from Bodmer JG, Marsh SGE, Albert ED, et al. Nomenclature for factors of the HLA system, 1998. *Hum Immunol.* 1999;60:361–95.)

Number of alleles at each HLA locus		
Locus		Number
Class I	A	147
	B	294
	C	81
	E	5
	F	1
	G	14
Total HLA Class I		**542**
Class II	DRB1	223
	DRB3	20
	DRB4	9
	DRB5	14
	DRB6	3
	DRB7	2
	DRA	2
	DRB	274
	DQA1	20
	DQB1	42
	DPA1	17
	DPB1	86
	DMA	4
	DMB	5
	DOA	8
Total HLA Class II		**729**

Fig. 19.37 Alleles: number at each HLA locus, as assigned by the WHO Nomenclature Committee for Factors of the HLA System, June 1999. (Prepared by Steven GE Marsh.)

Typing of human leucocyte antigens

HLA-A, -B and -C typing is usually carried out on peripheral blood lymphocytes. Originally, antigens of the D system were identified by non-reactivity in mixed lymphocyte culture (a lymphocyte reaction proliferation assay) against rare homozygous D-locus cells. There are over 30 genes that code for the antigens in this region (*Fig. 19.36*), with multiple alleles at each locus (*Fig. 19.37*). It is now possible to detect HLA-D region antigens serologically or by molecular biological techniques, including:

- Sequence-specific primer amplification (PCR-SSP);
- sequence-specific oligonucleotide probe (PCR-SSO);
- heteroduplex analysis;
- direct nucleotide sequencing;
- single-strand conformational polymorphism analysis (SSCPA); and
- double-stranded conformational analysis (DSCA; *Figs 19.38 and 19.39*).

The region is referred to as HLA-D and is subdivided serologically into three groups, DP, DQ and DR. A current list of HLA antigens is given in *Fig. 19.40*.

OTHER HUMAN LEUCOCYTE ANTIGENS

Human leucocytes carry a variety of antigens that are recognized by monoclonal antibodies. These various antigens are listed in Appendix 1, together with examples of antibodies that detect them. The use of these antibodies to define normal and malignant haemopoietic cell subpopulations is described in other chapters.

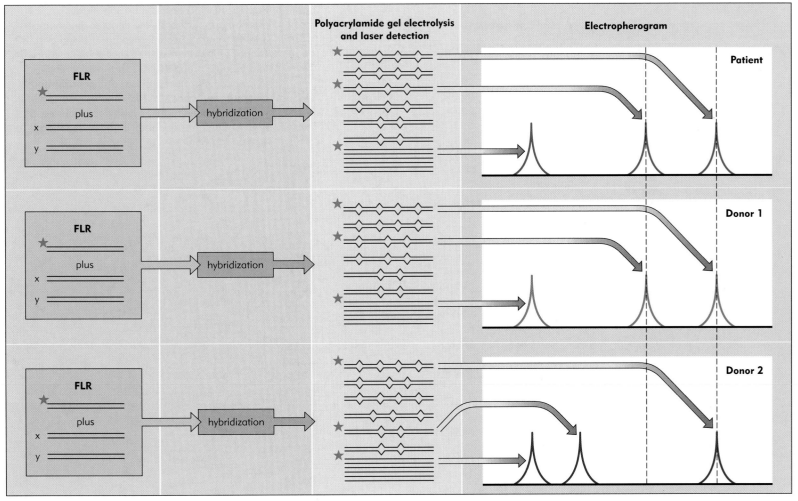

Fig. 19.38 Allogeneic bone marrow transplantation: reference-strand conformation analysis (RSCA) method. The locus-specific fluorescein-labelled reference (FLR) polymerase chain reaction (PCR) product contains a fluorescent Cy5 label on its sense strand (indicated by a star). The FLR is hybridized with the locus-specific PCR product from the sample to be tested. For heterozygous loci, two alleles are present (indicated as 'x' and 'y'). During hybridization the sense and antisense strands of the DNA strands present are initially separated by denaturation followed by re-annealing, whereby the sense and antisense strands can cross-hybridize to generate, in addition to the starting homoduplexes, heteroduplexes, two of which possess the Cy5-labelled sense strand of the FLR. The duplexes formed are separated by polyacrylamide gel electrophoresis, and those duplexes that possess a Cy5 label are detected with the laser. In this example, the patient and donor 1 have alleles with identical mobility, whereas donor 2 has one allele that differs. (Redrawn with permission from Arguello JR, Little AM, Pay AL, et al. Mutation detection and typing of polymorphic loci through double-strand conformational analysis. *Nat Genet*. 1998:18;192–4; courtesy of Prof. JA Madrigal.)

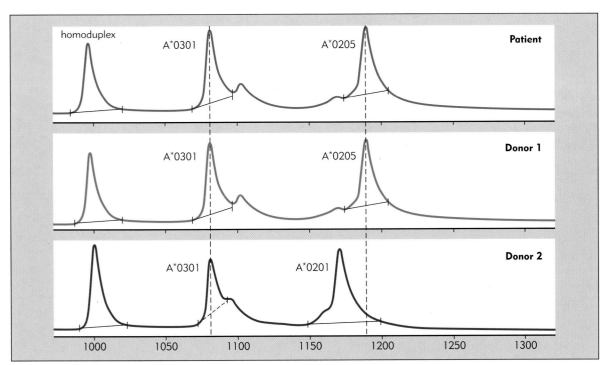

Fig. 19.39 Allogeneic bone marrow transplantation: electropherogram with results for HLA-A locus matching for a patient and two unrelated bone marrow donors. After electrophoresis the homoduplex peak is assigned an arbitrary value of 1000 on the horizontal scale. The vertical scale represents the homoduplex and heteroduplex peaks detected by laser. The patient and two potential donors were matched by serology for HLA-A2 and -A3. By RSCA analysis, the patient shares allele A*0301 with both potential donors, but only shares the second allele, A*0205, with donor 1. (Courtesy of Prof. JA Madrigal.)

Recognized HLA specificities						
A	**B**	**C**	**D**	**DR**	**DQ**	**DP**
A1	B5	Cw1	Dw1	DR1	DQ1	DPw1
A2	B7	Cw2	Dw2	DR103	DQ2	DPw2
A203	B703	Cw3	Dw3	DR2	DQ3	DPw3
A210	B8	Cw4	Dw4	DR3	DQ4	DPw4
A3	B12	Cw5	Dw5	DR4	DQ5(1)	DPw5
A9	B13	Cw6	Dw6	DR5	DQ6(1)	DPw6
A10	B14	Cw7	Dw7	DR6	DQ7(3)	
A11	B15	Cw8	Dw8	DR7	DQ8(3)	
A19	B16	Cw9(w3)	Dw9	DR8	DQ9(3)	
A23(9)	B17	Cw10(w3)	Dw10	DR9		
A24(9)	B18		Dw11(w7)	DR10		
A2403	B21		Dw12	DR11(5)		
A25(10)	B22		Dw13	DR12(5)		
A26(10)	B27		Dw14	DR13(6)		
A28	B2708		Dw15	DR14(6)		
A29(19)	B35		Dw16	DR1403		
A30(19)	B37		Dw17(w7)	DR1404		
A31(19)	B38(16)		Dw18(w6)	DR15(2)		
A32(19)	B39(16)		Dw19(w6)	DR16(2)		
A33(19)	B3901		Dw20	DR17(3)		
A34(10)	B3902		Dw21	DR18(3)		
A36	B40		Dw22			
A43	B4005		Dw23	DR51		
A66(10)	B41					
A68(28)	B42		Dw24	DR52		
A69(28)	B44(12)		Dw25			
A74(19)	B45(12)		Dw26	DR53		
A80	B46					
	B47					
	B48					
	B49(21)					
	B50(21)					
	B51(5)					
	B5102					
	B5103					
	B52(5)					
	B53					
	B54(22)					
	B55(22)					
	B56(22)					
	B57(17)					
	B58(17)					
	B59					
	B60(40)					
	B61(40)					
	B62(15)					
	B63(15)					
	B64(14)					
	B65(14)					
	B67					
	B70					
	B71(70)					
	B72(70)					
	B73					
	B75(15)					
	B76(15)					
	B77(15)					
	B78					
	B81					
	Bw4					
	Bw6					

Fig. 19.40 Recognized HLA specificities: established specificities are denoted by a number; and those not fully confirmed are prefixed by a 'w' (workshop). More restricted specificities are included in a broader group ('splits') shown in parentheses following the firmer specificity. Antigens Bw4 and Bw6 are very broad ('public') and include splits which have been further subdivided. (Courtesy of Prof. M Contreras and the North London Blood Transfusion Centre.)

Principal features of known cluster of differentiation of molecules

Principal features of known cluster of differentiation molecules				
CD	**Identity**	**Function**	**Cellular distribution**	**Ligands**
CD1a		Peptide and lipid antigen presentation	Thymocyte, LC, DC	Unknown
CD1b			Thymocyte, DC	Unknown
CD1c			Thymocyte, LC, DC B(sub)	Unknown
CD2	LFA-2, T11	T adhesion to target cells or APC	Thymocytes, T, NK	LFA-3, CD58, CD59
CD3		Signal transduction (ζ) and T activation	Thymocyte, T	Unknown
CD4		Helper activity	Thymocyte(sub), T(sub), Mo, Mφ	MHC Class II
CD5	Lue-1, Ly-1	Signal for T and thymocyte activation	Thymocyte, T, B(sub)	CD72
CD6		T activation and thymocyte–stromal interaction	Thymocyte, T	CD166
CD7		Signal transduction	SC, thymocyte, T	FcμR?
CD8		Maturation and positive selection of T	Thymocyte(sub), T(sub)	MHC Class I
CD9		Platelet activation and aggregation	Pre-B, platelet	CD41/CD61
CD10	CALLA, NEP	May limit activity of peptide hormones	BM	Unknown
CD11a/CD18	LFA-1, $\alpha_L\beta_2$	Leucocyte–leucocyte and leucocyte–endothelium interactions	Haemopoietic cells, most leucocytes, eosinophils	ICAM-1, -2, -3
CD11b/CD18	Mac-1, $\alpha_M\beta_2$, CR3	Adhesion of Mo/neutrophils to vascular endothelium	NK, most leucocytes	ICAM-1, ic3b, fibrinogen
CD11c/CD18	CR4, $\alpha_x\beta_2$, p150, 95	Adhesion of Gr to inflamed endothelium	NK, Gr	ic3b, fibrinogen
CDw12			Mo, Gr, platelet	
CD13		Aminopeptidase	Mo, Gr	
CD14		LPS-binding protein	Mo	
CD15		ELAM receptor	Gr	
CD16	FcγRIII	Phagocytosis and ADCC	Gr, NK, Mφ	Fcγ
CDw17		Lactosylceramide	Mo, Gr	
CD18		β-Chain of CD11	Leucocytes	
CD19	B4	B activation and proliferation	B	Unknown
CD20	B1, Bp35	Regulation of B activation and, proliferation	B	Unknown
CD21	CR2, EBVR, C3dR	Part of a signal–transduction complex	B, FDC	C3d, CD23, EBV
CD22	BL-CAM	B adhesion interactions	B Mat(sub)	Sialyl proteins, CD45
CD23	FcϵRI	B activation and IgE regulation	B, *Mφ, FDC, platelet	Fcϵ, CD21
CD24	HSA	Signalling and support of T growth	T, B, Gr	Unknown
CD25	IL-2 Rα	T growth	Thymocytes, *T, pre-B	IL-2
CD26	DPPIV	Binds and transports adenosine deaminase to the cell surface	*T, *B, Mw	Unknown
CD27		Co-stimulatory signal for T activation	Thymocyte, T	CD70
CD28		Co-stimulatory molecule	T(sub), *B	CD86, CD80
CD29	VLA β chain		Leucocytes	
CD30		Transduction of a signal for apoptosis	*T, *B	CD153
CD31	PECAM-1	Transendothelial migration of leucocytes	Mo, platelet, neutrophils, NK, endothelial and naive T	CD31, $\alpha_v\beta_3$
CD32	FcγRII		B, Mφ, Gr	Fcγ
CD33	My9		Mo, Mφ, mast cells	
CD34	My10	Adhesion	Progenitor cells, endothelial cells	CD62E?, CD62L?
CD35	CR1, C3b/C4b R	Inhibits complement activation	Erythrocytes, B, T(sub), phagocytes, eosinophils	C3b, C4b

Appendix 1 Cluster of differentiation (CD) molecules on haemopoietic cells. (APC, antigen-presenting cell; BM, bone marrow; T, T cell; B, B cell; NK, natural killer cell; Mo, monocyte; Mφ, macrophage; Gr, granulocyte; LC, Langerhans cell; DC, interdigitating dendritic cell; FDC, follicular dendritic cell; SC, stem cell; *, activated; Rest, resting; Mat, mature; (sub), subset; EBV, Epstein–Barr virus; ECM, extracellular matrix; VWF, von Willebrand's factor; adapted with permission from Roitt IM. *Essential Immunology*, 9th edn. Oxford: Blackwell Scientific; 1997.)

Principal features of known cluster of differentiation molecules

CD	Identity	Function	Cellular distribution	Ligands
CD36	GPIIIb, MFGM, PAS IV	Adhesion molecule	Endothelial cells, platelet, Mo, megakaryocytes	Thrombospondin, collagen
CD37		B activation and proliferation	B, T	Unknown
CD38	T10	Unknown	B(sub), *T	Unknown
CD39	gp80		B(sub), *NK(sub), *T(sub)	
CD40		B activation, proliferation, differentiation	B, Mo, DC	CD1
CD41/CD61	$\alpha_{IIb}\beta_3$, GPIIb IIIa complex	Platelet aggregation	The major integrin on platelet plasma membrane, megakaryocytes	VWF, fibrinogen, fibronectin
CD42	GP IX (CD42a), GP Ibα (CD42b), GP Ibβ (CD42c), GP V (CD42d), GP Ib–IX–V complex	Platelet adherence and aggregation at sites of vascular damage	Platelets, megakaryocytes, vascular tonsillar endothelial cells	VWF, thrombin
CD43	Leucosialin, gp115	Haemopoietic progenitor cell proliferation	Leucocytes	ICAM-1 (CD54)
CD44	H-CAM, Pgp-1, HERMES	Cell–cell and cell–ECM adhesion	Haemopoietic cells, B and T, Mo, neutrophils, epithelial cells	Hyaluronate
CD45	LCA	Signalling in B and T	Leucocytes	CD22
CD45RA	Restricted LCA		T(sub), B, Gr(sub), Mo	
CD45RB	Restricted LCA		T(sub), B, Gr, Mo	
CD45RC	Restricted LCA			
CD45RO	Restricted LCA		T(sub), Gr, Mo	
CD46	Membrane co-factor protein (MCP)		Widespread	
CD47	Integrin-associated protein (IAP)	Associated with vitronectin receptor	Broad	
CD48	Blast-1, OX-45, BCM1	T adhesion to target cells and APC	Haemopoietic and non-haemopoietic tissues	CD2 (rodent)
CD49a/CD29	VLA-1, $\alpha_1\beta_1$	Receptor for the E1 domain of laminin and a region of collagen I and IV	Fibroblasts, capillary endothelial cells, NK cells, *T	Laminin, collagen I and IV
CD49b/CD29	VLA-2, $\alpha_2\beta_1$	Regulates the expression of MMP-1 collagen Type I	Fibroblasts, endothelial cells, platelets, B and T, keratinocytes	Collagen I–IV, laminin
CD49c/CD29	VLA-3, $\alpha_3\beta_1$	Cell–cell interaction	Fibroblasts, keratinocytes, epithelial cells, B	Fibronectin, collagen
CD49d/CD29	VLA-4, $\alpha_4\beta_1$	Leucocyte rolling, adhesion and migration	Widespread	VCAM-1, fibronectin
CD49e/CD29	VLA-5, $\alpha_5\beta_1$	Cell adhesion, cell migration and matrix assembly	Fibroblasts, epithelial and endothelial cells, muscle cells, platelets	Fibronectin and L1
CD49f/CD29	VLA-6, $\alpha_6\beta_1$	Cell adhesion, spreading and migration	Widespread	Laminin
CD50	ICAM-3	Signalling and co-stimulatory molecule on T	Mo, neutrophils, lymphocytes	$\alpha_d\beta_2$, LFA-1
CD51/CD61	$\alpha_v\beta_3$, vitronectin receptor	Recruitment, distribution and retention of cells via ECM molecules	Endothelial cells, Mo, platelets, osteoclasts, tumour cells, some B, T	CD31, laminin, fibrinogen, fibronectin
CD52	Campath-1		Leucocytes	
CD53	MEM-53	Activation	Leucocytes	
CD54	ICAM-1	Leucocyte adhesion to endothelium in inflammation	Endothelial cells, dendritic cells, epithelial cells, Mo, B	LFA-1, MAC-1, CD43
CD55		Delay accelerating factor (DAF)	Most cells	
CD56	NCAM, D2-CAM, Leu-19, NKH1	Developmental of normal tissue architecture	Neurons, astrocytes, myoblasts, myotubes, *T, NK	CD56, heparan sulphate
CD57	HNK-1, Leu-7	MHC non-restricted cytotoxicity after activation	NK, T(sub), B(sub), Mo	Unknown
CD58	LFA-3	Interactions of APC and target cells with T	Leucocytes, erythrocytes, endothelial cells, epithelial cells, fibroblasts	CD2
CD59		Protects from complement-mediated lysis	Widespread	CD2
CDw60	NeuAc–NeuAc–Gal		T(sub), platelets	
CD61	Vitronectin receptor β		Platelets	
CD62E	E-Selectin, ELAM-1	Tethering and rolling of leucocytes on cytokine-activated endothelium	Endothelial cells	ESL-1
CD62L	L-Selectin, Leu-8	Tethering and rolling of lymphocytes on LN HEV and leucocytes on endothelium	Leucocytes; is down-regulated on activation by endoproteolysis (shedding)	CD34, MAdCAM, GlyCAM-1, sLe^x
CD62P	P-Selectin, GMP-140, PADGEM	Adhesion of platelet to Mo and neutrophils, and leucocytes to endothelium	Thrombin/histamine *platelet and endothelium; stored in granules prior to activation	PSGL-1
CD63	LIMP, ME491		*Platelet, Mo	
CD64	FcγRI		Mo	Fcγ
CD65	Lew^x poly-N-acetyl-lactosamine	Unknown	Mo	Unknown
CD65s	sLew^x poly-N-acetyl-lactosamine	Unknown	Mo, neutrophils	Unknown

Principal features of known cluster of differentiation molecules

CD	Identity	Function	Cellular distribution	Ligands
CD66 series	Carcinoembryonic antigen (CEA) gene		Gr	
CD67	CANCELLED (now CD66b)			
CD68	Microsialin		Mo, Mφ, *platelet	Oxidized LDL
CD69	AIM, Leu-23	Activation, signal transduction	Early *T, early *B, Mφ	
CD70	Ki-24		*T(sub), *B(sub)	CD27
CD71		Transferrin receptor	*T, *B, *NK, *Mo, Mφ, SC	
CD72		B activation and proliferation	B	CD5
CD73		Ecto-5' nucleotidase	T(sub), B(sub)	
CD74		MHC Class II invariant chain	B, Mo, LC	
CDw75		Unknown	B, T(sub)	CD22?
CDw76			B(sub), T(sub), endothelial cells	CD22?
CD77		Globotriaosylceramide	B	
CDw78	Ba		B, Mφ(sub)	
CD79a	Igα, mb1	Signal transduction as part of B receptor	B	Unknown
CD79b	Igβ, B29	Signal transduction as part of B receptor	B	Unknown
CD80	B7.1, BB1	Binding regulates IL-2 gene expression	B(sub)	CD28, CD152
CD81	TAPA-1	Cross-linking induces effects consistent with a role in signal transduction	T, B	Unknown
CD82	R2	Largely unknown (signal transduction?)	Leucocytes	Unknown
CD83	HB15	Unknown (antigen presentation?)	*T, *B, DC	Unknown
CD84	2G7		Mo, Mφ, platelet, B	
CD85		Unknown	B, Mo	Unknown
CD86	B7.2	Regulates IL-2 expression	B, Mo	CD28, CD152
CD87	Urokinase plasminogen activator protein	Receptor	Mo, Mw, Gr, *T, endothelial cells	Vitronectin
CD88	C5a receptor	Complement receptor	Gr, Mo, Mφ, mast cells	C5a
CD89	Fcα receptor	Fc receptor	Gr, Mo, Mφ, B(sub), T(sub)	IgA1, IgA2
CD90	Thy-1	Lymphocyte recirculation and T activation	Thymocyte, T (mouse)	Unknown
CD91	α₂-Macroglobulin receptor LDRL-related protein	Receptor	Mo, Mφ	α₂-Macroglobulin
CDw92	VIM15		Gr, Mo, platelet, endothelial cells	
CD93	p120		Mo, Gr, endothelial cells	
CD94	kp43	Inhibition/activation of cytotoxicity	T(sub), NK	Some HLA Class I molecules
CD95	Fas, APO-1	Transduces an apoptic signal	Widespread	Fas-L
CD96	Tactile		*T, *NK	
CD97	p74/80/89		Gr, Mo, *T, *B	CD55
CD98	4F2	Modulates intracellular Ca^{2+} levels	T, B, NK, Gr	Unknown
CD99	E2, MIC2	T and red-cell rosette formation	Thymocyte, T, B	Unknown
CD100		Proliferation of PBMCs	Leucocytes	Unknown
CD101		Type I transmembrane protein	Gr, Mo, Mφ, DC, *T	Unknown
CD102	ICAM-2	Lymphocyte recirculation and trafficking	Endothelial cells, HEVs, lymphocytes, Mo, NK, platelet	LFA-1
CD103	α$_E$β$_7$, M290/β$_7$, integrin, HML-1	Heterotypic adhesion of mucosal lymphocytes to epithelial cells	Most intra-epithelial T and 50% of lamina propria lymphocytes, absent from PBLs	E-cadherin
CD104	Integrin β$_4$ chain	Adhesion molecule with integrin α$_6$ chain		Laminin, epiligrin
CD105	Endoglin		*Mo, endothelial cells	
CD106	VCAM-1	Leucocyte migration and recruitment to sites of inflammation	APC, BM stromal cells, vascular endothelial cells	VLA-4, α$_4$β$_7$
CD107a	LAMP-1		*Platelet	
CD107b	LAMP-2		*Platelet	
CDw108	GPI-gp80		*T	
CD109	Sialomucin	Unknown	Endothelial cells, stromal cells, some myeloid cells	Unknown
CD114	G-CSFR, IL-10R	Proliferation and differentiation of human B	Gr, Mo, platelet	IL-10, G-CSF
CD115	CSF-1R	Cytokine receptor	Mo, Mφ	M-CSF
CD116	GM-CSF Rα	Unknown	Mo, Gr	GM-CSF
CD117	c-kit, SCF-R	Signal transduction, regulation of adhesion	Haemopoietic progenitors, mast cells	SCF

Principal features of known cluster of differentiation molecules

CD	Identity	Function	Cellular distribution	Ligands
CDw119	IFNγR	Cytokine receptor	Mo, Gr	IFN-γ
CD120a	TNF receptor type I	Cytokine receptor	Broad	TNFα, lymphotoxin (TNFβ)
CD120b	TNF receptor type II	Cytokine receptor	Broad	TNFα, lymphotoxin (TNFβ)
CD121a	IL-1RI	Stimulates T growth	Thymocytes, T, fibroblasts, endothelial cells	IL-1α, β, ra
CD121b	IL-1RII		B, T, Mo, Mφ	IL-1α, β, ra
CD122	IL-2Rβ	Unknown	T, NK	IL-2
CDw123	IL-3Rα	Unknown	Not determined	IL-3
CD124	IL-4Rα	Proliferative activity in pre-activated B and T	T and B, haemopoietic precursors, fibroblasts	IL-4
CD125	IL-5Rα	Growth and differentiation of eosinophils	Eosinophils, basophils	IL-5
CD126	IL-6Rα	Differentiation and proliferation of haemo-poietic precursors and acute phase response	*B, plasma cells, T, Mo, epithelial cells, fibroblasts, neural cells	IL-6
CD127	IL-7Rα	Proliferation of pro- and pre-activated B and T	Immature thymocytes, hepatocytes, pre-B, T Mat	IL-7
CDw128	IL-8R	Cytokine receptor	Gr, T(sub), Mo	IL-8
CD129	IL-9R	Growth-promoting activity for T tumours	T and B, macrophages, megakaryoblasts	IL-9
CD130	gp130	Signal transduction	Not determined	IL-6, IL-11, LIF, OSM, CNTF, CT-1
CDw131	Common β chain	B growth	Mo, Gr, eosinophils, human B, basophils, mouse B	IL-3, IL-5, GM-CSF
CD132	Common γ chain	B/T growth	T and B, haemopoietic precursors, fibroblasts	IL-2, -4, -7, -9, -15
CD134	OX40	Adhesion of *T to vascular endothelial cells	Expressed on *T	OX40 ligand, gp34
CD135	Flt3/Flk2	Receptor, tyrosine kinase	CD34 cells, carcinoma cells	Flt3/Flk2 ligand
CD136	MSP R, RON	Receptor, tyrosine kinase	Not determined	Macrophage stimulating protein
CDw137	4-1BB	Co-stimulatory molecule for T activation	T	4-1BB ligand
CD138	Syndecan-1	Heparan sulphate proteoglycan	B(sub)	Collagen Type 1
CD139	Unknown	B	Unknown	
CD140a	PDGF Rα	Tyrosine kinase	Unknown	PDGF A or B
CD140b	PDGF Rβ	Tyrosine kinase	Endothelial cells, stromal cells, mesangial cells	PDGF B
CD141	Thrombomodulin	Down-regulates coagulation	Myeloid cells, endothelial cells, smooth muscle cells	Thrombin
CD142	Tissue factor	Induces coagulation	Mo, endothelial cells, keratinocytes, endothelial cells	Factor VII
CD143	ACE	Peptidylpeptidase	Endothelial cells, epithelial cells, Mφ	N/A
CD144	VE-cadherin	Adhesion molecule	Endothelial cells	Unknown
CDw145			Endothelial cells	
CD146	MUC18, S-endo	Extravasation/homing of *T	Endothelial cells, FDC, *T	Unknown
CD147	Neurothelin, basigin, TCSF, EMMPRIN, M6	Adhesion molecule?	Endothelial cells, myeloid cells, lymphoid cells	Type IV collagen? Fibronectin? Laminin?
CD148	HPTP-eta, DEP-1	Contact inhibition of cell growth	Haemopoietic cells	Unknown
CD149	MEM133	Unknown	Lymphocytes, Mo	Unknown
CDw150	SLAM	Signalling molecules	T(sub), B(sub), thymocytes	Unknown
CD151	PETA3	Signalling complex with FcR IIa?	Platelets, Gr, endothelial cells, smooth muscle cells, epithelial cells	Integrins? HLA-DR?
CD152	CTLA-4	Negative regulator for T co-stimulation	*T	CD80, CD86
CD153	CD30L	Co-stimulatory for T	*T, Gr, B, Mφ	CD30
CD154	CD40L, gp39	Co-stimulatory molecule	*T, *B, NK, mast cells	CD40
CD155	Polio virus R	Unknown	Mo, macrophages, thymocytes, CNS neurons	CD44?
CD156	ADAM8	Unknown	Mo, macrophages, Gr	Unknown
CD157	Bst-1	ADP-ribose cyclase	Mo, neutrophils, endothelial cells, FDC	Unknown
CD158a	p58.1, p50.1	Inhibition of cytotoxicity	T, NK	HLA-CW2, -CW4, -CW5, -CW6
CD158b	p58.2, p50.2	Inhibition of cytotoxicity	T, NK	HLA-CW1, -CW3, -CW7, -CW8
CD161	NKRP1A	Regulation of NK-cell-mediated cytotoxic activity	NK, Mo, T(sub)	Negative charged CHOs
CD162	PSGL-1	Leucocyte rolling on activated endothelium	Mo, Gr, T, subset of B	P-Selectin
CD163	M130	Unknown	Mo, some Mφ	Unknown
CD164	MGC-24	Adhesion of haemopoietic progenitor cells to stromal cells	Myeloid cells, T, epithelial cells, BM stromal cells, haemopoietic progenitor cells, certain carcinoma cells	Unknown
CD165	AD2, gp37	Adhesion of thymocytes to thymic epithelium	T, NK, platelet, thymocytes, thymic epithelium, CNS neurons	Unknown
CD166	ALCAM	Activated leucocyte adhesion molecule	Activated B and T, eosinophils, thymic epithelium, fibroblasts, endothelial cells, keratinocytes	CD6

Provisional WHO classification of neoplastic diseases of the lymphoid and haemopoietic tissues

Provisional WHO classification of neoplastic diseases of the lymphoid and haemopoietic tissues (continued from Figure 11.58)

Immunodeficiency-related lymphoproliferative disorders*†

Congenital immunodeficiency-associated lymphoproliferative disorders†
atypical lymphoproliferative disorders
diffuse large B-cell lymphoma

Post-transplantation and other iatrogenic lymphoproliferative disorders
polymorphic B-cell lymphoproliferative disorders
diffuse large B-cell lymphoma
plasmacytoma (+/– multiple myeloma)
peripheral T-cell lymphomas (cytotoxic, NK/T)
Hodgkin lymphoma

AIDS-associated lymphoproliferative disorders
Burkitt and atypical Burkitt lymphoma
diffuse large B-cell lymphoma
immunoblastic lymphoma (with plasmacytoid differentiation)
primary effusion lymphoma

Histiocytic/dendritic-cell neoplasms and related disorders)

Macrophage/histiocyte related
histiocytic sarcoma (mainly localized)
malignant histiocytosis (generalized, may be related to acute monocytic leukaemia)

Dendritic-cell related
Langerhan cell histiocytosis
  localized
  generalized
Langerhan cell sarcoma
interdigitating dendritic cell sarcoma
follicular dendritic cell sarcoma/tumour

Myeloid neoplasms‡

Myeloproliferative diseases
chronic myelogenous leukaemia, Philadelphia chromosome (Ph1) [t(9;22)(qq34;q11), BCR/ABL]+
chronic neutrophilic leukaemia
hypereosinophilic syndrome/chronic eosinophilic leukaemia
chronic idiopathic myelofibrosis
polycythaemia vera
essential thrombocythaemia
myeloproliferative disease, unclassifiable

Myelodysplastic/myeloproliferative diseases
chronic myelomonocytic leukaemia (CMML)
atypical chronic myelogenous leukaemia, BCR/ABL-(aCML)
juvenile myelomonocytic leukaemia (JMML)

Myelodysplastic syndromes
refractory anaemia (RA)
refractory anaemia with ringed sideroblasts (RARS)
refractory cytopenia with multilineage dysplasia (RCMD)
refractory anaemia with excess blasts (RAEB)
5q-syndrome
myelodysplastic syndrome, unclassifiable

Acute myeloid leukaemias

Acute myeloid leukaemias with recurrent cytogenetic translocations
AML with features of t(8;21)(q22;q22),AML1(CBFa)/ETO
AML with features of t(15;17)(q11–12),PML/RARα and variants (promyelocytic leukaemia)
AML with features of inv(16)(p13q22),CBFb/MYH11 and variants
AML with 11q23 (MLL) abnormalities

Acute myeloid leukaemia with myelodysplasia-related features
AML with multilineage dysplasia
AML arising in a previous MDS

Acute myeloid leukaemia, NOS/unspecified
AML minimally differentiated (M_0)
AML without maturation (M_1)
AML with maturation (M_2)
acute myelomonocytic leukaemia (M_4)
acute monocytic leukaemia (M_5)
acute erythroid leukaemia (M_6)
acute megakaryocytic leukaemia (M_7)
acute basophilic leukaemia
acute panmyelosis with myelofibrosis

Acute myeloid leukaemia, therapy related
alkylating agent related
epipodophyllotoxin related (some may be lymphoid)
other types

Acute biphenotypic leukaemias

*The disorders listed are seen with increased frequency in immunodeficiency states. This list is not intended to imply an independent classification scheme for immunodeficiency-associated lymphoproliferative disorders. Those disorders that occur without known immunodeficiency are listed as well, with the above B- and T-cell neoplasms.

‡Only major disease categories are listed.

†The congenital immunodeficiencies most commonly associated with lymphoprolifeative disorders include Wiskott–Aldrich syndrome, common variable immunodeficiency, ataxia telangiectasia, severe combined immunodeficiency, X-linked lymphoproliferative disorder and hyper-IgM syndrome. Each form of immunodeficiency disorder is associated with its own risk factors, which affect the pattern of lymphoproliferative disorder encountered. Consequently, the lymphoproliferative disorders vary by type and frequency according to the form of underlying immune deficiency.

Appendix 2 Provisional WHO classification of neoplastic diseases of the haemopoietic and lymphoid tissues (*see also* Fig. 11.58 for complete classification of lymphoid disorders). (Courtesy of Drs ES Jaffe, NL Harris, J Diebold, K Muller–Hermelink, G Flandrin, J Vardiman.)

Index

Note: Where a subject in the index appears in the text, and that text contains a pointer to figure(s) on the same or following page(s), usually only page references for the text are given.

Abbreviations: ALL, acute lymphoblastic leukaemia; AML, acute myeloid leukaemia; CLL, chronic lymphocytic leukaemia; CML, chronic myeloid leukaemia.